Pahrump Community Library
701 East Street
Pahrump, NV 89048

Master the
Nursing School &
Allied Health
Entrance Exams

19th Edition

Marion F. Gooding, RN, Ph.D.

Professor of Nursing
North Carolina Central University
Durham, North Carolina

CONTRIBUTING EDITORS

Mattie Moss, Ed.D.
Mathematics

Duana A. Dreyer, Ph.D.
Anatomy and Physiology

Charles R. George, Ph.D.
Biology

Doris E. Wilson, B.A.
Language Arts

James M. Schooler, Ph.D.
Chemistry

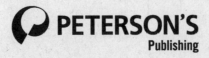
PETERSON'S
Publishing

Pahrump Community Library
701 East Street
Pahrump, NV 89048

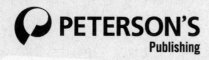

About Peterson's Publishing

Peterson's Publishing provides the accurate, dependable, high-quality education content and guidance you need to succeed. No matter where you are on your academic or professional path, you can rely on Peterson's print and digital publications for the most up-to-date education exploration data, expert test-prep tools, and top-notch career success resources—everything you need to achieve your goals.

Visit us online at www.petersonspublishing.com and let Peterson's help you achieve your goals.

For more information, contact Peterson's, 2000 Lenox Drive, Lawrenceville, NJ 08648; 800-338-3282 Ext. 54229; or find us online at www.petersonspublishing.com.

Peterson's makes every reasonable effort to obtain from reliable sources accurate, complete, and timely information about the tests covered in this book. Nevertheless, changes can be made in the tests or the administration of the tests at any time and Peterson's makes no representation or warranty, either expressed or implied as to the accuracy, timeliness, or completeness of the information contained in this book.

© 2012 Peterson's, a Nelnet company

Facebook® and Facebook logos are registered trademarks of Facebook, Inc. Facebook, Inc. was not involved in the production of this book and makes no endorsement of this product.

Bernadette Webster, Director of Publishing; Ray Golaszewski, Publishing Operations Manager; Linda M. Williams, Composition Manager; Developed by Practical Strategies, LLC

ALL RIGHTS RESERVED. No part of this work covered by the copyright herein may be reproduced or used in any form or by any means—graphic, electronic, or mechanical, including photocopying, recording, taping, Web distribution, or information storage and retrieval systems—without the prior written permission of the publisher.

For permission to use material from this text or product, complete the Permission Request Form at http://www.petersons.com/permissions.

ISBN-13: 978-0-7689-3618-6
ISBN-10: 0-7689-3618-7

Printed in the United States of America

10 9 8 7 6 5 4 3 2 1   14 13 12

Nineteenth Edition

By printing this book on recycled paper (40% post-consumer waste) 163 trees were saved.

Petersonspublishing.com/publishingupdates

Check out our Web site at www.petersonspublishing.com/publishingupdates to see if there is any new information regarding the tests and any revisions or corrections to the content of this book. We've made sure the information in this book is accurate and up-to-date; however, the test format or content may have changed since the time of publication.

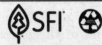

Certified Chain of Custody

60% Certified Fiber Sourcing and
40% Post-Consumer Recycled

www.sfiprogram.org

*This label applies to the text stock.

Sustainability—Its Importance to Peterson's, a Nelnet company

What does sustainability mean to Peterson's? As a leading publisher, we are aware that our business has a direct impact on vital resources—most especially the trees that are used to make our books. Peterson's Publishing is proud that its products are certified by the Sustainable Forestry Initiative (SFI) and that all of its books are printed on paper that is 40% post-consumer waste.

Being a part of the Sustainable Forestry Initiative (SFI) means that all of our vendors—from paper suppliers to printers—have undergone rigorous audits to demonstrate that they are maintaining a sustainable environment.

Peterson's Publishing continuously strives to find new ways to incorporate sustainability throughout all aspects of its business.

OUR PROMISE
SCORE HIGHER. GUARANTEED.

Peterson's Publishing, a Nelnet company, focuses on providing individuals and schools with the best test-prep products—books and electronic components that are complete, accurate, and up-to-date. In fact, we're so sure this book will help you improve your score on this test that we're guaranteeing you'll get a higher score. If you feel your score hasn't improved as a result of using this book, we'll refund the price you paid.

Guarantee Details:

If you don't think this book helped you get a higher score, just return the book with your original sales receipt for a full refund of the purchase price (excluding taxes or shipping costs or any other charges). Please underline the book price and title on the sales receipt. Be sure to include your name and mailing address. This offer is restricted to U.S. residents and to purchases made in U.S. dollars. All requests for refunds must be received by Peterson's within 120 days of the purchase date. Refunds are restricted to one book per person and one book per address.

Send to:
Peterson's Publishing, a Nelnet company
Customer Service
2000 Lenox Drive
Lawrenceville, NJ 08648

This guarantee gives you the limited right to have your purchase price refunded only if you are not satisfied that this book has improved your ability to score higher on the applicable test. If you are not satisfied, your sole remedy is to return this book to us with your sales receipt (within 120 days) so that we may refund the amount you paid for the book. Your refund is limited to the manufacturer's suggested retail price listed on the back of the book. This offer is void where restricted or prohibited.

Contents

Contents

Before You Begin

Now that you've decided on a career in nursing or in one of the allied healthcare fields, you'll need to take an entrance exam for the coursework and degree or certificate that you want. *Peterson's Master the Nursing School and Allied Health Entrance Examinations* can help you prepare for your test. This book provides review and practice in a variety of subjects and skills that you will need to do well on whichever test you are required to take.

HOW THIS BOOK IS ORGANIZED

Peterson's Master the Nursing School and Allied Health Entrance Examinations is divided into five parts to facilitate your study and review for whichever test you will be taking.

- **Part I** provides an overview of the different tests and how to apply to take the one that fits your career interests. You'll also find an overview of the tests and potential question types.

- **Part II** offers a diagnostic test to help you identity your strengths and those areas where you will need to spend more time preparing. The test is divided into three parts, one for those planning to test for registered nursing school, one for those planning to test for allied healthcare, and one for those planning to test for entrance to practical/vocational nursing school. For your ease in identifying the areas that you need to spend more time on while preparing for your test, the topic of each content area question is noted at the end of each answer explanation.

- **Part III** focuses on the types of information and questions typically found on nursing school entrance exams. Review and practice exercises prepare you to answer questions testing your verbal ability, mathematics, science, and reading comprehension skills.

- **Part IV** offers practice for allied health school entrance exams. Questions are provided in the areas of verbal ability, quantitative ability, science knowledge, and reading comprehension. The content review provided in Part III is appropriate for Part IV as well.

- **Part V** tackles review and practice for the practical nursing and vocational nursing school entrance exams. Here you'll find review material and practice exercise for verbal skills, arithmetic and mathematics, health and science, and reading comprehension.

- The special word power review provides lists of common roots, prefixes, and suffixes that will help all test-takers with the verbal sections of their tests (See pages 71–76).

SPECIAL STUDY FEATURES

Peterson's Master the Nursing School and Allied Health Entrance Examinations has several features that will help you get the most from your study time.

Overview

Review units begin with a listing of the major topics in that chapter followed by an introduction that explains what you will be reviewing in the chapter.

Bonus Information

You will find three types of notes in the margin of the *Peterson's Master the Nursing School and Allied Health Entrance Examinations* to alert you to important information about the test.

Note

Margin notes marked "Note" highlight information about the test structure itself.

Tip

A note marked "Tip" points out valuable advice for taking the *Nursing School & Allied Health Exams.*

Alert

An "Alert" identifies pitfalls in the testing format or question types that can cause mistakes in selecting answers.

YOU ARE WELL ON YOUR WAY TO SUCCESS

You have made the decision to apply to nursing school and have taken a very important step in that process. Peterson's *Master the Nusring School & Allied Health Entrance Exams* will help you score high on the exam and prepare you for everything you'll need to know on the day of your exam. Good Luck!

FIND US ON FACEBOOK

Join the conversation by liking us on Facebook at facebook.com/petersonspublishing. Here you'll find additional test-prep tips and advice. Peterson's resources are available to help you do your best on these important exams—and others in your future.

GIVE US YOUR FEEDBACK

Peterson's publishes a full line of books—test prep, education exploration, financial aid, and career preparation. Peterson's publications can be found at high school guidance offices, college libraries and career centers, and your local bookstore or library. Peterson's books are now also available as eBooks.

We welcome any comments or suggestions you may have about this publication.

TOP 10 STRATEGIES TO RAISE YOUR SCORE

Many people become anxious about taking a test, especially a standardized test or a computer-based test. To help you deal with your anxiety, first, realize that anxiety can be productive. Anxiety can be energizing if you direct the energy toward your goals and away from negative thinking such as "I hate tests. I never do well on tests." Remember that admissions tests are only one thing that committees look at in determining to whom to offer admission. One way to lower your anxiety level is to prepare for the test you will be taking. Practicing ahead of time will boost your confidence. The following are ten strategies to help you feel confident and do well on your entrance exam.

1. **Use the Diagnostic Test as a tool.** Taking the test and studying answers will help you identify the content that you need to spend the most time reviewing. The answer explanations include the topics and specific content for the math and science questions, so you will have a quick-and-easy way to decide which topics to spend more time on.

2. **Schedule your study time.** Between now and the time you take your exam, set aside time each day except Sunday to study. Try to give the same amount of time each day. Find a place that is conducive to studying.

3. **Budget your time on the topics.** Don't move too quickly through the material, but don't get bogged down and spend too much time on one or two topics. Be sure that you are comfortable with each topic before you move on to the next one, but avoid spending too much time early in your schedule on just a couple of topics and then having to rush through the end of your review.

4. **Memorize basic math rules.** Be sure that you know basic rules so that you have a firm grasp of what the basic rules are and how to apply them. This will help reduce your stress level.

5. **PRACTICE, PRACTICE, PRACTICE.** Practice may not get you a perfect score, but it will help you score better. Take the Diagnostic Test, and complete each set of exercises in each unit.

6. **Establish a pacing schedule for taking each subtest.** Before you take the Diagnostic Test, work out what you think will be a reasonable pacing plan so that you can answer every question. Then set the timer and take the test. After you finish the test, see if your plan allowed you to answer all the questions without having to rush at the end. Make adjustments as needed and time yourself as you work through each set of practice tests.

Before the Test

7. **Find the location of the test center.** If you aren't familiar with the location of the test site, take a trial run to find it and find out how long it takes to get there. If you're driving, locate a parking lot or garage. This may seem like overkill, but who wants to arrive at the testing site with five minutes to spare and out of breath because you got lost on the way or spent 20 minutes trying to find a parking lot that turned out to be eight blocks away?

8. **Organize what you need for the test.** The night before the test, lay out on your bureau, the table by the door, or wherever you will see them, the forms of identification that you are going to need, your admission ticket, and anything else you may need. The confirmation you received reserving your seat will tell what you need and what you may not

bring. If it doesn't, check the Web site for the test. Organizing ahead of time may seem unnecessary, but you don't want to waste time the day of the test by rooting around for a utility bill or a library card to prove you are who you say you are (**No calculators allowed on any of these tests…***)

During the Test

9. **Use the features that are given to you.** If you are taking a computer-based test, follow along as the monitor explains the functions that are available for your use. Take any tutorial that is offered and be sure that you understand the program before you begin the test.

10. **Use these four general strategies as you work through the test.**

    - Use your pacing plan.

    - Skip and return to questions that you aren't sure about.

    - Eliminate answer choices that you know are incorrect.

    - Use educated guessing to rule out answers you aren't sure about.

PART I

INFORMATION ABOUT NURSING AND ALLIED HEALTH PROGRAMS AND ENTRANCE EXAMINATIONS

About the Nursing Profession

About the Nursing Profession

OVERVIEW

- Getting on the path to a career in the nursing and allied health professions
- Selecting a nursing program
- Selecting an allied health program
- Financial aid resources
- About the examinations
- How to apply to take an entrance examination
- Administration of the examinations
- Reducing Test Anxiety

Nursing and allied healthcare are in-demand careers as the 78.2 million baby boomers age. By the end of the first decade of this century, there were some 2.6 million registered nurses, and the projected growth is much faster than average. Between 2008 and 2018, the Bureau of Labor Statistics (BLS) projects 1 million job openings for registered nurses. The demand for licensed practical nurses and licensed vocational nurses is also projected to be high. In 2008, there were 754,000 LPNs and LVNs, and the projected growth for this career is also much faster than average. Between 2008 and 2018, there will be an estimated 391,300 job openings. Generally, allied health professionals are either technicians, that is, assistants, or therapists or technologists. In all, there are some 200 different allied health careers in such varied jobs as cardiovascular technologist, radiologic technician, chemotherapy technician, and respiratory therapist. Job openings for allied healthcare professionals are also expected to have faster than average growth between now and 2018.

GETTING ON THE PATH TO A CAREER IN THE NURSING AND ALLIED HEALTH PROFESSIONS

As you can see from this section, the nursing and allied health fields have many opportunities. For careers in allied health, the path to a fulfilling career is less defined than the nursing career because of the multiplicity of choices available. According to the Web site explorehealthcareers. org, "there are 5 million allied health care providers in the U.S. who work in more than 80 different professions and represent approximately 60% of all health care providers."

The type of training and degree or certificate required for an allied health career varies by career. The best strategy to determine the program you will need to realize your career ambitions is to talk to a career counselor, attend career fairs, and search the Web for information about potential careers in your area of interest. Look particularly for professional organizations and associations for healthcare providers. Check whether your specialty will require licensing. Once you have narrowed your choice down to a particular type of job or jobs, begin to search college, community college, and vocational school Web sites, depending on your potential career choice, for information on career preparation and coursework.

For those interested in a career in nursing, there are four kinds of programs that provide preparation for a nursing career:

1. The practical-nurse programs are usually offered in vocational schools, hospitals, and community colleges. The programs vary from nine to eighteen months. The courses include the basic sciences and medical-surgical, pediatric, and obstetrical nursing. Some mental health concepts are included. The major focus is on technical skills. A practical nurse works under the supervision of a registered nurse (RN).

2. The associate-degree nurse is a graduate of a two-year college program that is designed with a balance between clinical nursing courses (medical, surgical, psychiatric, obstetrical, and pediatric nursing) and general education courses (biological and physical sciences, behavioral sciences, humanities, and electives) to provide a background for making important judgments about patient care. The graduate is prepared for technical expertise in the assessment, planning, and delivery of direct patient care in the hospital setting.

3. The graduate of the hospital-based diploma program functions on the nursing team in the same manner as the associate-degree nurse. Most diploma programs are twenty-four to thirty months in length, and the non-nursing courses may be offered through a college.

4. The baccalaureate nursing program is four years in length and is offered in senior colleges and universities. The required courses in the biological, physical, and behavioral sciences are both basic and advanced. These general education requirements, along with courses that provide a broad liberal arts background, are taken during the first two years. The major clinical courses are offered in the third and fourth years and include the five clinical areas previously identified, with an emphasis on community health nursing and the role of the professional nurse as manager. Most nursing programs offering the professional baccalaureate degree admit graduates from the diploma and associate-degree programs with varying degrees of advanced standing.

The graduates of all four programs take a licensing examination. At the present time, there are two kinds of licenses: the practical-nurse license and the registered-nurse license for graduates of the diploma, associate-degree, and baccalaureate-degree programs.

A nurse may continue studies to receive a master's degree and a doctorate with a major in clinical specialties, teaching, administration, or research, depending on his or her career choice. There is a great demand for nurses in hospitals, schools, clinics, public health agencies, and many other settings throughout the world. Nurses may become anesthetists, enter the military, or become writers, consultants, or private practitioners. Nursing provides a foundation for many career opportunities and, more importantly, a personally and financially satisfying vocation.

Regardless of which kind of nursing program you choose to enter, you will have opportunities to provide an important service. You may enter nursing at one level and expand your skills through practice and additional education. Advancement within the nursing profession comes about in several ways. A practical nurse may decide to become a registered nurse, an upward move. A registered nurse may decide to move from the hospital setting into community-based care, a lateral move that expands the types of services a nurse can provide. A registered nurse who does not have a baccalaureate degree may decide to earn one in order to step up to a management position.

SELECTING A NURSING PROGRAM

The first factor you should consider when selecting a nursing program is your career goal. Do you plan to work in a hospital or as a member of the health team? Is your ultimate goal to function as a manager or an administrator? Are you primarily interested in teaching? Do you want to specialize in a specific clinical area? Are you planning to work in a community setting, providing services to families? Is your ultimate goal to become an entrepreneur?

The rapidly moving trend in nursing today is to license two levels of nursing for entry into the professional services. The assistant level will be represented by graduates of the associate-degree nursing programs; the professional level, by graduates of the baccalaureate nursing programs. Baccalaureate education in nursing forms the foundation for graduate education in nursing, where specialization as a clinical practitioner, administrator, and teacher occurs. Other types of graduates (practical nurse and diploma) will achieve these credentials through career mobility programs.

A second factor to consider is cost. The demands of full-time study and the length of the program may necessitate resigning from your current job.

A third factor is your qualification for admission. As the levels of performance increase, so do the academic requirements.

Once you have matched your career goals with a program, you should use the following guidelines to finalize your program choice.

- Is the program approved by the state regulating body?

- Is the program accredited by a voluntary agency?

- What is the program's reputation in terms of graduate performance?

- How does the social and academic environment meet your needs?

SELECTING AN ALLIED HEALTH PROGRAM

Occupations related to allied health are rapidly expanding. The criteria for selecting a program are similar to those for nursing:

- If a license is required to practice, be certain that the program is approved by the regulating body.

- Check to see if the program is accredited by the appropriate voluntary agency.

- Find out how well the graduates are performing on the licensing examination.

- Consider how well the program meets your short- and long-term career goals.

FINANCIAL AID RESOURCES

Federal financial aid has not kept pace with the increasing cost of post-secondary education. Therefore, it is important to be familiar with the sources of funding, the eligibility requirements, and the application procedures. It is also important to apply as early as possible to a variety of programs.

To initiate the application process, get the Free Application for Federal Student Aid form (FAFSA) from your local high school counseling office, the school to which you are seeking admission, or online from the Department of Education. The online FAFSA can be accessed, completed, and submitted at www.fafsa.ed.gov. If you opt to use the paper copy of the FAFSA, the form must be completed and mailed to the address on the form. In a few days (if you applied online) or in approximately six weeks (if you applied using the paper copy), a report is sent back that identifies whether or not you are eligible for financial aid. The schools you identified when filling out the FAFSA receive similar reports so that the amount of aid for which you are eligible and the amount you will have to pay out-of-pocket can be determined.

The amount of money a recipient can receive is dependent upon the need analysis derived from the financial aid form and the financial aid program in which the nursing school, college, or university is participating. The school usually prepares a financial aid package that includes a combination of financial sources to make up the difference between the amount the student and his or her family can contribute and the total costs of the nursing program.

Some financial aid funding sources are loans, which must be paid back at a low interest rate over a prolonged period of time. Other funding sources are grants and scholarships, which do not have to be paid back. The obligation for debt payment requires serious thought on the part of the student, since a default on a loan can affect his or her credit rating.

When shopping for financial aid, check the accreditation status of the nursing program and the institution's eligibility for aid. Most accredited nursing programs are eligible for federal funding, but some institutions have limited federal sources due to high default rates.

Federal Sources

Pell Grants are awarded to undergraduate students who have not previously earned a degree. The grant does not have to be repaid and may be supplemented by other funds. Eligibility is based on need, which is calculated by a formula. The amounts of the awards vary yearly and depend on program funding. The maximum award for 2011–2012 was $5,550 per year. You do not have to be a full-time student; however, the amount you receive as a part-time student will be proportionate to your attendance.

Academic Competitiveness Grants (ACG) can only be awarded to citizens of the United States who receive a Pell Grant in the same year and are enrolled full-time in degree- or certificate-granting programs. The ACG can only be received in the first academic year ($750) and the second academic year ($1,300). Eligibility is based on having completed a course of rigorous academic study in high school.

Stafford Loans

Stafford loans are of two types: Direct Subsidized Loans and Direct Unsubsidized Loans. Direct Subsidized Loans are awarded on the basis of need and do not accrue interest before the repayment period begins as long as you are at least a half-time student or during periods of deferent. Direct Unsubsidized Loans are not based on need and accrue interest from the time of disbursement. Dependent undergraduate students may borrow $5,500 for the first year, $6,500 for the second year, and $7,500 for the third year and beyond. Independent students and dependent students whose parents are unable to obtain PLUS Loans may borrow $9,500, $10,500, and $12,500 for years 1, 2, 3, and beyond respectively.

PLUS Loans

PLUS loans enable parents with stable credit histories to borrow for the education expenses of each dependent child who is an undergraduate student enrolled at least half-time. The annual maximum is equal to the cost of attendance minus any additional financial aid the student receives.

Consolidation Loans

These loans are designed to help students and parents simplify loan repayment by consolidating several types of federal loans into one loan with one repayment schedule. Student loans cannot be consolidated until they enter repayment.

Campus-Based Programs (Administered by Financial Aid Office)

Federal Supplemental Educational Opportunity Grants (SEOG) are for undergraduates with exceptional financial need; students who received Federal Pell Grants are given priority in awarding these grants. Students can receive between $100 to $4,000 per year depending on student need, the funding at the school, and the school's financial aid policies.

Federal Work Study provides a work-study program for undergraduate and graduate students in financial need. Students are able to earn money through community service and work related to their course of study.

The Federal Perkins Loans are low-interest loans for both undergraduate and graduate students with exceptional financial need. The school is the lender, and the loan must be repaid to the school, but the loan is made with funding from the federal government. Loans may be granted in the amount of $5,500 for each year of undergraduate study, up to a total of $27,500, and $8,000 for each year of graduate study to a total of $60,000.

For additional information on federal loans and other aid, call 1-800-FED-AID or download *Funding Your Education Beyond High School: The Guide to Federal Student Aid* online at **http://studentaid. ed.gov/students/publications/student_guide/index/html**.

Other Sources of Financial Aid

Peterson's Scholarships, Grants, & Prizes is a helpful source for information on foundations, religious organizations, fraternities and sororities, and civic groups that provide scholarships and/or loans for educational purposes. In addition, the military offers scholarships through its ROTC Program and through the G. I.Bill for former members of the Armed Services. You should also seek out resources from the organizations related to your field of interest.

ABOUT THE EXAMINATIONS

Registered nursing programs, practical/vocational nursing programs, and allied health programs all require different entrance examinations. The following listing provides contact information for applying for each test and a description of each exam.

Registered Nursing Entrance Exams

For registered nursing programs, you may be required to take the Pre-Admission Examination-RN (PAX-RN), the PSB-Nursing School Aptitude Examination (RN), the Nurse Entrance Test (NET), or the Test of Essential Academic Skills (TEAS). All the exams evaluate the academic ability of applicants in key areas of the basic nursing curriculum.

For information about the **Pre-Admission Examination (PAX-RN),** contact:

National League for Nursing
61 Broadway
33rd Floor
New York, NY 10006
212-363-5555
www.nln.org

- The Pre-Admission Examination-RN is computer-based.

- The test has three sections and lasts 3 hours.

- Calculators may not be used.

The exam has the following three multiple-choice tests:

TEST SECTION	CONTENT	TIME
Verbal Ability	Multiple-choice covering: Word Knowledge Reading Comprehension	One Hour
Mathematics	Multiple-choice covering: Basic Calculations Word Problems Algebra Geometry Conversions Graphs Applied Mathematics	One Hour
Science	Multiple-choice covering: General Biology Chemistry Physics Earth Science	One Hour

NOTE: Experimental items are also included but do not affect your test score.

For more information about the **PSB-Registered Nursing School Aptitude Examination (RN)**, contact:

Psychological Services Bureau, Inc,
977 Seminole Trail
PMB 317
Charlottesville, VA 22901
www.psbtests.com

- The PSB-Registered Nursing School Aptitude Examination is computer-based or paper-and-pencil, depending on the test site.

- The test contains 360 questions.

- Calculators may not be used, but scratch paper is available.

The PSB-Nursing School Aptitude Examination (RN) contains the following five tests:

TEST SECTION	CONTENT	# OF QUESTIONS
Academic Aptitude (3 subtests)	Verbal: Emphasizes vocabulary-related questions	30 Questions
	Arithmetic: Focuses on skill and computational speed with arithmetic	30 Questions
	Non-Verbal: Deals with recognizing relationships and differences between objects; measures mental manipulation and reasoning	30 Questions
Spelling	Measures written expression or communication skills	50 Questions
Reading Comprehension	Determines ability to interpret passages, understand direct statements, infer ideas and purposes, and derive author's intent	40 Questions
Information in the Natural Sciences	Tests understanding of biology, chemistry, health, safety, etc., at an elementary level	90 Questions
Vocational Adjustment Index	Ascertains an individual's characteristic lifestyle by examining his or her educational and occupational adjustment	90 Questions

For more information about the **Test of Essential Academic Skills (TEAS)** for entrance into practical/vocational nursing programs, contact:

Assessment Technologies, Inc. (ATI)
7500 W. 160th Street
Stilwell, KS 66085
800-667-7531
www.atitesting.com

- TEAS is a computer-based test.

- The test contains 170 multiple-choice questions.

- Calculators may not be used.

TEAS covers the following four general areas:

1. Math: whole numbers, metric conversion, fractions and decimals, algebraic equations, percentages, and ratio/proportion

2. Reading: paragraph comprehension, passage comprehension, and inferences/conclusions

3. English: punctuation, grammar, sentence structure, contextual words, and spelling

4. Science: science reasoning, science knowledge, biology, chemistry, anatomy and physiology, basic physical principles, and general science

Allied Health School Entrance Exams

Allied health program entrance exams measure academic ability and scientific knowledge. You may be required to take the PSB-Health Occupations Aptitude Examination or the Test of Essential Academic Skills.

For more information about the **PSB-Health Occupations Aptitude Examination**, contact:

Psychological Services Bureau, Inc.

977 Seminole Trail

PMB 317

Charlottesville, VA 22901

www.psbtests.com

- The PSB-Health Occupations Aptitude Exam is computer-based or paper-and-pencil, depending on the test site.

- The test contains 380 questions.

- Calculators may not be used, but scratch paper is available.

The exam has the following five tests:

TEST SECTION	CONTENT
Academic Aptitude (3 subtests)	Verbal: Emphasizes vocabulary-related questions (30 questions) Arithmetic: Focuses on skill and computational speed with arithmetic (30 questions)
	Non-Verbal: Deals with recognizing relationships and differences between objects; measures mental manipulation and reasoning (30 questions)
Spelling	Measures written expression or communication skills relative to spelling skills (60 questions)
Reading Comprehension	Measures the ability to understand direct statements, interpret written content, understand text intent, organize ideas, and extract information (50 questions)
Information in the Natural Sciences	Determines understanding of biology, chemistry, health, safety, hygiene, etc., at an elementary level (90 questions)
Vocational Adjustment Index	Ascertains an individual's characteristic lifestyle by examining his or her educational and occupational adjustment (90 questions)

Practical/Vocational Nursing Entrance Exams

The entrance exams for practical/vocational nursing programs assess knowledge of areas essential to the basic practical/vocational nursing curriculum. You may be required to take either the Pre-Admissions Examination-PN or the PSB-Aptitude for Practical Nursing Examination.

For more information about the **Pre-Admission Examination-PN (PAX-PN)**, contact:

National League for Nursing
61 Broadway, 33rd Floor
New York, NY 10006
212-363-5555
www.nln.org

- PAX-PN is computer-based test, but may also be taken as a paper-and-pencil test.

- The test contains multiple-choice questions.

- Calculators may not be used.

PAX-PN covers the following three areas:

Practical Nursing Entrance Exams

The Pre-Admission Examination-PN (PAX-PN) has the same test format as the registered nursing exam; however, its contents are at a level appropriate for applicants to practical/vocational programs. The test format is as follows:

TEST SECTION	CONTENT	TIME
Verbal Skills	Multiple-choice covering: Word Knowledge Reading Comprehension	One Hour
Mathematics	Multiple-choice covering: Basic Calculations Word Problems Algebra Geometry Conversions Graphs Applied Mathematics	One Hour
Science	Multiple-choice covering: Biology Chemistry Physics Earth Science	One Hour

Note: Exams contain experimental items (not included in the examinees' scores) for purposes of future test development.

For more information about the PSB-Aptitude for Practical Nursing Examination, contact:

Psychological Services Bureau, Inc.
977 Seminole Trail PMB 317
Charlottesville, VA 22901

The PSB-Aptitude for Practical Nursing Examination contains five tests and three subtests, and takes about two hours and fifteen minutes to complete. The test format is as follows:

TEST SECTION	CONTENT
Academic Aptitude (3 subtests)	Verbal: Emphasizes vocabulary-related questions Arithmetic: Focuses on skill and computational speed with arithmetic Non-Verbal: Deals with recognizing relationships and differences between objects; measures mental manipulation and reasoning
Spelling	Measures written expression or communication skills
Judgement and Comprehension in Practical Nursing Situations	Evaluates the judgement of the nurse as student and as practitioner in working situations
Information in the Natural Sciences	Tests understanding of biology, chemistry, health, safety, etc., at an elementary level
Vocational Adjustment Index	Ascertains an individual's characteristic lifestyle by examining his or her educational and occupational adjustment

HOW TO APPLY TO TAKE AN ENTRANCE EXAMINATION

Different institutions have different requirements and arrangements for testing. Admissions information for schools typically lists the exam that you need to take and contact information for the test-maker or test administrator if the latter is different. Typically, you will need to register online to take the entrance exam. Once at the site, you will be able to find the location of testing centers and testing windows. Register as soon as possible, because testing centers fill up on a first-come, first-served basis. Follow the registration instructions carefully and be sure to download the confirmation e-mail and admission ticket.

The site will also provide specific information about the format and makeup of the exam. Be sure to download this information as well.

ADMINISTRATION OF THE EXAMINATIONS

The entrance exams are administered by qualified persons at a testing center. Pay careful attention to the information on the testing center's Web site or in your confirmation e-mail about what you may or may not bring to the test site and what you may or may not have in the exam room with you. None of the tests, for example, allow the use of calculators, so there is no reason to bring one.

Specific instructions for taking the exam will be given by the proctor overseeing the exam administration. If there is a tutorial for the computer-based test, take it so you become familiar with the functions that the program has available to you. All tests are timed. Depending on the length of the test, you may or may not have a break. The proctor will tell you when to begin and when to stop.

Some of the computer-based exams provide a score report immediately. Others will have a report available within 24 to 48 hours. Information available from the test-maker will describe the process of reporting scores to the institutions you are applying to.

Answering Test Questions

Studying the more than 1,400 test questions in this book, which are similar to the questions included in the entrance examinations, enables you to review material you already know, gain new knowledge, and become familiar with the format of timed tests.

After completing the overview of a section, answer the sample test questions. Like the ones on the real exams, the questions in this book are multiple choice. You are not penalized for incorrect answers in these exams, so use educated guessing if you do not know the answer or aren't sure. A good strategy to use is to go through the entire test, answering the questions you know, and then go back and make educated guesses for the questions you don't know. Here's how to make an educated guess:

- Carefully read the question (the *stem*). Look for the clues or the main ideas in the stem that will lead you to the correct answer.

- Go through the entire examination, answering all the questions that you feel sure about. This will give you an overall idea of what the test is about and lessen the time pressure. You may even run across related information that will help you to answer the questions you don't know.

- Now go back to those items you didn't answer and use the test-taking techniques. First, look for the key word(s) or clue(s) in the stem. Keeping that in mind, try to eliminate the choices that do not relate to the clue. Look at the remaining choices to identify similarities and differences to the stem or clue. Compare the differences with the clue to see if you can eliminate another choice. Select the remaining choice.

Example:

Which of the following observations may be an indication of high blood pressure?
(A) Flushed skin
(B) Pale skin
(C) Cold skin
(D) Weak pulse

What is the clue?

Answer: high pressure

Can I eliminate any choices?

Answer: Yes. There is a direct relationship between pressure and force; therefore, choice (D) cannot be the correct answer.

What are the similarities and differences among choices (A), (B), and (C)?

Answer: They all relate to changes in skin characteristics. However, choices (B) and (C) are similar. As a matter of fact, if choice (B) were correct, choice (C) would also be correct.

The correct answer, then, is choice (A).

Now, let's assume that the following question is also on the test.

Why do some people with high blood pressure have flushed skin?

(A) The pulse weakens and blood pools in the skin.

(B) The skin temperature lowers and the skin blood vessels dilate.

(C) The increased pressure increases the volume of blood to the arteries.

(D) The increased pressure forces the arteries to dilate.

Based on your experience with the previous item, you would immediately eliminate choices (A) and (B). Looking at choices (C) and (D), you might think that both would cause reddened skin. However, you would either eliminate choice (D) because it contradicts the relationship between pressure and volume, or you would select choice (C) because it supports the relationship between pressure and volume.

PLEASE PRACTICE THIS TECHNIQUE WITH THE SAMPLE ITEMS!

A summary of the seven steps for preparing to take a nursing school entrance examination follows:

1. Study the concepts and principles presented in each section so that you will have a good base of knowledge.

2. Study one section at a time over a period of time—whatever is reasonable for your learning style. Do not cram!

3. Take the tests related to each section immediately after studying the explanatory materials.

4. Follow all directions for each test carefully.

5. Utilize the guidelines for test-taking as presented in this section.

6. Check your answers in order to diagnose your strengths and weaknesses.

7. Seek additional information from reliable resources in the areas in which you are weak.

REDUCING TEST ANXIETY

Anxiety results from a threat to our well-being that might be real or perceived. This threat makes us uncomfortable and affects our feelings of self-esteem. We then change our behavior in an attempt to seek relief.

Many people become anxious about taking a test because they anticipate that someone is going to make a judgment about them based on their test performance. Is your self-esteem strong enough for you to think, "I can pass this test!" Or, do you lack confidence in yourself and assume "I am going to fail."

What can you do to prevent this kind of negative thinking? First, you must realize that anxiety can be both productive and destructive. Anxiety can be energizing if you direct the energy toward your goals and away from the imagined threats. For example, you may have the idea that the admission test will determine your entire future. If you don't pass the test, you imagine that you won't be admitted to the program of your choice. The fact is that admission tests are used along with many other kinds of information to determine your eligibility for entering a program. Therefore, this is not a real threat. On the other hand, if you have made no effort to prepare for this test, then your chances for admission might be threatened.

The secret to success is confidence. You can gain that confidence by completing the practice tests in this book with a score of 80 percent or above in all areas. This should assure you that you can perform well on the admission test.

There are several things that you can do to relieve anxiety.

Set up a time-frame for studying this book. Schedule a few pages per day to avoid a last-minute rush.

Sharing your anxiety helps to reduce it. Talk to a friend. Explore the *'what if'* situations and the related options for achieving your career goals.

Provide an outlet for yourself—perhaps exercise or some other physical activity that you enjoy.

Think back to how you have handled stress and anxiety in your past experiences. Draw on those experiences.

Positive thinking is a must. Imagine yourself receiving the results of your test enclosed in a letter of congratulations that you share with your family and friends. Make plans for the next step toward achieving your career goals. Imagine the pleasurable feeling and comfort that comes from a job well done. You'll do just fine!

PART II
DIAGNOSING STRENGTHS AND WEAKNESSES

Diagnostic Test

The following Diagnostic Test is divided into three parts: one each for Registered Nursing, Allied Health, and Practical/Vocational Nursing. Each part is divided further into four sections: Verbal Ability or Verbal Skills, depending on the exam; Mathematics, Quantitative Ability, or Arithmetic and Mathematics, again depending on the exam; Science; and Reading Comprehension. The question types are similar to what you will find on each exam.

After each Part, you will find an Answer Key and Answer Explanations for that Part. At the end of each explanation, you will find the topic or theme assessed in that question. This information will help you identify areas that you should spend more time on as you study and prepare for your exam.

Each Part begins with directions and a time limit. Set a timer for that amount of time and see how you do answering all the questions in that amount of time. Knowing how long it takes you will help you determine a pacing plan for each section of the actual exam.

Choose the Part of the Diagnostic Test that matches the nursing career that you are pursuing and complete it to see your strengths and those areas that you need to improve on.

diagnostic

Part I: Registered Nursing School

Verbal Ability

1. Ⓐ Ⓑ Ⓒ Ⓓ   3. Ⓐ Ⓑ Ⓒ Ⓓ   5. Ⓐ Ⓑ Ⓒ Ⓓ   7. Ⓐ Ⓑ Ⓒ Ⓓ   9. Ⓐ Ⓑ Ⓒ Ⓓ
2. Ⓐ Ⓑ Ⓒ Ⓓ   4. Ⓐ Ⓑ Ⓒ Ⓓ   6. Ⓐ Ⓑ Ⓒ Ⓓ   8. Ⓐ Ⓑ Ⓒ Ⓓ   10. Ⓐ Ⓑ Ⓒ Ⓓ

Mathematics

1. Ⓐ Ⓑ Ⓒ Ⓓ   3. Ⓐ Ⓑ Ⓒ Ⓓ   5. Ⓐ Ⓑ Ⓒ Ⓓ   7. Ⓐ Ⓑ Ⓒ Ⓓ   9. Ⓐ Ⓑ Ⓒ Ⓓ
2. Ⓐ Ⓑ Ⓒ Ⓓ   4. Ⓐ Ⓑ Ⓒ Ⓓ   6. Ⓐ Ⓑ Ⓒ Ⓓ   8. Ⓐ Ⓑ Ⓒ Ⓓ   10. Ⓐ Ⓑ Ⓒ Ⓓ

Science

1. Ⓐ Ⓑ Ⓒ Ⓓ   3. Ⓐ Ⓑ Ⓒ Ⓓ   5. Ⓐ Ⓑ Ⓒ Ⓓ   7. Ⓐ Ⓑ Ⓒ Ⓓ   9. Ⓐ Ⓑ Ⓒ Ⓓ
2. Ⓐ Ⓑ Ⓒ Ⓓ   4. Ⓐ Ⓑ Ⓒ Ⓓ   6. Ⓐ Ⓑ Ⓒ Ⓓ   8. Ⓐ Ⓑ Ⓒ Ⓓ   10. Ⓐ Ⓑ Ⓒ Ⓓ

Reading Comprehension

1. Ⓐ Ⓑ Ⓒ Ⓓ   3. Ⓐ Ⓑ Ⓒ Ⓓ   5. Ⓐ Ⓑ Ⓒ Ⓓ   7. Ⓐ Ⓑ Ⓒ Ⓓ   9. Ⓐ Ⓑ Ⓒ Ⓓ
2. Ⓐ Ⓑ Ⓒ Ⓓ   4. Ⓐ Ⓑ Ⓒ Ⓓ   6. Ⓐ Ⓑ Ⓒ Ⓓ   8. Ⓐ Ⓑ Ⓒ Ⓓ   10. Ⓐ Ⓑ Ⓒ Ⓓ

Allied Health School

Verbal Ability

1. Ⓐ Ⓑ Ⓒ Ⓓ   3. Ⓐ Ⓑ Ⓒ Ⓓ   5. Ⓐ Ⓑ Ⓒ Ⓓ   7. Ⓐ Ⓑ Ⓒ Ⓓ   9. Ⓐ Ⓑ Ⓒ Ⓓ
2. Ⓐ Ⓑ Ⓒ Ⓓ   4. Ⓐ Ⓑ Ⓒ Ⓓ   6. Ⓐ Ⓑ Ⓒ Ⓓ   8. Ⓐ Ⓑ Ⓒ Ⓓ   10. Ⓐ Ⓑ Ⓒ Ⓓ

Quantitative Ability

1. Ⓐ Ⓑ Ⓒ Ⓓ   3. Ⓐ Ⓑ Ⓒ Ⓓ   5. Ⓐ Ⓑ Ⓒ Ⓓ   7. Ⓐ Ⓑ Ⓒ Ⓓ   9. Ⓐ Ⓑ Ⓒ Ⓓ
2. Ⓐ Ⓑ Ⓒ Ⓓ   4. Ⓐ Ⓑ Ⓒ Ⓓ   6. Ⓐ Ⓑ Ⓒ Ⓓ   8. Ⓐ Ⓑ Ⓒ Ⓓ   10. Ⓐ Ⓑ Ⓒ Ⓓ

Science

1. Ⓐ Ⓑ Ⓒ Ⓓ   3. Ⓐ Ⓑ Ⓒ Ⓓ   5. Ⓐ Ⓑ Ⓒ Ⓓ   7. Ⓐ Ⓑ Ⓒ Ⓓ   9. Ⓐ Ⓑ Ⓒ Ⓓ
2. Ⓐ Ⓑ Ⓒ Ⓓ   4. Ⓐ Ⓑ Ⓒ Ⓓ   6. Ⓐ Ⓑ Ⓒ Ⓓ   8. Ⓐ Ⓑ Ⓒ Ⓓ   10. Ⓐ Ⓑ Ⓒ Ⓓ

Reading Comprehension

1. Ⓐ Ⓑ Ⓒ Ⓓ   3. Ⓐ Ⓑ Ⓒ Ⓓ   5. Ⓐ Ⓑ Ⓒ Ⓓ   7. Ⓐ Ⓑ Ⓒ Ⓓ   9. Ⓐ Ⓑ Ⓒ Ⓓ
2. Ⓐ Ⓑ Ⓒ Ⓓ   4. Ⓐ Ⓑ Ⓒ Ⓓ   6. Ⓐ Ⓑ Ⓒ Ⓓ   8. Ⓐ Ⓑ Ⓒ Ⓓ   10. Ⓐ Ⓑ Ⓒ Ⓓ

answer sheet

Practical/Vocational Nursing School

Verbal Ability

1. Ⓐ Ⓑ Ⓒ Ⓓ   3. Ⓐ Ⓑ Ⓒ Ⓓ   5. Ⓐ Ⓑ Ⓒ Ⓓ   7. Ⓐ Ⓑ Ⓒ Ⓓ   9. Ⓐ Ⓑ Ⓒ Ⓓ
2. Ⓐ Ⓑ Ⓒ Ⓓ   4. Ⓐ Ⓑ Ⓒ Ⓓ   6. Ⓐ Ⓑ Ⓒ Ⓓ   8. Ⓐ Ⓑ Ⓒ Ⓓ   10. Ⓐ Ⓑ Ⓒ Ⓓ

Arithmetic and Mathematics

1. Ⓐ Ⓑ Ⓒ Ⓓ   3. Ⓐ Ⓑ Ⓒ Ⓓ   5. Ⓐ Ⓑ Ⓒ Ⓓ   7. Ⓐ Ⓑ Ⓒ Ⓓ   9. Ⓐ Ⓑ Ⓒ Ⓓ
2. Ⓐ Ⓑ Ⓒ Ⓓ   4. Ⓐ Ⓑ Ⓒ Ⓓ   6. Ⓐ Ⓑ Ⓒ Ⓓ   8. Ⓐ Ⓑ Ⓒ Ⓓ   10. Ⓐ Ⓑ Ⓒ Ⓓ

Science

1. Ⓐ Ⓑ Ⓒ Ⓓ   3. Ⓐ Ⓑ Ⓒ Ⓓ   5. Ⓐ Ⓑ Ⓒ Ⓓ   7. Ⓐ Ⓑ Ⓒ Ⓓ   9. Ⓐ Ⓑ Ⓒ Ⓓ
2. Ⓐ Ⓑ Ⓒ Ⓓ   4. Ⓐ Ⓑ Ⓒ Ⓓ   6. Ⓐ Ⓑ Ⓒ Ⓓ   8. Ⓐ Ⓑ Ⓒ Ⓓ   10. Ⓐ Ⓑ Ⓒ Ⓓ

Reading Comprehension

1. Ⓐ Ⓑ Ⓒ Ⓓ   3. Ⓐ Ⓑ Ⓒ Ⓓ   5. Ⓐ Ⓑ Ⓒ Ⓓ   7. Ⓐ Ⓑ Ⓒ Ⓓ   9. Ⓐ Ⓑ Ⓒ Ⓓ
2. Ⓐ Ⓑ Ⓒ Ⓓ   4. Ⓐ Ⓑ Ⓒ Ⓓ   6. Ⓐ Ⓑ Ⓒ Ⓓ   8. Ⓐ Ⓑ Ⓒ Ⓓ   10. Ⓐ Ⓑ Ⓒ Ⓓ

REGISTERED NURSING SCHOOL

Verbal Ability

10 Questions • 5 Minutes

Directions: In each of the sentences below, one word is italicized. Following each sentence are four words or phrases. For each sentence, choose the word or phrase that most nearly corresponds in meaning with the italicized word.

1. The *adverse* publicity about the mayor's decision caused him to reverse it.
   - **(A)** affirmative
   - **(B)** unfavorable
   - **(C)** anxious
   - **(D)** conspicuous

2. The patient's *florid* complexion was a sign of a high fever.
   - **(A)** flamboyant
   - **(B)** challenging
   - **(C)** flushed
   - **(D)** impressive

3. She was so happy at being accepted into school that she broke into an *impromptu* dance by the mailbox.
   - **(A)** accidental
   - **(B)** incongruous
   - **(C)** spontaneous
   - **(D)** funny

Directions: In each of the following questions, select the word opposite in meaning to the word printed in capital letters.

4. BLAMELESS
   - **(A)** culpable
   - **(B)** honest
   - **(C)** irreproachable
   - **(D)** upright

5. MINISTER TO
   - **(A)** official
   - **(B)** delegate to
   - **(C)** ignore
   - **(D)** tend to

6. FIERCE
   - **(A)** tame
   - **(B)** vehement
   - **(C)** aggressive
   - **(D)** intense

7. ADMONISH
   - **(A)** admission
   - **(B)** rebuke
   - **(C)** censure
   - **(D)** compliment

Directions: In the following questions, determine the relationship between the first pair of capitalized words and then decide which of the answer choices shares a similar relationship with the third capitalized word.

8. LOYAL : TRAITOROUS :: BENEVOLENT :
   - **(A)** ungenerous
   - **(B)** disloyal
   - **(C)** advantageous
   - **(D)** congratulatory

9. SURGEON : OPERATING ROOM :: ACTOR :
   - **(A)** dressing room
   - **(B)** theater
   - **(C)** stage
   - **(D)** audition

10. MASON : BRICKLAYING :: CARPEN-
TER :
    (A) building
    (B) hammer
    (C) laying pipe
    (D) wiring

Mathematics

10 Questions • 10 Minutes

Directions: Each problem requires logical reasoning and thinking in addition to simple computations to find the solution. Read each questions carefully and choose the correct answer from the four choices that follow.

1. Sally receives a 15% commission on all the pharmaceuticals she sells. In the month of July, she sold $14,500 worth of pharmaceuticals. What was the value of her commission?
   (A) $2,000
   (B) $2,175
   (C) $2,375
   (D) $2,565

2. $3 + 5(0.4 - 0.1)(4)^2 =$
   (A) 18
   (B) 21
   (C) 22
   (D) 27

3. 18 is what percent of 72?
   (A) 25%
   (B) 18%
   (C) 5%
   (D) 4%

4. Dr. Sarah Johnson bought an old house and wants to fix it up. The first project she wants to do is paint the walls of the family room. If the room is 8 feet high, 13 feet wide, and 18 feet long, how much paint would she need to do two coats, if the paint covers 300 square feet per gallon?
   (A) 2.2
   (B) 3
   (C) 3.3
   (D) 4

5. Jack Anderson recently financed the purchase of a new house. He bought the house for $132,000. The mortgage is for 80%. What is the amount of his mortgage?
   (A) $132,000
   (B) $80,000
   (C) $16,400
   (D) $105,600

6. Which of the following is true about two perpendicular lines?
   (A) They never cross.
   (B) The angles created by their crossing are acute.
   (C) The angles created by their crossing are obtuse.
   (D) The angles created by their crossing are right angles.

7. A triangle has an area of 196. What is its height, if the base is 16?

    (A) 6.125

    (B) 12.25

    (C) 24.5

    (D) 49

8. 516 sets of scrubs at $3,512 per hundred will cost

    (A) $18,121.92

    (B) $21,154.74

    (C) $10,342.84

    (D) $32,749.02

Directions: For questions 9 and 10, two quantities are given: one in Column A and one in Column B. Compare the two quantities to determine the correct answer. Your options (A) through (D) are shown with each question.

9.

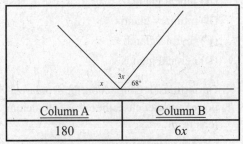

Column A	Column B
180	6x

    (A) if quantity A is greater.

    (B) if quantity B is greater.

    (C) if the two quantities are equal.

    (D) if the relationship cannot be determined from the information given.

10.

$xy = 15$	
Column A	Column B
$(3x)(4y)$	180

    (A) if quantity A is greater.

    (B) if quantity B is greater.

    (C) if the two quantities are equal.

    (D) if the relationship cannot be determined from the information given.

Science

10 Questions • 10 Minutes

Directions: Read each question carefully and consider all possible answers. There is only one best answer for each question.

1. The cellular organelle in which cellular respiration takes place is the
   (A) ribosomes.
   (B) endoplasmic reticulum.
   (C) mitochondria.
   (D) Golgi apparatus.

2. The fusion of two gametes of different size and structure is called
   (A) isogamy.
   (B) ansiogamy.
   (C) conjugation.
   (D) oogamy.

3. Which process of human cellular metabolism releases carbon dioxide during the reaction?
   (A) Krebs cycle
   (B) Glycolysis
   (C) Oxidative phosphorylation
   (D) Photosynthesis

4. Which type of nucleic acid matches a specific amino acid to its codon?
   (A) mRNA
   (B) rRNA
   (C) tRNA
   (D) DNA

5. Which two ions play a role in the transmission of sensory information to the brain?
   (A) Na^+ and Ca^{2+}
   (B) Na^+ and K^+
   (C) K^+ and Ca^{2+}
   (D) H^+ and K^+

6. Which structure of the respiratory system is encircled by rings of cartilage to ensure that air can always pass through?
   (A) Bronchioles
   (B) Pharynx
   (C) Diaphragm
   (D) Trachea

7. Blood is classified into a specific type by its
   (A) erythrocyte antigens.
   (B) plasma antigens.
   (C) plasma antibodies.
   (D) platelet antibodies.

8. Metabolic processes in the body are regulated by hormones produced in the
   (A) pineal gland.
   (B) pituitary gland.
   (C) thyroid gland.
   (D) adrenal glands.

9. During muscle contraction, the depolarization of muscle causes the release of calcium ions from
   (A) neurotransmitters.
   (B) the sacroplasmic reticulum.
   (C) the endoplasmic reticulum.
   (D) the actin filaments.

10. In a simple food chain, humans are classified as
    (A) parasites.
    (B) producers.
    (C) consumers.
    (D) decomposers.

Reading Comprehension

10 Questions • 20 Minutes

> **Directions:** Carefully read the following paragraphs and then answer the accompanying questions, basing your answer on what is stated in the paragraphs. There is only one best answer for each question.

Some Therapies for Asthma Sufferers

A

There are a number of treatments available for asthma sufferers, but some are more effective for certain types of use than others. For example, short-acting best agonists (bronchodilators) and oral and intravenous corticosteroids are best for rapid relief. They are not for long-term use. However, they can be beneficial for those who have exercise-induced asthma if used before commencing exercise.

B

Inhaled corticosteroids provide long-term control of asthma symptoms. Sometimes, combining medications with both a beta-2 agonist and an inhaled steroid is useful for long-term control. Those who have allergy-induced asthma may be prescribed a course of shots for desensitization, that is, a course of specific immunotherapy related to the allergen.

C

Controversial therapies include the use of leukotriene modifiers. These prevent symptoms for up to 24 hours. However, there are a number of recorded side effects. Patients taking this class of drugs have experienced hallucinations, agitations, aggressive behavior, and even thoughts of suicide. Among unproven methods for relief of asthma are breathing techniques, including so-called "yoga breathing," and the ingestion of herbal remedies such as gingko.

1. Oral and intravenous corticosteroids are best for
   - **(A)** long-term control of asthma symptoms.
   - **(B)** preventing symptoms up to 24 hours.
   - **(C)** rapid relief of symptoms.
   - **(D)** desensitizing those who have allergy-induced asthma.

2. Which statement is supported by paragraph C?
   - **(A)** Techniques such as yoga breathing are controversial.
   - **(B)** Leutokriene modifiers combine several medications to be most effective.
   - **(C)** Ginkgo is prescribed for controlling asthma symptoms in the short term.
   - **(D)** Doctors prescribing leukotriene modifiers should monitor their patients closely.

Obesity in Children

A

Obesity is a problem that affects children as well as adults. Since the 1970s, childhood obesity has been on the rise among U.S. children. Like their parents, obese children face a series of health problems. These include hypertension, high cholesterol, and Type 2 diabetes, as well as discrimination from less overweight peers. The latter can lead to depression and poor self-esteem. Some children may be able to overcome their weight as adults, but the evidence *belies* this for most obese children. An obese child has a 70 percent chance of being obese as an adult.

B

It's never too late to help children eat healthful meals and snacks, but parents have to be willing to eat healthfully themselves. That means following the U.S. Department of Agriculture's Food Plate to ensure that they and their children have the right amount of fruits, vegetables, grains, protein, and dairy while reducing the amount of oils, sugar, and fats in their diet. Cooking oils are major ingredients in foods such as cookies, cakes, chips, and donuts. Other foods have what dieticians call empty calories because they have few or no nutrients. These foods include sodas and energy, sports, and fruit drinks; cheese, pizza; ice cream; sausage; hot dogs; bacon; and ribs. Cheese, pizza, ice cream, and ribs may seem less appetizing when you think of them as solid fat. The added sugar in ice cream also adds to its being unhealthful.

C

One way to get around the problem with some of these foods is to buy low-fat or sugar-free versions. For example, you can buy low-fat hot dogs and low-fat cheese as well as plain water and sugar-free sodas. Other foods to look for are unsweetened applesauce, cereals, and gelatin; extra lean ground meat; and fat-free milk. Drinking plain water is also a good antidote to the empty calories in sodas, flavored waters, and sports drinks.

D

But it's not just parents who need to help children maintain a healthy weight. Schools have to be willing to forego some of their revenue from allowing companies to stock school vending machines with candy bars and sugary drinks, including flavored waters high in sugar content. Owners of stores near schools that sell snacks to students need to be willing to substitute healthful snacks for bags of potato chips, candy bars, and popsicles.

E

Schools have another responsibility, but ultimately it can come down to taxpayers. It's important that children and adolescents get at least 60 minutes or more of physical activity daily according to the FDA. This moderate to vigorous activity should include muscle strengthening and bone strengthening. Much of this is done, or could be done, outside of school, but an active physical education program in schools is also an important component. However, when faced with budget deficits and increased pressure on passing state academic tests, districts choose to cut physical education programs to the detriment of their students, especially urban students with no place to play after school.

3. Which of the following would be a better title for this passage?
   (A) Helping Children Maintain Healthy Weight
   (B) Schools Have a Responsibility in the Childhood Obesity Trend
   (C) Stores That Sell Snacks Need to Change
   (D) Parents Need Education on How to Fight Obesity

4. The word *belie* in paragraph A means
   (A) contradicts.
   (B) proves.
   (C) interprets.
   (D) expresses.

5. According to the passage, parents can buy a healthful alternative to which of the following foods?

    (A) Donuts

    (B) Hot dogs

    (C) Pizza

    (D) Cookies

6. Empty-calorie foods are foods that

    (A) are good to eat because they fill a person up without adding weight.

    (B) leave a person hungry after eating them.

    (C) have little or no nutritional value.

    (D) have a lot of air in them.

7. What kind of activities should children and adolescents have daily?

    (A) A physical education program

    (B) Running and jumping

    (C) Vigorous exercise

    (D) Bone-strengthening and muscle-strengthening activities

Making the Decision to Move

A

Are you going to be the caregiver for your parents or for other older relatives like a beloved aunt? Where do they live now? How old are they? Have they or you given any thought to having them move close to you? How *feasible* will it be to take time off and fly or even drive several hours if the person falls and breaks a hip or has a heart attack? How long can you take off from work to be with the person? Will you need to come home and then go back when the person is ready to come home from the hospital or from rehab? These are questions facing many adult children today whose family member or members they will be caring for in later years.

B

And "later" for some of these adult children is right around the corner—or even now. According to the 2010 Census, there were more than 40 million Americans 65 and older. This is 13 percent of the total population. By 2050, the percentage is expected to grow to 21 percent. Of the more than 40 million 65 and older, less than half—43 percent or 17 million—are men. The trend line for the percentage as well as real number of Americans 65 and older has moved steadily upward since 1900. The other notable fact between 2000 and 2010 is that the population of those 65 years and over grew at a faster rate than the total population. While women over 65 still outnumber men in that age group, the number of males over 65 increased faster than the number of women.

C

All increase in population also means more people needing care. There are various solutions to the problem. One is for the family member or members to move close to the potential caregiver while still young enough to do it on their own and still able to get around, make new friends, and experience what their new locales offer in the way of entertainment, hobbies, and life-long learning. Another is to stay where the older person currently lives, but to move into a community with step-up care, that is, a community that provides a continuum of care from totally independent housing to assisted living to nursing facilities. In this way, the potential caregiver is relieved of worry about the person while also being relieved of day-to-day direct care responsibilities.

8. What does the word *feasible* mean in paragraph A?
   (A) Possible
   (B) Impractical
   (C) Unworkable
   (D) Capable

9. In 2010, what was the percentage of the total U.S. population 65 and older?
   (A) 40
   (B) 43
   (C) 13
   (D) 21

10. What can a new locale offer older persons who move on their own?
   (A) Day-to-day direct care
   (B) Proximity to their families
   (C) A nursing home
   (D) New friends and experiences

ANSWER KEY AND EXPLANATIONS

Verbal Ability

1. B	3. C	5. C	7. D	9. C
2. C	4. A	6. A	8. A	10. A

1. **The correct answer is (B).** *Adverse* means "unfavorable." Choice (A) is incorrect because *affirmative* means "approval or agreement," and if the publicity had been good, the mayor would not have reversed his decision. *Affirmative* is an antonym for *adverse*, not a synonym. Choice (C) is incorrect because the mayor may have been *anxious*, but the word has no relation to *adverse*. Choice (D) is incorrect because although the publicity may have been *conspicuous*, that is, obvious and easy to notice, which may have helped the mayor decide, it would have been the type of publicity—negative—that motivated him to change his mind. **(Synonyms)**

2. **The correct answer is (C).** *Florid* means "*flushed*, ruddy, reddish," but the word may also mean "flowery" and "ornate, flamboyant." However, in this context, choice (A) is incorrect and choice (C) is correct. Choice (B) is incorrect because while getting a high fever down may be *challenging*, the word has no relation to *florid*, and neither does choice (D), *impressive*. **(Synonyms)**

3. **The correct answer is (C).** *Impromptu* and *spontaneous* are synonyms. The dance may have been *accidental*, in that she hadn't planned on doing it, but *accidental* doesn't have the same positive connotation as *impromptu*, so choice (A) is incorrect. Choice (B) is incorrect because *incongruous* means "incompatible, improper." Choice (D) is incorrect because while the dance may have been *funny*, it is not a synonym for *impromptu*. **(Synonyms)**

4. **The correct answer is (A).** The opposite of *blameless* is *culpable*, or blameworthy. Choice (B) is incorrect because *honest* is a

synonym for *blameless*, as are choice (C), *irreproachable*, and choice (D), *upright*. **(Antonyms)**

5. **The correct answer is (C).** To *minister to* someone is "to *tend to* someone," so choice (D) is incorrect because you need an antonym. Choice (A) is incorrect because *official* is a noun and the question requires a verb. Choice (B) is incorrect because *delegate to* is "to give someone else a task or authority to get something done. That leaves only choice (C), *ignore*. **(Antonyms)**

6. **The correct answer is (A).** The opposite of *fierce* is *tame*. Choices (B), (C), and (D), *vehement, aggressive,* and *intense*, are similar in meanings to *fierce*, rather than being antonyms. **(Antonyms)**

7. **The correct answer is (D).** To *admonish* is "to *rebuke*" or "to *censure*," meaning "to warn, caution, or discourage against someone or something," so choices (B) and (C) are incorrect. Choice (A), *admission*, which may be a confession of guilt or of wrongdoing, is a noun and the question requires a verb. That leaves only choice (D), *compliment*, meaning "praise." **(Antonyms)**

8. **The correct answer is (A).** This is an antonym analogy. *Traitorous* is the opposite of *loyal*, so you need an answer that is the opposite of *benevolent*, meaning "generous, giving willingly." The opposite of this is choice (A), *ungenerous*. Choice (B) is incorrect because *disloyal* is the opposite of *loyal* in the first pair of words. Choices (C) and (D) are incorrect because *advantageous* and *congratulatory* are not antonyms for *benevolent*. **(Antonym Analogy)**

9. **The correct answer is (C).** This is a person/worker-to-place analogy. A *surgeon* works in an *operating room* and an *actor* works on a *stage*. Choice (A) is incorrect because an actor's natural place of work is the *stage*, not the *dressing room* where the actor prepares to work. Choice (B) is incorrect because *theater* is too general a term; it would have fit if the first pair had been *surgeon* to *hospital*. Choice (D) is incorrect because an *audition* is not a place. **(Person/worker-to-place Analogy)**

10. **The correct answer is (A).** In this person/worker-to-occupation analogy, a *mason lays brick* and a *carpenter builds*. Choice (B) is incorrect because a *hammer* is a tool, not an occupation. Choice (C) is incorrect because a plumber *lays pipe*. Choice (D) is incorrect because an electrician handles *wiring*. **(Person/worker-to-occupation Analogy)**

Mathematics

1. B	3. A	5. D	7. C	9. A
2. D	4. C	6. D	8. A	10. C

1. The correct answer is (B).

$$15\%\big(\$14,500\big) = 0.15\big(\$14,500\big)$$
$$= \$2,175$$

(Percentages)

2. The correct answer is (D).

$$3 + 5\big(0.4 - 0.1\big)\big(4\big)^2 = 3 + 5\big(0.3\big)\big(4\big)^2$$
$$= 3 + 5\big(0.3\big)\big(16\big)$$
$$= 3 + 24$$
$$= 27$$

(Order of Operations, Decimals)

3. The correct answer is (A).

$$\frac{18}{72} = 0.25, \text{ or } 25\%$$

(Percentages)

4 The correct answer is (C).

$$\text{one coat} = 2\big(8 \times 13\big) + 2\big(8 \times 18\big)$$
$$= 2\big(104\big) + 2\big(144\big)$$
$$= 208 + 288$$
$$= 496$$

$$\text{two coats} = 2\big(496\big)$$
$$= 992$$

$$\frac{992}{300} = 3.30$$

(Order of Operations; Problem Solving)

5. The correct answer is (D).

$$80\%\big(\$132,000\big) = 0.8\big(\$132,000\big)$$
$$= \$105,600$$

(Percentages)

6. The correct answer is (D).

Perpendicular lines by definition are lines that intersect to form right angles.

(Geometry Definitions)

7. The correct answer is (C).

$$\text{area of a triangle} = \frac{1}{2}\big(\text{base}\big)\big(\text{height}\big)$$
$$196 = \frac{1}{2}\big(16\big)\big(x\big)$$
$$196 = 8x$$
$$\frac{196}{8} = x$$
$$24.5 = x$$

(Area)

8. The correct answer is (A).

$$\$3,512 \div 100 = \$35.12$$

$$\$35.12\big(516\big) = \$18,121.92$$

(Multiplication, Division, Decimals; Problem Solving)

9. **The correct answer is (A).**

$$x + 3x + 68 = 180$$
$$4x = 112$$
$$x = 28$$
$$6(28) = 168$$

(One Variable)

10. **The correct answer is (C).**

$$(3x)(4y) = 12xy$$
$$= 12(15)$$
$$= 180$$

(Two Variables)

Science

1. C	3. A	5. B	7. A	9. B
2. D	4. C	6. D	8. C	10. C

1. **The correct answer is (C).** Mitochondria are important organelles in the cell in which cellular respiration occurs. Macromolecules such as carbohydrates, fats, and proteins are oxidized resulting in the release of ATP, a form of usable energy that all cells require. Choice (A) is incorrect because ribosomes are the organelles that synthesize proteins from mRNA templates. Choice (B) is incorrect because the endoplasmic reticulum is active in the synthesis and transport of proteins. Choice (D) is incorrect because the Golgi apparatus functions in the synthesis, modification, sorting, and secretion of cell products. Products of the ER are modified and stored in the Golgi and then sent to other destinations. **(The Cell)**

2. **The correct answer is (D).** Heterogamy is a mechanism of sexual reproduction involving the fusion of gametes that differ in size and/or structure, and oogamy is a type of heterogamy that involves gametes that differ in size and structure. Choice (A) is incorrect because isogamy is a mechanism of sexual reproduction involving the fusion of gametes of identical size and structure. Choice (B) is incorrect because ansiogamy is a type of heterogamy that involves motile gametes that differ only in size. Choice (C) is incorrect because conjugation is a mechanism of sexual reproduction that involves the temporary union of cells to allow for the exchange or transmission of genetic information. **(Reproduction)**

3. **The correct answer is (A).** During two different steps of the Krebs cycle, or citric acid cycle, CO_2 is released as a by-product of a reaction step. Choice (B) is incorrect because the glycolysis reaction that takes place in the cytosol in the absence of oxygen releases H_2O, but does not release CO_2. Choice (C) is incorrect because the process of oxidative phosphorylation also releases H_2O, but not CO_2. Choice (D) is incorrect because although photosynthesis requires CO_2 as a reactant, it releases O_2, and also, it takes place only in green plants, not humans. **(Metabolism)**

4. **The correct answer is (C).** Transfer RNA, or tRNA, matches each specific amino acid to its codon on an mRNA strand. The codon is a three-nucleotide sequence that is specific for only one of the 26 amino acids. Thus, tRNA molecules are able to pick up a specific amino acid and deliver it to a specific amino acid codon. Choice (A) is incorrect because messenger RNA, or mRNA, is the template for amino acid synthesis and contains the codon sequences. Choice (B) is incorrect because ribosomal RNA, or rRNA, is the key component of ribosomes. Choice (D) is incorrect because DNA contains genetic information, but is not directly involved in protein synthesis. **(Nucleic Acids)**

5. **The correct answer is (B).** The transmission of nerve impulse is electrical in nature and involves a difference in the concentration of certain ions, in particular sodium (Na^+) and potassium (K^+). The difference in concentration forms a gradient along the nerve fibers. Choice (A) is incorrect because Ca^{2+} ions do not play a role in the transmission of sensory information. Choice (C) is incorrect because Ca^{2+} does not play a role in the transmission of sensory information. Choice (D) is incorrect because protons, H^+, do not play a role in the transmission of sensory information. **(Nervous System)**

6. **The correct answer is (D).** The trachea, or windpipe, is encircled by rings of cartilage so that it always remains open. Choice (A) is incorrect because the bronchi are two branches that connect the trachea to the lungs and they are also encircled by

cartilage, but the bronchioles are smaller, narrower tubes through which air is distributed around the lungs. They are not surrounded by cartilage. Choice (B) is incorrect because the pharynx, or throat, is made of soft tissue, not cartilage. Choice (C) is incorrect because the diaphragm is a muscle in the lower portion of the respiratory system; thus, it is composed of muscle tissue, not cartilage. **(Respiratory System)**

7. **The correct answer is (A).** Blood is classified into one of the four blood types based on the antigens found on red blood cells, or erythrocytes. Choice (B) is incorrect because blood is classified based on antigens found on the surface of red blood cells. Antigens are not present in blood plasma. Choice (C) is incorrect because although plasma contains antibodies, it is the antigens that are used to classify blood by type. Choice (D) is incorrect because platelets are small fragments in the blood that are important for clotting. They do not contain antibodies. **(Circulatory System)**

8. **The correct answer is (C).** The thyroid gland produces thyroxine (T4) and tri-iodothryonine (T3) that stimulate and maintain metabolic processes. Choice (A) is incorrect because the pineal gland is a small pea-sized gland near the center of the brain that synthesizes and secretes melatonin. Melatonin links biorhythms with environmental light (daily and seasonal). Choice (B) is incorrect because one lobe of the pituitary gland secretes hormones made in the hypothalamus, including oxytocin and antidiruretic hormone. The other lobe of the pituitary gland makes and secretes hormones into the bloodstream. These hormones do not play a role in metabolism. Choice (D) is incorrect because the adrenal glands are located above the kidneys and secrete hormones in response to stress on the body. **(Endocrine System)**

9. **The correct answer is (B).** During the process of muscle contraction, the depolarization of the muscle causes the release of calcium ions from the sacroplasmic reticulum. The sacroplasmic reticulum stores calcium ions that are released upon the arrival of a stimulus from the action potential of nerve cells surrounding the muscle. Choice (A) is incorrect because neurotransmitters are released by neurons sending an impulse. The neurotransmitters are released onto the muscle cells. Choice (C) is incorrect because the endoplasmic reticulum is a cellular organelle that is responsible for the synthesis and processing of proteins. It does not release calcium ions. Choice (D) is incorrect because the actin filaments act in muscle contraction by sliding past the myosin filaments, but they do not release calcium ions. **(Musculoskeletal System)**

10. **The correct answer is (C).** Consumers are organisms in a food chain, or food web, that either eat producers or other consumers to obtain energy. Humans are classified as consumers. In particular, humans are omnivores because they eat both producers (plants) and consumers (animals). Choice (A) is incorrect because parasites are organisms that live on a host organism and obtain nourishment while harming the health of the host. Choice (B) is incorrect because producers are organisms that are able to use energy from the sun to make complex organic molecules from simple inorganic substances such as nitrogen and phosphorous in their environment. Plants are producers that carry out the process of photosynthesis. Choice (D) is incorrect because decomposers are organisms that rely upon nonliving organic matter as a source of energy and material for growth. Fungi are examples of decomposers. **(Energy in Ecosystems)**

Reading Comprehension

1. C	3. A	5. B	7. D	9. C
2. D	4. A	6. C	8. A	10. D

1. **The correct answer is (C).** The answer is stated in paragraph A, sentence 2.

2. **The correct answer is (D).** This answer requires an inference. You can infer from the side effects listed in paragraph C, sentence 3, that patients taking leukotriene modifiers would require monitoring.

3. **The correct answer is (A).** The title of a piece of writing typically reflects the main idea or theme of the piece. Only choice (A) expresses the general idea, which is about ways to help children maintain a healthy weight. Choices (B) and (C) are too specific; each addresses only one factor discussed in the passage. Choice (D) is incorrect because the need for parental education is not addressed as such in the passage, only that parents need to eat healthfully also.

4. **The correct answer is (A).** *Belie* means "to contradict." Choice (B) is incorrect because *proves* is an antonym. Choices (C) and (D) are incorrect because *interprets* and *expresses* have no relation to *belie*.

5. **The correct answer is (B).** The answer is stated in paragraph C, sentence 2.

6. **The correct answer is (C).** The answer is stated in paragraph B, sentence 4. Choice (B) may be true in that eating these foods high in fat and sugar may leave a person hungry, but that's not why they are called empty calories, so eliminate choice (B). In addition, this information is not stated in the passage and you should base your answers on only what is in the passage.

7. **The correct answer is (D).** The answer is stated in paragraph E, sentence 3. Choice (C) is incorrect because the answer would need to include moderate as well as vigorous activities to be correct.

8. **The correct answer is (A).** *Feasible* means "possible." Choices (B) and (C) are incorrect because both *impractical* and *unworkable* are antonyms of *feasible*. Choice (D) is incorrect because *capable* means "suited, adequate, able."

9. **The correct answer is (C).** The answer is stated in paragraph B, sentence 3.

10. **The correct answer is (D).** The answer is stated in paragraph C, sentence 3.

ALLIED HEALTH SCHOOL

Verbal Ability

10 Questions • 5 Minutes

Directions: In each of the sentences below, one word is italicized. Following each sentence are four words or phrases. For each sentence, choose the word or phrase that most nearly corresponds in meaning with the italicized word.

1. The doctor asked the lab to *verify* the results because they were so atypical for the symptoms.
   - **(A)** stabilize
   - **(B)** test
   - **(C)** validate
   - **(D)** concern

2. The *infrequent* news from the earthquake site was very upsetting to families with loved ones in the area.
   - **(A)** abundant
   - **(B)** sporadic
   - **(C)** balanced
   - **(D)** unnecessary

3. The *sly* fox going after other animals and children to eat is a well-known figure in fairy tales from around the world.
   - **(A)** tricky
   - **(B)** cultured
   - **(C)** worldly
   - **(D)** foolish

4. The student was *stunned* by the grade on her report. She had never gotten such a low grade before.
   - **(A)** sensitized
   - **(B)** shocked
   - **(C)** unconscious
   - **(D)** concluded

5. *Prompted* by his wife, the man complained to the landlord about the dirty hallway.
   - **(A)** prohibited
   - **(B)** persuasion
   - **(C)** suggestion
   - **(D)** urged

Directions: In each of the following questions, select the word opposite in meaning to the word printed in capital letters.

6. PUGNACIOUS
   - **(A)** belligerent
   - **(B)** aggressive
   - **(C)** peace-loving
   - **(D)** hot-tempered

7. DISORDERLY
   - **(A)** noisy
   - **(B)** interfering
   - **(C)** controllable
   - **(D)** raucous

8. SUCCINCT
   - **(A)** long-winded
   - **(B)** loud
   - **(C)** admiring
   - **(D)** brief

9. RUDE
   - **(A)** stubborn
   - **(B)** courteous
   - **(C)** difficult
   - **(D)** insolent

10. INGENIOUS
    - **(A)** unimaginative
    - **(B)** brilliant
    - **(C)** originate
    - **(D)** personable

Quantitative Ability

10 Questions • 20 Minutes

Directions: Read each question carefully and consider all possible answers. There is only one best answer for each question.

1. $\frac{1}{8} + \frac{3}{5} + 2\frac{3}{20} =$

    (A) $2\frac{7}{33}$

    (B) $2\frac{7}{8}$

    (C) $\frac{7}{8}$

    (D) 6

2. If it takes $5\frac{1}{2}$ bricks to fill a square foot, how many bricks are needed to build a 220-square foot plaza?

    (A) 1,210
    (B) 225
    (C) 1,500
    (D) 1,230

3. Tastey Pastries are sold by the case to the supermarket. A case costs $171.36. If each case holds 12 boxes and each box holds 12 pastries, at what price does the supermarket need to sell each pastry in order to break even?

    (A) $1.99
    (B) $1.29
    (C) $1.19
    (D) $0.99

4. When you multiply $3\frac{4}{9}$ by $6\frac{1}{3}$, the answer is

    (A) $\frac{589}{27}$

    (B) $\frac{13}{2}$

    (C) 4

    (D) $\frac{137}{17}$

5. If $3(x + 2) = 19$, then $x = ?$

    (A) 5
    (B) 6.33
    (C) 13
    (D) 4.33

6. Mary Kipple owns three dogs and a cat. If it costs $0.30 to feed the cat for a day, and $0.42 to feed a dog for a day, how much does Mary Kipple pay to feed her dogs for a week?

    (A) $2.94
    (B) $8.82
    (C) $6.30
    (D) $15.12

7. What is the answer to $\frac{1}{2} \div \frac{2}{3}$?

    (A) $\frac{3}{4}$

    (B) $\frac{3}{2}$

    (C) $\frac{1}{2}$

    (D) $\frac{2}{6}$

Directions: For questions 8, 9, and 10, two quantities are given: one in Column A and one in Column B. Compare the two quantities to determine the correct answer.

8.

$x > 0$	
$y > 0$	
Column A	Column B
xy	z

(A) if quantity A is greater.

(B) if quantity B is greater.

(C) if the two quantities are equal.

(D) if the relationship cannot be determined from the information given.

9.

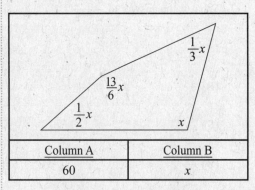

Column A	Column B
60	x

(A) if quantity A is greater.

(B) if quantity B is greater.

(C) if the two quantities are equal.

(D) if the relationship cannot be determined from the information given.

10.

Column A	Column B
The length of one side of an isosceles triangle	The perimeter of an isosceles triangle divided by 3

(A) if quantity A is greater.

(B) if quantity B is greater.

(C) if the two quantities are equal.

(D) if the relationship cannot be determined from the information given.

Science

10 Questions • 8 Minutes

Directions: Read each question carefully and consider all possible answers. There is only one best answer for each question.

1. Which cellular organelle is responsible for transporting proteins to the cell membrane for export?
   - **(A)** Mitochondria
   - **(B)** Golgi apparatus
   - **(C)** Nucleus
   - **(D)** Ribosome

2. Skin, nail, and hair are part of which body system?
   - **(A)** Musculoskeletal system
   - **(B)** Immune system
   - **(C)** Integumentary system
   - **(D)** Endocrine system

3. Individuals with type AB blood have which type of antibodies in their red blood cells?
   - **(A)** Anti-A
   - **(B)** Anti-B
   - **(C)** Anti-A and anti-B
   - **(D)** None

4. Chemicals produced in the body to block virus replication are called
   - **(A)** basophils.
   - **(B)** natural killer cells.
   - **(C)** interferons.
   - **(D)** cytotoxic T-cells.

5. During the process of digestion, most nutrients are absorbed into the bloodstream in which location?
   - **(A)** Small intestine
   - **(B)** Large intestine
   - **(C)** Stomach
   - **(D)** Liver

6. Which type of muscle cells are found in the lining of blood vessels?
   - **(A)** Striated muscles
   - **(B)** Cardiac muscles
   - **(C)** Smooth muscles
   - **(D)** Vessel muscles

7. Nerve cells that receive information from the PNS and send it to the brain are called
   - **(A)** sensory neurons.
   - **(B)** motor neurons.
   - **(C)** brain cells.
   - **(D)** interneurons.

8. Which of the following hormones stimulates activity in the ovaries AND the testes?
   - **(A)** LH
   - **(B)** FSH
   - **(C)** Estrogen
   - **(D)** Testosterone

9. Which type of weight loss plan may make it difficult for the body to absorb certain vitamins?
   - **(A)** Low-carbohydrate diet
   - **(B)** Low-fat diet
   - **(C)** Glycemic index diet
   - **(D)** Formula diet

10. Which type of hormone does the body release in response to stress?
    - **(A)** Estrogen
    - **(B)** Testosterone
    - **(C)** Cortisol
    - **(D)** Thryoxine

diagnostic test

Reading Comprehension

10 Questions • 20 Minutes

Directions: Carefully read the following paragraphs and then answer the accompanying questions, basing your answer on what is stated in the paragraphs. There is only one best answer for each question.

At the conclusion of World War II, Japan became an occupied nation. The occupation lasted from 1945 until 1952. Most occupying forces were from the U.S. During the occupation, the U.S. military government achieved its two main goals. It brought democracy to Japan and also helped lay the foundation for Japan's economic recovery.

The occupation government helped Japan draft a new constitution. The document removed political power from the emperor, a parliamentary system was put into place, and basic rights were guaranteed for all. Women for the first time were given the right to vote. The constitution also stated that the Japanese army would be limited to a size only large enough for national defense.

In addition to political changes, economic changes were introduced. The right of workers to unionize was written into the constitution. Land reforms were introduced. The chief beneficiaries were tenant farmers. They were allowed to buy land, leading to a new class of independent farmers. The Americans tried to disband the large business corporations that existed in Japan, called zaibatsu. This was unsuccessful because Japan believed it needed the corporations to compete with other nations. Although a small number of companies were dismantled, the system remained. The business experience that existed because of the zaibatsu became a positive factor in Japan's economic growth.

After the occupation ended, Japan experienced extraordinary economic growth. A number of factors contributed to this success. During World War II, many Japanese cities and factories had been destroyed. However, this destruction turned out to be beneficial. The Japanese had to build new factories, which were more productive, efficient, and state-of-the-art than were older factories in other manufacturing centers. This included the United States.

In addition to new manufacturing facilities, Japan was able to take advantage of cheap oil prices in the 1950s and 1960s. Japan also had a large workforce, providing cheap labor for factories. The Japanese had a long tradition of saving money, so banks had money to lend to new businesses. Because Japan had few natural resources, it turned to manufacturing products for export. By the 1970s, Japan was a leader in electronics and began producing high-quality automobiles for export. Japan's economic growth was not just due to its technological and manufacturing advances. The Japanese government's protectionist trade policies also helped Japan become an economic superpower.

1. What factor outside of Japan helped it become a manufacturing power?
   - **(A)** Its large supply of natural resources
   - **(B)** Cheap oil in the 1950s and 1960s
   - **(C)** A large cheap labor force
   - **(D)** Bombed-out factories in other nations

2. What were two goals of the occupation?
   - **(A)** Make Japan democratic and write a new constitution
   - **(B)** Give women the right to vote and enable farmers to own their own land
   - **(C)** Make Japan democratic and begin Japan's economic recovery
   - **(D)** Begin Japan's economic recovery and set up a protectionist trade policy for it

3. What are zaibatsu?
   - **(A)** Tenant farmers
   - **(B)** Large business corporations
   - **(C)** Factory centers
   - **(D)** The name given to Japanese trade policies

4. Beneficiaries are
   (A) people who give something away.
   (B) advantages.
   (C) people who gain in some way.
   (D) participants.

5. Which of the following would be a good title for this passage?
   (A) "Japan: On the Road to Recovery"
   (B) "Japan's Miracle Recovery"
   (C) "Japan's Progress"
   (D) "Progress and Reform"

Proteins and You

Proteins are the most complex and diverse macromolecules in any living organism. They are polymers composed of linear chains of monomers called amino acids. A protein macromolecule typically contains between 200 and 300 amino acids. However, the largest can contain nearly 27,000 amino acids on a single chain. These chains are typically found in the skeletal system and cardiac muscle.

Proteins are responsible for an amazing variety of processes within your body. Enzymes are proteins in your body that make chemical reactions occur up to a million times faster. Without enzymes, these chemical reactions either would not occur or would happen too slowly for bodily functions to take place.

Proteins also keep your body safe. Antibodies are proteins that function within your immune system to help you fight disease. Other proteins help your blood form clots so you don't bleed to death when you get a cut. If you ever find yourself needing to flee from a scary situation, you can thank the proteins in your muscles that help you move. Much of the muscle mass in your body is made of proteins.

Transportation is another important job for proteins. Proteins transport materials in fluids throughout your body. For example, hemoglobin is a protein in your blood that carries oxygen from your lungs to your cells.

The most abundant protein in all the animal kingdom is collagen. The body uses it for strength and support. Collagen surrounds and contains all of your body's cells and organs, and it is in your teeth and bones. Another protein, keratin, provides strength for your hair and fingernails.

The same proteins that help your body function are also at work in animals. Like your hair and fingernails, feathers, fur, wool, and cashmere are all made of keratin. So are animal hooves. Leather, which is derived from animal skin, contains collagen and keratin. Silk, a fiber produced by special caterpillars, is also made of protein.

6. Protein is made up of
   (A) amino acids.
   (B) enzymes.
   (C) antibodies.
   (D) hemoglobin.

7. From the final paragraph, you can assume that
   (A) proteins don't protect animals the way they do humans.
   (B) proteins have different results in different animals, including humans.
   (C) keratin is a protein found in animals.
   (D) collagen also surrounds animal organs.

8. Which of the following is found in both human hair and horses' hooves?
   (A) Keratin
   (B) Antibodies
   (C) Collagen
   (D) Enzymes

Mutations

Suppose you pick what you think is a juicy Red Delicious apple to eat. Then you notice that half the apple is yellow. This is an example of a mutation. It is the result of a change in an organism's DNA. Mutations in nature are random, that is, they are not related to how useful they will be to an organism. Most mutations are neutral or harmless. But some mutations can be helpful to organisms. Still others can be dangerous or even fatal.

When a cell divides normally, it makes a perfect copy of its DNA. However, sometimes a cell will not copy perfectly. There may be an addition or subtraction of nucleotides. There could also be a substitution of nucleotides. All of these changes result in a mutation.

Mutations can be inherited and acquired. There are two ways that a mutation is acquired. A cell's DNA may make a mistake when copying itself. Most often, cells can repair themselves, but not always. The result is a mutation. Mutations can also happen when an organism is exposed to certain chemicals or to radiation. This can cause the DNA to break down.

The addition or subtraction of a nucleotide can cause different proteins to be made. Both can also cause a cell to stop protein production. In either case, the result is usually a harmful mutation. The substitution of one nucleotide for another may not lead to a harmful effect. However, it could alter a protein, so that it cannot function normally.

Mutations that are harmful include diseases such as PKU. It is due to a single mutation on chromosome 12 in both parents. If left untreated, it can lead to brain damage and mental retardation. Doctors now regularly test newborns for the mutant gene.

Other mutations can be beneficial and help species evolve. An example is the panda's wrist bone that has evolved into a thumb. This mutation enables pandas to get a better grip on bamboo, which is a major part of their diet. Sickle cell is a mutation that is both harmful and beneficial. People with one sickle cell gene are resistant to malaria, a dangerous disease. But if a person inherits the gene for sickle cell from both parents, the mutation may result in sickle cell anemia, a fatal disease.

9. Which of the following probably results in a mutation that is not harmful?

  (A) Substitution of a nucleotide

  (B) Addition of a nucleotide

  (C) Subtraction of a nucleotide

  (D) Exposure to chemicals

10. Which of the following most accurately describes mutations?

  (A) They can be harmful or beneficial.

  (B) They are seldom neutral, but mostly harmful.

  (C) They can be harmful, beneficial, or harmful and beneficial at the same time.

  (D) They are seldom beneficial, but mostly harmful.

ANSWER KEY AND EXPLANATIONS

Verbal Ability

1. C	3. A	5. D	7. C	9. B
2. B	4. B	6. C	8. A	10. A

1. **The correct answer is (C).** To *verify* is "to *validate*" or "to confirm." Choice (A) is incorrect because *stabilize* means "to make something stable, to make it steady." Choice (B) is incorrect because to *test* the results is not the same as confirming the results. Choice (D) is incorrect because *concern* means "something of interest or anxiety" as a noun or "to worry about, be mindful of" as a verb.

2. **The correct answer is (B).** *Infrequent* and *sporadic* are synonyms. Choice (A) is incorrect because having lots of news coverage wouldn't be upsetting to people with family in a dangerous place. Common sense would indicate that they would want to know as much as they could. This also rules out choice (D) *unnecessary*. Choice (C), *balanced*, doesn't make sense either in context.

3. **The correct answer is (A).** *Sly*, meaning "cunning, clever," and *tricky* are synonyms. Choice (B) is incorrect because *cultured* means "refined, mannerly, educated." Choice (C) is incorrect because *worldly* has no relation to *sly*. Choice (D) is incorrect because *foolish* is closer in meaning to an antonym for *sly*.

4. **The correct answer is (B).** *Stunned* and *shocked* are synonyms. Choice (A) is incorrect because *sensitized* is an antonym to *stunned*; *desensitized* would the synonym. Choice (C) is incorrect because *unconscious* has no relation to *stunned*, and neither does choice (D), *concluded*, meaning "determined that" or "ended."

5. **The correct answer is (D).** *Prompted* and *urged* are synonyms. Choice (A) is incorrect because *prohibited* means "forbidden, prevented." Choice (B) is incorrect because

persuasion is a noun and the question requires an adjective. This also rules out choice (C), *suggestion*. Look for this kind of clue in eliminating answer choices.

6. **The correct answer is (C).** *Pugnacious* is the same as *belligerent, aggressive,* and *hot-tempered,* so you can eliminate choices (A), (B), and (D), leaving choice (C), *peace-loving* as the answer.

7. **The correct answer is (C).** Someone who is *disorderly* is out of control, so *controllable* is the antonym. Choice (A) is incorrect because *noisy* is a synonym for *disorderly,* as is choice (D), *raucous*. Choice (B) is incorrect because *interfering* has no relation to *disorderly*.

8. **The correct answer is (A).** A *succinct* description is brief, so eliminate choice (D), and select choice (A), *long-winded,* as the antonym for *succinct*. Choices (B) and (C) are incorrect because *loud* and *admiring* have no relation to *succinct*.

9. **The correct answer is (B).** A person who is *rude* is impolite, uncivil, and discourteous, so *courteous* is the antonym for *rude*. Choice (A) is incorrect because *stubbornness* may be a characteristic of a rude person, but it is not an antonym. Choice (C) is incorrect because *difficult* may also be a characteristic of a rude person, but is not an antonym. Choice (D) is incorrect because *insolent* is a synonym for *rude*.

10. **The correct answer is (A).** The opposite of being *ingenious* is being *unimaginative*. Choice (B) is incorrect because *brilliant* is a synonym for *ingenious*. Choice (C) is incorrect because *originate* has no relation to *ingenious*, and neither has choice (D), *personable*.

Quantitative Ability

1. B	3. C	5. D	7. A	9. B
2. A	4. A	6. B	8. D	10. C

1. **The correct answer is (B).**

$$\frac{1}{8} + \frac{3}{5} + 2\frac{3}{20} = 5\left(\frac{1}{8}\right) + 8\left(\frac{3}{5}\right) + 2\left(\frac{43}{20}\right)$$

$$= \frac{5}{40} + \frac{24}{40} + \frac{86}{40}$$

$$= \frac{115}{40}$$

$$= \frac{23}{8}$$

$$= 2\frac{7}{8}$$

$\frac{1}{8} + \frac{3}{5} + 2\frac{3}{20}$

$5\left(\frac{1}{8}\right) + 8\left(\frac{3}{5}\right) + 2\left(\frac{43}{20}\right)$

$\frac{5}{40} + \frac{24}{40} + \frac{86}{40}$

$\frac{115}{40}$

$\frac{23}{8}$

$2\frac{7}{8}$

(Addition of Fractions)

2. **The correct answer is (A).**

$220(5.5) = 1,210$

(Multiplication)

3. **The correct answer is (C).**

$$\frac{171.36}{12(12)} = \frac{171.36}{144}$$

$$= 1.19$$

(Problem Solving: Multiplication, Division)

4. **The correct answer is (A).**

$$3\frac{4}{9} \times 6\frac{1}{3} = \frac{31}{9} \times \frac{19}{3}$$

$$= \frac{589}{27}$$

(Multiplication of Complex Fractions)

5. **The correct answer is (D).**

$$3(x + 2) = 19$$
$$3x + 6 = 19$$
$$3x = 13$$
$$x = 4.33$$

(Solving Equations)

6. **The correct answer is (B).**

$7(3)(\$0.42) = \$8.82$

(Problem Solving: Multiplication)

7. **The correct answer is (A).**

$$\frac{1}{2} \div \frac{2}{3} = \frac{1}{2} \times \frac{3}{2}$$

$$= \frac{3}{4}$$

(Division of Fractions)

8. The correct answer is (D).

There is no information given about z, so no relationship can be determined.

(Problem Solving)

9. The correct answer is (B).

$$\frac{1}{3}x + \frac{13}{6}x + \frac{1}{2}x + x = 360$$

$$\frac{2}{6}x + \frac{13}{6}x + \frac{3}{6}x + x = 360$$

$$\frac{18}{6}x + x = 360$$

$$3x + x = 360$$

$$4x = 360$$

$$x = 90$$

(Geometry: Area: Algebra: Solving Equations)

10. The correct answer is (C).

By definition, an isosceles triangle is made up of three even sides.

(Geometry Definitions)

Science

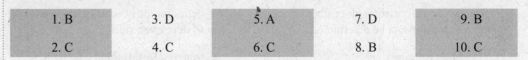

1. B	3. D	5. A	7. D	9. B
2. C	4. C	6. C	8. B	10. C

1. **The correct answer is (B).** The Golgi apparatus, or Golgi body, plays a role in protein synthesis by making modifications to proteins, processing and sorting them, and then packaging the final protein product in a small sac called a vesicle. The vesicle leaves the Golgi body and transports the protein to the cell membrane where it can leave the cell to carry out its function in the body. Choice (A) is incorrect because the mitochondria are the organelles in which energy from organic molecules is converted to ATP. Choice (C) is incorrect because the nucleus is the organelle that contains the genetic information of the cell. Choice (D) is incorrect because the ribosomes are the site of protein synthesis in the cell. **(The Cell)**

2. **The correct answer is (C).** The integumentary system is composed of skin, hair, nails, and sweat and sebaceous glands. It functions to protect the body from injury and dehydration, to maintain a constant temperature in the body, to produce vitamin D, to excrete waste materials and toxins, and to react to microorganisms and chemicals. Choice (A) is incorrect because the musculoskeletal system is only composed of muscles, bones, joints, ligaments, cartilage, and tendons. Choice (B) is incorrect because the immune system is composed of cells that help to fight infection. In particular, these are white blood cells. Choice (D) is incorrect because the endocrine system is made up of organs that produce and secrete hormones and steroids. **(Integumentary System)**

3. **The correct answer is (D).** Type AB blood contains A and B antigens and no antibodies. Individuals with type AB can only donate blood to AB individuals, but they can receive blood of all blood types. Choices (A), (B), and (C) are incorrect because type AB blood does not contain antibodies against any type of blood cells. **(Cardiovascular System)**

4. **The correct answer is (C).** Interferons and cytokines are chemicals in the immune system that are released to block viruses from replicating and to activate surrounding cells that have antiviral functions. Choice (A) is incorrect because basophils are cells that release chemicals that respond to inflammation at the site of an infection. Choice (B) is incorrect because natural killer cells are released to attack foreign antigens in the body. Choice (D) is incorrect because cytotoxic T-cells act to recognize and kill infected cells. **(Immune System)**

5. **The correct answer is (A).** The small intestine is a long, muscular tube of narrow diameter where most chemical digestion takes place and most nutrients are absorbed. After nutrients are broken down, they are absorbed into the bloodstream. Choice (B) is incorrect because by the time food reaches the large intestine, most of the nutrients have already been absorbed. In the large intestine, water and vitamins are absorbed. Choice (C) is incorrect because in the stomach, acids and enzymes act to break down proteins and to kill bacteria. Absorption occurs in the small intestine. Choice (D) is incorrect because the liver functions in the digestive system to produce bile, which breaks down fats. **(Digestive System)**

6. **The correct answer is (C).** Smooth muscle is found in the lining of blood vessels and the lining of organs such as the stomach, intestines, and bladder. Smooth muscle functions to help move materials, such as blood and food, through the body. Smooth muscle is involuntary. Choice (A) is incorrect because striated muscle can undergo voluntary contractions and is found attached to bones for movement of

the body. Choice (B) is incorrect because cardiac muscle is the tissue that makes up the heart, not blood vessels. Choice (D) is incorrect because there are only three muscle types: smooth, striated, and cardiac.

7. **The correct answer is (D).** Interneurons, or association neurons, are neurons that link sensory neurons to motor neurons. They are found in the brain and the spinal cord. They receive information from the sensory neurons of the peripheral nervous system and transport this signal to the brain and then to motor neurons for the output signal. Choice (A) is incorrect because sensory neurons receive sensory information from a stimulus; the signal is sent to interneurons before it reaches the brain. Choice (B) is incorrect because motor neurons receive an output signal from interneurons leaving the brain and translate that signal into a motor response. Choice (C) is incorrect because brain cells do not directly receive a signal from the PNS. The signal passes through interneurons before it is received by the brain. **(Nervous System)**

8. **The correct answer is (B).** Follicle-stimulating hormone, or FSH, plays a role in stimulating the activity of the ovaries in females and the testes in males. Choice (A) is incorrect because the function of luteinizing hormone, LH, is to release an ovum in females and produce testosterone in males. Choice (C) is incorrect because the main function of estrogen is to promote female secondary sex characteristics, thicken the endometrial lining, and promote oogenesis. Choice (D) is incorrect because the main function of testosterone is to promote male secondary sex characteristics and spermatogenesis. **(Reproductive System)**

9. **The correct answer is (B).** Low-fat diets can lack sufficient amounts of fatty acids and protein that may make it difficult for the body to absorb fat-soluble vitamins. Choice (A) is incorrect because a low-carbohydrate diet contains fat, so that both fat-soluble and water-soluble vitamins can be absorbed by the body easily. Choice (C) is incorrect because a glycemic index diet aims to lower blood sugar levels, but does not restrict fat intake; therefore, there is no danger that fat-soluble vitamins would not be absorbed. Choice (D) is incorrect because a formula diet has a carefully calculated balance between protein, fat, and carbohydrate, so that all vitamins would be absorbed by the body without difficulty. **(Nutrition)**

10. **The correct answer is (C).** The nervous system triggers the endocrine system. The endocrine system releases hormones and other chemical signals to the bloodstream. Some key hormones released in response to stress are cortisol and epinephrine. Choice (A) is incorrect because estrogen is a sex hormone and is not released during stress. Choice (B) is incorrect because testosterone is a male sex hormone and is not released in direct response to stress. Choice (D) is incorrect because thyroxine is a hormone released by the thyroid gland to stimulate the metabolism. **(Factors Affecting Health)**

answers diagnostic test

Reading Comprehension

1. B	3. B	5. B	7. B	9. A
2. C	4. C	6. A	8. A	10. C

1. **The correct answer is (B).** The answer is stated in the last paragraph, sentence 1. The key is the word *outside* in the question stem.

2. **The correct answer is (C).** The answer is stated in paragraph 1, sentence 5.

3. **The correct answer is (B).** The answer is stated in paragraph 3, sentence 6.

4. **The correct answer is (C).** Beneficiaries are people who gain something. Think of the word *benefit*.

5. **The correct answer is (B).** A title should reflect the main idea, or theme, of a piece of writing. It needs to be general enough to touch on all the main points in the passage. Choice (A) is incorrect because it describes just the first part of the passage and doesn't include the idea that Japan became an economic power after the occupation. Choice (C) is incorrect for the same reason. It doesn't include what happened to Japan after the occupation. Choice (D) is incorrect because it stops with progress and doesn't include the idea of a recovered Japan. Only choice (B) implies through the use of the word *miracle* that the passage is about both how Japan recovered and what the recovery was like.

6. **The correct answer is (A).** The answer is stated in paragraph 1, sentence 2.

7. **The correct answer is (B).** The final paragraph contrasts what keratin and collagen do in humans and in animals, and the results are different, so it is credible to assume, or infer, that proteins have different results in different animals.

8. **The correct answer is (A).** The answer is stated in the final paragraph, sentences 2 and 3.

9. **The correct answer is (A).** The answer is stated in paragraph 4, sentence 4.

10. **The correct answer is (C).** The answer can be pulled together from information in paragraph 1, sentences 6, 7, and 8, and paragraph 6, sentence 4.

PRACTICAL/VOCATIONAL NURSING SCHOOL

Verbal Ability

10 Questions • 5 Minutes

Directions: In each of the sentences below, one word is italicized. Following each sentence are four words or phrases. For each sentence, choose the word or phrase that most nearly corresponds in meaning with the italicized word.

1. The mother was *anxious* that her son would be upset if he didn't make the team.
   - (A) elated
   - (B) worried
   - (C) eager
   - (D) certain

2. The senator wanted *a reform* of the tax code, but others wanted to throw it out entirely.
   - (A) a mending
   - (B) a remodeling
   - (C) an improvement
   - (D) an announcement

3. The man was a *credible* witness, and the prosecutor seemed pleased with his testimony.
   - (A) unfortunate
   - (B) lamentable
   - (C) rehabilitated
   - (D) believable

Directions: In each of the following questions, select the word opposite in meaning to the word printed in capital letters.

4. SUPERFICIAL
   - (A) complete
   - (B) casual
   - (C) serious
   - (D) artificial

5. OBLIQUE
   - (A) translucent
   - (B) implied
   - (C) honest
   - (D) indirect

6. PERSISTENT
   - (A) lasting
   - (B) constant
   - (C) intermittent
   - (D) continuous

7. TIMIDITY
   - (A) boldness
   - (B) shyness
   - (C) uncertainty
   - (D) doubtfulness

Directions: Select the word that belongs in the blank space in the sentence.

8. He did all the exercises _____ the deep knee bends.
   - (A) except
   - (B) accept

9. For the end of her speech, she _____ the poem to make it fit the situation.
   - (A) adopted
   - (B) adapted

10. I was told to _____ to the conference room where the others were already meeting.
    - (A) proceed
    - (B) precede

facebook.com/petersonspublishing

Arithmetic and Mathematics

10 Questions • 10 Minutes

Directions: Read each question carefully and decide which is the best answer.

1. What is the answer when the following fractions are added together: $\frac{1}{3}$, $\frac{5}{6}$ and $\frac{7}{12}$?

   (A) $1\frac{1}{4}$

   (B) $1\frac{1}{2}$

   (C) $1\frac{3}{4}$

   (D) $2\frac{3}{4}$

2. What is the product of 5.36 and 2.91?
   (A) 10.8396
   (B) 15.5976
   (C) 12.96
   (D) 17.1236

3. What is the difference of 76.8342 from 428.64?
   (A) 321.8058
   (B) 274.9806
   (C) 422.37
   (D) 351.8058

4. When 18.032 is divided by 0.04, the answer is
   (A) 0.4508
   (B) 4.508
   (C) 45.08
   (D) 450.8

5. Express 36% as a fraction and reduce it to its lowest terms.

   (A) $\frac{9}{25}$

   (B) $\frac{18}{25}$

   (C) $\frac{18}{50}$

   (D) $\frac{36}{100}$

6. Write $\frac{3}{16}$ as a ratio.
   (A) 3.16
   (B) 3:16
   (C) 16:3
   (D) 16.3

7. What is the difference between $\frac{3}{8}$ and $\frac{3}{24}$?

   (A) 0

   (B) $\frac{1}{8}$

   (C) $\frac{1}{6}$

   (D) $\frac{1}{4}$

8. If an IV drop has 15 parts per 1,000 ml, how many parts would there be in 430 ml?
   (A) 5.97
   (B) 6.45
   (C) 6.73
   (D) 7.29

9. A yard of concrete includes $1\frac{1}{4}$ tons of sand, $1\frac{1}{3}$ tons of crushed stone, and $\frac{1}{5}$ of a ton of water. How many tons of material are used in a ton of concrete?

(A) $2\frac{3}{15}$

(B) $2\frac{3}{12}$

(C) $2\frac{47}{60}$

(D) $2\frac{3}{60}$

10. If there are 432 nurses at City General Hospital and 7/8 of them are female, how many male nurses work at City General?

(A) 46

(B) 54

(C) 378

(D) 432

Science

10 Questions • 10 Minutes

Directions: Read each question carefully and consider all possible answers. There is only one best answer for each question.

1. Oxygen is passed from the lungs into cells via which structures?
   (A) Arteries
   (B) Bronchioles
   (C) Capillaries
   (D) Veins

2. The upper chambers of the heart are called
   (A) atria.
   (B) ventricles.
   (C) arteries.
   (D) valves.

3. In order to attack pathogens in the body, lymph nodes contain
   (A) bone marrow.
   (B) B-lymphocytes.
   (C) cytotoxic T-cells.
   (D) red blood cells.

4. Bile stored in the gall bladder aids in the digestion of
   (A) proteins.
   (B) carbohydrates.
   (C) sugars.
   (D) fats.

5. Three components of urine are
   (A) uric acid, ammonia, and creatinine.
   (B) urea, ammonia, and glucose.
   (C) urea, uric acid, and creatinine.
   (D) urea, uric acid, and glucose.

6. The strong, flexible strands of connective tissue that connect bones to one another are
   (A) joints.
   (B) ligaments.
   (C) muscles.
   (D) cartilages.

7. In a developing fetus, bones and joints form during the
   (A) first trimester.
   (B) second month.
   (C) second trimester.
   (D) eighth month.

8. Which of the following is a list of functions that contribute to the basal metabolic rate?
   (A) Breathing, heartbeat, cell maintenance
   (B) Heartbeat, striated muscular movements, talking
   (C) Breathing, walking, sleeping
   (D) Heartbeat, sleeping, eating

9. Which of the following is an essential fatty acid?
   (A) Phosphorous
   (B) Tocopherol
   (C) Biotin
   (D) Omega-3

10. High LDL levels can lead to which of the following health effects?
    (A) Clogged arteries
    (B) Paralysis
    (C) Obesity
    (D) Blood clots

Reading Comprehension

10 Questions • 20 Minutes

Directions: Carefully read the following paragraphs and then answer the accompanying questions, basing your answer on what is stated in the paragraphs. There is only one best answer for each question.

Listening to Music
Through the Years

Listen to music today and you are most likely listening to it on an MP3 player, but the first audiences for music were in the streets, music halls, theaters, and clubs. By the late 1800s and early 1900s, musicians had begun recording their music in recording studios. Fans bought the music on disks that were played on phonograph machines, one disk at a time. The disks were called records. By the 1920s, the records were made of vinyl, a type of plastic. Over the years, companies produced them in different sizes and speeds: 78s, 45s, and 33 1/3. The larger records held several songs. Companies soon figured out how to build phonograph machines that could stack several records at a time.

Phonograph machines were large, and many phonographs were actually built into pieces of furniture. Even smaller phonographs sat on tables or cabinets. There was nothing portable about phonographs until around the 1940s when companies began making them in little suitcases.

During the 1970s, audiotapes replaced records. Each tape could hold ten or so songs. Fans listened to tapes in cassette players. Some players were large "boom boxes," but they could be carried around by a handle. Others were personal tape players like the Walkman™. In the 1980s, compact disks (CDs) replaced tapes, and CD players replaced tape players. Instead of walking around with earphones for tape players, people were plugged into personal CD players.

The first MP3 players for sale were produced in the late 1990s. Soon people were walking around with earbuds for MP3 players in their ears. These new music players are so small they can fit into a pocket or hook onto a belt. Around the same time as MP3 players were being invented, people began using cell phones more and more. Now people download their music to MP3 players and their cell phones as well as their desktops, laptops, and tablets. Download music? Instead of buying music in a "record store," many people buy it from a "music store" on the Web.

Today, musicians still record in studios, but how we listen to their music has greatly changed since the first records.

1. A problem with early phonograph players was that
   (A) they were expensive.
   (B) only one record could be played at a time.
   (C) the carrying handles were not strong enough.
   (D) they could hold only ten songs.

2. When were the first MP3 players sold?
   (A) Early 1900s
   (B) 1920s
   (C) 1980s
   (D) 1990s

3. What replaced boom boxes?
   (A) MP3 players
   (B) CDs
   (C) Cassette tapes
   (D) Phonograph records

From: *Green Jobs for a New Economy*, Peterson's Publishing

Once upon a time—actually, just a few years ago—if you were looking for a job, you'd read the want ads in the newspaper or in trade and association publications. Today, most job listings have *migrated* to the Internet where you will find hundreds of job boards. How do you decide which ones to search and what to look for? Here are a few ideas to help you concentrate your search in the best places.

Remember that job boards are not just for searching when you are looking for a job. They can be helpful when you are deciding on a career to pursue. Analyzing job titles related to your interests; the regions of the country where particular jobs are most common, for example, the Southwest and Southeast where many people are retiring; types of employers such as public or private, nonprofit, small companies, or large corporations; and salaries can help direct your career choice.

Major Internet sites for jobs are monster. com, careerbuilder.com, and hotjobs.yahoo.com. Type in your job area, such as "licensed practical nurse," and see what jobs come up. You can search for jobs in a specific city or nationwide and for specific industries such as hospitals, correctional institutions, and community clinics. You can also search for full-time, part-time, per diem, and temporary employment.

You can also look at the Web sites of professional organizations and unions that represent licensed practical nurses. Many of them will have job boards, and their postings will be the most closely <u>aligned</u> with the group's specialties. Don't overlook your school's career counseling and job placement offices.

4. The word *migrated* means
   (A) moved
   (B) shown up
   (C) survived
   (D) are found

5. In which part of the country are there likely to be more nursing jobs because of more retirees?
   (A) Northeast
   (B) Midwest
   (C) Southeast
   (D) Mid-Atlantic

6. A good title for this article is
   (A) "Where to Look for Jobs"
   (B) "The Job Hunt"
   (C) "Finding a Job"
   (D) "Using The Internet for a Job Search"

7. *Aligned* means
   (A) cooperated
   (B) in a straight line
   (C) adjusted to
   (D) produced

Potential Relief for Alzheimer's Patients

There is an ongoing debate about the effectiveness of the drugs used to treat Alzheimer's disease. At this time, there are no drugs available that will cure or even stop the disease's progression. However, available drugs can lessen symptoms. But should a particular patient be prescribed a drug? If so, when? For how long? Does the patient actually have Alzheimer's or is the patient suffering from dementia? The problem is the inability to diagnose Alzheimer's because there is no firm diagnosis until a patient is dead and an autopsy can be performed. Patients may be assumed to have the disease because of the symptoms they present. Some patients may actually have dementia rather than Alzheimer's disease.

There are two classes of drugs available at present to treat the Alzheimer's: a glutamate regulator and cholinesterase inhibitors. The former blocks the death of brain cells and the latter improves symptoms, or possibly only reduces unwanted behaviors. The glutamate regulators are prescribed to patients in moderate to severe stages of Alzheimer's, and cholinesterase inhibitors are given to patients in early to moderate stages. Both drugs have some side effects, though they are considered minor. *Ironically*, a potential side effect of the class of glutamate regulators is confusion.

8. Why is it difficult to decide if a patient should be given drug therapy for Alzheimer's?

(A) There are too many questions to be answered.

(B) Drugs don't cure the disease.

(C) The disease cannot be diagnosed while a patient is alive.

(D) The drugs are expensive.

9. *Ironically* in the last sentence means

(A) absurd.

(B) usual.

(C) formal.

(D) specific.

10. Glutamate regulators are prescribed in which stage of the disease?

(A) Onset

(B) Early

(C) Late

(D) Moderate

ANSWER KEY AND EXPLANATIONS

Verbal Ability

1. B	3. D	5. C	7. A	9. B
2. C	4. C	6. C	8. A	10. A

1. **The correct answer is (B).** *Anxious* and *worried* are synonyms. You can eliminate choice (A), *elated*, because a mother wouldn't be happy that her son would be upset, nor would she be *eager* to see her son upset, choice (C). Choice (D) is incorrect because although *certain* makes sense, it isn't a synonym for *anxious*.

2. **The correct answer is (C).** *Reform* and *improvement* are synonyms. Choice (A) is incorrect because *mending* isn't used in the context of laws, and neither is choice (B), *remodeling*. Choice (D) is incorrect because *announcement* is not a synonym for *reform*.

3. **The correct answer is (D).** *Believable* is another word for *credible*. Choice (A) is incorrect because *unfortunate* isn't a synonym for *credible*. If you weren't sure, try it out in the sentence and you'll see that it doesn't make sense. Choice (B) is incorrect because *lamentable* means "unfortunate, tragic." Choice (C) is incorrect because *rehabilitated* is not a synonym for *credible*.

4. **The correct answer is (C).** *Superficial* means "obvious, what's on or near the surface" or "silly, frivolous," so an antonym is *serious*. Choice (A) is incorrect because *complete* has no relation to *superficial*. Choice (B) is incorrect because *casual* is closer in meaning to *superficial* than to an antonym for it. Choice (D) is incorrect because *artificial* has no relation to *superficial*.

5. **The correct answer is (C).** *Oblique* means "being slanted or sloping" or "indirect, misleading, dishonest," so *honest* is its antonym. Choice (A) is incorrect because *translucent* means "clear" or "allowing light to shine through" and is used to describe things such as curtains and shades. Choice (B) is incorrect because *implied* means "indirect," but not in the sense of being misleading. Choice (D) is incorrect because *indirect* is a synonym for *oblique*.

6. **The correct answer is (C).** *Persistent* means "never giving up, persevering," so *intermittent*, meaning "random, sporadic, now and then," is an antonym. Choice (A) is incorrect because *lasting* is similar in meaning to *persistent*. The same goes for *constant*, choice (B). Choice (D) is incorrect because *continuous* means "uninterrupted, continuing."

7. **The correct answer is (A).** *Timidity* means "shyness, uncertainty, and doubtfulness," so choices (B), (C), and (D) are synonyms, not antonyms. Choice (A), *boldness*, is the opposite.

8. **The correct answer is (A).** *Except* means "but, with the exception of." *Accept* means "to take, to receive" and doesn't make sense in the sentence.

9. **The correct answer is (B).** To *adopt* is "to take on" or "to select to choose," whereas to *adapt* is "to change." Only *adapt* makes sense in the sentence.

10. **The correct answer is (A).** To *proceed* is "to go forward, to move ahead," and to *precede* is "to go ahead of someone, to be in front." Context tells you that *proceed* is the correct.

Arithmetic and Mathematics

1. C	3. D	5. A	7. D	9. C
2. B	4. D	6. B	8. B	10. B

1. **The correct answer is (C).**

$$\frac{1}{3} + \frac{5}{6} + \frac{7}{12} = \frac{4}{12} + \frac{10}{12} + \frac{7}{12}$$

$$= \frac{21}{12}$$

$$= 1\frac{9}{12}$$

$$= 1\frac{3}{4}$$

(Addition of Fractions)

2. **The correct answer is (B).**

$$
\begin{array}{r}
5.36 \\
\times \quad 2.91 \\
\hline
536 \\
4824 \\
1072 \\
\hline
15.5976
\end{array}
$$

(Multiplication of Decimals)

3. **The correct answer is (D).**

$$
\begin{array}{r}
428.6400 \\
- \quad 76.8342 \\
\hline
351.8058
\end{array}
$$

(Subtraction of decimals)

4. **The correct answer is (D).**

$$0.04\overline{)18.032} = 4\overline{)1803.2}^{\,450.8}$$

$$
\begin{array}{r}
450.8 \\
4\overline{)1803.2} \\
16 \\
\hline
20 \\
20 \\
\hline
032 \\
32 \\
\hline
0
\end{array}
$$

(Division of Decimals)

5. **The correct answer is (A).**

$$\frac{36}{100} = \frac{36 \div 4}{100 \div 4} = \frac{9}{25}$$

(Conversion of Percentage to Fraction in Lowest Terms)

6. **The correct answer is (B).**

$$\frac{3}{16} = 3:16$$

(Conversion of Fractions to Ratios)

7. **The correct answer is (D).**

$$\frac{3}{8} - \frac{3}{24} = \frac{9}{24} - \frac{3}{24}$$

$$= \frac{6}{24}$$

$$= \frac{1}{4}$$

(Subtraction of Fractions)

answers diagnostic test

8. **The correct answer is (B).**

$$\frac{15}{1000} = \frac{x}{430}$$

$$\frac{15(430)}{1000} = x$$

$$\frac{6450}{1000} = x$$

$$6.54 = x$$

(Arithmetic: Proportions, Problem Solving)

9. **The correct answer is (C).**

$$1\frac{1}{4} + 1\frac{1}{3} + \frac{1}{5} = \frac{5}{4} + \frac{4}{3} + \frac{1}{5}$$

$$= \frac{75}{60} + \frac{80}{60} + \frac{12}{60}$$

$$= \frac{167}{60}$$

$$= 2\frac{47}{60}$$

(Addition of Complex Fractions)

10. **The correct answer is (B).**

$$\frac{x}{432} = \frac{1}{8}$$

$$x = \frac{432}{8}$$

$$x = 54$$

(Proportions: Problem Solving)

Science

1. C	3. B	5. C	7. C	9. D
2. A	4. D	6. B	8. A	10. A

1. **The correct answer is (C).** The oxygen-rich blood in the lungs leaves via capillaries and enters cells in the body. The oxygen gas molecules can pass through the thin walls of the capillaries and into the cells. Choice (A) is incorrect because the function of arteries is to carry blood away from the heart to the rest of the body. Choice (B) is incorrect because the bronchioles are small branching structures in the lungs through which air travels. Choice (D) is incorrect because veins are the blood vessels that carry blood from all over the body back to the heart. **(Respiratory System)**

2. **The correct answer is (A).** The upper chambers of the heart are the right and left artia. The left atrium receives oxygen-rich blood from the lungs and the right atrium receives oxygen-poor blood from the body. Choice (B) is incorrect because the ventricles are the two lower chambers of the heart. Choice (C) is incorrect because arteries are blood vessels that carry blood away from the heart. Choice (D) is incorrect because valves are structures that separate the upper and lower chambers of the heart to ensure that blood does not flow from the lower chamber back into the upper chamber. **(Cardiovascular System)**

3. **The correct answer is (B).** Infection-fighting white blood cells called B-lymphocytes are found in lymph nodes. When bacteria or other pathogens cause an infection, the number of B-lymphocytes increases. Pathogens are destroyed by the B-lymphocytes. Choice (A) is incorrect because bone marrow is found in the center of bones and is the site where blood cells are produced. Choice (C) is incorrect because although cytotoxic T-cells attack and kill cells infected with pathogen, they are not found in lymph nodes. Choice (D) is incorrect because it is the white blood cells, in particular the B-lymphocytes, that

are stored in the lymph nodes in order to attack pathogens in the body. **(Lymphatic System)**

4. **The correct answer is (D).** The liver produces and releases a mixture called bile, which is stored in the gall bladder. The bile acts to break down fats into small droplets. Choice (A) is incorrect because bile breaks down fat into small easily digestible droplets. It does not break down proteins. Choice (B) is incorrect because fats, not carbohydrates, are broken down by bile stored in the gall bladder. Choice (C) is incorrect because fats, not sugars are broken down by bile. **(Digestive System)**

5. **The correct answer is (C).** Urine is made up of urea, uric acid, and creatinine. Urea is a waste product formed from the breakdown of amino acids (proteins). Uric acid is a waste product from the breakdown of nucleic acids (DNA and RNA), and creatinine is a waste product formed by muscle metabolism. Choice (A) is incorrect because although ammonia can be formed by the breakdown of proteins, the component of urine in humans is urea, not ammonia. Choice (B) is incorrect because ammonia and glucose are not components of urine. Choice (D) is incorrect because urine from humans contains creatinine, not glucose. **(Excretory System)**

6. **The correct answer is (B).** Ligaments are tough flexible strands of connective tissue that connect bones to one another. Ligaments hold joints between bones together and allow for movement and flexibility of the body. Choice (A) is incorrect because joints are the places where ligaments connect bones to each other, but the connective tissue forms ligaments. Choice (C) is incorrect because muscles surround joints and ligaments, but it is the ligament that attaches one bone to another. Choice (D)

answers diagnostic test

is incorrect because although cartilage is also made of strong flexible connective tissue, it is found at the ends of bones and does not form a connection between two bones. **(Musculoskeletal System)**

7. **The correct answer is (C).** The second trimester spans months four through six of development. During the second trimester, bones and joints begin to form. Muscles develop and the fetus becomes stronger. Choice (A) is incorrect because organs form, but bone is still undeveloped. Choice (B) is incorrect because the second month of pregnancy is still part of the first trimester when bones have not yet formed. Choice (D) is incorrect because in the eighth month, which is part of the third trimester, bones have already formed and are growing as the fetus grows. **(Reproduction)**

8. **The correct answer is (A).** The number of kilocalories that a resting body requires to maintain functions such as cellular maintenance, breathing, heartbeat, and regulation of body temperature is called the basal metabolic rate (BMR). Choice (B) is incorrect because the voluntary movement of striated muscles requires additional calories because voluntary movement is not a basic body function. Choice (C) is incorrect because walking expends additional kilocalories beyond the basal metabolic rate. Choice (D) is incorrect because eating expends kilocalories in addition to the basal metabolic rate. **(Nutrition–Chemical Energy)**

9. **The correct answer is (D).** Essential fatty acids include omega-3 and omega-6 fatty acids as well as linoleic acid. Choice (A) is incorrect because phosphorous is an essential mineral, not an essential fatty acid. Choice (B) is incorrect because tocopherol is an essential vitamin, also known as Vitamin E. Choice (C) is incorrect because biotin is an essential vitamin, not an essential fatty acid. **(Nutrition)**

10. **The correct answer is (A).** High LDL levels contribute to clogged arteries. Clogged arteries, in turn, can lead to high blood pressure and cardiovascular disease. Choice (B) is incorrect because high LDL cholesterol levels do not lead to paralysis. Choice (C) is incorrect because obesity is a risk factor of cardiovascular disease, but it is not caused by high LDL cholesterol level. Choice (D) is incorrect because blood clots are formed by the buildup of plaque or platelets in blood vessels. **(Factors Affecting Health)**

Reading Comprehension

1. B	3. B	5. C	7. C	9. A
2. D	4. A	6. A	8. C	10. D

1. **The correct answer is (B).** Sentence 3 in paragraph 1 states that phonograph records could be played on early phonographs only one record at a time. You can infer that this would be a problem because songs are short and people would have to get up after each record to put on a new one. Choice (A) is incorrect because price is not mentioned in the passage. Choice (C) is incorrect because early phonographs did not have carrying handles. Choice (D) is incorrect because it was audiotapes that could only hold ten or so records.

2. **The correct answer is (D).** The answer is stated in paragraph 4, sentence 1.

3. **The correct answer is (B).** The chronology, or timeline, described in paragraph 3, sentence 6 states that CDs replaced tapes, which were played on boom boxes (sentence 4), so you can infer that CDs replaced boom boxes. Choice (C) is incorrect because cassette tapes were played on boom boxes. Choice (A) is incorrect because CDs and CD players came after boom boxes/cassette tapes and before MP3 players. Choice (D) is incorrect because phonograph records came before any of the other answers.

4. **The correct answer is (A).** *Migrated* means "moved."

5. **The correct answer is (C).** The answer is stated in paragraph 2, sentence 3.

6. **The correct answer is (A).** A title reflects the main idea, or theme, of a piece of writing, so it must be broad enough to include the main points of the passage. Only choice (A) accomplishes this. Choice (B) is incorrect because it is too general. You don't know from the title that the passage is specifically about where to look for jobs. Choice (C) is incorrect because it doesn't indicate that the passage is about where to look for jobs. The passage might include anything related to looking for a job such as completing the job application or preparing for an interview. You might have been tempted by choice (D), but the passage is about more than just using the Internet; reread the final paragraph.

7. **The correct answer is (C).** *Aligned* means "adjusted to" in the sense of "made to agree with."

8. **The correct answer is (C).** The answer is stated in paragraph 1, sentence 8.

9. **The correct answer is (A).** *Ironically* means "absurd, contrary, the opposite of what is expected."

10. **The correct answer is (D).** The answer is stated in paragraph 2, sentence 3.

facebook.com/petersonspublishing

answers diagnostic test

PART III

PRACTICE FOR REGISTERED NURSING SCHOOL ENTRANCE EXAMINATIONS

Unit 1: Verbal Ability

Unit 2: Mathematics

Unit 3: Science

Unit 4: Reading Comprehension

Verbal Ability

OVERVIEW

- **What is verbal ability?**
- **Measuring verbal ability**
- **Extending your vocabulary**
- **Etymology—key to word recognition**
- **Know your roots (or stems)**
- **Prefixes and suffixes**
- **Increased word power from beginning to end**
- **Synonyms**
- **Synonyms test**
- **Answer key and explanations**
- **Antonyms**
- **Antonyms test**
- **Answer key and explanations**
- **Skill with verbal analogies**
- **Analogy Relationships**
- **Answer key and explanations**
- **Verbal Analogies test**
- **Answer key and explanations**
- **Let's put you to the test**
- **Final Verbal Ability examination**
- **Answer key and explanations**

The purpose of this section is to provide you with practice exercises representative of the three most common kinds of verbal-ability test items: synonyms, antonyms, and verbal analogies. This section covers these question types in three separate subsections.

An explanation of each kind of test item, helpful study hints, and test-taking strategies precede each subsection. Subsections also include a 75-question, multiple-choice test. An answer key follows each sample test to help you immediately evaluate your performance and determine areas of weakness. You may wish to use these answer keys to compile a word study list.

Remember that this section is not meant for easy reading. It is a guide to a program of study that will prove invaluable if you do your part. Do not try to absorb too much at one time. If you can put in a half-hour every day, your study will yield better results.

unit 1

After you have done your preliminary work and have a better idea of how words are formed in English, attempt the various vocabulary tests we have provided. They cover a wide variety of the vocabulary questions commonly encountered on examinations. These lengthy tests are not meant to be taken all at once. Space them out. Adhere closely to the directions, which differ depending on the test. Keep an honest record of your scores. Study your corrected mistakes and look them up in your dictionary. Concentrate closely on each sample test, and watch your scores improve.

WHAT IS VERBAL ABILITY?

Verbal ability may be defined as skill with word usage and comprehension. It is often evaluated in the form of written vocabulary tests. These vocabulary tests measure the test-taker's ability to recall and produce *lexical units*. A lexical unit is a word or group of words possessing a specific meaning. A single word can have a variety of meanings in different contexts (that is, phrases or sentences). For this reason, a single word may represent several lexical units. Consider the following example:

Her answer to the question was *right*.

She handed the paper to the person on her *right*.

She has a *right* to know the results of the test.

She felt compelled to help *right* the wrong that was done.

MEASURING VERBAL ABILITY

Measurement of verbal skill encompasses many elements. Although vocabulary test items may or may not appear on your test, it is advisable to study and practice with the kind of material presented in this verbal ability section. Words and their meanings are vital for good scores on tests of reading comprehension, effective writing, and current usage. Expanding your vocabulary will result in a marked improvement in your scores in these and similar subjects.

The vocabulary test usually includes words from your *active* vocabulary—words that you see, hear, and use frequently—and words from your *passive* vocabulary—words that you have heard and seen, and might comprehend, but that you rarely, if ever, use. It also includes words that may be common in written language but are not often used in spoken expression, and vice versa.

EXTENDING YOUR VOCABULARY

A good command of words is essential to most aspects of your life. Words can broaden your horizons and reveal new interests in your daily environment and activities. Such discoveries may never be accessible to you if your vocabulary remains restricted or too specialized.

Effective expression is essential to making and maintaining meaningful social relationships. An extensive vocabulary will help you to convey ideas, desires, and information. If you are enrolled in school, regardless of the level, you will learn faster and enjoy the process more if you are "fortified" with a large, effective vocabulary. Your comprehension of a broad range of words will help you to determine what you do *not* understand and will help you remedy the situation by posing intelligent questions.

Your word power directly affects your work. If you are seeking to improve your occupational status through a job change or a promotion from your present position, a better command of words will undoubtedly help you to succeed. This fact has been proven time and again through scientific studies conducted by educators, psychologists, sociologists, and personnel specialists. Many employers require a battery of tests, the results of which are used in determining which applicants are best suited to an available position. Frequently these tests incorporate a number of items designed to measure verbal ability.

Attaining a leadership role depends on, among other things, the extent of your vocabulary. Leadership tasks demand that you get your ideas across, that you speak and are heard. You will need to use all your expressive powers to voice your opinion with conviction. Articulation can furnish you with an astonishing amount of persuasive power. A larger vocabulary will help you feel secure and competent in every undertaking.

Let's explore the means by which this vocabulary may be acquired. The following strategies are designed to increase your vocabulary and help you achieve word mastery. Word mastery implies reaching a level of verbal ability at which you can both recognize and comprehend words—and use them frequently and appropriately.

- **Read as much as you can, taking care not to confine yourself to one kind of reading material.** Seek variety in what you read—periodicals, newspapers, nonfiction, novels and other fiction, poetry, prose, essays, etc. Reading from a broad range of material will accelerate your vocabulary growth. You will learn the meaning of words by context. This means that at times you will not know the definition of an isolated word, but the words or phrase within which this word appears will be familiar and therefore provide a clue to its meaning.

- **Take vocabulary tests.** There are many practice books containing word tests. These tests are challenging and make an enjoyable leisure-time activity. More importantly, they are fast vocabulary builders.

- **Listen to lectures, discussion, and talks given by people who speak well.** TV and radio are excellent means of learning new terminology coming into common usage in the English language. A word of caution: You cannot always rely on a speaker's pronunciation. Always check your dictionary for proper pronunciation.

- **Use a dictionary when you are not certain of a word's meaning.** If you do not have access to a dictionary when you encounter the word, make a note of it (and its context) and research it at your earliest convenience. Find out how it is pronounced, what words are related to it, its finer shades of meaning, and its correct usage. A good dictionary is a must!

- **Crossword puzzles, anagrams, and similar word games provide a relaxing method of acquiring new vocabulary.** Most of these puzzles are published in varying degrees of difficulty. Start with the easy level and progress to the expert level. You will find it a challenging learning experience.

- **Review the etymological charts and diagrams in this book, which explain word derivations.** A knowledge of roots, or stems, of words will enable you to infer the meaning of new words having roots similar to words you already know.

- **Study words by central ideas.** It is difficult to study and retain isolated words. Even context clues sometimes are not enough to help you remember a word, its meaning, or its appropriate use. Studying vocabulary by central idea encourages you to consider groups of related words. As you learn each term, you associate it with some other word. For example: The words *ingest, devour, consume, voracious, edible, delectable,* and *palatable* are all tied to the principle idea of eating. The central idea strategy of studying words will not only provide you with a basis for remembering the word but will also motivate you to use the word in your everyday oral and written expression. Frequent use of the word will in turn ensure your ability to recall its meaning in a testing situation. This word study method also fosters comprehension of jargon or word usage particular to specific fields. A number of workbooks and study materials present words according to a central idea and feature exercises formatted to this method. Such books may be found in the "study aids" section of most bookstores.

Be sure to record all new words in a notebook dedicated to that purpose. Make notes alongside each entry that include a simple definition or synonym, finer shades of meaning, related forms, and sample sentences of the word in context. Finally, make these words your own. Use them in your writing and speaking. Remember—verbal ability is a skill you can improve at any age.

ETYMOLOGY—KEY TO WORD RECOGNITION

Etymology is the study of the history and origin of words. It explains how a word came into being, the place of its beginning, and how it has been used through the ages. The etymology of a word also outlines alterations in its meaning, usage, and spelling through the years.

Although the term *etymology* sounds somewhat complex and weighty, the science itself is not difficult to understand. Etymologies may be simple and concise or lengthy and intricate. To find them, use your dictionary. Etymologies are usually found at the beginning of a definition of a principal entry (the word you are looking up, usually printed in bold type), enclosed in brackets and placed directly before the definition.

> **arris** ar ə s\n, pl arris or **arrises** [probably modif. of MF *areste,* lit., fishbone, fr LL *arista,* ear of grain]: the sharp edge or salient angle formed by the meeting of two surfaces, esp. in moldings.

You should familiarize yourself with the abbreviations used to denote the origin of words. Consult the front pages of your dictionary where you will find a guide to the use of that particular publication. Look for a heading that refers to etymologies or abbreviations and symbols used in etymologies. These keys will help you interpret a word's entry. For instance, the entry on the previous page uses the abbreviations MF and LL indicating that the entry *arris* is derived from Middle French or Late Latin.

Many English words have their origin in Greek and Roman myths and legends. If you are well-read, you may already have an edge in using the etymological method of determining word meaning. For instance, if you have read the story of the mythical king Tantalus, you would understand the derivation of the verb *tantalize.* King Tantalus, after his death, was punished for his wickedness by being placed in water up to his chin. When he stooped to drink, the water would recede out of reach. Above his head, branches laden with fruit bobbed out of his reach. So from the name Tantalus came the word *tantalize,* meaning "to tease."

A great many of the words we use daily came into our language from the Latin and Greek. Approximately half the words in the dictionary are derived from Latin. Many Latin words and phrases have been borrowed and adopted by other languages. European languages such as French and Spanish came directly from Latin and are known as Romance languages. Consequently, if you are or have been a student of Latin, you will find it easier to build your vocabulary.

Many foreign terms were absorbed into English as parts of several different words related in meaning to each other. These parts of words fall into three groups.

Roots (or stems)—These carry the basic meaning and are combined with each other and with prefixes and suffixes to create other words with related meanings.

Prefixes—Letter combinations with their own particular meaning that appear at the beginning of a word.

Suffixes—Letter combinations with their own particular meaning that appear at the end of a word.

The lists of roots, prefixes, and suffixes in this section are accompanied by words in which the letter combinations appear. Use the dictionary to look up any words that are not clear in your mind.

KNOW YOUR ROOTS (OR STEMS)

The root, or stem, is that part of the word that conveys the basic meaning of the word. For example, in the word *introduction, duct* is the root. It means "lead." *Intro-* means *within, into,* and *-tion* is a noun ending. Hence, the meaning of introduction—a "leading into."

Below is a chart of common stems. See how well you "know your roots."

Common Stems

Stem	Meaning	Example
ag, ac	do	agenda, action
agri	farm	agriculture
aqua	water	aquatic
auto	self	automatic
biblio	book	bibliography
bio	life	biography
cad, cas	fall	cadence, casual
cap, cep, cept	take	captive, accept
capit	head	capital, decapitate
ced, cede, ceed, cess	go	intercede
celer	speed	accelerate
chrom	color	monochromatic
chron	time	chronological

TIP

Take the time to learn these roots and their meaning.

Stem	Meaning	Example
cide, cis	cut	incision
clude, clud, clus	close, close in	include, cluster
cog, cogn	knowledge of	recognize
cur, curs	run	recur, cursive
ded	give	dedicate
dent, dont	tooth	dental
duce, duct	lead	induce, deduct
fact, fect, fict	make, do	perfect, fiction, factory
fer, late	carry	refer, dilate, transfer, translate
flect, flex	bend, turn	reflect
fring, fract	break	infringe, refract
graph, gram	picture, writing	graphic, telegram
greg	group, gather	gregarious, congregation
gress, grad	step, walk	progress, degrade
hydr	water	hydrate
ject	throw	inject
jud	right	judicial
junct	join	conjunction
juris	law, justice	jurist
lect, leg	read, choose	collect, legible
logue	speech, speaking	dialogue
logy	study of	psychology
loq, loc	speak	elocution
lude, lus	play, perform	elude, ludicrous
manu	by hand	manuscript
mand	order	demand
mar	sea	maritime
med	middle	intermediate
ment, mem	mind, memory	mention
meter	measure	thermometer
micro	small	microscope
min	lessen	miniature
mis, miss, mit	send	remit, dismiss
mot, mov	move	remote, remove
mute	change	commute, mutation
naut	sailor, sail	nautical
nounce, nunci	declare, state	announce, enunciate
ped, pod	foot	pedal
pel, pulse	drive, push	dispel, impulse
pend, pense	hang	depend, dispenser
plac	please	placate
plic	fold	implicate

Stem	Meaning	Example
port	carry	portable
pose, pone	put, place	depose, component
reg, rect	rule	regulate, direct
rupt	break	disruption
sec, sect	cut	bisect
sed	remain	sedentary
sert	weave, bind	insert
serve	keep, save	preserve
scend, scent	climb	ascent
scribe, script	write	describe, transcript
sist	stand, set	insist
spect	look	inspect
spire, spirat	breath, breathe	perspire
strict	tighten	restrict
tain	hold	detain
term	end	terminate
tract	draw, drag	detract
tort	twist	distort
vene, vent	come	intervene, invent
vict	overcome, conquer	evict
volve, volu	roll, turn	evolve, evolution

PREFIXES AND SUFFIXES

Prefixes and suffixes are the "beginning and end." A prefix is a letter-combination attached to the beginning of a word; it usually carries a meaning independent of the word to which it is attached. For example, the prefix *semi* means "half." It can be added to many words—*semicircle, semilunar, semiprofessional, semiformal*. Attaching a prefix sometimes requires the placement of a hyphen between the prefix and the root word. A hyphen is used when the prefix is attached to a proper noun: *all-American, pro-British, anti-Fascist, un-Christian*.

A suffix is a combination of letters attached to the end of a word and usually possesses a meaning separate from the word to which it is affixed, for example, *-less* (without)—*careless, hopeless, meaningless*. Usually, affixing a suffix to a word changes its part of speech, for example, *assert* (verb)—*assertion* (noun), *beautiful* (adjective)—*beautifully* (adverb).

Study the following prefix and suffix charts to increase your understanding of related words and inflected (changed) forms.

Prefixes

Prefix	Meaning	Example
a	not	amoral
ab, a	away from	absent
ad, ac, ag, at	to	advent, accrue, attract, aggressive
an	without	anarchy
ante	before	antedate
anti	against	antipathy
aud, audit	hear	auditor
bene	well	beneficent
bi	two	bicameral
cap, capt, cept	take, seize, hold	capture
ced, cess	go, yield	rescind, recess
circum	around	circumspect
com, con, col	together	commit, confound, collate
contra	against	contraband
cred, credit	believe	credible
de	from, down	descend
dic, dict	say	dictionary
dis, di	apart	distract, divert
dom	home, rule	domicile, dominate
duc, duct	lead	induce
ex, e	out	exit, emit
extra	beyond	extracurricular
fac, fact	make	facsimile
in, im, ir, il, un	not	inept, irregular, illegal
in, im	in, into	interest, imbibe
inter	between	interscholastic
intra, intro	within	intramural
mal	bad	malcontent
mis	wrong	misnomer
non	not	nonentity
ob	against	obstacle
omni	all	omnivorous
per	through	permeate
peri	around	periscope
poly	many	polytheism
post	after	postmortem
pre	before	premonition
pro	forward	propose
re	again	review

Prefix	Meaning	Example
se	apart	seduce
semi	half	semicircle
sub	under	subvert
sui	self	suicide
super	above	superimpose
sur	on, upon	surcharge
trans	across	transpose
un	not	unwelcome
vice	instead of	vice-president

Suffixes

Suffix	Meaning	Example
able, ible	capable of being	capable, reversible
age	state of	storage
al	pertaining to	instructional
ance	relating to	reliance
ary	relating to	dictionary
ate	act	confiscate
ation	action	radiation
cy	quality	democracy
ed	past action	subsided
ence	relating to	confidence
er, or	one who	adviser, actor
ic	pertaining to	democratic
ing	present action	surmising
ious	full of	rebellious
ish	like, as	childish
ive	having the quality of	creative
ize	to make like	harmonize
less	without	hopeless
ly	the quality of	carefully
ment	result	amusement
ness	the quality of being	selfishness
ty	condition	sanity

INCREASED WORD POWER FROM BEGINNING TO END

Using the etymological approach can simplify the process by which you attack the monumental feat of learning medical terminology. By knowing that the suffix *itis* implies inflammation and *ectomy* means "the cutting out or removal of," you can easily deduce that the term *appendicitis* means "inflammation of the appendix" and *appendectomy* means "the cutting out or removal of the appendix."

Now that you have studied the various letter combinations or word components, see if you can make an educated guess at the meanings of the terms listed below. Start with the root or stem. Next, add the suffix and/or prefix to the interpretation in the order that provides a clear definition. The result will be increased word power from "beginning to end." It's as challenging as a jigsaw puzzle! Be sure to compare your definitions with those in the dictionary.

decapitate	colloquy	emissary	aggregation	incursion
retractable	involuted	implacable	convocation	celerity

SYNONYMS

The Name's the Same

Synonyms are words that share meanings. The English language abounds in synonyms. In your effort to acquire word mastery, you must learn to express your ideas without redundancy and constant use of overworked words. Effective writing and speaking may be achieved through the precise use of synonyms.

Words such as *brave* and *courageous,* which may allude to an identical quality, can be used interchangeably. Some synonyms, however, differ in definition or usage. For example, *fewer* refers to number, while *less* refers to quantity: John has *fewer* books and *less* money than his brother. These words are indeed similar in meaning, but one cannot be substituted for the other.

The adjectives *beautiful* and *handsome* both describe someone or something attractive or pleasing to the eye. Nevertheless, you would not usually speak of a "beautiful man" or a "handsome young lady." In our society, common usage would cause one to reverse these expressions to a "beautiful young lady" and a "handsome man."

A study of the finer shades of the meaning of synonyms will help you be more precise when you convey your feelings or mental picture of an object or scene. For instance, if you were to say, "The *bottom* of the lamp is made of Indian brass and features intricate carvings," one might simply envision the underside of the lamp. However, if you were to substitute *base* for the word *bottom,* one would instead get a visual image of something highly decorative that supports the upper structure of the lamp. So even though the "name" appears to be the same, an investigation into finer shades of definition will assist you in distinguishing variations in usage.

Familiar Surroundings?

The most common way of testing vocabulary on a standardized test is in context, that is, to present the items in a sentence or phrase so that you can see how a word is used. You can then determine whether the word is used as a noun, a verb, an adjective, etc. The test, therefore, is designed to encourage the extraction of word meaning from context; however, the context will not be so explicit that you can easily infer the meaning of a word.

More specifically, the synonym test item is usually a multiple-choice item that appears in one of three formats:

Type A

Given an underlined or italicized word in a complete sentence, the test-taker is required to identify which of the four other words is a synonym for the underlined or italicized word.

Example

The disinterested witness was able to give a *candid* account of the incident.
- **(A)** complete
- **(B)** impartial
- **(C)** biased
- **(D)** candescent

Type B

Given an underlined or italicized word in a phrase, the test-taker is required to identify which of the four other words is a synonym for the underlined or italicized word.

Example

The *emaciated* patient
- **(A)** discharged
- **(B)** emancipated
- **(C)** emotional
- **(D)** shriveled

Type C

Given a sentence with a missing word, the test-taker is required to identify which of the four other words best completes the sentence.

Example

An *apology* is appropriate when a person feels
- **(A)** sorry.
- **(B)** apathetic.
- **(C)** rejected.
- **(D)** elated.

OR

Example

He is a *staunch* supporter of the presidential candidate. Staunch means

    (A) stubborn.

    (B) faithful.

    (C) inflexible.

    (D) hopeful.

Context Clues

Examining the various types of context clues is another means of understanding how to extract the meaning of a word from the words surrounding it. The fourteen sample sentences below illustrate the different kinds of context clues.

1. Since the *litigation* would be costly, the lawyers advised that such a suit should be settled out of court. (**DEFINITION**)

2. The crumbling *edifice,* a building located on the north side of town, is targeted for implosion early in June. (**DEFINITION**)

3. He exhibits his *sloth* by resting on the couch while his wife and elderly father shovel snow. (**DESCRIPTION**)

4. She had indeed turned into a *shrew* with her screaming, nagging, and quarrelsome manner. (**DESCRIPTION**)

5. Tyler was anything but *amenable* to the proposal of another coed dorm on campus; on the contrary, he vehemently protested the board's recommendation for such action. (**CONTRAST**)

6. Crestville was a *quaint,* little town until the relocation of several large corporations turned it into a bustling metropolis. (**CONTRAST**)

7. Charles, like his brave and *dauntless* father, was fearless in the face of trouble. (**COMPARISON**)

8. She was stricken with the disease at an early age; her daughter likewise was *infirm* while very young. (**COMPARISON**)

9. The sentence of five years in prison hardly seemed adequate *retribution* for this dreadful crime. (**EXAMPLES**)

10. Peas and beans are two kinds of *legumes*. (**EXAMPLES**)

11. The disease is considered *infectious,* or contagious. (**SYNONYMS**)

12. The *cardiologist,* or heart specialist, ordered several tests for his patient. (**SYNONYMS**)

13. Karin was *elated* at the news of her job transfer; however, her mother appeared sad. (**ANTONYMS**)

14. The *arid* climate was a welcome change from the dampness I experienced in London. (**ANTONYMS**)

Especially Special: Scientific Terms

When preparing for an entrance exam for programs leading to science-related careers, it is beneficial to familiarize yourself with the specialized vocabulary of this discipline. Remember, even though the general public considers scientific jargon confusing, technical terms are imperative for scientific communication. If you plan to study science, your ability to comprehend the terminology of the field could indicate how well you will do in the related course work. Your entrance exam may measure your scientific vocabulary skills.

Mastery of specialized vocabulary—or any vocabulary for that matter—can best be achieved by learning words as you encounter them in your reading. However, when preparing for an entrance exam, you may want to employ the following nine strategies:

1. Review "Know Your Roots (or Stems)" and "Prefixes and Suffixes" on pages 71-75 of this publication.

2. Read a variety of scientific articles, science textbook chapters, etc.

3. Try to understand the unfamiliar words that you encounter in these readings as they are used in context.

4. If you cannot grasp the meaning from context, then put your knowledge of roots and affixes to work. Take the word apart and see if you can determine a meaning that fits the context (or if you are in the testing situation, a meaning that comes close to one of the multiple-choice items).

5. If Step 4 does not yield a reasonable definition, then check the footnotes, glossary, or index of the text you are reading. If you find the word in the index, skim the pages listed for that word, checking for either its definition or its contextual usage.

6. If you cannot find a definition of the word in the material that you are reading, look it up in a dictionary. It would be best to use a scientific dictionary or encyclopedia. There are dictionaries that are for specific areas of study, such as geography, modern history, politics, and biology.

7. Once you have come up with a definition for the word, you may want to write it on an index card (word on one side, definition on the other). After accumulating a number of these vocabulary cards, carry them in your pocket or book bag. Flip through them when you have a spare moment (commuting by train or bus, sitting in the waiting room of the dentist or doctor, etc.).

8. Become accustomed to recognizing words that stand for concepts rather than facts. To a scientist, a concept is a generalization or an idea based on information or knowledge that explains a phenomenon. Read the following paragraph and underline those words which you feel represent scientific concepts. *Karotyping is a process that enables scientists to study the chromosomes of human beings. Sometimes the study can be made even before birth. Chromosomes can best be observed during metaphase in mitosis. At this point they are coiled. Skin cells are good to use in making a Karyotype because they divide frequently. Some genetic disorders can be identified just by looking at the Karyotype of a person.* If you underlined *Karyotype process, metaphase, mitosis,* and *genetic disorders,* you would be correct. These words represent ideas.

They cannot be touched and they have no exact physical form or boundaries, yet they are real because they represent scientific facts.

9. Finally, learn to connect symbols to words. A scientific symbol is an abbreviation that stands for a word or concept.

Example

$C_6H_{12}O_6$ represents glucose, a chemical compound.

You will have the opportunity to practice your use of these vocabulary expansion strategies as you encounter scientific terms on the verbal ability tests in this book. The answers to several of the questions in the reading comprehension test involve scientific terms. These questions are indicated by asterisks.

In completing a synonym test item, remember to look for a word that means the same, or almost the same, as the target word in the item (the underlined or italicized word). Do not be distracted by a word that is a look-alike, that is, one that looks similar or begins with the same three or four letters but is unrelated in meaning. When possible, apply the etymological approach of interpreting roots, prefixes, and suffixes.

SYNONYMS TEST ANSWER SHEET

1. Ⓐ Ⓑ Ⓒ Ⓓ	16. Ⓐ Ⓑ Ⓒ Ⓓ	31. Ⓐ Ⓑ Ⓒ Ⓓ	46. Ⓐ Ⓑ Ⓒ Ⓓ	61. Ⓐ Ⓑ Ⓒ Ⓓ
2. Ⓐ Ⓑ Ⓒ Ⓓ	17. Ⓐ Ⓑ Ⓒ Ⓓ	32. Ⓐ Ⓑ Ⓒ Ⓓ	47. Ⓐ Ⓑ Ⓒ Ⓓ	62. Ⓐ Ⓑ Ⓒ Ⓓ
3. Ⓐ Ⓑ Ⓒ Ⓓ	18. Ⓐ Ⓑ Ⓒ Ⓓ	33. Ⓐ Ⓑ Ⓒ Ⓓ	48. Ⓐ Ⓑ Ⓒ Ⓓ	63. Ⓐ Ⓑ Ⓒ Ⓓ
4. Ⓐ Ⓑ Ⓒ Ⓓ	19. Ⓐ Ⓑ Ⓒ Ⓓ	34. Ⓐ Ⓑ Ⓒ Ⓓ	49. Ⓐ Ⓑ Ⓒ Ⓓ	64. Ⓐ Ⓑ Ⓒ Ⓓ
5. Ⓐ Ⓑ Ⓒ Ⓓ	20. Ⓐ Ⓑ Ⓒ Ⓓ	35. Ⓐ Ⓑ Ⓒ Ⓓ	50. Ⓐ Ⓑ Ⓒ Ⓓ	65. Ⓐ Ⓑ Ⓒ Ⓓ
6. Ⓐ Ⓑ Ⓒ Ⓓ	21. Ⓐ Ⓑ Ⓒ Ⓓ	36. Ⓐ Ⓑ Ⓒ Ⓓ	51. Ⓐ Ⓑ Ⓒ Ⓓ	66. Ⓐ Ⓑ Ⓒ Ⓓ
7. Ⓐ Ⓑ Ⓒ Ⓓ	22. Ⓐ Ⓑ Ⓒ Ⓓ	37. Ⓐ Ⓑ Ⓒ Ⓓ	52. Ⓐ Ⓑ Ⓒ Ⓓ	67. Ⓐ Ⓑ Ⓒ Ⓓ
8. Ⓐ Ⓑ Ⓒ Ⓓ	23. Ⓐ Ⓑ Ⓒ Ⓓ	38. Ⓐ Ⓑ Ⓒ Ⓓ	53. Ⓐ Ⓑ Ⓒ Ⓓ	68. Ⓐ Ⓑ Ⓒ Ⓓ
9. Ⓐ Ⓑ Ⓒ Ⓓ	24. Ⓐ Ⓑ Ⓒ Ⓓ	39. Ⓐ Ⓑ Ⓒ Ⓓ	54. Ⓐ Ⓑ Ⓒ Ⓓ	69. Ⓐ Ⓑ Ⓒ Ⓓ
10. Ⓐ Ⓑ Ⓒ Ⓓ	25. Ⓐ Ⓑ Ⓒ Ⓓ	40. Ⓐ Ⓑ Ⓒ Ⓓ	55. Ⓐ Ⓑ Ⓒ Ⓓ	70. Ⓐ Ⓑ Ⓒ Ⓓ
11. Ⓐ Ⓑ Ⓒ Ⓓ	26. Ⓐ Ⓑ Ⓒ Ⓓ	41. Ⓐ Ⓑ Ⓒ Ⓓ	56. Ⓐ Ⓑ Ⓒ Ⓓ	71. Ⓐ Ⓑ Ⓒ Ⓓ
12. Ⓐ Ⓑ Ⓒ Ⓓ	27. Ⓐ Ⓑ Ⓒ Ⓓ	42. Ⓐ Ⓑ Ⓒ Ⓓ	57. Ⓐ Ⓑ Ⓒ Ⓓ	72. Ⓐ Ⓑ Ⓒ Ⓓ
13. Ⓐ Ⓑ Ⓒ Ⓓ	28. Ⓐ Ⓑ Ⓒ Ⓓ	43. Ⓐ Ⓑ Ⓒ Ⓓ	58. Ⓐ Ⓑ Ⓒ Ⓓ	73. Ⓐ Ⓑ Ⓒ Ⓓ
14. Ⓐ Ⓑ Ⓒ Ⓓ	29. Ⓐ Ⓑ Ⓒ Ⓓ	44. Ⓐ Ⓑ Ⓒ Ⓓ	59. Ⓐ Ⓑ Ⓒ Ⓓ	74. Ⓐ Ⓑ Ⓒ Ⓓ
15. Ⓐ Ⓑ Ⓒ Ⓓ	30. Ⓐ Ⓑ Ⓒ Ⓓ	45. Ⓐ Ⓑ Ⓒ Ⓓ	60. Ⓐ Ⓑ Ⓒ Ⓓ	75. Ⓐ Ⓑ Ⓒ Ⓓ

answer sheet

SYNONYMS TEST

75 Questions • 35 Minutes

Directions: In each of the sentences below, one word is italicized. Following each sentence are four words or phrases. For each sentence, choose the word or phrase that most nearly corresponds in meaning with the italicized word.

1. The *diction* acceptable in speech is usually more informal than that required in writing.
   (A) conviction
   (B) language
   (C) discourse
   (D) denunciation

2. It is apparent that Gina Smith is the most *sedulous* and active member of the group.
   (A) hideous
   (B) generous
   (C) infirm
   (D) industrious

3. During the hockey game several *altercations* took place.
   (A) fracases
   (B) substitutions
   (C) alterations
   (D) plays

4. The carrot is a perfect illustration of a *biennial*.
   (A) occurring quarterly
   (B) occurring once in two years
   (C) perennial
   (D) bisection

5. He has run the *gamut* of clerical jobs in this office.
   (A) periphery
   (B) margin
   (C) range
   (D) imperception

6. His deeds amounted to nothing more than those of a *sanctimonious* hypocrite.
   (A) parsimonious
   (B) perpetual
   (C) intrinsic
   (D) self-righteous

7. He displayed the manners of an *urbane* gentleman.
   (A) suave
   (B) poignant
   (C) spasmodic
   (D) pensive

8. The *slogan* is appropriate for both the product and its service.
   (A) catchword
   (B) sample
   (C) design
   (D) passage

9. The man was *vociferous* in his complaints about his dinner.
   (A) strident
   (B) muted
   (C) insistent
   (D) importunate

10. He was determined to *foil* the scheme of his opponent.
    (A) heighten
    (B) secure
    (C) disencumber
    (D) thwart

11. The examiner *purported* to be an official representative.
    (A) addressed
    (B) claimed
    (C) propitiated
    (D) conciliated

12. The ships carried happy vacationers *bent* on having a good time.
    (A) flexible
    (B) determined
    (C) inclined
    (D) endowed

13. The child could not *recollect* the incident.
    (A) remember
    (B) doubt
    (C) interrogate
    (D) illumine

14. The governor *rescinded* the state of emergency as soon as the roads were cleared of snow.
    (A) negated
    (B) maneuvered
    (C) revoked
    (D) accepted

15. The implementation of the plan was given *scant* consideration.
    (A) audacious
    (B) fervid
    (C) little
    (D) clothed

16. The key speaker, in his lengthy presentation, *scoffed at* the notion of marketing as a public service.
    (A) exonerated
    (B) amplified
    (C) confuted
    (D) mocked

17. She completed the *sprint* with a sudden surge of energy.
    (A) relaxation
    (B) adventure
    (C) run
    (D) convergence

18. The content of the message was *urgent*.
    (A) privileged
    (B) amendable
    (C) pressing
    (D) absolved

19. A *simulated* rescue mission was conducted by the forest rangers.
    (A) pretended
    (B) superficial
    (C) stimulated
    (D) simultaneous

20. Through the course of the day, she became more *agitated* by the noise of the demolition and less focused on her work.
    (A) worried
    (B) upset
    (C) convulsed
    (D) composed

21. Her quickening gait seemed regulated by the *pulse* of the big city.
    (A) utility
    (B) pace
    (C) reverence
    (D) solace

22. The language of the publication is *unsophisticated* but informative.
    (A) ponderous
    (B) elaborate
    (C) simple
    (D) artificial

23. All the evidence presented pointed to *willful* execution of a crime.
    - (A) deliberate
    - (B) eminent
    - (C) amicable
    - (D) remorseful

24. There is no *provision* for deadlines in the contract.
    - (A) improvement
    - (B) convenience
    - (C) aggregation
    - (D) stipulation

25. The furnishings *impart* an air of elegance to the room.
    - (A) communicate
    - (B) indemnify
    - (C) reinforce
    - (D) disguise

26. She exhibited great *valor* in handling the emergency.
    - (A) ingeniousness
    - (B) courage
    - (C) discretion
    - (D) optimism

27. Various courses were *fused* in the revision of the curriculum.
    - (A) required
    - (B) implicated
    - (C) combined
    - (D) involved

28. He was able to *duplicate* his work even though his hard drive with all his data had died.
    - (A) replicate
    - (B) synthesize
    - (C) fixate
    - (D) replenish

29. The task of choosing one from so many qualified applicants *bewildered* the employer.
    - (A) perplexed
    - (B) aggravated
    - (C) subdued
    - (D) infuriated

30. The revision of the city plan incorporated adjustments in the projected *modes* of transportation.
    - (A) increments
    - (B) expenditures
    - (C) means
    - (D) modifications

31. The politician sought to *aggrandize* himself at the expense of the people.
    - (A) exhaust
    - (B) subjugate
    - (C) sacrifice
    - (D) enrich

32. The newcomer made an effort to *mingle* with the crowd.
    - (A) argue
    - (B) mix
    - (C) disrupt
    - (D) flout

33. If an organization's programs were described as *philanthropic*, the programs would be
    - (A) primitive.
    - (B) deleterious.
    - (C) extraneous.
    - (D) benevolent.

34. If the traits of a nation's leader were *covetous*, they were
    - (A) greedy.
    - (B) exemplary.
    - (C) disparate.
    - (D) adventitious.

35. Rabbits *breed* offspring rapidly.
    (A) raise
    (B) gather
    (C) propagate
    (D) destroy

36. He *reiterated* the need to document the procedures in the experiment.
    (A) adjusted
    (B) defended
    (C) fermented
    (D) repeated

37. A shadow of a man *loomed* ominously in the dimly lit corridor.
    (A) asserted
    (B) yielded
    (C) appeared
    (D) rebuffed

38. Alcohol consumption often exerts *an adverse* influence on an individual.
    (A) an ecstatic
    (B) an injurious
    (C) a luminous
    (D) a gloomy

39. The girl is reported to have left of her own *volition*.
    (A) flight
    (B) will
    (C) repudiation
    (D) recognizance

40. The one-sided score was *an anomaly* in a Division 1 game.
    (A) an anachronism
    (B) a change
    (C) an embarrassment
    (D) an aberration

41. The *similitude* between the original painting and the reproduction is remarkable.
    (A) incongruity
    (B) connection
    (C) resemblance
    (D) relationship

42. A *prudent* individual will save some portion of his or her wage.
    (A) judicious
    (B) terse
    (C) audacious
    (D) laconic

43. His decision to return home was *instinctive*.
    (A) spontaneous
    (B) turgid
    (C) premeditated
    (D) irrelevant

44. It seemed as if the sky opened and a *torrent* of rain poured down on unprepared pedestrians.
    (A) slide
    (B) avalanche
    (C) deluge
    (D) air

45. The self-portrait *embodies* the true spirit of the artist.
    (A) combats
    (B) eliminates
    (C) abjures
    (D) symbolizes

46. Her sudden decision is typical of her *impetuous* behavior.
    (A) contemptible
    (B) sophisticated
    (C) impulsive
    (D) fallacious

47. It is fitting that we *eulogize* one who has contributed so greatly to our society.
- **(A)** promulgate
- **(B)** praise
- **(C)** denigrate
- **(D)** append

48. The convention hall swelled with the *vociferation* of various campaign groups.
- **(A)** clamor
- **(B)** taciturnity
- **(C)** oblivion
- **(D)** discernment

49. The blackmailer has placed her in a *precarious* position.
- **(A)** mellifluous
- **(B)** intrusive
- **(C)** unusual
- **(D)** unstable

50. Her neighbor's display of so much fine china was too *ostentatious*.
- **(A)** pretentious
- **(B)** inconspicuous
- **(C)** ascribable
- **(D)** candid

51. To *manifest* interest
- **(A)** conceal
- **(B)** diminish
- **(C)** augment
- **(D)** display

52. *Banter* and laughter
- **(A)** discourse
- **(B)** singing
- **(C)** toasting
- **(D)** raillery

53. *Aesthetic* value
- **(A)** practical
- **(B)** artistic
- **(C)** monetary
- **(D)** estimable

54. Confirmed his *apostasy*
- **(A)** defiance
- **(B)** defection
- **(C)** belief
- **(D)** inference

55. The *cryptic* message
- **(A)** cynical
- **(B)** mysterious
- **(C)** critical
- **(D)** censorious

56. New witnesses *emerged*
- **(A)** deviated
- **(B)** divested
- **(C)** declined
- **(D)** appeared

57. The *contumacious* youngster
- **(A)** exuberant
- **(B)** rebellious
- **(C)** awkward
- **(D)** mischievous

58. *Cognizant* of the ill will
- **(A)** ignorant
- **(B)** aware
- **(C)** insensitive
- **(D)** remorseful

59. *Glacial* region
- **(A)** glass-like
- **(B)** illiberal
- **(C)** frigid
- **(D)** reticent

60. *Instigated* the rebellion
- **(A)** quelled
- **(B)** incited
- **(C)** assisted
- **(D)** depressed

61. A fight *ensued*
- **(A)** followed
- **(B)** terminated
- **(C)** was avoided
- **(D)** culminated

62. *Retrospect* of events
    (A) review
    (B) concept
    (C) knowledge
    (D) awareness

63. *Malice* toward my friend
    (A) adoration
    (B) sympathy
    (C) ill will
    (D) apathy

64. *Saturated* with moisture
    (A) void (of)
    (B) mixed
    (C) soaked
    (D) replaced

65. *Debilitating* to people
    (A) invigorating
    (B) stimulating
    (C) tolerable
    (D) weakening

66. Ten years' *servitude*
    (A) freedom
    (B) lethargy
    (C) vicissitude
    (D) bondage

67. *Relish* the thought
    (A) enjoy
    (B) dread
    (C) spread
    (D) implant

68. A *lackadaisical* attitude
    (A) enthusiastic
    (B) complacent
    (C) profound
    (D) indifferent

69. To *hoist* the sails
    (A) cast
    (B) raise
    (C) prepare
    (D) repair

70. *Asperse* the family's good name
    (A) slander
    (B) fathom
    (C) extol
    (D) palliate

71. *Sordid* details
    (A) bizarre
    (B) wretched
    (C) primordial
    (D) exaggerated

72. Sudden *alienation*
    (A) agitation
    (B) inception
    (C) subsistence
    (D) isolation

73. *Dereliction* of duty
    (A) neglect
    (B) expansion
    (C) attainment
    (D) fulfillment

74. *Accede* to the request
    (A) attend
    (B) refer
    (C) adjust
    (D) agree

75. The *proximity* of the lake
    (A) worthlessness
    (B) nearness
    (C) level
    (D) ebullition

STOP

IF YOU FINISH BEFORE TIME IS CALLED, YOU MAY CHECK
YOUR WORK ON THIS SECTION ONLY. DO NOT TURN TO ANY
OTHER SECTION IN THE TEST.

facebook.com/petersonspublishing

ANSWER KEY AND EXPLANATIONS

1. B	16. D	31. D	46. C	61. A
2. D	17. C	32. B	47. B	62. A
3. A	18. C	33. D	48. A	63. C
4. B	19. A	34. A	49. D	64. C
5. C	20. B	35. C	50. A	65. D
6. D	21. B	36. D	51. D	66. D
7. A	22. C	37. C	52. D	67. A
8. A	23. A	38. B	53. B	68. D
9. A	24. D	39. B	54. B	69. B
10. D	25. A	40. D	55. B	70. A
11. B	26. B	41. C	56. D	71. B
12. B	27. C	42. A	57. B	72. D
13. A	28. A	43. A	58. B	73. A
14. C	29. A	44. C	59. C	74. D
15. C	30. C	45. D	60. B	75. B

1. **The correct answer is (B).** *Diction* and *language* are synonyms. Choice (A) is incorrect because *conviction* makes no sense and is not a synonym. Choice (C) is incorrect because *discourse* means "conversation, expressing one's self in writing or speaking" and isn't specific enough to be a synonym in this case. Choice (D) is incorrect because while *denunciation* might tempt you into thinking it has something to do with words, it means "a public condemnation or accusation of someone" and has nothing to do with language.

2. **The correct answer is (D).** *Sedulous* and *industrious* both mean "hard working" and so are synonyms. Choices (A), (B), and (C), *hideous, generous,* and *infirm,* have no relation to sedulous.

3. **The correct answer is (A).** An *altercation* is a fight, quarrel, or argument, and a *fracas* is a noisy fight or quarrel. Choice (B) is incorrect, but might tempt you because *substitutions* makes sense in the sentence; however, it is not a synonym for *altercation.* Choice (C) might also look like the answer if you think of *alterations* as changes, but remember you're looking for the synonym for *altercations*, not what makes sense in the sentence. Choice (D) is incorrect because *plays* is not a synonym.

4. **The correct answer is (B).** If you didn't know what *biennial* means, remember that *bi-* means "two," which narrows the choices to choice (B). Choice (A) is incorrect because a biennial blooms once every two years, not once a quarter. Choice (C) is incorrect because a plant can't be a biennial and a *perennial*, which is a plant that blooms every year. Choice (D) is incorrect because *bisection* has no relation to *biennial.*

5. **The correct answer is (C).** *Gamut* means "range or extent," so *range* is a synonym. Choice (A) is incorrect because *periphery* means "outside boundary." Choice (B) is incorrect because *margin,* meaning "a boundary line," is a synonym for *periphery,* not *gamut.* Choice (D) is incorrect because *imperception* means "lack of perception."

6. **The correct answer is (D).** *Sanctimonious* means "making a show of being holy or pious," so *self-righteous,* meaning "excessively or hypocritically pious," is a synonym. Choice (A) is incorrect because *parsimonious* means "stingy, miserly." Choice (B) is incorrect because *perpetual* means "for all eternity" or "lasting for an indefinite period." Choice (C) is incorrect because *intrinsic* means "essential to something, belonging to something by its nature."

7. **The correct answer is (A).** *Urbane* means "characterized by sophistication" or "polite, refined," and *suave* means "having sophistication and charm" or "urbane, courteous." Choice (B) is incorrect because *poignant* means "very moving, distressing." Choice (C) is incorrect because *spasmodic* means "intermittently," "relating to a spasm," or "excitable," none of which indicate that *spasmodic* is a synonym for *urbane.* Choice (D) is incorrect because *pensive* means "very thoughtful, serious."

8. **The correct answer is (A).** A slogan is a phrase used in advertising to describe a product or service; groups and organizations may also have slogans. A *catchword* is a favorite saying of a group. *Sample, design,* and *passage* all make sense if they were substituted into the sentence, but none are correct because none is a synonym for *slogan.*

9. **The correct answer is (A).** *Vociferous* means "very loud, noisy, vehement," and *strident* means "loud, vehement." Choice (B) is incorrect because *muted,* meaning "silent," is the opposite. Choice (C) is incorrect because *insistent,* meaning "demanding," has no relation to *vociferous.*

Choice (D) is incorrect because *importunate* means "insistent, demanding."

10. **The correct answer is (D).** To *foil* is "to stop, prevent," which are meanings of *thwart.* Choice (A) is incorrect because *heighten* has no relation to *foil,* nor does choice (B), *secure.* Choice (C) is incorrect because *disencumber* means "to relieve of burdens" or "to free from difficulties."

11. **The correct answer is (B).** *Purported* means "to have claimed to be something, usually falsely," so *claimed* is a synonym. Choice (A) is incorrect because it is not a synonym for *purported.* If you tried substituting the word in the sentence if you weren't sure, you see that it doesn't fit ("addressed to be an official"). Choice (C) is incorrect because *propitiated* means "to make peace with someone, to appease." Choice (D) is incorrect because *conciliated* means "to overcome distrust, to appease," so *propitiated* and *conciliated* are synonyms for each other, but not *purported.*

12. **The correct answer is (B).** *Bent* in this context means "determined, disposed to," so *determined* is a synonym. Choice (A) is incorrect because *flexible* means "able to be bent," which is not the same as being *determined.* Choice (C) is incorrect because *inclined* does not relate to this meaning of *bent.* Choice (D) is incorrect because *endowed* means "having been given certain qualities or abilities."

13. **The correct answer is (A).** *Remember* is a synonym for *recollect.* None of the other words makes sense in the context. *Illumine,* choice (D), means "to shed light on" and might tempt you, but it doesn't have the same or a similar meaning as *recollect.* Sometimes, the simplest answer is the right answer.

14. **The correct answer is (C).** To *rescind* is "to *revoke.*" Choice (A) is incorrect because typically an official order such as a declaration of a state of emergency is *revoked,* not *negated.* Choice (B), *maneuver,* means "to carry out a military action," "to change tactics," or "to alter

the placement of troops," none of which are synonyms of *rescind*. Choice (D) is incorrect because the governor is ending the state of emergency, not *accepting* it.

15. **The correct answer is (C).** *Scant* means "little." Choice (A) is incorrect because *audacious* means "bold, fearless, spirited." Choice (B) is incorrect because *fervid* means "impassioned, intense emotion." Choice (D) is incorrect because *clothed* makes no sense, even in a metaphorical sense.

16. **The correct answer is (D).** To *scoff at* is "to mock or make fun of." Choice (A) makes no sense because *exonerate* is "to free someone from blame or responsibility." Choice (B) is incorrect because *amplify* is "to increase," "to exaggerate," or "to make complete." Choice (C), *confute*, is "to prove something or someone wrong."

17. **The correct answer is (C).** *Run* and *sprint* can be synonyms and are in this case. Choice (A) makes no sense because you don't need a surge of energy to *relax*. Choice (B) is incorrect because while *adventure* makes some sense, it is not a synonym for *run*. Choice (D), *convergence*, meaning "where two things come together," makes no sense.

18. **The correct answer is (C).** *Pressing* means "demanding immediate attention," in other words, *urgent*. Choice (A), *privileged*, meaning "confidential," isn't correct. Choice (B), *amendable*, meaning "capable of being changed," is also incorrect. Choice (D), *absolved*, meaning "pronounced not guilty," is also incorrect.

19. **The correct answer is (A).** *Simulated* is something made to resemble something else; in other words, it is *pretended*. Choice (B) is incorrect because something *superficial* is something that may be frivolous, perfunctory, or on the surface, none of which are the same as *simulated*. Choice (C) is incorrect because *stimulated* means "aroused or excited emotionally." Choice (D) is incorrect because *simultaneous* means "at the same time."

20. **The correct answer is (B).** Both *worried* and *upset* can be synonyms of *agitated*, but in this sentence, *upset* fits the context better. Choice (C) is incorrect because *convulsed* means "shaking violently"; it can be a synonym of *agitate*, but not in this context. Choice (D) is incorrect because *composed*, meaning "calm," is the opposite of *agitated*.

21. **The correct answer is (B).** A *pulse* is beat or *pace*. Choice (A) is incorrect because *utility* means either "usefulness" or "a power company." Choice (C) is incorrect because *reverence* is a feeling of profound awe or respect and makes no sense; it is also not a synonym of *pulse*. Choice (D) is incorrect because *solace* is the same as comfort, not a *pulse*.

22. **The correct answer is (C).** One synonym for *unsophisticated* is *simple*. Choice (A) is incorrect because *ponderous* means "heavy, dull, tedious," none of which is the same as *unsophisticated*. Choice (B) is incorrect because *elaborate* tends to the opposite of *unsophisticated*. Choice (D) is incorrect because *artificial* means "contrived, inauthentic, forced, affected," in other words, the opposite of *unsophisticated*.

23. **The correct answer is (A).** *Willful* and *deliberate* are synonyms. Choice (B) is incorrect because *eminent* means "prominent, great, well-known"; don't confuse it with *imminent*, meaning "about to happen." Choice (C), *amicable*, means "friendly" and makes no sense. Choice (D) is incorrect because *remorseful* means "sorry," and while someone caught for a crime may feel remorseful, it is not a synonym for *willful* and makes no sense.

24. **The correct answer is (D).** *Stipulation* is a synonym for *provision*, meaning "arrangement or plan." Choice (A) is incorrect because *improvement* is not the same as a *stipulation* and doesn't fit the sense. Choice (B) is incorrect because *convenience* means "benefit, advantage" or "suitability." Choice (C) is incorrect

because *aggregation* means "a collection of several things taken as a whole."

25. The correct answer is (A). *Impart* and *communicate* are synonyms. Choice (B) is incorrect because *indemnify* means "to protect against damage or loss." Choice (C), *reinforce,* may seem like a good choice, and in terms of context could work except that *impart* and *reinforce* aren't synonyms. Choice (D) is incorrect because *disguise* isn't a synonym for transmitting information, in this case, a feeling or sense of style.

26. The correct answer is (B). *Valor* and *courage* are the same thing. Choice (A) is incorrect because *ingeniousness* is cleverness, inventiveness, and creative thinking. Choice (C) is incorrect because *discretion* is tactfulness. Choice (D) is incorrect because *optimism* means "expecting that the best will happen."

27. The correct answer is (C). To *fuse* is "to mix together," but also "to unite, to join," and among the answer choices, *combine* is the closest in meaning. Choice (A) is incorrect because *required* is not a synonym for joining, though courses can be required. Choice (B) is incorrect because *implicated,* meaning "to involve or incriminate someone," makes no sense. Choice (D) is incorrect because while *involved* may make sense in the context, it is not a synonym for *fuse.*

28. The correct answer is (A). To *duplicate* is "to *replicate*" or "to make an exact copy." Choice (B) is incorrect because *synthesize* means "to combine pieces to form something new." Choice (C) is incorrect because "to *fixate*" is "to make something stable" or "to focus attention on something or someone." Choice (D), *replenish,* means "to make something full or complete again."

29. The correct answer is (A). To *bewilder* is "to *perplex*," meaning "to confuse." Choice (B) is incorrect because *aggravated* means "made angry" or "made something worse." Choice (C) is incorrect because *subdued*

means "conquered, brought under control." Choice (D) is incorrect because *infuriated* means "angry, enraged."

30. The correct answer is (C). *Means* can be a synonym of *modes* when they both mean "method, way, or variety," which fits the context of the sentence. Choice (A) is incorrect because *increments* means "the process of increasing in number, size, or quantity." Choice (B) is incorrect because *expenditures* refers to the disbursement of money. Choice (D) is incorrect because *modifications* refers to changes.

31. The correct answer is (D). One meaning of *aggrandize* is "to *enrich* one's self." Choice (A) is incorrect because *exhaust,* "to tire," is not a synonym and doesn't make sense since the politician would be exhausting himself, not the people. Choice (B) is incorrect because *subjugate* means "to conquer, to make subservient" and is not only not a synonym, but the politician isn't about to subjugate himself. Choice (C) is incorrect because *sacrifice* is not a synonym and a politician aggrandizing himself is the opposite of one sacrificing himself for his constituents.

32. The correct answer is (B). To *mingle* is "to *mix*." Choice (A) is incorrect because *argue* is not the same as *mingle.* Choice (C) is incorrect because to *disrupt* is "to interrupt" or "to break up." Choice (D) is incorrect because to *flout* is "to show contempt for" or "to brush off, to ignore."

33. The correct answer is (D). *Philanthropic* programs are *benevolent,* meaning "generous in helping others, showing kindness." Choice (A) is incorrect because *primitive* means "basic, simple." Choice (B) is incorrect because *deleterious* means "harmful," the opposite of *philanthropic.* Choice (C) is incorrect because *extraneous* means "not essential, unnecessary."

34. The correct answer is (A). A *covetous* person is a *greedy* person. Choice (B) is incorrect because *exemplary* means "worthy of being imitated, a model." Choice (C) is incorrect because *disparate* means "something that is very different, unlike." Choice (D) is incorrect because *adventitious* means "added to something by chance or accidentally."

35. **The correct answer is (C).** To *breed* is "to *propagate*," or reproduce. Choice (A) is incorrect because *raise* is not the same as reproduce. Choice (B), *gather*, is not only not a synonym, but makes no sense. Choice (D), *destroy*, is the opposite of breeding.

36. **The correct answer is (D).** To *reiterate* is "to *repeat*." Choice (A) is incorrect because *adjusted* is not a synonym for *reiterate*, nor is choice (B), *defended*, even though it would make sense in the sentence. Choice (C) is incorrect because *fermented* means "having been broken down into simpler substances."

37. **The correct answer is (C).** To *loom* is "to appear in one's view, seemingly threateningly," so *appeared* is a synonym. Choice (A) is incorrect because *assert* means "to state something positively, to insist." Choice (B) is incorrect because *yield* means "to give up, to give in." Choice (D) is incorrect because *rebuff* means "to reject" or "to drive back."

38. **The correct answer is (B).** *Adverse* means "harmful, *injurious*." Choice (A) is incorrect because *ecstatic* means "joyful, feeling great delight." Choice (C) is incorrect because *luminous* means "full of light, radiant." Choice (D) is incorrect because *gloomy* is not a synonym for *adverse*.

39. **The correct answer is (B).** *Volition* means "conscious decision, doing something willingly," so *will* is a synonym. Choice (A) is incorrect because *flight* has no relation to *volition* and doesn't make sense in the sentence either. Choice (C) is incorrect because *repudiation* means "rejection or disowning something as invalid." Choice (D) is incorrect because *recognizance* means "an obligation entered into as a result of court order, typically to go free on condition of appearing in court for a hearing."

40. **The correct answer is (D).** An *anomaly* is a departure from the normal, or something that is abnormal or irregular, and an *aberration* is a departure from the normal or typical. Choice (A) is incorrect because an *anachronism* is someone or something that seems to belong to another time period. It's similar to *anomaly*, but *aberration* is closer in meaning to *anomaly* in this sentence. Choice (B) is incorrect because a *change* is not the same as an *anomaly*. Choice (C) is incorrect because the score may have been an embarrassment, but *embarrassment* is not a synonym for *anomaly*.

41. **The correct answer is (C).** *Similitude* means "similarity in appearance," so *resemblance* is a synonym. Choice (A) is incorrect because *incongruity* means "lacking congruity," that is, "being unsuitable or inappropriate." Choice (B) is incorrect because a *connection* is not the same as being similar. Choice (D) is incorrect because a similarity in appearance shows some *relationship* between things, but it's not a synonym.

42. **The correct answer is (A).** *Prudent* means "wise, careful and sensible, using good judgement," so *judicious,* meaning "prudent, showing good judgement," is a synonym. Choice (B) is incorrect because *terse* means "brief, to the point." Choice (C) is incorrect because *audacious* means "bold, fearless, spirited" and can be considered an antonym for *prudent*. Choice (D) is incorrect because *laconic* means "using few words, terse, to the point" and is a synonym for *terse*, but not *prudent*.

43. **The correct answer is (A).** *Instinctive* means "impulsive, *spontaneous,* and unthinking." Choice (B) is incorrect because *turgid* means "pompous, lofty in style." Choice (C) is incorrect because *premeditated* means "thought out in advance," making it an antonym for *instinctive*. Choice (D) is incorrect because *irrelevant* means "not important, not having a connection with something."

44. **The correct answer is (C).** A *torrent* is "a fast-flowing stream or water" or "a

deluge, a heavy downpour," so *deluge* is a synonym. Choice (A) is incorrect because a *slide* has no relation to a torrent. Choice (B) is incorrect because an *avalanche* is a fall or slide of snow, not water. Choice (D) is incorrect because *air* has no relation to *torrent*.

45. **The correct answer is (D).** To *embody* is "to represent or express something" or "to symbolize something," so *symbolize* is a synonym. Choice (A) is incorrect because *combat* has no relation to *embody*, nor has choice (B), *eliminate*. Choice (C) is incorrect because *abjure* means "to renounce, to repudiate."

46. **The correct answer is (C).** To be *impetuous* is "to be *impulsive*." Choice (A) is incorrect because *contemptible* means "worthy of contempt, shameful, despicable." Choice (B) is incorrect because *sophisticated* means "refined or cultured in tastes and habits" as well as "complex." Choice (D) is incorrect because *fallacious* means "deceptive" or "erroneous."

47. **The correct answer is (B).** *Eulogize* means "to praise, acclaim, usually in a speech," so *praise* is a synonym. Choice (A) is incorrect because *promulgate* means "to make known, to announce, to proclaim." Choice (C) is incorrect because *denigrate* is the opposite of *eulogize*. Choice (D) is incorrect because *append* means "to add, to attach." Think of an *appendix* to a book.

48. **The correct answer is (A).** *Vociferation* means "a loud outcry, often in protest," so *clamor* meaning "a loud outcry" or "a vehement expression of protest" is a synonym. Choice (B) is incorrect because *taciturnity* means "silent, a habit of not being communicative," so this can be considered an antonym. Choice (C) is incorrect because *oblivion* means "the condition of being forgotten or disregarded." Choice (D) is incorrect because *discernment* means "evidence of keen judgement or insight."

49. **The correct answer is (D).** To be *precarious* is "to be *unstable*." Choice (A) is incorrect because *mellifluous* means "pleasing

to the ear." Choice (B) is incorrect because *intrusive* means "tending to intrude, to interfere." Choice (C) is incorrect because *unusual* has no relation to *precarious*.

50. **The correct answer is (A).** *Ostentatious* means "showy, pretentious, meaning to attract attention and impress others," so *pretentious* is a synonym. Choice (B) is incorrect because *inconspicuous* means "not very noticeable," so it's actually an antonym. Choice (C) is incorrect because *ascribable* means "able to be attributed to something" or "able to assign a quality or characteristic to someone." Choice (D) is incorrect because *candid* means "frank, outspoken, open, unreserved."

51. **The correct answer is (D).** To *manifest* interest is to show, that is, to *display*, interest. Choice (A) is incorrect because *conceal* is an antonym for *manifest*. Choice (B) is incorrect because to *diminish* is to lessen. Choice (C) is incorrect because to *augment* is to add.

52. **The correct answer is (D).** *Banter* is good-natured teasing, which is also what *raillery* is. Choice (A) is incorrect because *discourse* is conversation. Choices (B) and (D) are incorrect because *singing* and *toasting* are not synonyms for *banter*.

53. **The correct answer is (B).** *Aesthetic* means "artistic" as well as "characterized by an appreciation of beauty." Choices (A) and (C) are incorrect because neither *practical* nor *monetary* relate to *aesthetic*. Choice (D) is incorrect because *estimable* means "admirable."

54. **The correct answer is (B).** *Apostasy* means "abandoning one's faith, political party, or similar loyalty," so *defection*, meaning "abandonment of principles, duty, and the like," is a synonym. Choice (A) is incorrect because *defiance* means "boldly resisting." Choice (C) is incorrect because *belief* is what an apostate abandons, not the act of abandonment. Choice (D) is incorrect because an *inference* is "a conclusion reached by interpreting information."

55. **The correct answer is (B).** *Cryptic* means "having a hidden meaning," in other words, *mysterious.* Choice (A) is incorrect because *cynical* means "believing the worst of people, distrustful." Choice (C) is incorrect because *critical* is not related to *cryptic.* Choice (D) is incorrect because *censorious* means "highly critical, fault finding" and is a synonym for *critical,* but not *cryptic.*

56. **The correct answer is (D).** To *emerge* is "to *appear.*" Choice (A) is incorrect because *deviated* means "to have departed or moved away from the norm or purpose." Choice (B) is incorrect because *divested* means "to have disposed of" or "to have taken something away from someone." Choice (C) is incorrect because *declined* means "to have refused politely."

57. **The correct answer is (B).** *Contumacious* means "disobedient, rebellious," so *rebellious* is a synonym. Choice (A) is incorrect because *exuberant* means "unrestrained, high-spirited." Choices (C) and (D) are incorrect because *awkward* and *mischievous* have no relation to *contumacious.*

58. **The correct answer is (B).** *Cognizant* means "aware" and "having knowledge," so *aware* is a synonym. Choice (A) is incorrect because *ignorant* is the opposite of *cognizant.* Choice (C) is incorrect because *insensitive* has no relation to *cognizant.* Choice (D) is incorrect because *remorseful* means "feeling sorrow or pain for having done something."

59. **The correct answer is (C).** A *glacial* region is one that has a glacier, making it *frigid.* Choice (A) is incorrect because *glass-like* may be tempting, but *frigid* is closer in meaning to *glacial.* Choice (B) is incorrect because *illiberal,* meaning not liberal, has no relation to glacial. Choice (D) is incorrect because *reticent* means "reluctant, unwilling" or "reserved, quiet."

60. **The correct answer is (B).** *Instigate* means the same as *incite,* "to stir up, to urge, to provoke." Choice (A) is incorrect because to *quell* is "to stop, to put down a rebellion." Choice (C) is incorrect because

while *assisted* is close in meaning, *incite* is the same meaning, so it's a better choice. Choice (D) is incorrect because *depressed,* meaning either "gloomy, dejected" or "to press down," doesn't fit as a synonym.

61. **The correct answer is (A).** *Ensued* means "*followed.*" Choice (B) is incorrect because *terminated* means "ended." Choice (C) is incorrect because *was avoided* is the reverse of *ensued.* Choice (D) is incorrect because *culminated* means "ended in" and is a synonym for *terminated,* rather than *ensued.*

62. **The correct answer is (A).** *Retrospect* means "*review,* contemplation of past events." Choice (B) is incorrect because a *concept* is a general idea, usually an abstract idea. Choices (C) and (D), *knowledge* and *awareness,* are incorrect because they have no relation to *retrospect.*

63. **The correct answer is (C).** *Malice* means "*ill will,* desire to harm." Choice (A) is incorrect because *adoration* is the opposite. Choice (B) is incorrect because *sympathy,* meaning "sharing another's feeling or emotions," has no relation to *malice.* Choice (D) is incorrect because *apathy* means "lack of interest, feelings, or emotion,"

64. **The correct answer is (C).** *Saturated* means "*soaked.*" Choice (A) is incorrect because *void of* means "empty of." Choices (B) and (D), *mixed* and *replaced,* are incorrect because neither have any relation to *saturated.*

65. **The correct answer is (D).** *Debilitating* means "draining the strength from, *weakening.*" Choice (A) is incorrect because *invigorating,* meaning "giving energy or strength, making lively," is an antonym. Choice (B) is incorrect because *stimulating* means "exciting or invigorating someone," so it's a synonym for *invigorating* and another antonym for *debilitating.* Choice (C) is incorrect because *tolerable* means "able to be tolerated or endured" and has no relation to *debilitating.*

66. The correct answer is (D). *Servitude* is similar to *bondage* in the sense of forced labor—slavery or serfdom. Choice (A) is incorrect because *freedom* is the opposite. Choice (B) is incorrect because *lethargy* means "slowness, sluggishness" or "being inactive." Choice (C) is incorrect because *vicissitude* means "sudden change in circumstances."

67. The correct answer is (A). *Relish* in this sense means *enjoy*. Choice (B) is incorrect because *dread* means "fear, terror." Choices (C) and (D), *spread* and *implant*, have no relation to *relish*.

68. The correct answer is (D). *Lackadaisical* means "lazy" and "lacking in liveliness," so *indifferent* is a synonym. Choice (A) is incorrect because *enthusiastic* is an antonym. Choice (B) is incorrect because *complacent* means "self-satisfied, pleased with one's self." Choice (C) is incorrect because *profound* means "intense" and "showing great intellectual depth."

69. The correct answer is (B). To *hoist* is "to *raise*." None of the other answers, *cast, prepare,* or *repair,* are synonyms.

70. The correct answer is (A). *Asperse* is "to spread false rumors," and *slander* means "to spread false information." Choice (B) is incorrect because *fathom* means "to understand"; it is also a unit of measurement. Choice (C) is incorrect because *extol* means "to praise greatly," so it's an antonym. Choice (D) is incorrect because *palliate* means "to relieve pain, make pain less intense."

71. The correct answer is (B). *Sordid* means "dirty, filthy," and *wretched* means "miserable, in pitiful circumstances." Of the entries in the list, *wretched* is the nearest in meaning. Choice (A) is incorrect because *bizarre* means "odd, unusual." Choice (C) is incorrect because *primordial* means "fundamental, existing from the beginning." Choice (D) is incorrect because *exaggerated* has no relation to *sordid*.

72. The correct answer is (D). *Alienation* means "*isolation,* a turning away." Choice (A) is incorrect because *agitation* means "being in a state of excitement or worry." Choice (B) is incorrect because *inception* means "the beginning of something." Choice (C) is incorrect because *subsistence* means "means of surviving, the least needed to live on."

73. The correct answer is (A). *Dereliction* of duty is *neglect* of duty. Choice (B) is incorrect because *expansion* may make sense, but is not a synonym. Both choices (C) and (D), *attainment* and *fulfillment,* are antonyms of *dereliction*.

74. The correct answer is (D). *Accede* means "to *agree*." Choices (A, (B), and (C), *attend, refer,* and *adjust,* have no relation to *accede*.

75. The correct answer is (B). *Proximity* means "*nearness*." Choice (A) is incorrect because *worthlessness* has no relation to *proximity*. Choice (C) is incorrect because although *level* makes sense, it is not a synonym. Choice (D) is incorrect because *ebullition* means either "a sudden outburst" or "the process of boiling."

ANTONYMS

The Turnabouts

Thus far, emphasis has been placed on synonyms, or words with similar or identical meanings. You are now ready to increase your word power from a contrasting point of view. Antonyms are words that are opposite in meaning. Some simple examples are: *hot/cold, strong/weak, sit/stand, night/day,* and *lazy/industrious*.

Antonyms are extremely useful to express contrast. The use of certain antonyms can result in the verbal creation of a universal portrait or concept. For instance, everyone associates the name "Scrooge" with *penny-pinching* or *miserly* traits. The Dickens character was anything but philanthropic, a term that characterizes people or agencies who devote themselves to helping and giving to humanity. Therefore, if you read that "a former Scrooge has transformed himself into a philanthropist," you would surmise that the person being described has had a complete change of heart. The term *philanthropist* has been contrasted with a symbol of *miserly* and *penny-pinching* traits.

When taking a test measuring your comprehension of verbal contrasts, be certain to select a response that is the same part of speech as the term in question. Although *discourtesy* and *insolent* share the same shade of meaning, one could not be substituted for the other—the former is a noun and the latter an adjective. Therefore, they could not play identical roles in a sentence.

If you are stumped by any one test item, move on quickly to the next. When you have completed the test, and if time permits, return to any test item(s) you have skipped. Mentally put the various word choices, including the test item, in a sentence. Then remove the test item again.

Example

Polite

    (A) desperate

    (B) discourtesy

    (C) insolent

    (D) discriminate

For the above example, make up a sentence using the word *polite* and then substitute the choices, such as "The boy is *discourtesy*" and "The boy is *insolent*." Obviously, *insolent* is the correct response, as it is the word opposite in meaning to *polite* and best fits the sentence pattern "The boy is . . ."

Using Prefixes

Another helpful technique in taking antonym tests is the close examination of prefixes. Review the etymological information before attempting the sample antonym test, and pay special attention to prefixes. Prefixes can often be the key to contrast in meaning. For example, the prefixes *un, im,* and *in* frequently denote the opposite meaning of the word to which they are affixed: *happy/unhappy; adequate/inadequate; polite/impolite*. These examples make it apparent that the actual meaning of the prefixes is "not." The prefixes *in* and *ex* are opposite in meaning. *In* means, "in," "into," "inside"; and *ex* means "out," "outside of."

If the target word is *internal,* which of the following words would you select as its antonym?

    (A) interior

    (B) ephemeral

    (C) illegal

    (D) external

Of course, *external* is the correct response. Study the list of contrasting prefixes below. Then try your hand at making the "turnabout."

Contrasting Prefixes

ad, ac, ag, at (to)	*ab, a* (away from)
ante (before)	*post* (after)
anti, contra (against)	*pro* (for)
bene (well, good)	*mal* (bad)
corn, con, col (together)	*dis, di* (apart)
con, com (with)	*an* (without)
eu (good)	*dys* (bad)
in, im (in)	*e, ex* (out)
hypo (under)	*hyper* (over)
pro (forward)	*retro* (backward)
sub (under)	*super, sur.* (above)

ANTONYMS TEST ANSWER SHEET

1. Ⓐ Ⓑ Ⓒ Ⓓ	16. Ⓐ Ⓑ Ⓒ Ⓓ	31. Ⓐ Ⓑ Ⓒ Ⓓ	46. Ⓐ Ⓑ Ⓒ Ⓓ	61. Ⓐ Ⓑ Ⓒ Ⓓ
2. Ⓐ Ⓑ Ⓒ Ⓓ	17. Ⓐ Ⓑ Ⓒ Ⓓ	32. Ⓐ Ⓑ Ⓒ Ⓓ	47. Ⓐ Ⓑ Ⓒ Ⓓ	62. Ⓐ Ⓑ Ⓒ Ⓓ
3. Ⓐ Ⓑ Ⓒ Ⓓ	18. Ⓐ Ⓑ Ⓒ Ⓓ	33. Ⓐ Ⓑ Ⓒ Ⓓ	48. Ⓐ Ⓑ Ⓒ Ⓓ	63. Ⓐ Ⓑ Ⓒ Ⓓ
4. Ⓐ Ⓑ Ⓒ Ⓓ	19. Ⓐ Ⓑ Ⓒ Ⓓ	34. Ⓐ Ⓑ Ⓒ Ⓓ	49. Ⓐ Ⓑ Ⓒ Ⓓ	64. Ⓐ Ⓑ Ⓒ Ⓓ
5. Ⓐ Ⓑ Ⓒ Ⓓ	20. Ⓐ Ⓑ Ⓒ Ⓓ	35. Ⓐ Ⓑ Ⓒ Ⓓ	50. Ⓐ Ⓑ Ⓒ Ⓓ	65. Ⓐ Ⓑ Ⓒ Ⓓ
6. Ⓐ Ⓑ Ⓒ Ⓓ	21. Ⓐ Ⓑ Ⓒ Ⓓ	36. Ⓐ Ⓑ Ⓒ Ⓓ	51. Ⓐ Ⓑ Ⓒ Ⓓ	66. Ⓐ Ⓑ Ⓒ Ⓓ
7. Ⓐ Ⓑ Ⓒ Ⓓ	22. Ⓐ Ⓑ Ⓒ Ⓓ	37. Ⓐ Ⓑ Ⓒ Ⓓ	52. Ⓐ Ⓑ Ⓒ Ⓓ	67. Ⓐ Ⓑ Ⓒ Ⓓ
8. Ⓐ Ⓑ Ⓒ Ⓓ	23. Ⓐ Ⓑ Ⓒ Ⓓ	38. Ⓐ Ⓑ Ⓒ Ⓓ	53. Ⓐ Ⓑ Ⓒ Ⓓ	68. Ⓐ Ⓑ Ⓒ Ⓓ
9. Ⓐ Ⓑ Ⓒ Ⓓ	24. Ⓐ Ⓑ Ⓒ Ⓓ	39. Ⓐ Ⓑ Ⓒ Ⓓ	54. Ⓐ Ⓑ Ⓒ Ⓓ	69. Ⓐ Ⓑ Ⓒ Ⓓ
10. Ⓐ Ⓑ Ⓒ Ⓓ	25. Ⓐ Ⓑ Ⓒ Ⓓ	40. Ⓐ Ⓑ Ⓒ Ⓓ	55. Ⓐ Ⓑ Ⓒ Ⓓ	70. Ⓐ Ⓑ Ⓒ Ⓓ
11. Ⓐ Ⓑ Ⓒ Ⓓ	26. Ⓐ Ⓑ Ⓒ Ⓓ	41. Ⓐ Ⓑ Ⓒ Ⓓ	56. Ⓐ Ⓑ Ⓒ Ⓓ	71. Ⓐ Ⓑ Ⓒ Ⓓ
12. Ⓐ Ⓑ Ⓒ Ⓓ	27. Ⓐ Ⓑ Ⓒ Ⓓ	42. Ⓐ Ⓑ Ⓒ Ⓓ	57. Ⓐ Ⓑ Ⓒ Ⓓ	72. Ⓐ Ⓑ Ⓒ Ⓓ
13. Ⓐ Ⓑ Ⓒ Ⓓ	28. Ⓐ Ⓑ Ⓒ Ⓓ	43. Ⓐ Ⓑ Ⓒ Ⓓ	58. Ⓐ Ⓑ Ⓒ Ⓓ	73. Ⓐ Ⓑ Ⓒ Ⓓ
14. Ⓐ Ⓑ Ⓒ Ⓓ	29. Ⓐ Ⓑ Ⓒ Ⓓ	44. Ⓐ Ⓑ Ⓒ Ⓓ	59. Ⓐ Ⓑ Ⓒ Ⓓ	74. Ⓐ Ⓑ Ⓒ Ⓓ
15. Ⓐ Ⓑ Ⓒ Ⓓ	30. Ⓐ Ⓑ Ⓒ Ⓓ	45. Ⓐ Ⓑ Ⓒ Ⓓ	60. Ⓐ Ⓑ Ⓒ Ⓓ	75. Ⓐ Ⓑ Ⓒ Ⓓ

answer sheet

ANTONYMS TEST

75 Questions • 35 Minutes

Directions: For each of the following questions, select the word opposite in meaning to the word printed in capital letters.

1. DEFACE
   (A) defame
   (B) embellish
   (C) vilify
   (D) disfigure

2. SUPERFLUOUS
   (A) coarse
   (B) transient
   (C) insufficient
   (D) abundant

3. ASSUAGE
   (A) presume
   (B) agitate
   (C) alleviate
   (D) absorb

4. AUGURY
   (A) gentility
   (B) relentlessness
   (C) supremacy
   (D) science

5. TERMINATE
   (A) withhold
   (B) construe
   (C) repel
   (D) initiate

6. VITIATE
   (A) liquidate
   (B) revive
   (C) validate
   (D) slander

7. JUBILANT
   (A) lugubrious
   (B) irrepressible
   (C) discernible
   (D) jocular

8. HOSTILE
   (A) affable
   (B) awkward
   (C) judicious
   (D) politic

9. TACITURN
   (A) tactful
   (B) talkative
   (C) crucial
   (D) impetuous

10. LAGGARDLY
    (A) laboriously
    (B) languidly
    (C) briskly
    (D) cowardly

11. PHLEGMATIC
    (A) vital
    (B) apparent
    (C) conversant
    (D) apprehensive

12. LOATHSOME
    (A) alluring
    (B) mournful
    (C) indifferent
    (D) preposterous

13. EXALT
    (A) degrade
    (B) gratify
    (C) expose
    (D) desiderate

14. PACIFY
    (A) conciliate
    (B) palliate
    (C) quell
    (D) exasperate

15. SUBSEQUENT
    (A) worthless
    (B) inactive
    (C) preceding
    (D) demeaning

16. ULTIMATE
    (A) initial
    (B) equitable
    (C) irrefutable
    (D) turbid

17. LEEWAY
    (A) relevance
    (B) restriction
    (C) protection
    (D) satisfaction

18. PRETENTIOUS
    (A) flagrant
    (B) diabolical
    (C) officious
    (D) modest

19. QUANDARY
    (A) certainty
    (B) mediocrity
    (C) ruthlessness
    (D) criterion

20. SAGACIOUS
    (A) obtuse
    (B) scurrilous
    (C) indulgent
    (D) impertinent

21. SAVANT
    (A) uncivilized
    (B) master
    (C) neophyte
    (D) constituent

22. SQUALID
    (A) staunch
    (B) stately
    (C) avaricious
    (D) equivocal

23. EXQUISITE
    (A) exorbitant
    (B) obscure
    (C) extraneous
    (D) ordinary

24. FACILITATE
    (A) falsify
    (B) delude
    (C) hinder
    (D) assimilate

25. FLAWLESS
    (A) pertinent
    (B) conventional
    (C) defective
    (D) complacent

26. RECOMPENSE
    (A) renovate
    (B) embezzle
    (C) retribution
    (D) sanction

27. FERVENT
    (A) nonchalant
    (B) lenient
    (C) meager
    (D) liable

28. AVERT
    (A) pursue
    (B) forestall
    (C) reject
    (D) relinquish

29. ARID
    (A) fragrant
    (B) moist
    (C) parched
    (D) odoriferous

30. IMPERATIVE
    (A) conceptive
    (B) illustrative
    (C) speculative
    (D) optional

31. SUCCINCT
    (A) corporeal
    (B) graphic
    (C) princely
    (D) loquacious

32. JEOPARDY
    (A) security
    (B) discernment
    (C) curiosity
    (D) tedium

33. SOMBER
    (A) insipid
    (B) congruous
    (C) festive
    (D) voluminous

34. EXOTIC
    (A) inveterate
    (B) erotic
    (C) common
    (D) harmonious

35. AFFILIATE
    (A) annihilate
    (B) disassociate
    (C) proffer
    (D) disparage

36. SINISTER
    (A) auspicious
    (B) immaculate
    (C) fanatical
    (D) transitory

37. INEXTRICABLE
    (A) intricate
    (B) judicious
    (C) disentangled
    (D) desperate

38. PROFLIGATE
    (A) insolvent
    (B) virtuous
    (C) redundant
    (D) incessant

39. TURBULENT
    (A) diaphanous
    (B) tranquil
    (C) formidable
    (D) diffident

40. UNWARRANTED
    (A) justifiable
    (B) baneful
    (C) depleted
    (D) contemplated

41. PLAINTIVE
    (A) embellished
    (B) poignant
    (C) rational
    (D) gleeful

42. ORNATE
    (A) unadorned
    (B) deft
    (C) subtle
    (D) conspicuous

43. ABROGATE
    (A) ratify
    (B) reconcile
    (C) abridge
    (D) alleviate

44. ABASE
    (A) cede
    (B) dignify
    (C) repudiate
    (D) engulf

45. RENOUNCE
    (A) claim
    (B) deride
    (C) conceive
    (D) alienate

46. SABOTAGE
    (A) compensate
    (B) reinforce
    (C) restrain
    (D) release

47. OBLIVIOUS
    (A) latent
    (B) integrant
    (C) repugnant
    (D) cognizant

48. SUBMISSIVE
    (A) offensive
    (B) tactless
    (C) incompliant
    (D) manifest

49. NURTURE
    (A) distinguish
    (B) impart
    (C) neglect
    (D) disclose

50. PRUDENCE
    (A) compunction
    (B) dilemma
    (C) anticipation
    (D) recklessness

51. LAMENT
    (A) rejoice
    (B) acclaim
    (C) surmise
    (D) deceive

52. GRUELING
    (A) relaxing
    (B) satisfying
    (C) taming
    (D) suppressing

53. TRIVIAL
    (A) nugatory
    (B) ungainly
    (C) critical
    (D) solicitous

54. ZENITH
    (A) vitality
    (B) rage
    (C) reverence
    (D) nadir

55. UNOBTRUSIVE
    (A) rcsonant
    (B) prominent
    (C) controlled
    (D) subjective

56. REFRACTIVE
    (A) cryptic
    (B) interruptive
    (C) applicable
    (D) direct

57. REBUFF
    (A) exclusion
    (B) disturbance
    (C) recall
    (D) encouragement

58. ADVERSARY
    (A) opponent
    (B) administrator
    (C) accomplice
    (D) enemy

59. OPTIMIST
    (A) rival
    (B) pessimist
    (C) analyst
    (D) protagonist

60. PERVASIVE
    (A) limited
    (B) universal
    (C) ubiquitous
    (D) common

61. ERUDITE
    (A) contagious
    (B) inadvertent
    (C) benevolent
    (D) ignorant

62. PARAMOUNT
    (A) admissible
    (B) inconsequential
    (C) tolerable
    (D) supreme

63. SURREPTITIOUS
    (A) authoritative
    (B) candid
    (C) vulnerable
    (D) subjugated

64. MENDACIOUS
    (A) meddlesome
    (B) incomparable
    (C) malicious
    (D) creditable

65. UNCTUOUS
    (A) awkward
    (B) dubious
    (C) furtive
    (D) disputable

66. IMPETUOUS
    (A) subdued
    (B) unmitigated
    (C) substantial
    (D) egregious

67. PENURIOUS
    (A) frugal
    (B) extravagant
    (C) plausible
    (D) absurd

68. ODIOUS
    (A) attentive
    (B) considerate
    (C) acceptable
    (D) unascertained

69. OSTENSIBLE
    (A) hidden
    (B) preliminary
    (C) authentic
    (D) unsuitable

70. DELETERIOUS
    (A) distressing
    (B) beneficial
    (C) grievous
    (D) delirious

71. IGNOMINY
    (A) honor
    (B) aversion
    (C) perplexity
    (D) remoteness

72. COMPATIBLE
    (A) dexterous
    (B) culminating
    (C) incongruous
    (D) captivating

73. PREMEDITATED
    (A) devoted
    (B) condescending
    (C) improvised
    (D) supposed

74. PERNICIOUS
    (A) restorative
    (B) conclusive
    (C) tractable
    (D) capricious

75. UMBRAGE
    (A) pique
    (B) monstrous
    (C) reliance
    (D) amity

STOP

IF YOU FINISH BEFORE TIME IS CALLED, YOU MAY CHECK YOUR WORK ON THIS SECTION ONLY. DO NOT TURN TO ANY OTHER SECTION IN THE TEST.

ANSWER KEY AND EXPLANATIONS

1. B	16. A	31. D	46. B	61. D
2. C	17. B	32. A	47. D	62. B
3. B	18. D	33. C	48. C	63. B
4. D	19. A	34. C	49. C	64. D
5. D	20. A	35. B	50. D	65. A
6. C	21. C	36. A	51. A	66. A
7. A	22. B	37. C	52. A	67. B
8. A	23. D	38. B	53. C	68. C
9. B	24. C	39. B	54. D	69. A
10. C	25. C	40. A	55. B	70. B
11. A	26. B	41. D	56. D	71. A
12. A	27. A	42. A	57. D	72. C
13. A	28. A	43. A	58. C	73. C
14. D	29. B	44. B	59. B	74. A
15. C	30. D	45. A	60. A	75. D

1. **The correct answer is (B).** *Deface* means "to *disfigure*," so that makes choice (D) a synonym, not an antonym. Choice (B), *embellish*, means "to decorate, to beautify," so it's the antonym. Choice (A) is incorrect because *defame* means "to attack the reputation of someone, to accuse a person falsely with the intent to damage his or her good name." Choice (C) is incorrect because *vilify* means "to make vicious statements about someone, to degrade," which is similar to *defame*.

2. **The correct answer is (C).** *Superfluous* means "more than enough, *abundant*," so choice (D) is incorrect because it's a synonym. However, choice (C) is correct because *insufficient* is the opposite of *superfluous*. Choice (A) is incorrect because *coarse* has no relation to *superfluous*. Choice (B) is incorrect because *transient* means "for a short time" or "a person who

moves around a lot, who stays for just a short time."

3. **The correct answer is (B).** To *assuage* is "to soothe, to relieve," so *agitate*, meaning "to excite," is its opposite. Choice (A) is incorrect because *presume* is "to take something for granted" or "to take something as true without evidence." Choice (C) is incorrect because *alleviate* is similar in meaning to *assuage,* rather than being an antonym. Choice (D) is incorrect because *absorb* means "to soak up," "to occupy one's interest or attention," or "to take in, assimilate," none of which are antonyms for *assuage.*

4. **The correct answer is (D).** *Augury* is foretelling the future by means of signs. It is an art, not a *science*. Choice (A) is incorrect because *gentility* means "refinement, fine manners." Choice (B) is incorrect because *relentlessness*, meaning "never giving up,

being persistent," has no relation to *augury*, and neither does choice (C), *supremacy*, meaning "supreme power or authority."

5. **The correct answer is (D).** *Terminate* means "to end," so its antonym is *initiate*, meaning "to begin." Choice (A) is incorrect because *withhold* has no relation to *terminate*. Choice (B) is incorrect because *construe* means "to interpret, to make sense of." Choice (C) is incorrect because *repel* means "to force back," "to fight against," and "to reject."

6. **The correct answer is (C).** *Vitiate* means "to corrupt," "to undermine," and "to destroy the legal force of something," so its antonym is *validate*, meaning "to declare legally valid." Choice (A) is incorrect because *liquidate* means "to pay off as debts" and "to end business operations." Choice (B) is incorrect because *revive* means "to bring back to life" and "to restore to use." Choice (D) is incorrect because *slander* means "to spread false information."

7. **The correct answer is (A).** A *jubilant* person is an *irrepressible* person, so choice (B) is incorrect. *Irrepressible* means "impossible to control" in a happy, ebullient way, so it's a synonym of *jubilant*. Choice (A) is correct because a *lugubrious* person is a dismal, gloomy person, the opposite of *jubilant*. Choice (C) is incorrect because *discernible* means "able to be perceived, obvious." Choice (D) is incorrect because *jocular* means "joking."

8. **The correct answer is (A).** The opposite of *hostile* in this list is *affable*, meaning "pleasant, easy." Choice (B) is incorrect because *awkward* has no relation to *hostile*, and neither does choice (C), *judicious*, meaning "having good judgement." Choice (D) is incorrect because *politic* means "showing shrewdness or cunning" and "judicious," making it a synonym of *judicious*, but not an antonym of *hostile*.

9. **The correct answer is (B).** *Taciturn* means "not talkative by nature," so *talkative* is an antonym. Choice (A) is incorrect because *tactful* means "showing concern in deal-

ing with others, diplomatic, thoughtful." Choice (C) is incorrect because *crucial* means "very important." Choice (D) is incorrect because *impetuous* means "impulsive, lacking in thought, hasty."

10. **The correct answer is (C).** *Laggardly* means "hanging back, lingering," whereas *briskly* is the opposite. Choice (A) is incorrect because *laboriously* means "hard working, industrious." Choice (B) is incorrect because *languidly* means "listlessly" or "lacking energy." Choice (D) is incorrect because *cowardly* has no relation to *laggardly*.

11. **The correct answer is (A).** *Phlegmatic* means "calm, showing little emotion," whereas *vital* means "full of life, lively" in this case. Choice (B) is incorrect because *apparent* has no relation to *phlegmatic*. Choice (C) is incorrect because *conversant* means "knowledgeable, skilled in, familiar with." Choice (D) is incorrect because *apprehensive* means "anxious, fearful."

12. **The correct answer is (A).** *Loathsome* means "hateful, disgusting, revolting," so *alluring*, meaning "attractive" or "fascinating," is its opposite. Choices (B) and (C) are incorrect because *mournful*, meaning "sad," and *indifferent*, have no relation to *loathsome*. Choice (D) is incorrect because *preposterous* means "absurd, ridiculous."

13. **The correct answer is (A).** *Exalt* means "to glorify, to praise," or "to raise in rank or status," so *degrade*, which means "to reduce in rank or status or "to dishonor or disgrace," is an antonym. Choice (B) is incorrect because *gratify* means "to please or satisfy." Choice (C) is incorrect because *expose* has no relation to *exalt*. Choice (D) is incorrect because *desiderate* means "to wish for" or "to miss."

14. **The correct answer is (D).** *Pacify* means "to calm" or "in military terms to restore peace or order," so *exasperate*, meaning "to make angry," is an antonym. Choice (A) is incorrect because *conciliate* means "to reconcile" or "to overcome distrust" and is close in meaning to *pacify*. Choice

(B) is incorrect because *palliate* means "to make something less serious" or "to lessen physical pain." Choice (C) is incorrect because *quell* means "to pacify" or "to suppress or put down something like a riot," so it's a synonym, not an antonym.

15. **The correct answer is (C).** *Subsequent* means "following in order, succeeding," so *preceding*, meaning "previous," is an antonym. Choices (A) and (B) are incorrect because *worthless* and *inactive* have no relation to *subsequent*. Choice (D) is incorrect because *demeaning* means "lacking in honor or integrity" or "humiliating or shaming one's self."

16. **The correct answer is (A).** *Ultimate* means "last or final in a series" as well as "most significant," so *initial* is an antonym. Choice (B) is incorrect because *equitable* means "fair, just." Choice (C) is incorrect because *irrefutable* means "impossible to deny." Choice (D) is incorrect because *turbid* means "muddy."

17. **The correct answer is (B).** *Leeway* means "amount of freedom of movement, both physical and abstract, margin of error," so *restriction* is an antonym. Choice (A) is incorrect because *relevance* means "connection or relation to something." Choices (C) and (D) are incorrect because *protection* and *satisfaction* have no relation to *leeway*.

18. **The correct answer is (D).** *Pretentious* means "trying to be something that one isn't, claiming a distinction or importance that is not deserved," whereas *modest* is the opposite. Choice (A) is incorrect because *flagrant* means "outrageous, shocking." Choice (B) is incorrect because *diabolical* means "evil." Choice (C) is incorrect because *officious* means "unnecessarily or excessively eager" or "intruding in an offensive way."

19. **The correct answer is (A).** A *quandary* is something difficult to get out of, in other words, a predicament, but it can also be a state of uncertainty, so *certainty* is an antonym. Choice (B) is incorrect because

mediocrity means "ordinary, moderate to inferior." Choice (C) is incorrect because *ruthlessness* has no relation to *quandary*. Choice (D) is incorrect because a *criterion* is a standard or rule by which something is judged.

20. **The correct answer is (A).** A *sagacious* person is a wise person, and an *obtuse* person is one who is dull, slow, or stupid, sometimes deliberately. Choice (B) is incorrect because *scurrilous* means "using vulgar or abusive language." Choice (C) is incorrect because *indulgent* means "lenient, giving in to someone's wishes," or "easygoing." Choice (D) is incorrect because *impertinent* means "rude."

21. **The correct answer is (C).** A *savant* is a person of great learning, so a *neophyte,* one who is new to something, is an antonym. Choice (A) might tempt you, but *uncivilized* is an adjective and *savant* is a noun, so you can rule out *uncivilized* immediately. Choice (B) is incorrect because *master* is a near synonym of *savant*. Choice (D) is incorrect because *constituent,* meaning "a person represented by an elected official," has no relation to *savant*.

22. **The correct answer is (B).** A *squalid* place is filthy, often because of extreme poverty, so a *stately* place is its opposite. *Stately* means "impressive, large, and orderly in appearance." Choice (A) is incorrect because *staunch* means "dependable, loyal." Choice (C) is incorrect because *avaricious* means "greedy." Choice (D) is incorrect because *equivocal* means "doubtful" or "deliberately vague."

23. **The correct answer is (D).** *Exquisite,* meaning "unusually fine and delicate in design" as well as "very beautiful," and *ordinary* are opposites. Choice (A) is incorrect because *exorbitant* means "very expensive." Choice (B) is incorrect because *obscure* means "unclear, vague" or "hidden, secret." Choice (C) is incorrect because *extraneous* means "unnecessary, irrelevant."

24. **The correct answer is (C).** To *facilitate* is "to make easier" or "to be of use," so *hinder,* or "to get in the way of," is an antonym. Choice (A) is incorrect because *falsify* means "to misrepresent, to make a false statement." Choice (B) is incorrect because *delude* means "to mislead, to deceive." Choice (D) is incorrect because *assimilate* is "to incorporate."

25. **The correct answer is (C).** *Flawless* means "having no flaws or imperfections," whereas *defective* is the condition of having flaws or defects, that is, being faulty in some way. Choice (A) is incorrect because *pertinent* means "relevant." Choice (B) is incorrect because *conventional* means "generally agreed on," or "following accepted practice." Choice (D) is incorrect because *complacent* means "self-satisfied, pleased with one's self."

26. **The correct answer is (B).** To *recompense* someone is "to pay someone, to compensate a person" or "the payment itself." To *embezzle* is "to steal from someone," so choice (B) is an antonym. Choice (A) is incorrect because *renovate* is "to restore of good condition, to repair." Choice (C) is incorrect because *retribution* means "something given or demanded in payment"; it's a synonym for *recompense* used as a noun. Choice (D) is incorrect because a *sanction* is "authorization to do something" or "a penalty or punishment."

27. **The correct answer is (A).** *Fervent* means "showing great emotion," whereas *nonchalant* means "indifferent, unconcerned." Choice (B) is incorrect because *lenient* means "generous, not harsh." Choice (C) is incorrect because *meager* means "very little, stingy." Choice (D) is incorrect because *liable* means "legally responsible" or "likely, probable."

28. **The correct answer is (A).** To *avert* is "to prevent from happening," whereas to *pursue* is "to seek to do or get something." Choice (B) is incorrect because *forestall* is "to delay, hinder, or prevent," so it's a synonym, not an antonym. Choice (C) is incorrect because *reject* has no relation to

avert, and neither does *relinquish,* choice (D), meaning "to give up" or "surrender."

29. **The correct answer is (B).** Something that is *arid* is very dry, so *moist* is an antonym. Choice (A) is incorrect because *fragrant* has no relation to *arid,* and neither does choice (D), *odoriferous,* meaning "having an odor." Choice (C) is incorrect because *parched* is a synonym for *arid.*

30. **The correct answer is (D).** *Imperative* means "very urgent"; a person must do what is being ordered. On the other hand, *optional* indicates something that may or not be done; it's up to the person to decide. Choice (A) is incorrect because *conceptive* means "capable of conceiving." Choice (B) is incorrect because *illustrative* is "something used as an example." Choice (C) is incorrect because *speculative* means "not financially safe" or "not based on evidence."

31. **The correct answer is (D).** *Succinct* means "brief, concise," whereas *loquacious,* meaning "very wordy," is the opposite. Choice (A) is incorrect because *corporeal* means "of the body" or "something that is tangible, can be touched." Choice (B) is incorrect because *graphic* means "something described in great and vivid detail" or "relating to a representation, either written or pictorial." Choice (C) is incorrect because *princely* has no relation to *succinct.*

32. **The correct answer is (A).** *Jeopardy* means "in danger of injury, death, risk, loss, damage," so *security* is the opposite. Choice (B) is incorrect because *discernment* means "evidence of keen judgement or interest." Choice (C) is incorrect because *curiosity* has no relation to *jeopardy.* Choice (D) is incorrect because *tedium* means "boredom, monotony."

33. **The correct answer is (C).** *Somber* means "dark, gloomy" or "melancholy, grave," so *festive* is an antonym. Choice (A) is incorrect because *insipid* means "lacking in flavor" or "lacking in anything that excites or stimulates." Choice (B) is incorrect

because *congruous* means "appropriate, in harmony with, suitable." Choice (D) is incorrect because *voluminous* means "large in size, fullness, or number."

34. **The correct answer is (C).** *Exotic* means "foreign" or "very unusual, strange or bizarre beauty," so *common* is an antonym. Choice (A) is incorrect because *inveterate* means "deep-seated" or "habitual." Choice (B) is incorrect because *erotic* means "of or concerning sexual desire." Choice (D) is incorrect because *harmonious,* being in agreement, has no relation to *exotic.*

35. **The correct answer is (B).** To *affiliate* is "to associate or join with," so *disassociate* is an antonym. Choice (A) is incorrect because *annihilate* is to "kill all, to destroy." Choice (C) is incorrect because *proffer* is "to offer or propose something for acceptance or rejection." Choice (D) is incorrect because *disparage* is "to speak disrespectfully or in a belittling way about something or someone."

36. **The correct answer is (A).** *Sinister* means "evil, treacherous" or "ominous, foretelling harm," so *auspicious*, meaning "foretelling favorable conditions," is an antonym. Choice (B) is incorrect because *immaculate* means "spotless." Choice (C) is incorrect because *fanatical* means "beyond normal enthusiasm, intense devotion to something or someone." Choice (D) is incorrect because *transitory* means "temporary, lasting only a short time."

37. **The correct answer is (C).** *Inextricable* means "not able to untangle or escape from," so *disentangle* is an antonym. Choice (A) is incorrect because *intricate* means "complex, elaborate." Choice (B) is incorrect because *judicious* means "having good judgement, being prudent." Choice (D) is incorrect because *desperate* has no relation to *inextricable.*

38. **The correct answer is (B).** *Profligate* means "shamelessly immoral" or "extremely wasteful," and *virtuous* is the opposite. Choice (A) is incorrect because *insolvent* means "bankrupt, unable to pay one's debts," which is what a profligate person may be, but it's not an antonym. Choice (C) is incorrect because *redundant* means "more than is needed or required" or "repetitive." Choice (D) is incorrect because *incessant* means "having no interruption, continual."

39. **The correct answer is (B).** *Turbulent* and *tranquil* are opposites, unrest and disorder versus calm. Choice (A) is incorrect because *diaphanous* means "transparent, flimsy." Choice (C) is incorrect because *formidable* means "inspiring awe or admiration" or "arousing fear or dread." Choice (D) is incorrect because *diffident* means "timid, shy" or "reserved, modest."

40. **The correct answer is (A).** *Unwarranted* means "lacking authorization or justification," so *justifiable* is an antonym. Choice (B) is incorrect because *baneful* means "very harmful." Choice (C) is incorrect because *depleted* means "drained, used up, no longer sufficient." Choice (D) is incorrect because *contemplated* means "thought about, considered."

41. **The correct answer is (D).** *Plaintive* means "mournful" or "sorrowful," so *gleeful* is an antonym. Choice (A) is incorrect because *embellished* means "made more interesting or beautiful by adding decoration." Choice (B) is incorrect because *poignant* means "very moving or touching, at times causing painful feelings." Choice (C) is incorrect because *rational* has no relation to *plaintive.*

42. **The correct answer is (A).** Something that is *ornate* is highly decorated or adorned, so something that is *unadorned* is the opposite. Choice (B) is incorrect because *deft* means "skillful, expert." Choice (C) is incorrect because *subtle* means "not immediately obvious" or "the ability to perceive small differences." Choice (D) is incorrect because *conspicuous* means "obvious, easy to see," so it is an antonym for *subtle*, but not for *ornate.*

43. **The correct answer is (A).** To *abrogate* is "to do away with, revoke, cancel," so

ratify, to approve, is an antonym. Choice (B) is incorrect because *reconcile* means "to settle or resolve." Choice (C) is incorrect because *abridge* is "to cut short" or "reduce the length of a written work by rewriting." Choice (D) is incorrect because *alleviate* is "to relieve, lessen, especially pain."

44. **The correct answer is (B).** *Abase* means "to belittle, humiliate," so *dignify* is an antonym. Choice (A) is incorrect because *cede* means "to surrender, relinquish." Choice (C) is incorrect because *repudiate* means "to reject, refuse to acknowledge someone or something as legitimate or valid." Choice (D) is incorrect because *engulf* means "to overwhelm."

45. **The correct answer is (A).** To *renounce* is "to give up" or "to reject," whereas to *claim* is the opposite. Choice (B) is incorrect because *deride* is "to ridicule, to treat or speak about with contempt." Choice (C) is incorrect because *conceive* has no relation to *renounce*. Choice (D) is incorrect because *alienate* is "to arouse indifference or hostility in a former friend."

46. **The correct answer is (B).** To *sabotage* is "to destroy, to damage," whereas to *reinforce* is "to strengthen or give more support to." Choice (A) is incorrect because *compensate* is "to pay for." Choice (C) is incorrect because *restrain* is "to hold back, to control" or "to limit." Choice (D) is incorrect because *release* has no relation to *sabotage*.

47. **The correct answer is (D).** *Oblivious* means "forgetful, unaware," so *cognizant*, meaning "aware" or "having knowledge of," is the opposite. Choice (A) is incorrect because *latent* means "not obvious, concealed." Choice (B) is incorrect because *integrant* means "part of a whole, that is, integral." Choice (C) is incorrect because *repugnant* means "offensive, distasteful."

48. **The correct answer is (C).** *Submissive* means "willing to submit to another's wishes, obedient, passive," whereas *incompliant* means "not willing to comply or yield." Choices (A) and (B), *offensive* and *tactless*, are incorrect because they have no relation to *submissive*. Choice (D) is incorrect because *manifest* means "very apparent, obvious."

49. **The correct answer is (C).** To *nurture* is "to help grow" or "to help raise," whereas to *neglect* is an antonym. Choice (A) is incorrect because *distinguish* is "to notice as different" or "to see, to perceive." Choice (B) is incorrect because *impart* is "to communicate" or "to give." Choice (D) is incorrect because *disclose* has no relation to *nurture*.

50. **The correct answer is (D).** *Prudence* is discretion or caution, whereas *recklessness* is the lack of prudence and, thus, an antonym. Choice (A) is incorrect because *compunction* means "feeling of remorse or guilt." Choice (B) is incorrect because a *dilemma* may require prudence, but it is neither a synonym nor an antonym for *prudence*. Choice (C) is incorrect because *anticipation* has no relation to *prudence*.

51. **The correct answer is (A).** To *lament* is "to express grief, to mourn," so to *rejoice* is its opposite. Choice (B) is incorrect because *acclaim* is "to honor or praise." Choice (C) is incorrect because *surmise* is "to guess" or "to infer." Choice (D) is incorrect because *deceive* has no relation to *lament*.

52. **The correct answer is (A).** *Grueling* means "activity to the point of exhaustion," whereas *relaxing* is its opposite. Choices (B) and (C) are incorrect because *satisfying* has no relation to *grueling* or *taming*. Choice (D) is incorrect because *suppressing* means "putting an end to, often by force" or "restraining."

53. **The correct answer is (C).** *Trivial*, meaning "of little significance," and *critical*, meaning "essential," are antonyms. Choice (A) is incorrect because *nugatory* is a synonym for *trivial*. Choice (B) is incorrect because *ungainly* means "awkward." Choice (D) is incorrect because *solicitous*

means "anxious, concerned, showing anxiety or concern for someone."

54. **The correct answer is (D).** The *zenith* is the highest point, the peak of something such as a career, whereas the *nadir* is the lowest point. Choice (A) is incorrect because *vitality*, meaning "liveliness, full of life," has no relation to *zenith*. Choice (B) is incorrect because *rage* has no relation to *zenith*, nor does choice (C), *reverence*.

55. **The correct answer is (B).** *Unobtrusive* means "not noticeable, not easily seen," so the opposite is *prominent*, meaning "immediately noticeable, conspicuous." Choice (A) is incorrect because *resonant* means "bringing to mind, reminiscent" as well as "producing a deep, full sound." Choice (C) is incorrect because *controlled* has no relation to *unobtrusive*, nor does choice (D), *subjective*.

56. **The correct answer is (D).** *Refractive* means "capable of changing or bending the direction of light or sound," so *direct* is an antonym. Choice (A) is incorrect because *cryptic* means "hidden, secret." Choice (B) is incorrect because *interruptive* is not an antonym for *refractive*, nor does choice (C), *applicable*.

57. **The correct answer is (D).** A *rebuff* is a refusal or rejection, so *encouragement* is an antonym. Choice (A) is incorrect because *exclusion* means "a deliberate omission." Choices (B) and (C) are incorrect because *disturbance* and *recall* have no relation to *rebuff*.

58. **The correct answer is (C).** An *adversary* is an *opponent* and so is an *enemy,* so choices (A) and (D) are incorrect. Choice (C) is correct because an *accomplice* aids someone in committing a crime. Choice (B) is incorrect because *administrator* has no relation to an adversary.

59. **The correct answer is (B).** An *optimist* is a person who sees things in a favorable way, in other words, who believes that good things will happen, whereas a *pessimist* is just the opposite. Choices (A), (C), and (D) are all incorrect because a *rival* has no relation to an *optimist*, an *analyst*, or a *protagonist*. The last is the main character in a play or work of fiction or nonfiction.

60. **The correct answer is (A).** *Pervasive* means "widespread," so *limited* is an antonym. Choices (B) and (C) are incorrect because both *universal* and *ubiquitous* are synonyms for *pervasive*. Choice (D) is incorrect because *common* may also be a synonym for *pervasive*.

61. **The correct answer is (D).** *Erudite* means "learned, educated," so *ignorant* is an antonym. Choice (A) is incorrect because *contagious* has no relation to being educated or not. Choice (B) is incorrect because *inadvertent* means "not deliberate, occurring by chance." Choice (C) is incorrect because *benevolent* means "generous in helping others, showing kindness."

62. **The correct answer is (B).** *Paramount* means "of greatest importance, most significant," whereas *inconsequential* is the opposite. Choice (A) is incorrect because *admissible* means "something that can be allowed or accepted." Choice (C) is incorrect because *tolerable*, able to be tolerated or endured, has no relation to *paramount*. Choice (D) is incorrect because *supreme* is a synonym for *paramount*.

63. **The correct answer is (B).** *Surreptitious* means "secretive, done in secret or through improper means," so *candid*, meaning "frank, outspoken, open, unreserved," is an antonym. Choice (A) is incorrect because *authoritative* means "official" or "being true or reliable." Choice (C) is incorrect because *vulnerable* has no relation to *surreptitious*. Choice (D) is incorrect because *subjugated* means "conquered, under control."

64. **The correct answer is (D).** *Mendacious* means "untruthful, lying," whereas *creditable*, meaning "admirable, praiseworthy, honorable," is an antonym. Choice (A) is incorrect because *meddlesome* means "interfering." Choice (B) is incorrect because *incomparable* means "unequalled,

above comparison, unsurpassed." Choice (C) is incorrect because *malicious* means "spiteful, bitter, vicious."

65. **The correct answer is (A).** An *unctuous* person is one who has a slick charm or ease and suavity about him or her, whereas an *awkward* person is the opposite—clumsy, embarrassed, not elegant. Choice (B) is incorrect because *dubious* means "doubtful." Choice (C) is incorrect because *furtive* means "secretive, surreptitious." Choice (D) is incorrect because something that is *disputable* is something that can be argued over.

66. **The correct answer is (A).** An *impetuous* person is one who is impulsive, so a *subdued* person is the opposite—under control, quiet, passive. Choice (B) is incorrect because *unmitigated* means "not diminished, still severe or harsh." Choice (C) is incorrect because *substantial* has no relation to *impetuous*. Choice (D) is incorrect because *egregious* means "extremely bad, outrageously bad."

67. **The correct answer is (B).** *Penurious* means "stingy" and also "destitute, unable to buy basic necessities," whereas *extravagant* is the opposite. Choice (A) is incorrect because *frugal* means "thrifty, not spending much" and is a near synonym for one meaning of *penurious*. Choice (C) is incorrect because *plausible* means "likely, seemingly valid or truthful." Choice (D) is incorrect because *absurd* has no relation to *penurious*.

68. **The correct answer is (C).** *Odious* means "arousing strong dislike," so *acceptable* is an antonym. Choice (A) is incorrect because *attentive* has no relation to *odious*, and neither does Choice (B), *considerate*. Choice (D) is incorrect because *unascertained* means "not capable of being found out or decided."

69. **The correct answer is (A).** *Ostensible* means "apparent, seeming," so its antonym is *hidden*. Choice (B) is incorrect because *preliminary* means "happening before something else." Choice (C) is incorrect

because *authentic* means "real, genuine." Choice (D) is incorrect because *unsuitable* has no relation to *ostensible*.

70. **The correct answer is (B).** *Deleterious* means "injurious, harmful," whereas *beneficial* is the opposite. Choice (A) is incorrect because although a *deleterious* action may be *distressing*, the words are neither synonyms nor antonyms. Choice (C) is incorrect because *grievous* means "serious" or "causing great pain or suffering" and could be considered a near synonym for *deleterious*. Choice (D) is incorrect because *delirious* means "suffering from delirium, which affects mental functions."

71. **The correct answer is (A).** *Ignominy* means "public shame or humiliation," so *honor* is an antonym. Choice (B) is incorrect because *aversion* means "extreme dislike." Choice (C) is incorrect because *perplexity* means "puzzlement, confusion because of complexity of something or someone." Choice (D) is incorrect because *remoteness* means "distant in time or place" or "standoffishness, having withdrawn."

72. **The correct answer is (C).** To be *compatible* is "to be complementary," whereas to be *incongruous* is "to be incompatible, not in agreement with principles, inconsistent with." Choice (A) is incorrect because *dexterous* means "skillful, either with one's hands or one's mental faculties." Choice (B) is incorrect because *culminating* means "ending in" as well as "reaching the highest point or degree." Choice (D) is incorrect because *captivating* has no relation to *compatible*.

73. **The correct answer is (C).** *Premeditated* means "planned, marked by prior thought," so *improvised*, meaning "invented with little forethought or preparation," is its antonym. Choice (A) is incorrect because *devoted* has no relation to *premeditated*. Choice (B) is incorrect because *condescending* means "patronizing, treating others as though they are social or intellectual inferiors." Choice (D) is incorrect because *supposed* has no relation to *premeditated*.

74. The correct answer is (A). *Pernicious* means "deadly, tending to cause harm or injury," whereas *restorative* means "tending to restore." Choice (B) is incorrect because *conclusive* has no relation to *pernicious*. Choice (C) is incorrect because *tractable* means "easily manageable." Choice (D) is incorrect because *capricious* means "impulsive, unpredictable."

75. The correct answer is (D). *Umbrage* is "offense, resentment," whereas *amity* is "friendship." Choice (A) is incorrect because *pique* is a feeling of resentment and so is a synonym for *umbrage*. Choice (B) is incorrect because *monstrous* has no relation to *umbrage*, nor does choice (C), *reliance*, meaning "dependence."

SKILL WITH VERBAL ANALOGIES

The verbal analogy is one variation of the vocabulary question often encountered on nursing school tests. It tests your understanding of word meanings and your ability to grasp relationships between words and ideas. This practice in mental agility will help you do better with all the other questions on the test.

In addition to their simple meanings, words carry subtle shades of implication that depend in some degree upon the relationship they bear to other words. There are various classifications of relationship, such as similarity (synonyms) and opposition (antonyms). Careful students will try to examine each shade of meaning they encounter.

The ability to detect the exact nature of the relationship between words is a function of your intelligence. In a sense, the verbal analogy test is a vocabulary test. But it is also a test of your ability to analyze meanings, think things out, and see the relationships between ideas and words. In mathematics, this kind of situation is expressed as a proportion problem: 3:5::6:X. Sometimes, verbal analogies are written in this mathematical form:

CLOCK : TIME :: THERMOMETER :
- **(A)** hour
- **(B)** degrees
- **(C)** climate
- **(D)** temperature

Or the question may be put:

CLOCK is to TIME as THERMOMETER is to
- **(A)** hour
- **(B)** degrees
- **(C)** climate
- **(D)** temperature

The challenge is to determine which one of the lettered words has the same relationship to *thermometer* as *time* has to *clock*. The best way to determine the correct answer is to provide a word or phrase that shows the relationship between these words. In the above example, "measures" is a word expressing the relationship. However, this may not be enough. The analogy must be exact. *Climate* or *weather* would not be exact enough. *Temperature,* of course, is the correct answer.

You will find that many of the choices have some relationship to the third word. Select the one with a relationship that *best* approximates the relationship between the first two words.

Three Examples of Verbal Analogy Questions

Some standardized tests provide four answer choices (A,B,C,D) and some, five (A,B,C,D,E).

Example 1

From the four pairs of words that follow, select the pair related in the same way as are the words of the first pair.

SPELLING: PUNCTUATION ::

(A) pajamas : fatigue

(B) powder : shaving

(C) bandage : cut

(D) biology : physics

Spelling and *punctuation* are elements of the mechanics of English; *biology* and *physics* are two of the subjects that make up the field of science. The other choices do not possess this part : part relationship. Therefore, **(D)** is the correct answer.

Example 2

Another popular format gives two words followed by a third word. The latter is related to one word in a group of choices in the same way that the first two words are related.

WINTER : SUMMER :: COLD :

(A) wet

(B) future

(C) hot

(D) freezing

Winter and *summer* bear an opposite relationship. *Cold* and *hot* have the same kind of opposite relationship. Therefore, choice **(C)** is the correct answer.

Example 3

Still another analogy format has a variable construction. Any one of the four relationship elements may not be specified. From choices offered—regardless of position—you are to select the one choice that completes the relationship with the other three items. In this example, the third relationship element is not specified.

SUBMARINE: FISH :: ___ : BIRD

(A) kite

(B) limousine

(C) feather

(D) chirp

Both a *submarine* and a *fish* are usually found in the water; both a *kite* and a *bird* are customarily seen in the air. Consequently, choice **(A)** is the correct answer.

ANALOGY RELATIONSHIPS

1. Purpose Relationship

   GLOVE : BALL ::
   (A) hook : fish
   (B) winter : weather
   (C) game : pennant
   (D) stadium : seats

2. Cause-and-Effect Relationship

   RACE : FATIGUE ::
   (A) track : athlete
   (B) ant : bug
   (C) fast : hunger
   (D) walking : running

3. Part : Whole Relationship

   SNAKE : REPTILE ::
   (A) patch : thread
   (B) removal : snow
   (C) struggle : wrestle
   (D) hand : clock

4. Part : Part Relationship

   GILL : FIN ::
   (A) plasma display : electrodes
   (B) instrument : violin
   (C) sea : fish
   (D) salad : supper

5. Action : Object Relationship

   KICK : FOOTBALL ::
   (A) kill : bomb
   (B) break : pieces
   (C) question : team
   (D) smoke : pipe

6. Object : Action Relationship

   STEAK : BROIL ::
   (A) bread : bake
   (B) food : eat
   (C) pour : wine
   (D) spill : sugar

7. Synonym Relationship

   ENORMOUS : HUGE ::
   (A) rogue : rock
   (B) muddy : unclear
   (C) purse : kitchen
   (D) black : white

8. Antonym Relationship

   PURITY : EVIL ::
   (A) suavity : bluntness
   (B) north : climate
   (C) angel : horns
   (D) boldness : victory

9. Place Relationship

   MIAMI : FLORIDA ::
   (A) Chicago : United States
   (B) New York : Albany
   (C) United States : Chicago
   (D) Albany : New York

10. Degree Relationship

    WARM : HOT ::
    (A) glue : paste
    (B) climate : weather
    (C) fried egg : boiled egg
    (D) bright : genius

11. Characteristic Relationship

   SKILL : PRACTICE ::
   (A) blood : wound
   (B) money : dollar
   (C) schools : elevators
   (D) education : stupidity

12. Sequence Relationship

   SPRING : SUMMER ::
   (A) Thursday : Wednesday
   (B) Wednesday : Monday
   (C) Monday : Sunday
   (D) Wednesday : Thursday

13. Grammatical Relationship

   RESTORE : CLIMB ::
   (A) segregation : seem
   (B) into : nymph
   (C) precipice : although
   (D) overpower : seethe

14. Association Relationship

   DEVIL : WRONG ::
   (A) color : sidewalk
   (B) slipper : state
   (C) ink : writing
   (D) picture : bed

15. Numerical Relationship
   4 : 12 ::
   (A) 10 : 16
   (B) 9 : 27
   (C) 3 : 4
   (D) 12 : 6

ANSWER KEY AND EXPLANATIONS

1. A	4. A	7. B	10. D	13. D
2. C	5. D	8. A	11. A	14. C
3. D	6. A	9. D	12. D	15. B

1. **The correct answer is (A).** In this purpose relationship, a *glove* is used to catch a *ball* and a *hook* is used to catch a *fish*. Choice (B) is incorrect because *winter* is a season, not a type of *weather*. Choice (C) is incorrect because a single *game* is not a way to win a *pennant*, that is, a championship. Choice (D) is incorrect because the purpose of a *stadium* is not to provide *seats*, but to provide a place for events.

2. **The correct answer is (C).** In this cause-and-effect relationship, a person is *fatigued*, that is, tired, after running a *race*. A person is *hungry* as a result of *fasting*, that is, not eating. Choice (A) is incorrect because a *track* doesn't result in an *athlete*. Choice (B) is incorrect because an *ant* is a type of *bug*, or insect; there is no cause-and-effect relationship. Choice (D) is incorrect because *walking* and *running* are both types of activities; there is no cause-and-effect relationship between them.

3. **The correct answer is (D).** In this part-to-whole relationship, a *snake* is one of the category *reptile*, and a *hand* is part of a *clock*. Choice (A) is incorrect because a *patch* is not a type of *thread*. Choice (B) is incorrect because *removal* is not a part of *snow*, though it is a way to get rid of snow. A snowball would be a part of snow. Choice (C) is incorrect because *struggle* is not a part of *wrestle*; wrestle would be a part of sports.

4. **The correct answer is (A).** In this part-to-part relationship, a *gill* and a *fin* are both parts of a fish as a *plasma display* and *electrodes* are both parts of flat screen TVs. Choice (B) is incorrect because a *violin* is an *instrument*, not part of an instrument. Choice (C) is incorrect because a *sea*

is home to many *fish*; it's not a part of something shared with fish. Choice (D) is incorrect because *salad* is part of a *supper*, which is a whole, not a part.

5. **The correct answer is (D).** In this action-to-object relationship, *kicking* is the action and the object that is kicked is a *football*. The action is *smoking* and the object that is smoked is a *pipe*. Choice (A) is incorrect because the action is to *kill*, but the object is not a *bomb*; a bomb is a means to kill; people would be the object. Choice (B) is incorrect because the action is *breaking*, and *pieces* aren't the object, but the result. The object would be something like a plate or bowl. Choice (C) is incorrect because *question* and *team* aren't related. The object for question would be answer.

6. **The correct answer is (A).** This is the reverse of the previous question. *Steak* is what receives the action, *broiling*, in this object-to-action relationship, so the second analogy is *bread*, the object, to *baking*, the action. Choice (B) is incorrect because *food* is the object and *eat* is the action, but the analogy is set up backwards. The same is true for choices (C) and (D), *pour* and *wine*, and *spill* and *sugar*.

7. **The correct answer is (B).** In this synonym relationship, you're looking for the two words that are alike. *Enormous* means the same as *huge*, and *muddy* means the same as *unclear*. Choice (A) is incorrect because *rogue* is a deceitful and unreliable person, which has no relation to *rock*. Choice (C) is incorrect because *purse* and *kitchen* are not synonyms, and neither are *black* and *white*, choice (D).

8. **The correct answer is (A).** This question asks for an antonym pair. *Evil* is the op-

posite of *purity* as *bluntness* is the opposite of *suavity*, meaning "smoothly agreeable, graciously polite." Choice (B) is incorrect because *north* and *climate* have no relation. Choice (C) is incorrect because *angel* and *horns* have no relation; it would have to be *devil* rather than *horns* to be an antonym pair. Choice (D) is incorrect because *boldness* and *victory* have no relation.

9. **The correct answer is (D).** The place relationship is city to state—the city of *Miami* to its state of *Florida*. The only pair that follows this model is the city of *Albany* to its state of *New York*. This makes choice (B) incorrect because here, the relationship is reversed. Choices (A) and (C) are incorrect because the *United States* is not a state.

10. **The correct answer is (D).** *Warm* is a degree of, or step to being, *hot* in this degree relationship. *Bright* is a degree of, or step in being, a *genius*. Choice (A) is incorrect because *glue* and *paste* are comparable materials; there is no degree relationship between them. Choice (B) is incorrect because *climate* is not a degree of *weather*. Choice (C) is incorrect because a *fried egg* and a *boiled egg* have no degree relationship; both are cooked eggs.

11. **The correct answer is (A).** In this characteristic relationship, *skill* is a characteristic gained from *practice*. *Blood* is a characteristic of a *wound*, that is, a wound bleeds. Choice (B) is incorrect because a *dollar* is *money;* it's not a characteristic of money, such as, for example, value and portability. Choice (C) is incorrect because *schools* are not characteristics of *elevators*, though schools may have elevators. Choice (D) is incorrect because *education* is not a characteristic of *stupidity*.

12. **The correct answer is (D).** In this sequence relationship, *summer* follows *spring* and *Wednesday* follows *Thursday*. Choice (A) is incorrect because the sequence is reversed. Choice (B) is incorrect because the sequence is reversed and one day is missing between the days. Choice (C) is incorrect because the sequence is reversed.

13. **The correct answer is (D).** Both words— *restore* and *climb*—are verbs, so you need to find the answer with a pair of verbs. Only choice (D) includes two verbs—*overpower* and *seethe*. Choice (A) is incorrect because *segregation* is a noun and *seem* is a verb. Choice (B) is incorrect because *into* is a preposition and *nymph* is a noun. Choice (C) is incorrect because *precipice* is a noun and *although* is a conjunction.

14. **The correct answer is (C).** In this association relationship, *devil* is to *wrong* as *ink* is to *writing*. Choice (A) is incorrect because a *color* and a *sidewalk* have no relation. Choice (B) is incorrect because a *slipper* and a *state* have no relation. Choice (D) is incorrect because a *picture* and a *bed* have no relation.

15. **The correct answer is (B).** The connection in this numerical relationship is multiplication by 3: $4 \times 3 = 12$ and $9 \times 3 = 27$. Choice (A) is incorrect because $10 \times 3 = 30$, not 16. Choice (C) is incorrect because $3 \times 3 = 9$, not 4. Choice (D) is incorrect because $12 \times 3 = 36$, not 6.

Points to Remember

In many analogy questions, the incorrect choices may be related in some way to the first two words. Don't let this association mislead you. For example, in number four (part : part relationship), choice (A), *tube : antenna* is the correct answer. Choice (C), *sea : fish,* is incorrect, although these two latter words are associated in a general sense with the first two words (*gill : fin*).

Often, the relationship of the first two words may apply to *more than one* of the choices given. In such a case, you must narrow down the initial relationship in order to get the correct choice. For example, in number six (object: action relationship), a *steak* is something that you *broil*. Now let us consider the choices: *bread* is something that you *bake*; *food* is something that you *eat*; *wine* is something that you *pour;* and *sugar* is something that you (can) *spill*. Thus far, each choice seems correct. Let us now narrow down the relationship: a *steak* is something that you *broil* with *heat*. The only choice that fulfills this *complete* relationship is choice (A), *bread*—something that you bake with *heat*. It follows that choice **(A)** is the correct answer.

Remember that the keys to analogy success are:

Step One: Determine the relationship between the first two words.

Step Two: Find the same relationship among the choices that follow the first two words.

VERBAL ANALOGIES TEST ANSWER SHEET

Part A

1. Ⓐ Ⓑ Ⓒ Ⓓ   6. Ⓐ Ⓑ Ⓒ Ⓓ   11. Ⓐ Ⓑ Ⓒ Ⓓ   16. Ⓐ Ⓑ Ⓒ Ⓓ   21. Ⓐ Ⓑ Ⓒ Ⓓ
2. Ⓐ Ⓑ Ⓒ Ⓓ   7. Ⓐ Ⓑ Ⓒ Ⓓ   12. Ⓐ Ⓑ Ⓒ Ⓓ   17. Ⓐ Ⓑ Ⓒ Ⓓ   22. Ⓐ Ⓑ Ⓒ Ⓓ
3. Ⓐ Ⓑ Ⓒ Ⓓ   8. Ⓐ Ⓑ Ⓒ Ⓓ   13. Ⓐ Ⓑ Ⓒ Ⓓ   18. Ⓐ Ⓑ Ⓒ Ⓓ   23. Ⓐ Ⓑ Ⓒ Ⓓ
4. Ⓐ Ⓑ Ⓒ Ⓓ   9. Ⓐ Ⓑ Ⓒ Ⓓ   14. Ⓐ Ⓑ Ⓒ Ⓓ   19. Ⓐ Ⓑ Ⓒ Ⓓ   24. Ⓐ Ⓑ Ⓒ Ⓓ
5. Ⓐ Ⓑ Ⓒ Ⓓ   10. Ⓐ Ⓑ Ⓒ Ⓓ   15. Ⓐ Ⓑ Ⓒ Ⓓ   20. Ⓐ Ⓑ Ⓒ Ⓓ   25. Ⓐ Ⓑ Ⓒ Ⓓ

Part B

1. Ⓐ Ⓑ Ⓒ Ⓓ Ⓔ   6. Ⓐ Ⓑ Ⓒ Ⓓ Ⓔ   11. Ⓐ Ⓑ Ⓒ Ⓓ Ⓔ   16. Ⓐ Ⓑ Ⓒ Ⓓ Ⓔ   21. Ⓐ Ⓑ Ⓒ Ⓓ Ⓔ
2. Ⓐ Ⓑ Ⓒ Ⓓ Ⓔ   7. Ⓐ Ⓑ Ⓒ Ⓓ Ⓔ   12. Ⓐ Ⓑ Ⓒ Ⓓ Ⓔ   17. Ⓐ Ⓑ Ⓒ Ⓓ Ⓔ   22. Ⓐ Ⓑ Ⓒ Ⓓ Ⓔ
3. Ⓐ Ⓑ Ⓒ Ⓓ Ⓔ   8. Ⓐ Ⓑ Ⓒ Ⓓ Ⓔ   13. Ⓐ Ⓑ Ⓒ Ⓓ Ⓔ   18. Ⓐ Ⓑ Ⓒ Ⓓ Ⓔ   23. Ⓐ Ⓑ Ⓒ Ⓓ Ⓔ
4. Ⓐ Ⓑ Ⓒ Ⓓ Ⓔ   9. Ⓐ Ⓑ Ⓒ Ⓓ Ⓔ   14. Ⓐ Ⓑ Ⓒ Ⓓ Ⓔ   19. Ⓐ Ⓑ Ⓒ Ⓓ Ⓔ   24. Ⓐ Ⓑ Ⓒ Ⓓ Ⓔ
5. Ⓐ Ⓑ Ⓒ Ⓓ Ⓔ   10. Ⓐ Ⓑ Ⓒ Ⓓ Ⓔ   15. Ⓐ Ⓑ Ⓒ Ⓓ Ⓔ   20. Ⓐ Ⓑ Ⓒ Ⓓ Ⓔ   25. Ⓐ Ⓑ Ⓒ Ⓓ Ⓔ

Part C

1. Ⓐ Ⓑ Ⓒ Ⓓ Ⓔ   6. Ⓐ Ⓑ Ⓒ Ⓓ Ⓔ   11. Ⓐ Ⓑ Ⓒ Ⓓ Ⓔ   16. Ⓐ Ⓑ Ⓒ Ⓓ Ⓔ   21. Ⓐ Ⓑ Ⓒ Ⓓ Ⓔ
2. Ⓐ Ⓑ Ⓒ Ⓓ Ⓔ   7. Ⓐ Ⓑ Ⓒ Ⓓ Ⓔ   12. Ⓐ Ⓑ Ⓒ Ⓓ Ⓔ   17. Ⓐ Ⓑ Ⓒ Ⓓ Ⓔ   22. Ⓐ Ⓑ Ⓒ Ⓓ Ⓔ
3. Ⓐ Ⓑ Ⓒ Ⓓ Ⓔ   8. Ⓐ Ⓑ Ⓒ Ⓓ Ⓔ   13. Ⓐ Ⓑ Ⓒ Ⓓ Ⓔ   18. Ⓐ Ⓑ Ⓒ Ⓓ Ⓔ   23. Ⓐ Ⓑ Ⓒ Ⓓ Ⓔ
4. Ⓐ Ⓑ Ⓒ Ⓓ Ⓔ   9. Ⓐ Ⓑ Ⓒ Ⓓ Ⓔ   14. Ⓐ Ⓑ Ⓒ Ⓓ Ⓔ   19. Ⓐ Ⓑ Ⓒ Ⓓ Ⓔ   24. Ⓐ Ⓑ Ⓒ Ⓓ Ⓔ
5. Ⓐ Ⓑ Ⓒ Ⓓ Ⓔ   10. Ⓐ Ⓑ Ⓒ Ⓓ Ⓔ   15. Ⓐ Ⓑ Ⓒ Ⓓ Ⓔ   20. Ⓐ Ⓑ Ⓒ Ⓓ Ⓔ   25. Ⓐ Ⓑ Ⓒ Ⓓ Ⓔ

answer sheet

VERBAL ANALOGIES TEST

75 Questions • 30 Minutes

Directions: In the following questions, determine the relationship between the first pair of capitalized words and then decide which of the answer choices shares a similar relationship with the third capitalized word. Parts A and B of this test are written in mathematical form (expressed as proportion problems). Part A's questions have four answer choices, Part B and Part C's questions have five. Part C is written so that relationships are expressed with "is to" and "as."

Part A

25 Questions • 10 Minutes

1. GUN : SHOOTS :: KNIFE :
   (A) run
   (B) cuts
   (C) sharpen
   (D) poke

2. EAR : HEAR :: EYE :
   (A) table
   (B) hand
   (C) see
   (D) foot

3. FUR : MAMMAL :: FEATHERS :
   (A) bird
   (B) neck
   (C) feet
   (D) bill

4. HANDLE : HAMMER :: KNOB :
   (A) key
   (B) room
   (C) shut
   (D) door

5. SHOE : FOOT :: COAT :
   (A) hat
   (B) buttons
   (C) body
   (D) head

6. WATER : DRINK :: BREAD :
   (A) cake
   (B) coffee
   (C) eat
   (D) pie

7. FOOD : HUMAN :: GASOLINE :
   (A) lube
   (B) oil
   (C) automobile
   (D) spark

8. EAT : FAT :: STARVE :
   (A) thin
   (B) food
   (C) bread
   (D) thirsty

9. HUMAN : HOUSE :: BIRD :
   (A) tree
   (B) insect
   (C) limb
   (D) nest

10. GO : COME :: SELL :
    (A) leave
    (B) buy
    (C) money
    (D) pawn

11. PENINSULA : LAND :: BAY
    (A) boat
    (B) inlet
    (C) water
    (D) harbor

12. HOUR : MINUTE :: MINUTE :
    (A) hour
    (B) week
    (C) second
    (D) short

13. ABIDE : DEPART :: STAY :
    (A) over
    (B) home
    (C) play
    (D) leave

14. JANUARY : FEBRUARY :: JUNE :
    (A) July
    (B) May
    (C) month
    (D) year

15. BOLD : TIMID :: ADVANCE :
    (A) proceed
    (B) retreat
    (C) campaign
    (D) soldiers

16. ABOVE : BELOW :: TOP :
    (A) spin
    (B) bottom
    (C) surface
    (D) side

17. LION : ANIMAL :: ROSE :
    (A) smell
    (B) leaf
    (C) plant
    (D) thorn

18. TIGER : CARNIVOROUS :: HORSE :
    (A) cow
    (B) nervous

(C) omnivorous
(D) herbivorous

19. SAILOR : NAVY :: SOLDIER :
    (A) gun
    (B) cap
    (C) hill
    (D) army

20. PICTURE : SEE :: SOUND :
    (A) noise
    (B) music
    (C) hear
    (D) bark

21. SUCCESS : JOY :: FAILURE :
    (A) sadness
    (B) enthusiasm
    (C) fault
    (D) work

22. HOPE : DESPAIR :: HAPPINESS :
    (A) frolic
    (B) fun
    (C) joy
    (D) misery

23. PRETTY : UGLY :: ATTRACT :
    (A) fine
    (B) repel
    (C) nice
    (D) draw

24. PUPIL : TEACHER :: CHILD :
    (A) parent
    (B) doll
    (C) youngster
    (D) obey

25. CITY : MAYOR :: ARMY :
    (A) navy
    (B) soldier
    (C) general
    (D) private

Part B

25 Questions • 10 Minutes

1. REMUNERATIVE : PROFITABLE ::
   FRAUDULENT :
   (A) liar
   (B) slander
   (C) fallacious
   (D) plausible
   (E) reward

2. AX : WOODSMAN :: WRENCH :
   (A) cut
   (B) hew
   (C) technician
   (D) plumber
   (E) cobbler

3. SURGEON : SCALPEL :: BUTCHER :
   (A) mallet
   (B) cleaver
   (C) chisel
   (D) screwdriver
   (E) medicine

4. CAT : FELINE :: HORSE :
   (A) equine
   (B) tiger
   (C) quadruped
   (D) carnivore
   (E) vulpine

5. ADVERSITY : HAPPINESS :: VEHE-
   MENCE :
   (A) misfortune
   (B) gaiety
   (C) troublesome
   (D) petulance
   (E) serenity

6. NECKLACE : ADORNMENT ::
   MEDAL :
   (A) jewel
   (B) metal
   (C) bravery
   (D) bronze
   (E) decoration

7. MINER : SHOVEL :: PIRATE :
   (A) treasure
   (B) sword
   (C) ship
   (D) flag
   (E) gold

8. ARCHAEOLOGIST : ANTIQUITY ::
   ICHTHYOLOGIST :
   (A) theology
   (B) ruins
   (C) horticulture
   (D) marine life
   (E) mystic

9. SHOE : LEATHER :: HIGHWAY :
   (A) passage
   (B) road
   (C) asphalt
   (D) trail
   (E) journey

10. SERFDOM : FEUDALISM :: ENTRE-
    PRENEUR :
    (A) liberal
    (B) captain
    (C) radical
    (D) agriculture
    (E) capitalism

11. FIN : FISH :: PROPELLER :
    (A) wing
    (B) plane
    (C) air
    (D) water
    (E) canoe

12. SATISFIED : SATIETY :: POOR :
    (A) destitute
    (B) subsistence
    (C) sustainable
    (D) lesser
    (E) abandoned

13. SKIN : HUMAN :: HIDE :
    (A) scales
    (B) fur
    (C) animal
    (D) hair
    (E) fish

14. RAIN : DROP :: SNOW :
    (A) ice
    (B) cold
    (C) zero
    (D) flake
    (E) sleet

15. WING : BIRD :: HOOF :
    (A) dog
    (B) foot
    (C) horse
    (D) girl
    (E) horseshoe

16. CONSTELLATION : STAR :: ARCHI-
    PELAGO :
    (A) continent
    (B) peninsula
    (C) country
    (D) island
    (E) river

17. INTERNET : E-MAILING :: SMART-
    PHONE
    (A) fast
    (B) messaging
    (C) calling
    (D) landline
    (E) snail mail

18. ABSENCE : PRESENCE :: STABLE :
    (A) steady
    (B) secure
    (C) safe
    (D) changeable
    (E) influential

19. RUBBER : FLEXIBILITY :: PIPE :
    (A) iron
    (B) copper
    (C) pliability
    (D) elasticity
    (E) rigidity

20. SAFETY VALVE : BOILER :: SPARK
    PLUG :
    (A) engine
    (B) house
    (C) wire
    (D) city
    (E) factory

21. SCHOLARLY : UNSCHOLARLY ::
    LEARNED :
    (A) ignorant
    (B) wise
    (C) skilled
    (D) educated
    (E) literary

22. IMMIGRANT : ARRIVAL ::
    EMIGRANT :
    (A) departure
    (B) alienation
    (C) native
    (D) welcoming
    (E) travel

23. GOVERNOR : STATE :: GENERAL :
    (A) lieutenant
    (B) army
    (C) navy
    (D) captain
    (E) general

24. TROUBLESOME : DISASTROUS ::
    COSTLY :
    (A) cheap
    (B) extravagant
    (C) gorgeous
    (D) valuable
    (E) turbulent

25. WOOL : COAT :: COTTON
    (A) tablecloth
    (B) cover
    (C) washable
    (D) dress
    (E) cleaner

Part C

25 Questions • 10 Minutes

1. BOAT is to DOCK as AIRPLANE is to
   (A) wing
   (B) strut
   (C) engine
   (D) wind
   (E) hangar

2. OAT is to BUSHEL as DIAMOND is to
   (A) gram
   (B) hardness
   (C) usefulness
   (D) carat
   (E) ornament

3. MEDICINE is to EXAMINATION as
   LAW is to
   (A) jurist
   (B) court
   (C) interrogation
   (D) contract
   (E) suit

4. PARENT is to GUIDE as SOLDIER is to
   (A) serve
   (B) obedience
   (C) participate
   (D) fly
   (E) achieve

5. CAPTAIN is to VESSEL as DIRECTOR
   is to
   (A) football team
   (B) board
   (C) cheerleader squad
   (D) orchestra
   (E) musician

6. FATHER is to DAUGHTER as UNCLE
   is to
   (A) son
   (B) daughter
   (C) son-in-law
   (D) niece
   (E) aunt

7. PISTOL is to TRIGGER as MOTOR is to
   (A) wire
   (B) dynamo
   (C) amperes
   (D) barrel
   (E) switch

8. CUBE is to PYRAMID as SQUARE is to
   (A) box
   (B) solid
   (C) pentagon
   (D) triangle
   (E) cylinder

9. PROFIT is to SELLING as FAME is to
   (A) buying
   (B) cheating
   (C) publicity
   (D) praying
   (E) loving

10. PRINTING is to BOOK as WELDING is to
    (A) door
    (B) tank
    (C) chair
    (D) wire
    (E) pencil

11. GYMNASIUM is to HEALTH as SCHOOL is to
    (A) sick
    (B) study
    (C) books
    (D) knowledge
    (E) library

12. RIGHT is to WRONG as SUCCESS is to
    (A) aid
    (B) profit
    (C) failure
    (D) error
    (E) gain

13. EIGHT is to OCTAGON as SEVEN is to
    (A) polygon
    (B) polyhedron
    (C) hexagon
    (D) quadrilateral
    (E) heptagon

14. IDIOM is to EXPRESSION as PARA-PHRASE is to
    (A) version
    (B) translation
    (C) statement
    (D) dialect
    (E) language

15. BOTTLE is to BRITTLE as TIRE is to
    (A) elastic
    (B) scarce
    (C) rubber
    (D) spheroid
    (E) automobile

16. SOPRANO is to HIGH as BASS is to
    (A) violin
    (B) good
    (C) low
    (D) fish
    (E) soft

17. OLFACTORY is to NOSE as TACTILE is to
    (A) tacit
    (B) bloody
    (C) finger
    (D) handkerchief
    (E) stomach

18. STREET is to HORIZONTAL as BUILD-ING is to
    (A) tall
    (B) brick
    (C) broad
    (D) vertical
    (E) large

19. ALLEGIANCE is to LOYALTY as TREA-SON is to
    (A) obedience
    (B) rebellion
    (C) murder
    (D) felony
    (E) homage

20. CANVAS is to PAINT as MOLD is to
    (A) clay
    (B) cloth
    (C) statue
    (D) art
    (E) aesthetic

21. ABRUPT is to SUDDEN as INCESSANT is to
    (A) ceaseless
    (B) occasional
    (C) irregular
    (D) brutal
    (E) concise

22. CONQUEST is to ASCENDANCY as DEFEAT is to
    (A) omission
    (B) frustration
    (C) censure
    (D) subjugation
    (E) mastery

23. SOLUTION is to MYSTERY as COMPLETION is to
    (A) puzzle
    (B) books
    (C) college
    (D) school
    (E) detective

24. ALUMNUS is to ALUMNA as PRINCE is to
    (A) castle
    (B) king
    (C) knight
    (D) country
    (E) princess

25. OCCULT is to OVERT as SECRET is to
    (A) abstract
    (B) outward
    (C) science
    (D) tarry
    (E) concealed

STOP

IF YOU FINISH BEFORE TIME IS CALLED, YOU MAY CHECK YOUR WORK ON THIS SECTION ONLY. DO NOT TURN TO ANY OTHER SECTION IN THE TEST.

ANSWER KEY AND EXPLANATIONS

Part A

1. B	6. C	11. C	16. B	21. A
2. C	7. C	12. C	17. C	22. D
3. A	8. A	13. D	18. D	23. B
4. D	9. D	14. A	19. D	24. A
5. C	10. B	15. B	20. C	25. C

1. **The correct answer is (B).** In this object-to-use analogy, a *knife cuts* as a *gun shoots*. Choice (C), *sharpen*, may tempt you, but sharpening is done to a knife, not done by a knife. A knife may be used to *poke* someone, but that is not the usual use for a knife, so eliminate choice (D).

2. **The correct answer is (C).** This is also an object-to-use analogy, an *eye sees* as an *ear hears*. None of the other answers makes sense with *eye*.

3. **The correct answer is (A).** In this object-to-use analogy, *feathers* cover *birds* and *fur* covers some *mammals*. None of the other answers makes sense with feathers.

4. **The correct answer is (D).** In this part-to-whole analogy, a *hammer* has a *handle* as a *door* has a *knob*. None of the other answers makes sense with a knob.

5. **The correct answer is (C).** In this object-to-use analogy, a *foot* wears a *shoe* as a *body* wears a *coat*. Don't be fooled by the typical use of *coat* and *hat* together as a phrase, so eliminate choice (A). A coat may have *buttons*, choice (B), but that relationship of whole to part is not the relationship set up in the question.

6. **The correct answer is (C).** This is another object-to-use analogy. *Water* is *drunk* as *bread* is *eaten*. You might have thought that the initial pair was setting up a relationship between near synonyms, water as a drink, but *bread* is not a *cake* or a *pie*, choices

(A) and (D), so that relationship couldn't be correct.

7. **The correct answer is (C).** In this object-to-use relationship, *food* fuels a *human* as *gasoline* fuels an *automobile*. Choices (A) and (B) are incorrect because *lube* and *oil* are what's done to an engine, but are not uses of gasoline. Neither is a *spark*, choice (D).

8. **The correct answer is (A).** This question sets up an action-to-quality relationship. *Eating* leads to being *fat*, and *starving* leads to being *thin*. Choices (B) and (C), *food* and *bread*, are things, not qualities. Choice (D) is a quality, but not *necessarily* related to starving.

9. **The correct answer is (D).** This is a person-to-place analogy. A *human* lives in a *house* and a *bird* lives in a *nest*. Birds may also be found in *trees* and on *limbs*, choices (A) and (B), but neither is as specific to birds as house is for humans. Choice (B) is a *meal*, not a place to live.

10. **The correct answer is (B).** This is an antonym analogy. The opposite of *go* is *come*, and the opposite of *sell* is *buy*. Choice (A) relates to the first pair in the question, not the second. Choice (C) is incorrect because *money* is what you hope to get when you sell something, but is not antonym for *sell*. Choice (D) is incorrect because it's a near synonym for *sell*, not an antonym.

11. **The correct answer is (C).** In this example-to-category analogy, a *peninsula* is a type

of *landform* and a *bay* is a type of *body of water.* Choice (A) is incorrect because a bay is not a *boat* type. Choices (B) and (D) are incorrect because both an *inlet* and a *harbor* are other types of bodies of water.

12. **The correct answer is (C).** In this whole-to-part analogy, a *minute* is part of an *hour* and a *second* is part of a *minute.* None of the other answer choices fits this whole-to-part relationship.

13. **The correct answer is (D).** You can tell by the first pair that this is an antonym relationship. "To *abide*" is "to remain or *stay,*" so *depart* is an antonym. An antonym for *stay* is *leave.* None of the other answer choices fit an antonym relationship.

14. **The correct answer is (A).** "*January* is to *February*" sets up a sequence relationship, so the missing month is *July,* that is, as "*June* is to *July.*" Choices (C) and (D) can't be correct because they are not the names of months. Choice (B) is incorrect because May precedes June, not follows it as February follows January.

15. **The correct answer is (B).** This is an antonym analogy. *Bold* and *timid* are antonyms, so you're looking for an antonym for *advance.* Instead of advancing, or moving forward, an army falls back, or *retreats.* Choice (A) is incorrect because although *proceed* also means "to move forward," it doesn't fit the military connotation of *advance.* Choice (C) is incorrect because a *campaign* is a series of military operations, not a single advance or retreat, and so doesn't fit the sense. Choice (D) is incorrect because *soldiers* are persons and this analogy requires an action.

16. **The correct answer is (B).** This is another antonym relationship. The opposite of *above* is *below,* and the opposite of *top* is *bottom.* Either choice (C) or choice (D) might tempt you, neither is the opposite of *top.*

17. **The correct answer is (C).** This is an example-to-category analogy. A *lion* is a type of *animal,* and a *rose* is a type of

plant. All the other choices characterize a rose, but each is a quality, not the category to which roses belong.

18. **The correct answer is (D).** Consider this an object-to-quality relationship. A *tiger* is *carnivorous,* that is, a meat eater, and a *horse* is *herbivorous,* a plant eater. You can fairly easily eliminate choices (A) and (B), but you may be stumped by choices (C) and (D). This is where prefixes help. *Omni-* means "all," so an animal that is an omnivore eats plants and animals. *Herb* is not a prefix, but think of herbs as green leafy plants to help you remember that herbivores are plant eaters.

19. **The correct answer is (D).** In this part-to-whole relationship, a *sailor* is part of the *navy* and a *soldier* is part of the *army.* None of the other answers fit this part-to-whole relationship.

20. **The correct answer is (C).** This is a form of an object-to-use analogy. You *see* a *picture,* and you *hear* a *sound.* A clue here is that *see* is a verb, and the only answer choice that is a verb is choice (C), *hear.*

21. **The correct answer is (A).** Consider this a cause-and-effect relationship. *Success* causes *joy,* and *failure* causes *sadness;* both are effects. Choice (C) may tempt you, yet a *fault* can be the cause of failure, but not an effect. It's also incorrect because *joy* is an abstract quality and a fault is not.

22. **The correct answer is (D).** In this antonym analogy, *hope* is the opposite of *despair,* so the opposite of *happiness* is *misery.* On a quick read if you're running out of time, you might be confused into choosing one of the other choices, which are synonyms for *happiness.* So remember to read quickly, but carefully.

23. **The correct answer is (B).** This is an antonym analogy with a twist. The first pair is adjectives, but *attract* is a verb, so you'll need to find the answer choice that is both an antonym and a verb. The only one that fits is choice (B); *repel* is the opposite of *attract.* Choice (A), *fine,* could

be a noun or a verb, but doesn't fit as an antonym for *attract*. Choice (D), *draw*, is a verb and may mean "to cause to move toward," but that would be a synonym for *attract*, not an antonym.

24. **The correct answer is (A).** This is another association analogy. A *pupil* and a *teacher* have a superior-subordinate relationship as a *child* and a *parent* have. Choice (B) is incorrect because a *doll* and a *child* may have a relationship, but it's not of the same superior-subordinate relationship and one part of the relationship isn't living. Choice (C) is incorrect because *child* and *youngster*

are synonymous. Choice (D) is incorrect because while *obey* indicates the type of relationship between a superior and a subordinate, it doesn't name a person.

25. **The correct answer is (C).** This is a person-to-occupation analogy. A *mayor* runs a *city,* and a *general* runs the *army.* None of the other answer choices fit the concept of operating or managing.

Part B

1. C	6. E	11. B	16. D	21. A
2. D	7. B	12. A	17. C	22. A
3. B	8. D	13. C	18. D	23. C
4. A	9. C	14. D	19. E	24. B
5. E	10. E	15. C	20. A	25. D

1. **The correct answer is (C).** This is a synonym analogy. *Remunerative* means "profitable, paying," so *profitable* is a synonym. *Fraudulent* means "deceitful," so *fallacious,* "tending to mislead or deceptive," is a synonym. Choices (A) and (B) are incorrect because both *liar* and *slander* are nouns, and the analogy requires an adjective. Choice (D) is incorrect because *plausible* means "likely, apparently reasonable." Choice (E) is incorrect because *reward* is both a noun and a synonym for *remunerative*, not *fraudulent.*

2. **The correct answer is (D).** This is a tool-to-worker analogy. A *woodsman* uses an *ax,* and a *plumber* uses a *wrench.* Choices (A) and (B), *cut* and *hew*, are actions that a woodsman might do, but you need a person to complete the partial analogy. Choice (C) is incorrect because a tech works on electronic equipment. Choice (E)

is incorrect because a *cobbler* is a person who mends shoes.

3. **The correct answer is (B).** This analogy reverses the tool-to-worker analogy in question 2 and is a worker-to-tool analogy. A *surgeon* uses a *scalpel* to cut and a *butcher* cuts with a *cleaver,* a large broadbladed knife or hatchet. Choices (A), (C), (D), and (E) are incorrect because a *mallet*, a *chisel*, a *screwdriver*, and *medicine* are not tools a butcher uses.

4. **The correct answer is (A).** The initial analogy sets up an example-to-category relationship. A *cat* belongs to the category of *feline* (or the family Felidae), and a *horse* belongs to the category of *equine* (or family Equidae). Even if you didn't know the Latin names, you might have recognized that a cat is a feline, so the missing word would be similar. Choice (B) is incorrect because a *tiger* isn't a horse. Choice (C) is incorrect because although

a horse has four legs and so does a cat, the first pair in the analogy isn't about leg number. Choice (D) is incorrect because horses aren't meat-eaters, the meaning of *carnivore*. Choice (E) is incorrect because *vulpine* means "resembling a fox."

5. **The correct answer is (E).** This analogy is looking for antonyms. *Adversity* means "misfortune, hardship," so *happiness* is an antonym. An antonym for *vehemence*, meaning "forcefulness, violence" as well as "energy, passion," is *serenity*, "great calmness." Choices (A) and (C) are incorrect because *misfortune* is a synonym for *adversity*, and *troublesome*, meaning "worrisome" and "turbulent, violent," is also a synonym. Choice (B) is incorrect because *gaiety* has no relation to *vehemence*. Choice (D) is incorrect because *petulance* means "characterized by being irritable, impatient, ill humored" and is closer in meaning to *vehemence* than an antonym.

6. **The correct answer is (E).** This is a characteristic relationship. A *necklace* is an *adornment* as a *medal* is a *decoration*. The correct answer is based on what is essential about a medal. A medal is still a medal whether it has a *jewel*, or is made of some *metal* including *bronze*, choices (A), (B), and (D). Choice (C) is incorrect because a medal may be given for *bravery*, but bravery is not an essential characteristic of medals.

7. **The correct answer is (B).** This is a worker-to-tool analogy. A *miner* uses a *shovel*, and a *pirate* uses a *sword* in his line of work. Both a miner and a pirate want *treasure* including *gold* possibly, but gold is not a tool, so choices (A) and (E) are incorrect. Choice (C) is incorrect because a pirate sails a *ship*, but it's not a tool in the same way that a sword is. Choice (D) is incorrect because although a pirate ship may fly a *flag*, a flag is not a tool for a pirate.

8. **The correct answer is (D).** This is a person-to-occupation relationship. An *archeologist* studies *antiquity*, and an *ichthyologist* studies *marine life*. If you

didn't know the answer, you could at least eliminate some answer choices as incorrect. Someone who studies *theology*, choice (A), is a theologian. Choice (B) is incorrect because *ruins* are what archeologists study; always check to make sure that an answer doesn't relate to the initial pair to confuse you. Choice (C) is incorrect because *horticulture* is studied by a horticulturalist. Choice (E) is incorrect because a *mystic* practices mysticism.

9. **The correct answer is (C).** In this characteristic analogy, you're looking for what *highways* are made of because *shoes* are made of *leather* (or at least some shoes are). Choices (A), (B), and (D), *passage*, *road*, and *trail*, can be near synonyms of *highway*, but this isn't what is required to answer the analogy. Choice (E) is incorrect because a *journey* is a trip and not a characteristic of a highway.

10. **The correct answer is (E).** *Serfdom* is a characteristic of the *feudal system*, and *entrepreneurship* is a characteristic of *capitalism*. None of the other answer choices relate to entrepreneurship.

11. **The correct answer is (B).** This is a part-to-whole analogy. A *fin* is part of a *fish* as a *propeller* is part of a *plane*. Choice (A) is incorrect because a *wing* is also part of a plane, not the whole plane. Choices (C) and (D) are incorrect because neither is the whole of which a propeller is part, though a propeller may be used in both. Choice (E) is incorrect because *canoes* don't have propellers.

12. **The correct answer is (A).** This is a quality-to-extreme, or degree, analogy. *Satiety* means "being full beyond just being satisfied," and *destitute* is more than being poor; it is being impoverished, without any resources. Choice (B) is incorrect because *subsistence* means "a small amount of resources needed to survive," whereas being destitute is having no resources. Choice (C) is incorrect because *sustainable* means "able to supply with resources," or "able to be maintained." Choice (D) is incorrect

because *lesser* has no relation with *poor,* and neither does choice (E), *abandoned.*

13. **The correct answer is (C).** This is a characteristic analogy. *Skin* is the external covering of *humans,* and *hide* is a similar external covering of *animals.* Choice (A) is incorrect because *scales* are the covering of fish. Choice (B) is incorrect because *fur* covers some animals' hides. Choice (D) is incorrect because *hair* covers some parts of humans' skin. Choice (E) is incorrect because a *fish* is not covered by a hide.

14. **The correct answer is (D).** This is a whole-to-part analogy. A *drop* is single particle of *rain,* and a *flake* is a single particle of *snow.* Choice (A) is incorrect because snow is not the same as *ice.* Choices (B) and (C) are incorrect because while it may be *cold,* even *zero* degrees, when it snows, neither are particles of snow. The same is true of choice (E), *sleet.*

15. **The correct answer is (C).** This is a part-to-whole analogy. A *wing* is part of a *bird,* and of the choices listed, only a *horse* has a *hoof.*

16. **The correct answer is (D).** This is another whole-to-part analogy. A *constellation* is a collection of *stars,* and an *archipelago* is a collection of *islands.* Choices (A), (B), and (C) are all landforms, but not the correct landform. Choice (E), *river,* has no relation to an archipelago.

17. **The correct answer is (C).** In this object-to-use relationship, the *Internet* is used for *e-mailing* and *smartphones* are used for *messaging.* Choice (A) is incorrect because *fast* doesn't parallel *e-mailing* in meaning. It's a characteristic, not a use. Choice (B) is incorrect because while you can make calls on a smartphone, it's not a similar innovative use of a smartphone as using the Internet is to send e-mails. Making calls is an old use for a new invention. Choice (D) is incorrect because *landlines* are things, not uses. Choice (E) is incorrect because smartphones don't send *snail mail.*

18. **The correct answer is (D).** This is an antonym analogy. Being *absent* is the opposite of being *present,* and *stable* is the opposite of *changeable.* Choices (A), (B), and (C), *steady, secure,* and *safe* are similar in meaning to *stable,* so all are incorrect. Choice (E) is incorrect because *influential* has no relation to *stable.*

19. **The correct answer is (E).** In this object-to-quality analogy, *flexibility* is a quality of *rubber,* and *rigidity* is a quality of a *pipe.* Choice (A) is incorrect because *iron* can be a type of pipe, but it is not a characteristic related to movement—or lack of movement. This is also true for choice (B), *copper.* Choices (C) and (D) are incorrect because both *pliability* and *elasticity* are qualities related to flexibility, which is not a quality of pipes.

20. **The correct answer is (A).** This is an part-to-whole analogy. A *safety valve* is part of a *boiler,* and a *spark plug* is part of an *engine.* None of the other choices relate to a *spark plug.*

21. **The correct answer is (A).** This is an antonym analogy. The opposite of *scholarly* is *unscholarly,* and the opposite of *learned* is *ignorant.* Choices (B), (C), and (D), *wise, skilled,* and *educated,* are incorrect because they are similar in meaning to *scholarly* rather than being antonyms. Choice (E) is incorrect because *literary* has no relation to *learned.*

22. **The correct answer is (A).** This is a person-to-behavior analogy. An *immigrant arrives,* and an *emigrant departs.* Choice (B) is incorrect because *alienation* means "state or condition of isolation." Choice (C) is incorrect because *native* has no relation to *emigrant.* If you weren't sure if choice (D) was incorrect, you can eliminate it because *welcoming* is an adjective and you need a noun to match the second word in the first pair, *arrival.* Choice (E) is incorrect because *travel* is not specific enough to an emigrant.

23. **The correct answer is (C).** This is a person-to-place analogy. A *governor* runs

a *state,* and an *admiral* runs the *navy.* Choices (A), (D), and (E) are incorrect because each is an officer in the military, and the analogy established by the first pair requires one of the armed services as the answer. Choice (B) is incorrect because an admiral runs the navy, not the army.

24. **The correct answer is (B).** This is a quality-to-extreme or degree analogy. *Disastrous* is an extreme form of *troublesome,* and *extravagant* is an extreme form of *costly.* Choice (A) is incorrect because *cheap* is an antonym for *extravagant,* not an extreme version of the word. Choice (C) is incorrect because *gorgeous* relates to looks, not price. Choice (D) is incorrect because *valuable* is not an extreme version of *costly.* Choice (E) is incorrect because *turbulent* has no relation to *costly.*

25. **The correct answer is (D).** This is a category analogy. A *coat* can be made out of *wool,* and a *dress* can be made out of *cotton.* Choice (A) is incorrect because a *tablecloth* isn't a piece of clothing. Choice (B) is incorrect because a *cover* isn't a specific type of clothing. Choice (C) is incorrect because *washable* is not a type of clothing, and neither is a *cleaner,* choice (E).

Part C

1. E	6. D	11. D	16. C	21. A
2. D	7. E	12. C	17. C	22. D
3. C	8. D	13. E	18. D	23. A
4. A	9. C	14. A	19. B	24. E
5. B	10. B	15. A	20. A	25. B

1. **The correct answer is (E).** This is a place analogy. A *boat* is kept at a *dock,* and an *airplane* is kept in a *hangar.* All the other answer choices are parts of a plane, not a place to keep one.

2. **The correct answer is (D).** In this association analogy, *oats* are measured in *bushels,* and *diamonds* are measured in *carats.* Choice (A) is incorrect because *gram* has no relation to diamonds. Choices (B), (C), and (E) are incorrect because they are characteristics or uses of diamonds, but not how diamonds are measured.

3. **The correct answer is (C).** In this characteristic analogy, an *examination* is a normal practice or part of *medicine,* and

an *interrogation* is a normal practice or part of *law.* All the other answer choices are things associated with the law, but are not a practice. For example, for choice (D) to be correct, the answer would need to be "write a contract," and for choice (E) to be correct, the answer would need to be "sue."

4. **The correct answer is (A).** This is a person-to-action analogy. A *parent guides* children, and a *soldier serves* in the army. Choice (B) is incorrect because *obedience* is a noun, and the answer, based on the first pair, requires a verb. Choice (C) is incorrect because *participate* in relation to a soldier in the army is not typical usage. Choice (D) is incorrect because the typical

job of a soldier is not *flying*. Choice (E) is incorrect because *achieve* is not typical usage with the word *soldier*.

5. **The correct answer is (B).** This is a person/worker-to-place analogy. A *captain* serves on a *vessel,* or ship, and a *director* serves on a *board.* Choice (A) is incorrect because a *football team* is led by a coach. Choice (C) is incorrect because a *cheerleading squad* is led by a captain. Choice (D) is incorrect because an *orchestra* has a conductor, not a director. Choice (E) is incorrect because a *musician* is not a director.

6. **The correct answer is (D).** This is a category-to-example relationship. Having a *daughter* (or son) makes a man a *father,* and having a *niece* (or nephew) makes a man an *uncle.* Choices (A) and (B) are incorrect because having a *son* or a *daughter* would make a man a father, not an uncle. Choice (C) is incorrect because a *son-in-law* has no bearing on whether a man is an uncle, and neither does having an *aunt,* choice (E).

7. **The correct answer is (E).** Pull the *trigger* and the *pistol* fires; turn the *switch* and the *motor* starts in this object-to-action analogy. Choices (A), (B), and (C) are incorrect because *wire, dynamo,* and *amperes* may all relate to some aspect of motors, but they are not to what turns it on. Choice (D) is incorrect because *barrel* relates to a gun, not a motor.

8. **The correct answer is (D).** This is a characteristic analogy. A *cube* is a three-dimensional figure based on a *square.* A *pyramid* is a three-dimensional figure based on a *triangle.* Choices (A) and (B) are incorrect because both a *box* and a *solid* are three-dimensional figures, but you are looking for a two-dimensional figure. Choice (C) is incorrect because even though a *pentagon* is a two-dimensional figure, it is not the base for a pyramid. Choice (E) is incorrect because a *cylinder* is a three-dimensional figure based on a circle.

9. **The correct answer is (C).** In this cause-and-effect analogy, *profit* is the end product of *selling* and *fame* is the end product, or result, of *publicity*. Choice (A) is incorrect because *buying* refers to the first pair in the analogy, not to *fame*. Choice (B) is incorrect because *cheating* has no relation to the analogy. Choices (D) and (E) are incorrect because *praying* and *loving* have no relation to the analogy.

10. **The correct answer is (B).** In this action-to-object relationship, a *book* is *printed* and a *tank* is *welded.* Choices (A), (C), and (E), *door, chair,* and *pencil,* have no relation to welding and are, therefore, incorrect. Choice (D) may tempt you, but if you think about it, *wires* aren't welded.

11. **The correct answer is (D).** This is a cause-and-effect analogy. The end product or result of going to the *gym* is being *healthy* and the end product of going to *school* is gaining *knowledge*. Choice (A) is incorrect because *sick* has no relation to *school*. Choices (B), (C), and (E) are incorrect because although they may relate to school, they are not the desired end product.

12. **The correct answer is (C).** This is a straightforward antonym analogy. The opposite of *right* is *wrong,* and the opposite of *success* is *failure.* Choices (A), (B), and (E), *aid, profit,* and *gain* are incorrect because they are somewhat similar in meaning to *success.* Choice (D) is incorrect because *error* is a synonym of *wrong,* not an antonym for *success.*

13. **The correct answer is (E).** This is a characteristic analogy. An *octagon* is an *eight-sided figure,* and a *heptagon* is a *seven-sided figure.* Knowledge of prefixes and geometry could help you answer this question. Choice (A), *polygon,* is a closed two-dimensional figure composed of line segments that are not curved; therefore, a heptagon is a polygon, but *polygon* is not as specific as heptagon, so it doesn't fit in the analogy as well as heptagon. Choice (B) is incorrect because a *polyhedron* is a three-dimensional solid with many faces. A heptagon is not a polyhedron because

it isn't three-dimensional. Choice (C) is incorrect because a *hexagon* has only six sides. Choice (D) is incorrect because a *quadrilateral* has four sides.

14. **The correct answer is (A).** This is a grammatical analogy. An *idiom* is an *expression,* and a *paraphrase* is a *version* of a piece of writing or speech. Choice (B) is incorrect because a *translation* is typically a near restatement of a piece of writing or speech from one language to another, whereas a paraphrase expresses the same idea in different word in the same language. Choice (C) is incorrect because a paraphrase is not a *statement,* but a restatement. Choice (D) is incorrect because a *dialect* is a set of usages and pronunciations used by a particular group or region. Choice (E) is incorrect because *language* is too broad a term to fit with *paraphrase.*

15. **The correct answer is (A).** This is an object-to-quality relationship. A *bottle* is *brittle,* or likely to break or snap, and a *tire* is flexible, or *elastic.* Choice (A) is incorrect because *scare* has no relation to *tire.* Choice (C) is incorrect, although it might confuse you into choosing it. Tires are made of *rubber,* but that is not a quality of a tire, and neither is *spheroid,* choice (D). Choice (E) is incorrect because while a tire is part of an *automobile,* that is not a quality of a tire.

16. **The correct answer is (C).** This is a person/worker-to-abstraction or quality relationship. A *soprano* has a *high* voice, and a *bass* has a *low* voice. None of the other answers have any relation to the voice of a bass. Don't be confused by choice (D), which wants you to think that *bass* is pronounced with a short "a" and is the name of a fish.

17. **The correct answer is (C).** This is a characteristic analogy. The sense of smell is characteristic of the *nose,* and *olfactory* relates to the sense of smell. The sense of touch is characteristic of the *finger,* and *tactile* relates to the sense of touch. Choice (A) is incorrect because *tacit* means "implied, understood, unspoken." None of the

other choices relate to a part of the body with the sense of touch.

18. **The correct answer is (D).** In this object-to-quality analogy, the missing word refers to direction. A *street* is *horizontal,* and a *building* is *vertical.* While the other choices may describe a building—*tall, brick, broad, large*—none of them relate to direction.

19. **The correct answer is (B).** This is a synonym analogy. *Allegiance* and *loyalty* are synonyms, just like *treason* and *rebellion* are synonyms. Choice (A) is incorrect because *obedience* is the opposite of *rebellion.* Choice (C) is incorrect because while treason may involve *murder,* murder doesn't necessarily involve treason, so it isn't a synonym for *treason.* For the same reason, choice (D), *felony,* is not a synonym. Choice (E) is incorrect because *homage* means "honor, respect paid to someone."

20. **The correct answer is (A).** In this association analogy, *paint* is used on a *canvas* and *clay* may be used in a *mold.* Choice (B) is incorrect because *cloth* has no relation to a mold. Choice (C) is incorrect because a *statue* may be the finished product of clay and a mold, but it doesn't fit the analogy. Paint is not a finished product of a canvas; a painting is. Choice (D) is incorrect because a clay figure may result in *art,* yet art is not an ingredient in a mold. Choice (E) is incorrect because *aesthetic* is the appreciation of art.

21. **The correct answer is (A).** The initial pair sets up a synonym relationship. *Incessant* means "uninterrupted, unending, unceasing," so *ceaseless* is a synonym. Choices (B) and (C) are incorrect because *occasional* and *irregular* are antonyms for *incessant.* Choice (D) is incorrect because *brutal* has no relation to *incessant,* and neither has *concise,* choice (E), meaning "brief, to the point."

22. **The correct answer is (D).** This is a sequence relationship. A *conquest* leads to *ascendancy,* or control, on one side, and

defeat on the other side leads to *subjugation*, or being controlled. Choice (A) is incorrect because *omission* has no relation to *defeat*. Choice (B) is incorrect because being defeated may be *frustrating*, but it's not a typical usage for the word. Choice (C) is incorrect because *censure* means "to strongly disapprove, criticize harshly." Choice (E) is incorrect because *mastery* means "having great skill, expertise."

23. **The correct answer is (A).** The first pair of words sets up an action-to-object analogy. A *solution* ends a *mystery,* and *completion* ends a *puzzle.* Choices (B), (C), and (D) are incorrect because completing a *book, college,* or *school* has no element of problem solving to them that both a mystery and a puzzle have. Choice (E) is incorrect because a *detective* isn't completed, which is how the analogy is set up.

24. **The correct answer is (E).** In this association analogy, an *alumnus,* a male graduate, and an *alumna,* a female graduate, are linked as equals, and a *prince* and

princess are linked because they belong to the same rank of royalty. Choice (A) is incorrect because a *castle* is a thing, and the answer requires a person. For the same reason, choice (D), *country,* is incorrect. Choice (B) is incorrect because a *king* is one rank above a prince; the answer also requires a woman. Choice (C) is incorrect because a *knight* is at a lower rank than a prince and a man.

25. **The correct answer is (B).** The first pair set up an antonym relationship. *Occult* means "hidden, not apparent to the senses, mysterious," whereas *overt* means "not hidden, able to be seen." Among the answer choices, only *outward* is the opposite of *secret.* Choice (A) is incorrect because *abstract* means "theoretical, difficult to understand." Choice (C) is incorrect because *science* has no relation to being secretive. Choice (D) is incorrect because *tarry* is "to delay." Choice (E) is incorrect because *concealed* is a synonym for *secret,* not an antonym.

LET'S PUT YOU TO THE TEST

Now that you have thoroughly reviewed the various kinds of verbal ability items and are familiar with the test-taking strategies associated with them, let's put you to the test.

Pay strict attention to the time allotted for each section of the test and do your best to adhere to these time limits. Read the directions for each part of the test before attempting to answer any of the questions.

This test has three parts: A—Synonyms; B—Antonyms; C—Verbal Analogies. The total time allotted for this test is 50 minutes. Have extra pencils available in case of point breakage, so as not to lose testing time.

An answer key is provided at the end of the test so that you can evaluate your performance. Remember, this is a simulation of the "real thing," so be honest with yourself and look at the answer key only after you have completed the test.

TIP

Remember to use the clock to keep up a steady pace in answering questions

FINAL VERBAL ABILITY EXAMINATION ANSWER SHEET

Part A: Synonyms

1. Ⓐ Ⓑ Ⓒ Ⓓ	8. Ⓐ Ⓑ Ⓒ Ⓓ	15. Ⓐ Ⓑ Ⓒ Ⓓ	22. Ⓐ Ⓑ Ⓒ Ⓓ	29. Ⓐ Ⓑ Ⓒ Ⓓ
2. Ⓐ Ⓑ Ⓒ Ⓓ	9. Ⓐ Ⓑ Ⓒ Ⓓ	16. Ⓐ Ⓑ Ⓒ Ⓓ	23. Ⓐ Ⓑ Ⓒ Ⓓ	30. Ⓐ Ⓑ Ⓒ Ⓓ
3. Ⓐ Ⓑ Ⓒ Ⓓ	10. Ⓐ Ⓑ Ⓒ Ⓓ	17. Ⓐ Ⓑ Ⓒ Ⓓ	24. Ⓐ Ⓑ Ⓒ Ⓓ	31. Ⓐ Ⓑ Ⓒ Ⓓ
4. Ⓐ Ⓑ Ⓒ Ⓓ	11. Ⓐ Ⓑ Ⓒ Ⓓ	18. Ⓐ Ⓑ Ⓒ Ⓓ	25. Ⓐ Ⓑ Ⓒ Ⓓ	32. Ⓐ Ⓑ Ⓒ Ⓓ
5. Ⓐ Ⓑ Ⓒ Ⓓ	12. Ⓐ Ⓑ Ⓒ Ⓓ	19. Ⓐ Ⓑ Ⓒ Ⓓ	26. Ⓐ Ⓑ Ⓒ Ⓓ	33. Ⓐ Ⓑ Ⓒ Ⓓ
6. Ⓐ Ⓑ Ⓒ Ⓓ	13. Ⓐ Ⓑ Ⓒ Ⓓ	20. Ⓐ Ⓑ Ⓒ Ⓓ	27. Ⓐ Ⓑ Ⓒ Ⓓ	34. Ⓐ Ⓑ Ⓒ Ⓓ
7. Ⓐ Ⓑ Ⓒ Ⓓ	14. Ⓐ Ⓑ Ⓒ Ⓓ	21. Ⓐ Ⓑ Ⓒ Ⓓ	28. Ⓐ Ⓑ Ⓒ Ⓓ	35. Ⓐ Ⓑ Ⓒ Ⓓ

Part B: Antonyms

1. Ⓐ Ⓑ Ⓒ Ⓓ	9. Ⓐ Ⓑ Ⓒ Ⓓ	17. Ⓐ Ⓑ Ⓒ Ⓓ	25. Ⓐ Ⓑ Ⓒ Ⓓ	33. Ⓐ Ⓑ Ⓒ Ⓓ
2. Ⓐ Ⓑ Ⓒ Ⓓ	10. Ⓐ Ⓑ Ⓒ Ⓓ	18. Ⓐ Ⓑ Ⓒ Ⓓ	26. Ⓐ Ⓑ Ⓒ Ⓓ	34. Ⓐ Ⓑ Ⓒ Ⓓ
3. Ⓐ Ⓑ Ⓒ Ⓓ	11. Ⓐ Ⓑ Ⓒ Ⓓ	19. Ⓐ Ⓑ Ⓒ Ⓓ	27. Ⓐ Ⓑ Ⓒ Ⓓ	35. Ⓐ Ⓑ Ⓒ Ⓓ
4. Ⓐ Ⓑ Ⓒ Ⓓ	12. Ⓐ Ⓑ Ⓒ Ⓓ	20. Ⓐ Ⓑ Ⓒ Ⓓ	28. Ⓐ Ⓑ Ⓒ Ⓓ	36. Ⓐ Ⓑ Ⓒ Ⓓ
5. Ⓐ Ⓑ Ⓒ Ⓓ	13. Ⓐ Ⓑ Ⓒ Ⓓ	21. Ⓐ Ⓑ Ⓒ Ⓓ	29. Ⓐ Ⓑ Ⓒ Ⓓ	37. Ⓐ Ⓑ Ⓒ Ⓓ
6. Ⓐ Ⓑ Ⓒ Ⓓ	14. Ⓐ Ⓑ Ⓒ Ⓓ	22. Ⓐ Ⓑ Ⓒ Ⓓ	30. Ⓐ Ⓑ Ⓒ Ⓓ	38. Ⓐ Ⓑ Ⓒ Ⓓ
7. Ⓐ Ⓑ Ⓒ Ⓓ	15. Ⓐ Ⓑ Ⓒ Ⓓ	23. Ⓐ Ⓑ Ⓒ Ⓓ	31. Ⓐ Ⓑ Ⓒ Ⓓ	39. Ⓐ Ⓑ Ⓒ Ⓓ
8. Ⓐ Ⓑ Ⓒ Ⓓ	16. Ⓐ Ⓑ Ⓒ Ⓓ	24. Ⓐ Ⓑ Ⓒ Ⓓ	32. Ⓐ Ⓑ Ⓒ Ⓓ	40. Ⓐ Ⓑ Ⓒ Ⓓ

Part C: Verbal Analogies

1. Ⓐ Ⓑ Ⓒ Ⓓ	6. Ⓐ Ⓑ Ⓒ Ⓓ	11. Ⓐ Ⓑ Ⓒ Ⓓ	16. Ⓐ Ⓑ Ⓒ Ⓓ	21. Ⓐ Ⓑ Ⓒ Ⓓ
2. Ⓐ Ⓑ Ⓒ Ⓓ	7. Ⓐ Ⓑ Ⓒ Ⓓ	12. Ⓐ Ⓑ Ⓒ Ⓓ	17. Ⓐ Ⓑ Ⓒ Ⓓ	22. Ⓐ Ⓑ Ⓒ Ⓓ
3. Ⓐ Ⓑ Ⓒ Ⓓ	8. Ⓐ Ⓑ Ⓒ Ⓓ	13. Ⓐ Ⓑ Ⓒ Ⓓ	18. Ⓐ Ⓑ Ⓒ Ⓓ	23. Ⓐ Ⓑ Ⓒ Ⓓ
4. Ⓐ Ⓑ Ⓒ Ⓓ	9. Ⓐ Ⓑ Ⓒ Ⓓ	14. Ⓐ Ⓑ Ⓒ Ⓓ	19. Ⓐ Ⓑ Ⓒ Ⓓ	24. Ⓐ Ⓑ Ⓒ Ⓓ
5. Ⓐ Ⓑ Ⓒ Ⓓ	10. Ⓐ Ⓑ Ⓒ Ⓓ	15. Ⓐ Ⓑ Ⓒ Ⓓ	20. Ⓐ Ⓑ Ⓒ Ⓓ	25. Ⓐ Ⓑ Ⓒ Ⓓ

FINAL VERBAL ABILITY EXAMINATION

100 Questions • 50 Minutes

Part A: Synonyms

35 Questions • 20 Minutes

Directions: In each of the sentences below, one word is in italics. Following each sentence are four words or phrases. For each sentence, select the word or phrase that best corresponds in meaning to the italicized word.

1. The chart *classifies* these organisms.
   - (A) fuses
   - (B) categorizes
   - (C) controls
   - (D) camouflages

2. On many teams, a player may face a *penalty* for irresponsible or unruly behavior.
   - (A) arrangement
   - (B) gratification
   - (C) punishment
   - (D) precaution

3. He used the *allotted* study time to complete his assignments.
   - (A) authorized
   - (B) designated
   - (C) agreed
   - (D) alerted

4. In examining the patient, the doctor noted his *pallor*.
   - (A) paleness
   - (B) ruddiness
   - (C) fever
   - (D) rigidity

5. It was apparent that he had attempted to *concoct* an alibi.
   - (A) inculcate
   - (B) conceal
   - (C) reveal
   - (D) fabricate

6. The City Council *sanctioned* as a responsible option the hiring of an outside firm to oversee the health department.
   - (A) positioned
   - (B) appeased
   - (C) rejected
   - (D) approved

7. The claim was *substantiated* by the evidence offered by the attorney.
   - (A) repealed
   - (B) ineffective
   - (C) applied
   - (D) supported

8. The soldiers retreated to a position of *comparative* safety.
   - (A) objective
   - (B) relative
   - (C) subjective
   - (D) scientific

9. Geologists *assure* us that our Earth is a few billion years old.
   - (A) guarantee
   - (B) instruct
   - (C) deny
   - (D) assail

10. It has been said that he is a *connoisseur* of fine wines.
   - (A) expert on
   - (B) taster of
   - (C) procurer of
   - (D) vendor of

11. He *spurned* the offer to run for office after the party's first three choices declined.
    (A) accepted
    (B) extolled
    (C) acclaimed
    (D) rejected

12. The well-dressed gentleman bowed *ceremoniously*.
    (A) without ritual
    (B) disrespectfully
    (C) serenely
    (D) formally

13. His diet was marked by *inordinate* amounts of carbohydrates and fats.
    (A) redundant
    (B) excessive
    (C) reasonable
    (D) exurberant

14. The annual parade *traversed* this magnificent city from the east to the west side.
    (A) was patronized
    (B) extended
    (C) crossed
    (D) augmented

15. *Enraptured* by the beauty of the mountains, they had not spoken for twenty minutes.
    (A) summoned
    (B) impeded
    (C) exonerated
    (D) entranced

16. The results of the experiment upheld the *contention* of those who supported the hypothesis.
    (A) realization
    (B) contiguity
    (C) argument
    (D) exhilaration

17. The *consensus* of the group
    (A) stipulation
    (B) regulation
    (C) conviction
    (D) collective opinion

18. Arthritis is a *chronic* disease that results from a faulty immune system.
    (A) long-lasting
    (B) serious
    (C) contagious
    (D) infectious

19. Mayan magnificence *abounds* in the small resort village of Kailuum.
    (A) is remote
    (B) is abundant
    (C) is significant
    (D) is inadequate

20. As enthusiasm for the project *waxed* under the direction of a newly appointed administrator, the level of excitement
    (A) stirred.
    (B) waned.
    (C) vanished.
    (D) increased.

21. *Void* of intellectual stimuli
    (A) composed
    (B) in excess
    (C) empty
    (D) full

22. The injuries sustained resulted in paralysis in two of the four *appendages*.
    (A) chambers
    (B) muscles
    (C) limbs
    (D) tubes

23. Security was *risked* to attain maximum career satisfaction.
    (A) ventured
    (B) squandered
    (C) exhausted
    (D) wasted

24. The fruit was *pared* and sliced for the salad.
    (A) divided
    (B) rinsed
    (C) peeled
    (D) sectioned

25. The hospital reorganization was an *initiative* of the new board chair.
    (A) enterprise
    (B) energy
    (C) zeal
    (D) leadership

26. The introduction *delineates* the book's content and format.
    (A) discredits
    (B) describes
    (C) disproves
    (D) endorses

27. The X-ray clearly showed the torn *cartilage* in the knee.
    (A) tissue
    (B) ligament
    (C) tendon
    (D) membrane

28. The receptionist *confirmed* the appointment.
    (A) canceled
    (B) rescheduled
    (C) verified
    (D) recorded

29. Her license was *invalidated* because she made a misstatement on her application.
    (A) authorized
    (B) canceled
    (C) contradicted
    (D) modified

30. If the engine was *malfunctioning* at the time, it was
    (A) operative.
    (B) operating incorrectly.
    (C) firing.
    (D) igniting.

31. The clients were shocked at the *fraudulent* practices of the contractors.
    (A) thorough
    (B) extensive
    (C) legal
    (D) deceitful

32. The employer questioned the *competence* of his staff. The employer was not sure about their
    (A) honesty.
    (B) punctuality.
    (C) credibility.
    (D) ability.

33. The reading list included an *anthology* by a famous author.
    (A) collection of literary selections
    (B) annotated bibliography
    (C) archaeological study
    (D) autobiography

34. Some bacteria are *mobile* because of their flagellum.
    (A) movement
    (B) deadly
    (C) migratory
    (D) motile

35. He smiled *wryly*.
    (A) deceptively
    (B) nastily
    (C) ironically
    (D) delightedly

Part B: Antonyms

40 Questions • 15 Minutes

Directions: For each of the following test items, select the word that is opposite in meaning to the term printed in capital letters.

1. IMPERIOUS
   (A) submissive
   (B) valuable
   (C) pointed
   (D) positive

2. CAPRICIOUS
   (A) whimsical
   (B) judicious
   (C) steadfast
   (D) tranquil

3. CANTANKEROUS
   (A) pleasant
   (B) dubious
   (C) effective
   (D) awkward

4. FORBEARANCE
   (A) indulgence
   (B) pliancy
   (C) politeness
   (D) impatience

5. HAPHAZARD
   (A) inefficient
   (B) premeditated
   (C) unsatisfactory
   (D) blundering

6. The *efficacy* of the procedure was in doubt until the study was completed.
   (A) ineffectiveness
   (B) efficiency
   (C) value
   (D) success

7. CHIMERICAL
   (A) philosophical
   (B) elite
   (C) factual
   (D) unimpressive

8. REPRESS
   (A) reserve
   (B) liberate
   (C) thrust
   (D) precipitate

9. ABOMINABLE
   (A) agreeable
   (B) loathsome
   (C) sufficient
   (D) degrading

10. UNETHICAL
    (A) vulgar
    (B) feasible
    (C) pompous
    (D) scrupulous

11. ANTECEDENT
    (A) previous
    (B) subsequent
    (C) foregoing
    (D) propitious

12. PONDEROUS
    (A) delicate
    (B) potent
    (C) supportive
    (D) massive

13. SUPPLICATION
    (A) worship
    (B) compassion
    (C) entreaty
    (D) disdain

14. POSITIVE
    (A) negative
    (B) sensitive
    (C) diplomatic
    (D) popular

15. RENEGADE
    (A) constant
    (B) extricate
    (C) loyal
    (D) heretical

16. DISREGARD
    (A) disown
    (B) attend to
    (C) revoke
    (D) recover

17. WRATH
    (A) delight
    (B) travail
    (C) frivolity
    (D) detriment

18. TEDIOUS
    (A) ungainly
    (B) imperative
    (C) stimulating
    (D) suitable

19. EMBODY
    (A) impel
    (B) fuse
    (C) dissociate
    (D) collect

20. DEFERRABLE
    (A) urgent
    (B) furtive
    (C) inclined
    (D) deniable

21. HOMOGENOUS
    (A) invariable
    (B) homosexual
    (C) importunate
    (D) heterogeneous

22. ADHERENT
    (A) disciple
    (B) repudiator
    (C) soothsayer
    (D) hypocrite

23. CRUDE
    (A) barbarous
    (B) refined
    (C) obscure
    (D) covetous

24. IRRATIONAL
    (A) cynical
    (B) sharp
    (C) prevalent
    (D) sensible

25. GRAPHIC
    (A) vague
    (B) illustrative
    (C) forcible
    (D) glacial

26. DEVASTATE
    (A) tolerate
    (B) obstruct
    (C) renovate
    (D) promote

27. STRINGENT
    (A) exacting
    (B) tough
    (C) influential
    (D) flexible

28. ACQUIESCE
    (A) contest
    (B) invest
    (C) dismiss
    (D) supply

29. BREVITY
    (A) abbreviation
    (B) length
    (C) ramification
    (D) delusion

30. FLAUNT
    (A) disavow
    (B) conserve
    (C) blight
    (D) astonish

31. CULTIVATE
    (A) restore
    (B) stifle
    (C) reinstate
    (D) nurture

32. DILATE
    (A) negate
    (B) abet
    (C) constrict
    (D) suspend

33. BEFITTING
    (A) enhancing
    (B) conciliatory
    (C) inappropriate
    (D) elegant

34. COHERENT
    (A) illogical
    (B) consecutive
    (C) cognizant
    (D) courtly

35. PALTRY
    (A) political
    (B) complaisant
    (C) clever
    (D) impressive

36. BUCOLIC
    (A) urban
    (B) gallant
    (C) valiant
    (D) functional

37. EXTRAVAGANT
    (A) coarse
    (B) superior
    (C) frugal
    (D) typical

38. LENIENCY
    (A) indulgence
    (B) severity
    (C) embroilment
    (D) inequality

39. MANIFEST
   (A) latent
   (B) oblivious
   (C) terminal
   (D) languid

40. PLEBEIAN
   (A) congenial
   (B) ignoble
   (C) scientific
   (D) patrician

Part C: Verbal Analogies

25 Questions • 15 Minutes

> **Directions:** In the following questions, determine the relationship between the first pair of capitalized words and then decide which of the choices share a similar relationship with the third capitalized word.

1. CAT is to DOG as CUP is to
   (A) knife
   (B) coffee
   (C) saucer
   (D) cream

2. SALTY is to SALINE as SUGARY is to
   (A) sweet
   (B) stale
   (C) bread
   (D) insipid

3. FLANNEL is to WOOL as BRICK is to
   (A) wood
   (B) clay
   (C) stone
   (D) mortar

4. CONTEMPORARY is to PRESENT as FUTURE is to
   (A) past
   (B) posterity
   (C) eventual
   (D) ancient

5. MOON is to EARTH as EARTH is to
   (A) space
   (B) moon
   (C) sky
   (D) sun

6. ACUTE is to CHRONIC as INTENSE is to
   (A) sardonic
   (B) tonic
   (C) persistent
   (D) pretty

7. PEAK is to MOUNTAIN as FLOOR is to
   (A) ceiling
   (B) canyon
   (C) river
   (D) cliff

8. EAST is to WEST as NORTHWEST is to
   (A) southeast
   (B) southwest
   (C) north
   (D) northeast

9. GASOLINE is to PETROLEUM as SUGAR is to
   (A) oil
   (B) cane
   (C) plant
   (D) sweet

10. DEFERENCE is to RESPECT as CONTEMPT is to
    (A) esteem
    (B) capitulation
    (C) discourtesy
    (D) tendency

11. SLOPE is to INCLINE as PLANE is to
    (A) dimensional
    (B) flat
    (C) square
    (D) rectangular

12. EDGE is to CENTER as EFFUSIVE is to
    (A) unemotional
    (B) exuberant
    (C) eclectic
    (D) eccentricity

13. PROCRASTINATOR is to DELAY as MENTOR is to
    (A) trusted
    (B) teacher
    (C) advice
    (D) measure

14. SOPHISTICATION is to FINESSE as INEPTITUDE is to
    (A) inefficiency
    (B) artistry
    (C) trickiness
    (D) insatiability

15. CAPTAIN is to STEAMSHIP as PRINCIPAL is to
    (A) interest
    (B) school
    (C) agent
    (D) concern

16. DIME is to SILVER as PENNY is to
    (A) mint
    (B) copper
    (C) currency
    (D) value

17. REVERT is to REVERSION as SYMPATHIZE is to
    (A) sympathetic
    (B) symposium
    (C) sympathy
    (D) sympathizing

18. REGRESSIVE is to REGRESS as STERILE is to
    (A) sterilization
    (B) sterilize
    (C) sterility
    (D) sterilizer

19. DOWN is to UP as AGE is to
    (A) year
    (B) youth
    (C) snow
    (D) date

20. I is to MINE as MAN is to
    (A) men
    (B) man's
    (C) his
    (D) hers

21. DISLOYAL is to FAITHLESS as IMPERFECTION is to
    (A) faithful
    (B) depression
    (C) foible
    (D) decrepitude

22. NECKLACE is to PEARLS as CHAIN is to
    (A) locket
    (B) prisoner
    (C) links
    (D) clasp

23. DRIFT is to SNOW as DUNE is to
    (A) hill
    (B) rain
    (C) sand
    (D) hail

24. BANK is to DEPOSITS as HOSPITAL is to

(A) blood

(B) care

(C) surgery

(D) tests

25. SCHOONER is to VESSEL as PERSIMMON is to

(A) machine

(B) fruit

(C) engine

(D) vehicle

STOP

IF YOU FINISH BEFORE TIME IS CALLED, YOU MAY CHECK YOUR WORK ON THIS SECTION ONLY. DO NOT TURN TO ANY OTHER SECTION IN THE TEST.

ANSWER KEY AND EXPLANATIONS

Part A: Synonyms

1. B	8. B	15. D	22. C	29. B
2. C	9. A	16. C	23. A	30. B
3. B	10. A	17. D	24. C	31. D
4. A	11. D	18. A	25. A	32. D
5. D	12. D	19. B	26. B	33. A
6. D	13. B	20. D	27. A	34. D
7. D	14. C	21. C	28. C	35. C

1. **The correct answer is (B).** *Classify* and *categorize* both mean "sort, file, arrange by class or category." Choice (A) is incorrect because *fuse* means "to merge, to combine." Choice (C) is incorrect because *control* is not a synonym for *classify*. Choice (D) is incorrect because *camouflage* means "to conceal by using a disguise or color."

2. **The correct answer is (C).** A *penalty* is a *punishment*. Choice (A), *arrangement*, has no relation to *penalty*. Choice (B) is incorrect because *gratification* means "the state of being satisfied, satisfaction." Choice (D) is incorrect because *precaution* is not a synonym for *penalty*.

3. **The correct answer is (B).** *Designated* means "allocated, assigned" and so is a synonym for *allotted*. Nothing indicates that someone gave the person permission to use his study time to do the assignment, so eliminate choice (A). Choice (C) can be eliminated because there is no indication that the person had *agreed* with someone to use the study time for the assignment. Choice (D) makes no sense.

4. **The correct answer is (A).** All of the answer choices make sense, but only *paleness* is an antonym for *pallor*. Choice (B), *ruddiness*, means "flushed, reddish" and is an antonym for *pallor*.

5. **The correct answer is (D).** *Concoct* means "to make up," and so does *fabricate*. Choice (A), *inculcate,* means "to instill or drill something into someone's mind by forceful repetition" and doesn't make sense. The same goes for choice (B), *conceal*, meaning "to hide." Choice (C), *reveal*, might be tempting, but the word is not a synonym for *concoct*.

6. **The correct answer is (D).** *Sanction* may mean "to approve" or it may mean "to penalize," though as the latter, *sanction* is typically used in terms of legal activity, especially international law. In this case, it means "to approve," so choice (D) is correct. Choice (A) is incorrect because *position* has no relation to *sanction*, and neither does *appease*, choice (B), meaning "to calm, to quiet." Choice (C) is incorrect because *reject* is the opposite of *approve*, so it's an antonym.

7. **The correct answer is (D).** To *substantiate* is "to *support,* to verify." Choice (A) is incorrect because *repeal* is used in reference to laws and legal orders, not evidence. Choice (B) is incorrect because the question requires a verb and *ineffective* is an adjective. Choice (C) is incorrect because *applied* is not a synonym and doesn't make sense in this sentence.

8. **The correct answer is (B).** *Comparative* means "relating to, based on, or involving

comparison," and one meaning of *relative* is "in comparison." Choices (A), (C), and (D) are incorrect because *objective, subjective,* and *scientific* have no relation to *comparative.*

9. **The correct answer is (A).** To *assure* is "to promise or guarantee." Choice (B) is incorrect because while *instruct* makes sense, it's not a synonym for *assure,* and neither is choice (C), *deny.* Choice (D) is incorrect because *assail* means "to attack with words, to criticize."

10. **The correct answer is (A).** A *connoisseur* is an *expert.* Choice (B) is incorrect because while a connoisseur *tastes* wine, it's not a synonym, and neither is choice (C), a *procurer,* meaning "a person who obtains things." Choice (D) is incorrect because a *vendor,* or seller of goods and services, not a synonym either.

11. **The correct answer is (D).** To *spurn* is "to reject, to refuse, to decline." Choice (A) is incorrect because *accept* is the opposite of *spurn.* Choice (B) is incorrect because *extol* means "to praise," as does choice (C), *acclaim.* If you're not sure about an answer, but two of the choices are similar in meaning, you can eliminate them both.

12. **The correct answer is (D).** *Ceremoniously* means "*formally,* with ceremony and ritual." Choice (A) is incorrect because *without ritual* is the opposite of *ceremoniously.* Choice (B) is incorrect because *disrespectfully* is closer in meaning to that of an antonym for *ceremoniously* than a synonym. Choice (C) is incorrect because *serenely* may describe someone who is acting ceremoniously, but it is not a synonym.

13. **The correct answer is (B).** *Inordinate* and *excessive* are synonyms. Choice (A) is incorrect because *redundant* means "more than is needed or required" or "repetitive." Choice (C) is incorrect because *reasonable* is the opposite of *inordinate.* Choice (D) is incorrect because *exuberant* is a synonym for *excessive,* depending on the context, but not for *inordinate.*

14. **The correct answer is (C).** To *traverse* is "to cross." Choice (A) is incorrect because *patronized* makes no sense and is not a synonym for *traverse,* and neither is choice (B), *extended.* Choice (D) is incorrect because *augment* means "to add to, to enlarge."

15. **The correct answer is (D).** Pronunciation may make all the difference in finding the correct answer. *Entranced* doesn't mean "entered" in this context; it means "in a trance," that is, "delighted, enchanted." Choices (A) and (B) are incorrect because *summoned* and *impeded* are not synonyms for *enraptured.* Choice (C) is incorrect because *exonerated* means "freed from blame, accusation, or suspicion."

16. **The correct answer is (C).** *Contention* and *argument,* meaning "a line of reasoning," are synonyms. Choice (A) is incorrect because *realization* is not a synonym for *contention.* Choice (B) is incorrect because *contiguity* means "being adjacent, being so near as to be touching." Choice (D) is incorrect because *exhilaration* means "feeling joyful."

17. **The correct answer is (D).** *Consensus* is the same as a *collective opinion.* Choice (A) is incorrect because *stipulation* means "a condition, an agreement reached by contending parties." Choice (B) is incorrect because *regulation* has no relation to *consensus.* Choice (C) is incorrect because *conviction,* meaning "strong belief," is not a synonym for *consensus.*

18. **The correct answer is (A).** A *chronic* disease is a *long-lasting* one. Choices (B), (C), and (D) are incorrect because although each one—*serious, contagious, infectious*—refers to diseases, none is a synonym for *chronic.*

19. **The correct answer is (B).** To *abound* is "to be abundant." Choice (A) is incorrect because *remote* means "far away, isolated." Choices (C) and (D), *is significant* and *is inadequate,* are not synonyms for *abounds.*

20. **The correct answer is (D).** To *wax* is "to *increase* in size, intensity, etc." Choice (A) is incorrect because although *stirred* can mean "to excite strong feelings" and, therefore, may confuse you, it's not a synonym for *wax*. Choice (B) is incorrect because *wane* means "to decrease gradually in size, intensity, etc.," so it is an antonym of *waxed*. Choice (C) is incorrect because *vanished* means "to disappear."

21. **The correct answer is (C).** Something that is *void* is *empty*. The other choices are antonyms for *void*.

22. **The correct answer is (C).** An *appendage* is a body part that extends from the body, that is, not an internal part. Answer choices (A), (B), and (D) are internal parts of the body.

23. **The correct answer is (A).** To *risk* is "to *venture*." Choice (B) is incorrect because *squander* is "to waste," choice (D), so both are incorrect. Choice (C) is incorrect because *exhausted* has no relation to *risk*.

24. **The correct answer is (C).** To *pare* is "to remove the outer skin," that is, to *peel* a fruit. The other choices all relate to preparing fruit for consumption, but they are not synonyms for *pare*. Note that choices (A) and (D) are themselves synonyms, and since both can't be right, both must be incorrect.

25. **The correct answer is (A).** An *initiative*, meaning "the opening or first step in a series of actions," and an *enterprise*, meaning "a readiness to begin a new venture," are near synonyms. Choices (B) and (D), *energy* and *leadership*, can be synonyms for *initiative*, but not in this context. Choice (C) is incorrect because *zeal*, meaning "enthusiasm," is not a synonym.

26. **The correct answer is (B).** *Delineate* means "to describe in great detail," so *describe* is its synonym. Choice (A) is incorrect because *discredit* means "to damage the reputation of someone" or "to cause distrust or disbelief." Choice (C) is incorrect because *disprove* means "to show

something to be in error or false." Choice (D) is incorrect because *endorses* means "to approve."

27. **The correct answer is (A).** *Cartilage* is *tissue*. None of the other choices—*ligament, tendon*, and *membrane*—though related to the body are the same as cartilage.

28. **The correct answer is (C).** To *confirm* is "to *verify*, to show to be true." Choices (A), (B), and (D), *canceled, rescheduled*, and *recorded*, can be done with appointments, but none are synonyms for *confirm*.

29. **The correct answer is (B).** To *invalidate* something is "to *cancel*" it. Choice (A) is incorrect because *authorize* means "to approve" and is the opposite of *invalidate*. Choice (C) is incorrect because *contradict* means "to deny something" or "to express the opposite." Choice (D) is incorrect because *modify* is "to change in some way," but is not the same as invalidating.

30. **The correct answer is (B).** A *malfunction* is a problem, so the correct synonym is "*operating incorrectly*." Choice (A) is incorrect because if the engine was not working properly, it probably wasn't *operative*. Choices (C) and (D), *firing* and *igniting*, can be applied to engines, but neither is a synonym for *malfunctioning*.

31. **The correct answer is (D).** *Fraudulent* means "*deceitful*." Choice (A) is incorrect because *thorough* has no relation to *fraudulent*, and neither does choice (B), *extensive*. Choice (C), *legal*, is the opposite of *fraudulent*.

32. **The correct answer is (D).** *Competence* and *ability* are synonyms. Choice (A) is incorrect because *honesty* has no relation to *competence*. Choice (B) is incorrect because *punctuality* refers to being on time. Choice (C) is incorrect because *credibility* refers to trustworthiness and reliability.

33. **The correct answer is (A).** An *anthology* is a *collection of literary selections*. An anthology may contain an *annotated bibliography*, choice (B), but that is not

an anthology. Choices (C) and (D) are not synonyms for *anthology*.

34. **The correct answer is (D).** *Mobile* and *motile*, meaning "having the power to move," are synonyms. Choice (A) is incorrect because *movement* is a noun, and the question requires an adjective. Choice (B) is incorrect because while bacteria can be *deadly*, that is not a synonym for *mobile*. Choice (C) is incorrect because *migratory* means "nomadic," and this is not correct usage for *mobile*.

35. **The correct answer is (C).** *Wryly* means "dryly humorous, often using *irony*." Choice (A) is incorrect because *deceptively*, meaning "dishonestly," is not a synonym. Choice (B) is incorrect because wry humor is not the same as being *nasty*. Choice (D) is incorrect because *delightedly*, meaning "very pleased," is not a synonym.

Part B: Antonyms

1. A	9. A	17. A	25. A	33. C
2. C	10. D	18. C	26. C	34. A
3. A	11. B	19. C	27. D	35. D
4. D	12. A	20. A	28. A	36. A
5. B	13. D	21. D	29. B	37. C
6. A	14. A	22. B	30. A	38. B
7. C	15. C	23. B	31. B	39. A
8. B	16. B	24. D	32. C	40. D

1. **The correct answer is (A).** *Imperious* means "overbearing, domineering," so the opposite is *submissive*, meaning "passive, compliant, obedient." None of the other choices has any relation to *imperious*.

2. **The correct answer is (C).** *Capricious* means "given to whims, unpredictable, unstable," so *steadfast*, meaning "steady, firm and dependable," is the opposite. Choice (A) is incorrect because *whimsical* is a synonym. Choice (B) is incorrect because *judicious* means "having good judgement, prudent." Choice (D) is incorrect because *tranquil* means "peaceful, serene."

3. **The correct answer is (A).** A *cantankerous* person is a disagreeable and difficult person, whereas the opposite is a *pleasant* person. Choice (B) is incorrect because *dubious* means "doubtful." Neither *effec-* tive nor *awkward*, choices (C) and (D), are antonyms.

4. **The correct answer is (D).** *Forbearance* means "tolerance, patience," so *impatience* is an antonym. Choice (A), *indulgence*, is incorrect because it's a synonym. Choice (B) is incorrect because *pliancy* means "easily influenced" or "adaptable." Choice (C) is incorrect because *politeness* has no relation to *forbearance*.

5. **The correct answer is (B).** Something that is *haphazard* is done without care, in a casual or careless way. The opposite is something that is *premeditated,* or done with purpose and at least some planning. Choice (A) is incorrect because *inefficient* means "unable to do something effectively or competently" and is closer in meaning to haphazard than to its opposite. Choice (C), *unsatisfactory*, is incorrect because

it may be the result of something done haphazardly, but it's not an antonym. Choice (D) is incorrect because *blundering* means "making a stupid and often serious mistake."

6. **The correct answer is (A).** *Efficacy* means "effectiveness, efficiency," so *ineffectiveness* is an antonym. Choice (B), *efficiency*, is incorrect because it's a synonym. Choices (C) and (D) are incorrect because *value* and *success* are near synonyms for *efficacy*.

7. **The correct answer is (C).** Something that is *chimerical* is highly imaginative or fanciful, and something that is *factual* is the opposite. Choice (A) is incorrect because *philosophical* has no relation to *chimerical*, and neither does *elite*, choice (B), meaning "a group of people with some superior quality or position in society." Choice (D) is incorrect because *unimpressive* has no relation to *chimerical*.

8. **The correct answer is (B).** To *repress* is "to restrain, to keep under control," so *liberate*, meaning "to free," is the opposite. Choice (A) is incorrect because *reserve* is "to keep back for future use" or "to set something apart for a particular use." Choice (C), *thrust*, means "to push with force" or "to impose on something." Choice (D) is incorrect because "to precipitate" is "to cause to happen."

9. **The correct answer is (A).** *Abominable* means "completely unpleasant or disagreeable," so *agreeable* is the opposite. Choice (B) is incorrect because *loathsome* is a synonym for *abominable*. Choice (C) is incorrect because *sufficient* has no relation to *abominable*, and neither does choice (D), *degrading*, meaning "humiliating someone, shaming."

10. **The correct answer is (D).** *Unethical*, that is, having no ethics or code of right and wrong, is the opposite of *scrupulous*, "having principles, being moral." Choice (A) is incorrect because *vulgar* means "crude, lacking good manners." Choice (B) is incorrect because *feasible* means

"possible, able to be achieved." Choice (C) is incorrect because *pompous* means "self-important, exaggerated sense of self."

11. **The correct answer is (B).** *Antecedent* as an adjective indicates something that comes before, and *subsequent* indicates something that comes after. Choice (A) is incorrect because *previous* indicates something occurring before. Choice (C) is incorrect because *foregoing* means "previous." Choice (D) is incorrect because *propitious* means "favorable."

12. **The correct answer is (A).** Something that is *ponderous* is heavy, awkward, and dull, so *delicate* is an antonym. Choice (B) is incorrect because *potent* means "powerful." Choice (C) is incorrect because *supportive* has no relation to *ponderous*. Choice (D) is incorrect because *massive* is a synonym for *ponderous*.

13. **The correct answer is (D).** *Supplication* means "a humble request, a plea," so *disdain*, meaning "scorn, a feeling or show of contempt" is an antonym. Choice (A) is incorrect because *worship* can be a near synonym for *supplication* when the latter means "prayer." Choice (B) is incorrect because *compassion* has no relation to *supplication*. Choice (C) is incorrect because *entreaty*, meaning "a plea," is a synonym for *supplication*.

14. **The correct answer is (A).** The opposite of *positive* is *negative*. None of the other choices has a relation to *positive*.

15. **The correct answer is (C).** *Renegade* as an adjective means "disloyal," so an antonym is *loyal*. Choice (A) is incorrect because *constant* has no relation to *renegade*. Choice (B) is incorrect because *extricate*, meaning "to disentangle, to get out of a difficulty," is a verb, and the answer requires an adjective. Choice (D) is incorrect because *heretical* is a near synonym for *renegade*.

16. **The correct answer is (B).** To *disregard* is "to pay no attention to, to ignore," so "to *attend to*" is an antonym. None of the other choices are antonyms for *disregard*.

17. **The correct answer is (A).** *Wrath* is anger, so *delight*, meaning "extreme pleasure or joy," is an antonym. Choice (B) is incorrect because *travail* means "very hard work." Choice (C) is incorrect because *frivolity* means "not being serious, silliness." Choice (D) is incorrect because detriment means "damage, harm" or "something that causes damage or harm."

18. **The correct answer is (C).** *Tedious* means "tiresome, boring, dull," so *stimulating* is an antonym. Choice (A) is incorrect because *ungainly* means "awkward." Choice (B) is incorrect because *imperative* means "urgent." Choice (D) is incorrect because *suitable* is not an antonym for *tedious*.

19. **The correct answer is (C).** To *embody* is "to be an example of, to give form to an idea," so *dissociate*, meaning "to separate, to differentiate," is the only possible antonym in the list. Choice (A) is incorrect because *impel* means "to force." Choice (B) is incorrect because *fuse* means "to merge, to combine." Choice (D) is incorrect because *collect* has no relation to *embody*.

20. **The correct answer is (A).** *Deferrable* means "able to be put off or postponed," so *urgent* is an antonym. Choice (B) is incorrect because *furtive* means "secretive." Choice (C) is incorrect because *inclined* means "having a preference or tendency." Choice (D) is incorrect because *deniable* means "possible to contradict, able to be denied."

21. **The correct answer is (D).** *Homogenous* means "consisting of elements that are all the same," whereas *heterogeneous* means "consisting of elements that are different." Choice (A) is incorrect because *invariable* means "unchanging." Choice (B) is incorrect because *homosexual* refers to a sexual orientation. Choice (C) is incorrect because *importunate* means "insistent, demanding."

22. **The correct answer is (B).** An *adherent* is a supporter or follower of a cause, whereas a *repudiator* is one who rejects authority. Choice (A) is incorrect because a *disciple* is a follower, so it is a synonym for *adherent*. Choice (C) is incorrect because a *soothsayer* is one who predicts the future. Choice (D) is incorrect because a *hypocrite* is a person who pretends to be something he or she is not or to hold beliefs and opinions that the person does not.

23. **The correct answer is (B).** The opposite of *crude* is *refined*. Choice (A) is incorrect because *barbarous* is similar to *crude*. Choice (C) is incorrect because *obscure* means "unclear, vague" or "secret, hidden." Choice (D) is incorrect because *covetous* means "greedy."

24. **The correct answer is (D).** The opposite of *irrational* is *sensible*. Choice (A) is incorrect because *cynical* means "believing the worst of people." Choice (B) is incorrect because *sharp* has no relation to *irrational*. Choice (C) is incorrect because *prevalent* means "widespread" or "predominant."

25. **The correct answer is (A).** *Graphic* has several meanings, but the one that works in this question is "describes in detail" because the only word that works as an antonym is *vague*. Choice (B) is incorrect because *illustrative* means "acting as an example or illustration of something," so it's similar in meaning to *graphic*, Choice (C) is incorrect because *forcible* has no relation to *graphic*. Choice (D) is incorrect because *glacial* refers to glaciers.

26. **The correct answer is (C).** To *devastate* is "to destroy," so "to *renovate*," meaning "to restore, to repair, to remodel," is an antonym. Choices (A), (B), and (D)—*tolerate, obstruct,* and *promote*—have no relation to *devastate*.

27. **The correct answer is (D).** *Stringent* means "exacting," so rule out choices (A) and (B), *exacting* and *tough*. Choice (C) is incorrect because *influential* has no relation to *stringent*. Choice (D), *flexible*, is the only possible answer.

28. **The correct answer is (A).** To *acquiesce* is "to agree," so *contest*, meaning "to argue, to dispute," is an antonym. Choice (B) is

incorrect because *invest* has no relation to *acquiesce*. Choice (C) is incorrect because *dismiss* means "to discharge, to let go." Choice (D) is incorrect because *supply* is not an antonym for *acquiesce*.

29. **The correct answer is (B).** *Brevity* refers to being concise or of short duration, so *length* is an antonym. Choice (A) is incorrect because an abbreviation is a shortened form of a word or phrase. Choice (C) is incorrect because *ramification* means "consequence of an action or event." Choice (D) is incorrect because *delusion* means "a misconception, mistaken idea or opinion."

30. **The correct answer is (A).** To *flaunt* is "to show off," whereas *disavow* is "to deny knowledge of something, to refuse to acknowledge." Choice (B) is incorrect because *conserve* is "to save." Choice (C) is incorrect because *blight* is "to have a bad effect on something." Choice (D) is incorrect because *astonish* is not an antonym for *flaunt*.

31. **The correct answer is (B).** *Cultivate* means "to grow" or "to nurture," so eliminate choice (D). Choice (B) is correct because *stifle* means "to smother, to suppress." Choice (A) is incorrect because *restore* has no relation to *cultivate*, and neither does choice (C), *reinstate*.

32. **The correct answer is (C).** The opposite of *dilate* is *constrict*. Choice (A) is incorrect because *negate* has no relation to *dilate*. Choice (B) is incorrect because *abet* means "to aid." Choice (D) is incorrect because *suspend* is not an antonym of *dilate*.

33. **The correct answer is (C).** *Befitting* means "appropriate," so *inappropriate* is an antonym. Choice (A) is incorrect because *enhancing* means "adding to, making greater by making more beautiful, valuable, or effective." Choice (B) is incorrect because *conciliatory* means "appeasing, overcoming distrust." Choice (D) is incorrect because *elegant* is not an antonym for befitting.

34. **The correct answer is (A).** To *be coherent* is "to be organized, clear, rational," so *illogical* is an antonym. Choice (B) is incorrect because *consecutive* means "following one after the other, successive." Choice (C) is incorrect because *cognizant* means "aware, knowledgeable." Choice (D) is incorrect because *courtly* means "mannerly."

35. **The correct answer is (D).** *Paltry* means "meager, insignificant," so *impressive* is an antonym. Choice (A) is incorrect because *political* has no relation to *paltry*. Choice (B) is incorrect because *complaisant* means "polite" or "willing to do favors." Choice (C) is incorrect because *clever* has no relation to *paltry*.

36. **The correct answer is (A).** *Bucolic* means "rustic, having to do with the country," so *urban*, having to with cities, is the opposite. Choice (B) is incorrect because *gallant* means "stylish" or "brave, courageous," which makes it a synonym for choice (C), *valiant*. Choice (D) is incorrect because *functional* means "useful, practical."

37. **The correct answer is (C).** *Extravagant* means "excessive, unrestrained, wasteful," so *frugal*, meaning "thrifty," is an antonym. Choice (A) is incorrect because *coarse* means "rough" or "crude, vulgar." Choice (B) is incorrect because *superior* has no relation to extravagant, and neither has choice (D), *typical*.

38. **The correct answer is (B).** *Leniency* means "mercifulness, compassion," so *severity* is an antonym. Choice (A) is incorrect because *indulgence* is a synonym for *leniency*. Choice (C) is incorrect because *embroilment* means "involvement in an argument." Choice (D) is incorrect because *inequality* has no relation to *leniency*.

39. **The correct answer is (A).** *Manifest* means "clearly apparent, obvious," so *latent*, meaning "not evident, potential," is an antonym. Choice (B) is incorrect because *oblivious* means "forgetful" as well as "unaware." Choice (C) is incorrect because *terminal* means "being at the end,

final." Choice (D) is incorrect because *languid* means "weak, lacking energy."

40. **The correct answer is (D).** *Plebeian* means "of the common people," whereas *patrician* refers to the aristocracy or elite, or having good manners and upbringing. Choice (A) is incorrect because *congenial* means "pleasant, easy to get along with."

Choice (B) is incorrect because *ignoble* means "common, not noble," so it's similar in meaning to *plebeian*. Choice (C) is incorrect because *scientific* has no relation to *plebeian*.

Part C: Verbal Analogies

1. C	6. C	11. B	16. B	21. C
2. A	7. B	12. A	17. C	22. C
3. B	8. A	13. C	18. B	23. C
4. C	9. B	14. A	19. B	24. B
5. D	10. C	15. B	20. C	25. B

1. **The correct answer is (C).** This is an association analogy. *Cat* and *dog* are often associated and so are *cup* and *saucer.* Choice (A) is incorrect because a *knife* is associated with a fork, but not a cup. Choices (B) and (D) are incorrect because *coffee* and *cream* may be found in a cup, but they are not associated with *cup* the way cats are with dogs.

2. **The correct answer is (A).** *Saline* is *salty* and *sugary* is *sweet* in this characteristic analogy. Choice (B) is incorrect because *stale* isn't a quality of sugar. Choice (C) is incorrect because the answer requires a quality, or adjective, and *bread* is a thing. Choice (D) is incorrect because *insipid*, meaning "not tasty," isn't a quality of associated with sugar.

3. **The correct answer is (B).** *Flannel* is made out of *wool,* and *bricks* are made out of *clay.* Choice (D) is incorrect because *mortar* is used to hold bricks in place, but bricks are not made of mortar. Choices (A) and (C), *wood* and *stone,* have no relation to bricks.

4. **The correct answer is (C).** This is a synonym analogy. *Contemporary,* meaning "current," is similar to *present,* and *future*

is similar to *eventual,* meaning "at some indefinite time in the future." Choice (A), *past,* is incorrect because this is not an antonym analogy. Choice (B) is incorrect because *posterity* means "future generations." Choice (D) is incorrect because *ancient* is past.

5. **The correct answer is (D).** The first pair sets up an analogy. The *moon* revolves around *Earth,* and *Earth* revolves around the *sun.* None of the other answer choices fulfills this association of Earth with an action.

6. **The correct answer is (C).** This is an antonym analogy. *Acute* pain is pain that begins abruptly and is of short duration, whereas *chronic* pain is long lasting. The word *intense* mirrors *acute,* so the answer must be similar to *chronic.* The only answer choice that is similar is *persistent.* Choice (A) is incorrect because *sardonic* means "bitterly mocking, sarcastic." Choice (B) is incorrect because *tonic* means "a kind of medicine" or "producing and restoring normal muscle or tissue tone." Choice (D) is incorrect because *pretty* has no relation to *intense.*

7. **The correct answer is (B).** This is a part-to-whole analogy. A *peak* is the top of a *mountain,* and a *floor* is the bottom of a *canyon.* Choice (A) is incorrect because a *ceiling* has nothing to do with topography, that is, physical geography. Choice (C) is incorrect because the bottom of a *river* is a riverbed. Choice (D) is incorrect because a *cliff* is a steep, rugged, high face of rock

8. **The correct answer is (A).** The first pair sets up an antonym analogy. *East* is the opposite of *west* as *northwest* is the opposite of *southeast.* Choice (D), *northeast,* is tempting, but not the better answer when compared to southeast, which is both south and east of northwest. Choice (B) is incorrect because *southwest* is only south of northwest. Choice (C) is incorrect because *north* is not as specific as the other answers.

9. **The correct answer is (B).** This is a cause-and-effect analogy. *Gasoline* is made from *petroleum,* and *sugar* is made from *cane,* that is, sugar cane. Choice (A) is incorrect because *oil* relates to petroleum, not sugar. Choices (C) and (D) are incorrect because although sugar comes from a *plant* and is *sweet,* there is no cause and effect involved in either answer.

10. **The correct answer is (C).** In this synonym analogy, *deference,* meaning "courtesy regard, submission or courteous compliance with another's wishes," and *respect* are synonyms. A synonym for *contempt* is *discourtesy.* Choice (A) is incorrect because *esteem,* meaning "holding someone in high regard," is a synonym for *deference* and an antonym for *contempt.* Choice (B) is incorrect because *capitulation* means "giving up, surrendering." Choice (D) is incorrect because *tendency* means "attitude, a leaning toward someone or something, an inclination."

11. **The correct answer is (B).** This is a characteristic or object-to-quality analogy. A *slope* has an *incline,* and a *plane* is *flat.* It is true that a plane is *dimensional,* choice (A), in that it is one-dimensional, but choice (B) is a better answer because

it is more specific to what a plane is—flat. Choice (C) is incorrect because a plane may be any of several one-dimensional shapes, including *square,* choice (D), and *rectangular,* choice (D).

12. **The correct answer is (A).** This is an antonym analogy. An *edge* is the opposite of a *center,* and *effusive,* meaning "unrestrained, exuberant," is the opposite of *unemotional.* Choice (B) is incorrect because *exuberant* is a synonym for *effusive.* Choice (C) is incorrect because *eclectic* means "choosing from a variety of ideas or styles." Choice (D) is incorrect because *eccentricity* means "unconventional behavior, nonconformity."

13. **The correct answer is (C).** The first pair sets up a person-to-action relationship. A *procrastinator delays* and a *mentor advises.* Choices (A) and (B) are incorrect because even though a mentor advises a *mentee* and may be a kind of *teacher,* the answer requires a verb, not a noun. Choice (D) is incorrect because *measuring* is not a particular action of a mentor.

14. **The correct answer is (A).** This is a synonym analogy. *Sophistication* means "worldliness, possessing finesse," and *finesse* means "skillful, tactful" as well as "elegant, polished in style and manners." Among the list, the only synonym for *ineptitude,* meaning "lacking in skill or ability, clumsiness, incompetence" is *inefficiency.* Choice (B) is incorrect because *artistry* might be considered an antonym for *ineptitude.* Choice (C) is incorrect because *trickiness* has no relation to *ineptitude.* Choice (D) is incorrect because *insatiability* means "impossible to satisfy."

15. **The correct answer is (B).** This is a straightforward person-to-occupation relationship. A *captain* runs a *ship,* and a *principal* runs a *school.* None of the other choices offer a valid site for a principal to manage.

16. **The correct answer is (B).** This is a characteristic analogy. A dime is made

out of silver and a penny is made out of *copper*. None of the other choices offer an ingredient, though all three—*mint, currency,* and *value*—relate to a penny in some way. Choice (A), *mint,* is where money is made.

17. **The correct answer is (C).** This is a grammatical analogy. *Reversion* is a noun related to the verb *revert,* meaning "to return to a former condition, practice, belief, etc." *Sympathy* is a noun related to the verb *sympathize.* Choice (A) is incorrect because *sympathetic* is an adjective, and the question requires a noun. Choice (B) is incorrect because *symposium,* meaning "conference," has no relation to *sympathize.* Choice (D) is incorrect because *sympathizing* is an adjective, and the question requires a noun.

18. **The correct answer is (B).** This is another grammatical analogy. *Regressive* is an adjective related to the verb *regress,* meaning "to go backward." *Sterile* is an adjective related to the verb *sterilize.* Choice (A) is incorrect because *sterilization* is a noun, just like choices (C) and (D), *sterility* and *sterilizer.*

19. **The correct answer is (B).** In this antonym analogy, *down* is the opposite of *up* and *age* is the opposite of *youth.* None of the other choices is related to age.

20. **The correct answer is (C).** In this grammar analogy, *mine* is the possessive pronoun for *I* and *his* is the possessive pronoun for *man.* Choice (A) is incorrect because *men* is a plural noun, and the question requires a possessive pronoun. Choice (B) is incorrect because *man's* could be a possessive adjective or a possessive noun, and the answer requires a possessive pronoun to parallel the first pair. Choice (D) is incorrect because *hers* is a possessive pronoun for a female antecedent, and the question offers a male antecedent in *man.*

21. **The correct answer is (C).** This is a synonym analogy. *Disloyal* and *faithless* are synonyms, and *imperfection* and *foible,* meaning "minor weakness of character, an

eccentricity" are synonyms. Choice (A) is incorrect because *faithful* has no relation to *imperfection,* and neither does choice (B), *depression.* Choice (D) is incorrect because *decrepitude* means "being worn out, deteriorated because of old age or use."

22. **The correct answer is (C).** This is an object-to-use analogy. A *necklace* is made of pearls, and a chain is made of *links.* Choice (B) is incorrect because a *prisoner* has no relation to a jewelry analogy. Choices (A) and (D) are incorrect because a locket and a clasp are found on a chain, but they are not what a chain is made of.

23. **The correct answer is (C).** This is a part-to-whole analogy. A *drift* is made of *snow,* and a *dune* is made of *sand.* Choice (A) is incorrect because a dune is a small *hill;* a dune isn't made out of a hill. Choices (B) and (D), *rain* and *hail,* have no relation to a dune.

24. **The correct answer is (B).** This is a purpose analogy. The primary purpose of a *bank* is to hold *deposits,* and the primary purpose of a *hospital* is to provide *care.* Choices (A), (C), and (D) are incorrect because *blood, surgery,* and *tests* are ways that hospitals provide care, which is the primary purpose.

25. **The correct answer is (B).** In this category-to-example analogy, a *schooner* is type of *vessel,* or ship, and a *persimmon* is a type of *fruit.* Choices (A), (C), and (D) are incorrect because a *machine,* an *engine,* and a *vehicle* have no relation to a persimmon. If you weren't sure what a persimmon is, you could figure out that because choices (A), (C), and (D) are similar, the odd answer must be the correct one.

Mathematics

OVERVIEW

This section's review of mathematics and the numerical ability tests include the following: basic quantitative problems involving addition, subtraction, multiplication, and division; calculations including decimals, fractions, percentages, and measurements; basic operations in algebra and geometry; and quantitative comparison questions. Throughout the exercises, emphasis is placed on verbal problems in order to prepare you for the interpretations and methods required for problem solving. The explanatory answers and problem solutions provide a variety of opportunities to review or to learn the numerical processes included on the pre-nursing examinations.

Study the guidelines listed below; they provide the major concepts needed for successful performance on your mathematics examination.

TIPS FOR STUDYING MATHEMATICS

In order to perform well on mathematics tests, it is important to be well prepared. To prepare, you must know what material will be covered on the test. The mathematics guidelines and practice exercises in this book provide a review of materials that are covered on the mathematics section of the nursing school entrance examination. You can maximize your performance on the test by following the eight steps below.

1. Choose a place to study where you won't be distracted.

2. Set aside adequate time to study. Try to set aside at least one hour for each study session. Study and practice each day if possible. Make a study schedule and stick to it.

3. Give your full focus and attention to your studies.

4. Read the explanatory material before doing any practice tests. Make sure that you understand what you're reading. Review information that you don't understand, and use other references when necessary.

5. Take the practice tests under test conditions. Read the instructions carefully. Complete tests in the amount of time suggested.

6. Compare your answers with those provided in the book. Carefully review answers to questions that you missed.

7. Seek help if you don't understand a problem after several tries.

8. Review regularly, and practice, practice, practice.

Test-Taking Tips

- Read test instructions carefully. Note the amount of time allotted for completion of the test and pace yourself accordingly.

- Read each problem carefully. Make sure you understand the concepts and terms being used. Try to restate the problem in your own words.

- Simplify the problem by breaking it down into smaller parts.

- Determine what information is given and what is to be solved.

- Determine whether there is sufficient information given to solve the problem.

- Eliminate extraneous information.

- Choose a strategy for solving the problem.

- Express your answer in the number of units requested. You may be asked to express your answer in terms of minutes, feet, or hours, or you may be asked to write your answer as a decimal or fraction.

- Check your solution to determine if it is reasonable. Does your answer appear to be unreasonably large or small?

- Don't spend too much time on a question that you find difficult. Move on to the next question and return to questions you have skipped after you complete the other test questions.

- Try an alternative strategy if the one you used didn't work.

- Review your answers if you finish before time is up. Check your computations very carefully.

MATHEMATICS REVIEW

Whole Numbers

Whole numbers have **place-value** based on units of ten (decimal system). Therefore, it is important that all whole numbers, including zeros, are lined up correctly in columns when adding and subtracting.

Example:

- Place values for the whole number 5,264 are illustrated below.

$5,264 = (5 \times 1,000) + (2 \times 100) + (6 \times 10) + (4 \times 1)$

- Numbers are lined up according to place values in the following **addition** and **subtraction** examples.

$$\begin{array}{r} 5,264 \\ +478 \\ \hline 5,742 \end{array} \qquad \begin{array}{r} 5,264 \\ -478 \\ \hline 4,786 \end{array}$$

Use **multiplication** to determine the value of several quantities with the same value if the value of one quantity is given.

Example: If one loaf of bread costs $0.80, how much will three loaves of bread cost? Multiply 3 times $0.80. The answer is $2.40.

When multiplying, be certain to include all zeros and to keep the columns in line.

Example:

$$\begin{array}{r} 3,600 \\ \times \quad 507 \\ \hline 25,200 \\ 0000 \\ 18,000 \\ \hline 1,825,200 \end{array}$$

Use **division** to determine the value of one quantity when the value of several quantities is given.

Example: Three loaves of bread cost $2.40. How much will one loaf cost? Divide 3 into $2.40. The answer is $0.80 (3 is the divisor, $2.40 is the dividend, and the quotient is $0.80).

Divisibility Tips

- If the last digit of a number is 0, 2, 4, 6, or 8, the number is divisible by 2.

- If the last digit of a number ends in 0 or 5, the number is divisible by 5.

- If the sum of the digits of a number is divisible by 3, the number is divisible by 3.

Example: The sum of the digits of 234 is $2 + 3 + 4 = 9$. Since 9 is divisible by 3, we know that 234 is also divisible by 3 ($234 \div 3 = 78$).

- If the sum of the digits of a number is divisible by 9, the number is divisible by 9. In the example above, it was shown that the sum of the digits of 234 is 9. By the above rule, we know that 234 is divisible by 9.

- If the number represented by the last two digits of a number is divisible by 4, the number is divisible by 4.

Example: 32 is the number represented by the last two digits of 232. Since 32 is divisible by 4, the number 232 is divisible by 4.

- Note that it is not possible to divide by zero.

- A **prime number** is any whole number other than 0 or 1 that is only divisible by itself and by 1.

Example: 17 is a prime number since it is only divisible by 1 and 17. The whole numbers 2, 3, 5, 7, and 11 are the first five prime numbers.

- Divisibility rules can be used to find the prime factors of whole numbers.

Example: 24 is divisible by 2 (last digit is 4) and is divisible by 3 (sum of digits is 6).

$$24 = 2 \times 2 \times 2 \times 3$$
$$= 2^3 \times 3$$

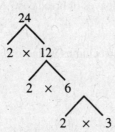

Two methods for determining the prime factors of a number are illustrated above. In each method, keep dividing until your quotient is a prime number.

- The **average** of a set of numbers is the sum of the numbers divided by the number of numbers added.

Example: The average of the numbers 10, 14, 17, and 23 is $\dfrac{10+14+17+23}{4} = \dfrac{64}{4} = 16$

- The **square** of a number is the product obtained when a number is multiplied by itself.

Example: $4^2 = 4 \times 4 = 16$

- The **square root** ($\sqrt{\ }$) of a given number is the number that yields the given number when multiplied by itself.

Example: $\sqrt{16} = 4$, since $4 \times 4 = 16$

- The square of any whole number is called a **perfect square.** Conversely, the square root of a perfect square is a whole number.

Example: $4^2 = 16$ (a perfect square); thus $\sqrt{16} = 4$.

- If a number is not a perfect square, you can **approximate the square root** of the number when a calculator is not available.

Example: Approximate the square root of 90 $(\sqrt{90})$.

1. Estimate the square root of the given number. Since 90 is between 81 and 100, the square root of 90 will be between 9 and 10. A possible estimate is 9.30.

2. Divide the given number by the estimated square root.

3. $90 \div 9.30 = 9.68$

4. Find the average of the resulting quotient and the estimated square root.

5. $\dfrac{9.68 + 9.30}{2} = 9.49$ (9.49 is the first approximation for $\sqrt{90}$)

6. Divide the given number by the average (first approximation) found above.

7. $90 \div 9.49 = 9.48$

8. Find the **average of the divisor** (first approximation) and the quotient found in step 4.

9. $\dfrac{9.49 + 9.48}{2} = 9.485$

10. The approximate square root of 90 is 9.485.

11. This process may be repeated to get a more accurate estimate of the square root of a number.

- To add or subtract **radicals** (numbers expressed as square roots), the **radicands** (numbers under the radical) must be the same.

Example: $4\sqrt{12} + 3\sqrt{12} = 7\sqrt{12}$

Example: If the radicands are not the same, simplify the radicals and then see if they can be combined.

$$3\sqrt{12} - 8\sqrt{3} = 3(\sqrt{4} \times \sqrt{3}) - 8\sqrt{3} \quad \text{(12 can be factored as 4 × 3)}$$
$$= 3 \times 2\sqrt{3} - 8\sqrt{3} \quad \text{(take } \sqrt{4}\text{, which equals 2)}$$
$$= 6\sqrt{3} - 8\sqrt{3}$$
$$= -2\sqrt{3}$$

Fractions

A fraction is a part of something. A fraction is expressed using two terms: a **numerator,** which is the number above the fraction line, and a **denominator**, which is the number below the fraction line.

In the fraction $\dfrac{3}{4}$, the numerator is 3 and the denominator is 4.

A **proper fraction** is one whose numerator is less than its denominator. An **improper fraction** has a numerator that is equal to or greater than its denominator.

$\dfrac{4}{5}$ is a proper fraction, and $\dfrac{7}{3}$ is an improper fraction.

An improper fraction can be expressed as a **mixed number,** which has both a whole and a fractional part. (Divide the denominator into the numerator to get the whole part. The remainder will be the numerator, and the divisor will be the denominator of the fractional part.)

Example: $\frac{7}{3} = 2\frac{1}{3}$

7 divided by 3 gives a quotient of 2 and a remainder of 1.

Reducing Fractions

Factor the numerator and denominator into prime factors and divide the numerator and denominator by the common factors. (The value of a fraction is unchanged when the numerator and denominator are multiplied or divided by the same number.)

Example: $\frac{35}{55} = \frac{7 \times 5}{11 \times 5} = \frac{7}{11}$

Note that the numerator and denominator were divided by 5.

Multiplying Fractions

To multiply two fractions, multiply the two numerators to get the numerator of the product of the two fractions, and multiply the two denominators to get the denominator of the product of the fractions. Then simplify the resulting fraction by reducing it to lowest terms and/or by changing it to a mixed number.

Example: $\frac{6}{9} \times \frac{3}{8} = \frac{18}{72} = \frac{\cancel{2} \times \cancel{3} \times \cancel{3}}{2 \times 2 \times \cancel{2} \times \cancel{3} \times \cancel{3}} = \frac{1}{4}$

Dividing Fractions

To divide two fractions, invert the divisor, then multiply the two fractions and simplify.

Examples: $\frac{9}{20} \div \frac{3}{4} = \frac{9}{20} \times \frac{4}{3} = \frac{36}{60} = \frac{\cancel{2} \times \cancel{2} \times \cancel{3} \times 3}{\cancel{2} \times \cancel{2} \times \cancel{3} \times 5} = \frac{3}{5}$

$2\frac{2}{3} \div 4 = \frac{8}{3} \times \frac{1}{4} = \frac{8}{12} = \frac{\cancel{2} \times \cancel{2} \times 2}{\cancel{2} \times \cancel{2} \times 3} = \frac{2}{3}$

Note that the mixed number $2\frac{2}{3}$ was changed to the improper fraction $\frac{8}{3}$, and the inversion of the whole number 4, which equals $\frac{4}{1}$, is $\frac{1}{4}$.

Adding and Subtracting Fractions

TIP

To add or subtract fractions quickly, remember that a sum can be found by adding the two cross-products and putting this answer over the denominator product.

To add or subtract fractions with the **same**, or common, denominator, keep the common denominator and add or subtract the numerators of the fractions.

Examples: $\frac{7}{9} + \frac{4}{9} = \frac{11}{9} = 1\frac{2}{9}$

$\frac{15}{32} - \frac{5}{32} = \frac{10}{32} = \frac{5}{16}$

To add or subtract fractions with different denominators, express the fractions as equivalent fractions with a common denominator. The **lowest common denominator (LCD)** is the smallest number that can be divided evenly by the denominators of the given fractions. To find the lowest common denominator (LCD) of two fractions, first express each denominator as a product of its prime factors. The lowest common denominator will be the number formed by multiplying each prime factor the largest number of times it occurs in the factorization of the denominators.

Example: $\frac{5}{9} + \frac{7}{12} = \frac{20}{36} + \frac{21}{36} = \frac{41}{36} = 1\frac{5}{36}$

Since $9 = 3 \times 3$ and $12 = 3 \times 4$, the lowest common denominator of 9 and 12 is

$3 \times 3 \times 4 = 36$.

Example: $\frac{7}{24} - \frac{9}{150}$

$150 = 2 \times 3 \times 5 \times 5$

$24 = 2 \times 2 \times 2 \times 3$

The largest number of times that 2 appears as a factor is 3 and the largest number of times that 5 appears as a factor is 2. 3 appears as a factor only once in each of the factorizations.

Thus, the lowest common denominator of the two fractions is 600.

$2 \times 2 \times 2 \times 3 \times 5 \times 5 = 600$

$\frac{7}{24} - \frac{9}{150} = \frac{7}{24} \times \frac{25}{25} - \frac{9}{150} \times \frac{4}{4} = \frac{175}{600} - \frac{36}{600} = \frac{139}{600}$

Thus, $\frac{7}{24} - \frac{9}{150} = \frac{175}{600} - \frac{36}{600} = \frac{139}{600}$

Example: $4\frac{2}{3} - 1\frac{3}{4} = 4\frac{8}{12} - 1\frac{9}{12}$

Since $\frac{9}{12}$ is greater than $\frac{8}{12}$, $4\frac{8}{12}$ is changed to $3 + 1 + \frac{8}{12}$.

(note that $1 = \frac{12}{12}$)

$= 3 + \frac{12}{12} + \frac{8}{12}$

$= 3 + \frac{20}{12}$ or $3\frac{20}{12}$

then $4\frac{2}{3} - 1\frac{3}{4}$

$= 4\frac{8}{12} - 1\frac{9}{12}$

$= 3\frac{20}{12} - 1\frac{9}{12}$

$= 2\frac{11}{12}$

Comparison of Fractions

To determine which of two fractions is larger, change the two fractions to equivalent fractions by expressing them as fractions with a common denominator and then comparing the numerators of the fractions. The fraction with the larger numerator is the larger fraction.

Example: Which is larger, $\frac{5}{6}$ or $\frac{7}{8}$?

24 is a common denominator for the two fractions, hence $\frac{5}{6} = \frac{20}{24}$ and $\frac{7}{8} = \frac{21}{24}$. Since

$\frac{21}{24}$ is larger than $\frac{20}{24}$, $\frac{7}{8}$ is larger than $\frac{5}{6}$.

Decimals

A common fraction can be expressed as a decimal. For example: $\frac{1}{2} = \frac{5}{10} = 0.5$. Each common fraction has an equivalent decimal form.

To change a common fraction to a decimal, divide the numerator of the fraction by the denominator.

Example: $\frac{3}{8} = .375$

$$
\begin{array}{r}
.375 \\
8\overline{)3.000} \\
\underline{24} \\
60 \\
\underline{56} \\
40 \\
\underline{40} \\
0
\end{array}
$$

When a decimal is changed to a fraction, the digits after the decimal point become the numerator. The denominator is 1 followed by as many zeros as there are decimal places. (The denominator can also be determined by raising 10 to a power. The power is the number of decimal places in the number.)

An alternate method for changing a decimal to a common fraction is to count the number of decimal places after the decimal. One decimal place represents tenths; two decimal places, hundredths; three decimal places, thousandths; and so on. The numerical part of the decimal indicates how many tenths, hundredths, thousandths, etc., there are.

Example: $0.540 = \frac{540}{1,000}$ (Note that $1,000 = 10^3$. There are 3 decimal places in the number so the power is 3.)

Example: $0.48 = \frac{48}{100}$ (There are 48 hundredths)

Adding and Subtracting Decimals

Arrange the decimals vertically with the decimal points aligned under each other. (Express whole numbers as decimals by appending a decimal point at the end of the number and adding as many zeros as desired, e.g., $23 = 23.0$.)

Example: Subtract 2.715 from 4

$$
\begin{array}{r}
4.000 \\
-\ 2.715 \\
\hline
1.285
\end{array}
$$

Example: Add $11.3 + 0.968 + 0.24 + 3$

$$
\begin{array}{r}
11.300 \\
.968 \\
.240 \\
+\ \ 3.000 \\
\hline
15.508
\end{array}
$$

Multiplying Decimals

To multiply decimals, multiply as you would with whole numbers. The number of decimal places in the product is the sum of the number of decimal places in the two numbers being multiplied.

Example: Multiply 2.47 times 0.315, that is,

$$
\begin{array}{r}
2.47 \\
.315 \\
\hline
1235 \\
247 \\
741 \\
\hline
.77805
\end{array}
$$

There are 2 decimal places in 2.47 and 3 in 0.315; therefore, there are 5 decimal places in the product of the two numbers. The product is 0.77805.

Dividing Decimals

When a decimal is divided by a whole number, the decimal point in the quotient should be aligned with the decimal point in the dividend. Divide as you would with whole numbers.

Example: 0.264 divided by 12

$$
\begin{array}{r}
.022 \\
12\overline{)\,.264} \\
24 \\
24 \\
24 \\
0
\end{array}
$$

To divide by a decimal, multiply the divisor by the multiple of 10 that will make the divisor a whole number, then multiply the dividend by the same multiple of 10. Divide as you would with whole numbers.

Example: 2.752 divided by 0.16

$$
.16\overline{)\,2.752}
$$

Multiply the divisor and dividend by 100 to get a new divisor of 16 and dividend of 275.2.

$$
\begin{array}{r}
17.2 \\
16\overline{)\,275.2} \\
16 \\
\hline
115 \\
112 \\
\hline
32 \\
32 \\
\hline
0
\end{array}
$$

Percents

Percent means "by the hundredths." A percent can be expressed as a fraction with a denominator of 100.

$$63\% = \frac{63}{100}$$

Converting decimals and fractions to percents and vice versa

Example: To convert a decimal to a percent, multiply the decimal by 100.

$$0.134 = 0.134 \times 100 = 13.4\%$$

Example: To convert a percent to a decimal, divide the percent by 100.

$$47\% = \frac{47}{100} = .47$$

To find a percent of a given number (the base), change the percent to a decimal and multiply the decimal times the base.

Example: 35% of 80 = 0.35 × 80 = 28

Example: The number of patients admitted to Get Well Hospital for drug overdoses was 24% higher in 2004 than in 2003. If 325 patients were admitted for drug overdoses in 2003, how many were admitted in 2004?

24% of 325 = .24 × 325 = 78

325 + 78 = 403

There were 78 more patients in 2004 than in 2003, making a total of 403 admitted for drug overdoses in 2004.

To determine the base when the percent and percentage are known, change the percent to a decimal and divide the percentage by the result. (Note that "is" can be interpreted as = and "of" as multiplication.)

Example: 32 is 20% of what number?

32 = 0.20 × B (B represents the base, which is the unknown number, and 32 is the percentage)

$$\frac{32}{.20} = B$$

160 = B

32 is 20% of 160.

To determine what percent a given percentage is of a base, divide the percentage by the base and change the resulting decimal to a percent.

Example: What percent of 60 is 15?

15 = P × 60 (60 is the base and 15 is the percentage.)

$$\frac{15}{60} = \frac{1}{4} = .25 = 25\%$$

Example: If a nurse with a salary of $40,000 receives a $2,000 bonus, what percent of his salary is his bonus? (That is, what percent of $40,000 is $2,000?)

$$2,000 = P \times 40,000$$

$$\frac{2,000}{40,000} = \frac{1}{20} = .05 \text{ or } 5\%$$

To find a percentage increase or percentage decrease in a word problem, write a fraction with the amount of increase or decrease as the numerator and the original amount as the denominator. Then change fraction to percentage.

Example: A patient's prescription was decreased from 2 grams to 1.5 grams. What is the percent of decrease of the new prescription?

The amount of decrease was 0.5 grams. What percent of 2 grams is 0.5 grams?

$$.5 = P \times 2$$

$$\frac{.5}{2} = .25 = 25\%$$

The dosage was decreased by 25%.

To determine discount in word problems, change the percentage to a fraction or decimal, multiply by the original cost, and deduct this amount from the original cost.

For word problems dealing with commission and taxes, multiply the total value of the goods or services by the percentage of tax or commission.

Ratios

A ratio is the comparison of two numerical quantities by division.

Example: A box contains 3 red balls and 2 blue balls. The ratio of blue to red balls in the box is 2 to 3, or $\frac{2}{3}$.

Proportions

A proportion is a statement that two ratios are equivalent.

Example: The ratio of 4 to x is equivalent to the ratio of 5 to 10.

$$\frac{4}{x} = \frac{5}{10}$$

Direct Proportions

In a direct proportion, one quantity increases ($\uparrow$) or decreases ($\downarrow$) as the other increases or decreases. In other words, the direction of the changes is the same for both factors. (x increases as y increases or x decreases as y decreases.)

Example: One orange sells for 15 cents. How much will six oranges cost?

$$\frac{1 \text{ orange}}{15¢} = \frac{6 \text{ oranges}}{y¢}$$

Cross-multiply: $1y = 6 \times 15$ $y = 90¢$

The total cost increases as the number of oranges sold increases.

Example: Six oranges cost 90 cents. How much would one orange cost?

$$\frac{6 \text{ oranges}}{90\text{¢}} = \frac{1 \text{ orange}}{y\text{¢}}$$

Cross-multiply: $6y = 90\text{¢}$ $y = 15\text{¢}$ (Divide both sides by 6.)

The cost decreases as the number of oranges purchased decreases.

Inverse Proportions

In an inverse proportion, one quantity increases (↑) as the other decreases (↓), and vice versa. In other words, the direction of the changes is opposite. (As x increases, y decreases; or as x decreases, y increases.)

Example: A 5-pound bag of dog food lasts one week when the dog is given 2 servings per day. How long would this bag last if the dog were to receive 3 servings per day?

$$\frac{3}{2} = \frac{7}{y}$$

$$3y = 14$$

$$y = 4.\overline{6} \text{ or } 4\frac{2}{3}$$

(As the number of meals increases, the number of days the dog food lasts decreases.)

Algebra

Algebra involves the use of letters and symbols as well as numbers. Some of the introductory concepts of algebra are reviewed in this section.

Operations with signed numbers

For operations with signed numbers (+ or –):

ADDITION

For numbers with the same sign, add and keep the same sign in the answer. For numbers with different signs, subtract and give the answer the sign of the higher number.

SUBTRACTION

Combine the two signs of the subtrahend, taking the subtraction sign as a negative sign, [– times – = +] [– times + = –]. Then use the rules for addition.

Examples: $-4 - (-2) = -4 + 2 = -2$
$-4 - (+2) = -4 - 2 = -6$

MULTIPLICATION

- The product of an odd number of negative numbers is negative.

- The product of an even number of negative numbers is positive.

Examples: $(-3)(-2)(-5) = -30$
$(-4)(-2)(-3)(-5) = 120$

DIVISION

If the two numbers have the same sign, the quotient is positive; if otherwise, the quotient is negative.

Algebraic Expressions

Algebraic expressions consist of a combination of variables and numbers connected by addition and subtraction signs. The parts of algebraic expressions connected by plus and minus signs are called **terms.**

COMBINING LIKE TERMS

Like terms are terms that contain the same variables. These variables have the same exponents.

$2xy^2$ and $5xy^2$ are like terms.

$3xy$ and $4x^2y$ are not like terms. The variable x in the two terms has different exponents.

Only like terms in an algebraic expression can be combined. To combine like terms, add their numerical coefficients.

Examples: $7x - 4x + 2 + 3 = 3x + 5$

$$2xy + 7x^2y - 4xy + 6y = 7x^2y - 2xy + 6y$$

Order of Operations

When simplifying an algebraic expression:

1. First remove grouping symbols (parentheses, brackets), starting with the innermost grouping symbols. (To remove grouping symbols, perform operations inside of symbols.)

2. Perform the operations of multiplication and division, moving from left to right.

3. Perform the operations of addition and subtraction, moving from left to right.

Example:
$$5x - 2\big[(3x - 1) + (4 - 2x)\big]$$
$$= 5x - 2\big[3x - 1 + 4 - 2x\big]$$
$$= 5x - 2\big[x + 3\big]$$
$$= 5x - 2x - 6$$
$$= 3x - 6$$

Evaluating Algebraic Expressions

Find the value of an algebraic expression for given values of the variable by substituting the value of the variables in the expression.

Example: Evaluate the expression $2x^2y + 3xy$ when $x = 2$ and $y = 3$.

$$2x^2y + 3xy = 2(2)^2(3) + 3(2)(3)$$
$$= 2(4)(3) + 3(2)(3)$$
$$= 2 \times 4 \times 3 + 3 \times 2 \times 3$$
$$= 24 + 18$$
$$= 42$$

Solving Equations with One Variable

An equation is a statement that two quantities are equal. An equation has one unknown if it has only one variable. Equations with one variable can be solved using inverse operations. One or more of the basic operations of addition, subtraction, multiplication, and division are used to solve equations.

Consider the equation $x - 7 = 3$.

7 has been subtracted from the variable; the inverse operation for subtraction is addition. To solve the equation, add 7 to both sides of the equation.

$$x - 7 = 3$$
$$x - 7 + 7 = 3 + 7$$
$$x = 10$$

Equivalent equations can be obtained by adding or subtracting the same number from both sides of the equation, or by multiplying or dividing both sides of the equation by the same number. (Do not divide by zero.)

Example:

$$3x + 5 = 17$$
$$3x + 5 - 5 = 17 - 5$$
$$3x = 12$$
$$\frac{3x}{3} = \frac{12}{3}$$
$$x = 4$$

Note that to solve an equation, it is necessary to get the variable on one side of the equation and the constant on the other side.

Example:

$$5x + 2 = x - 10$$
$$5x + 2 - 2 = x - 10 - 2$$
$$5x = x - 12$$
$$5x - x = x - 12 - x$$
$$4x = -12$$
$$\frac{4x}{4} = \frac{-12}{4}$$
$$x = -3$$

Solving Word Problems

The previously described methods can be used to solve word problems once they are translated into equations. The first step in translating a word problem into an equation is to represent the unknown quantity by a variable. Two equivalent algebraic expressions involving the variable are then written to represent information given in the problem. The two equivalent expressions form the equation.

Example: When 3 times a number is increased by 4, the result is 19.

Let N represent the unknown number.

$3N$ represents 3 times the number.

$3N + 4$ represents 3 times the number increased by 4.

(To increase a number means to add to it.)

Since the result is 19, the desired equation is

$3N + 4 = 19$.

$3N = 15$ (4 was subtracted from both.)

$N = 5$ (Both sides were divided by 3.)

The solution is 5.

Example:

A number decreased by $\frac{1}{2}$ of itself equals $\frac{3}{4}$. What decimal is equivalent to the resulting fraction?

Let y represent the unknown number.

$y - \frac{1}{2} y$ represents y decreased by $\frac{1}{2}$ of itself.

The desired equation is

$y - \frac{1}{2} y = \frac{3}{4}$

$\frac{1}{2} y = \frac{3}{4}$

Multiply both sides of the equation by 4 to get

$2y = 3$

$y = \frac{3}{2} = 1.5$

The solution is 1.5.

Formulas

An equation in which a variable is expressed in terms of another variable is called a formula.

$I = PRT$ is a formula for finding interest.
P represents the principal.
R represents the rate.
T represents the time.

$D = RT$ is the formula for finding distance.
R is the rate or speed.
T is the time.
$F = \frac{9}{5}C + 32$ is the formula for changing a temperature from Celsius to Fahrenheit.

$C = $ Celsius
$F = $ Fahrenheit

Example:

How long will it take to drive a distance of 330 miles traveling at a rate of 60 mph?

$$D = R \times T$$
$$330 = 60 \times T$$
$$\frac{330}{60} = T$$
$$5\frac{1}{2} = T$$

It will take $5\frac{1}{2}$ hours to drive the 330 miles at a rate of 60 mph.

Example: If a temperature reading on the Celsius scale is 40 degrees, what is the Fahrenheit reading?

$$F = \frac{9}{5}(40) + 32$$
$$F = \frac{360}{5} + 32 = 72 + 32 = 104 \text{ degrees Fahrenheit}$$

Inequalities

The symbols "<" and ">" are used to represent the inequalities "less than" and "greater than." Various statements of inequality are expressed as follows:

1. $a < b$ means a is less than b.
   $7 < 12$ means   7 is less than 12.
2. $a \le b$ means a is either less than or equal to b.
   $5 \le 9$ means   5 is less than or equal to 9.
3. $a > b$ means a is greater than b.
   $18 > 14$ means   18 is greater than 14.
4. $a \ge b$ means a is either greater than or equal to b.
   $3 \ge 3$ means   3 is greater than or equal to 3.
5. $a < b \le c$ means a is less than b, and b is less than or equal to c.
   $-1 < 3 \le 5$ means -1 is less than 3, and 3 is less than or equal to 5.
   $2 \le x < 5$ means   2 is less than or equal to x and x is less than 5.

Defined Functions

Certain questions may include a special sign such as "*" or "#" that is defined for you. The sign tells you to perform a specific function or operation. This kind of problem tests your ability to learn and apply a new concept.

Example: For all numbers, $a * b = \dfrac{a}{b} + 2$. What is $6 * 3$?

$$6 * 3 = \frac{6}{3} + 2$$
$$= 2 + 2$$
$$= 4$$

Geometry

Standard Measurements

The following are some standard units of measurement.

Linear
inches
feet (1 ft. = 12 in.)
yard (1 yd. = 3 ft.)
gallon (1 gal. = 4 qts.)

Capacity
ounces
pints (16 oz. = 1 pt.)
quart (1 qt. = 2 pts.)

Weight
ounces
pounds (1 lb. = 16 oz.)

Area is expressed in square units and volume is expressed in cubic units (square feet, cubic inches, etc.).

For **literal expressions** (problems with letters instead of numbers), use the same processes as you would for numbers.

Example: How many inches are in y yards and x feet?

$$y \text{ yd.} \times \frac{36 \text{ in.}}{\text{yd.}} = 36y \text{ in.} \quad x \text{ ft.} \times \frac{12 \text{ in.}}{\text{ft.}} = 12x \text{ in.}$$

Metric Measurements

Metric measurements are based on powers of 10. The basic metric units of measure are:

Length—Meter

Volume—Liter

Weight—Gram

Temperature—Celsius

The chart below illustrates the relationship between metric units.

MILLI	CENTI	DECI	UNIT	DEKA	HECTO	KILO
.001	.01	.1	1	10	100	1,000

Example:

$$1 \text{ gram} = 1,000 \text{ milligrams}$$
$$2 \text{ liters} = 2,000 \text{ milliliters}$$
$$1 \text{ hectometer} = 100 \text{ meters}$$

Computations in the metric system involve multiplication and division by powers of 10. Problems involving metric measurements (other than conversions within the metric system) are solved using the same techniques as problems with English measurement units.

Parallel and Perpendicular Lines

- Parallel lines are two lines that do not intersect (have no points in common). The slopes of two parallel lines are equal.

- Perpendicular lines are two lines that intersect at right angles. The slopes of two perpendicular lines have a product of -1.

Polygons

A polygon is a simple closed plane figure made up of line segments.

Polygons with three sides are called **triangles.** If the lengths of two sides of a triangle are equal, the triangle is called an isosceles triangle. When all three sides of a triangle have the same length, the triangle is called an **equilateral** triangle.

Polygons with four sides are called quadrilaterals. A **square** is a quadrilateral with all four sides equal. A **rectangle** is a quadrilateral with opposite sides equal and parallel.

Perimeter

To find the **perimeter (P)** of a figure, add the lengths of all its sides.

Triangle $P = $ sum of the three sides, or $P = a + b + c$

Rectangle $P = 2 \times \text{Length} + 2 \times \text{Width}$, or $P = 2L + 2W$

Square $P = 4 \times S$, where $S = $ length of each side.

Circle   The circumference (C) is the distance around a circle.

                The circumference of a circle is equal to $\pi \times$ the diameter:

                $C = \pi \times d$

In the drawing below, point O is the center of the given circle. Points P, R, and S are points on the circle.

A **chord** of a circle is any segment with its two end points on the circle. $\overline{MN}$ is a chord of the given circle.

A **radius** of a circle is a segment from the center of the circle to any point on the circle. $\overline{OP}$ is a radius of the circle.

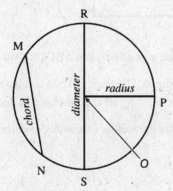

A **diameter** of a circle is a chord that passes through the center of a circle. $\overline{RS}$ is a diameter of the given circle.

All radii of a circle have the same length. A diameter of a given circle is always twice the radius of the circle.

Example:

If the length of radius $\overline{OP} = 7$ cm., the diameter $\overline{RS} = 14$ cm.

Area

To find the **area (A) of plane figures:**

Square $A = (\text{side})^2$, or $A = S^2$

Rectangle $A = \text{length} \times \text{width}$, or $A = L \times W$

Triangle $A = \frac{1}{2} \text{Base} \times \text{Height}$, or $A = \frac{1}{2}bh$

Circle $A = \pi \times (\text{radius})^2$, or $A = \pi r^2$

To find the **areas of other polygons,** divide the polygon into nonoverlapping triangles and/or quadrilaterals (squares, rectangles), and then add the areas of the triangles and quadrilaterals.

Nonoverlapping triangles and quadrilaterals may be obtained by drawing diagonals of the polygon. A **diagonal** of a polygon is a line segment joining two nonconsecutive vertices of a polygon. $\overline{BE}$ is a diagonal of polygon ABCDE below.

Example: Given polygon ABCDE with the measurements indicated, draw diagonal BE to divide the polygon into triangle BAE and rectangle BEDC.

Area of triangle BAE = $\frac{1}{2} \times 10 \times 4 = 20$ sq. in.

Area of rectangle BEDC = $2 \times 10 = 20$ sq. in.

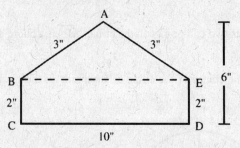

Since 20 + 20 = 40, the area of polygon ABCDE = 40 sq. in.

Similar triangles have the same shape. The angles of one similar triangle are equal to the angles of the other. The ratios of corresponding sides of similar triangles are equal.

Example: The two given triangles are similar (measures of corresponding angles are equal). Therefore $\frac{8}{x} = \frac{y}{5}$

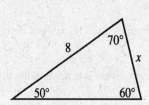
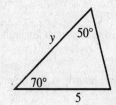

A **right triangle** is a triangle with a right angle. The side of the triangle that is opposite the right angle is called the **hypotenuse.**

Pythagorean theorem: The square of the hypotenuse of a triangle is equal to the sum of the squares of the other two sides.

$c^2 = a^2 + b^2$

Example: Find the hypotenuse of the right triangle given below.

The two sides of the triangle are 5 and 12. The hypotenuse, *c*, can be found with the use of the Pythagorean theorem.

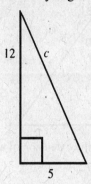

$$c^2 = 5^2 + 12^2$$
$$c^2 = 25 + 144$$
$$c^2 = 169 \quad \text{(To find } c, \text{ take the square root of 169.)}$$
$$c = 13$$

Units of measurement for angles are called **degrees.** An acute angle has a measure that is less than 90°.

A **right angle** has a measure of exactly 90°. (Perpendicular lines form right angles.)

An **obtuse angle** has a measure that is greater than 90° and less than 180°.

Two angles are **complementary** if the sum of their measures is 90°.

Two angles are **supplementary** if the sum of their measures is 180°.

If the exterior sides of a pair of adjacent angles form a straight line, the two adjacent angles are supplementary.

Example: If AB ⊥ DC (AB is perpendicular to DC), then

∠ABF and ∠FBC are complementary angles.

(The sum of the measures of ABF and ∠FBC = 90°.)

∠EBD and ∠EBC are supplementary angles.

(The sum of ∠EBD and ∠EBC = 180°.)

∠FBC is an acute angle. ∠ABC is a right angle.

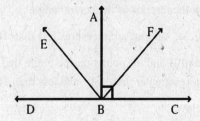

The sum of the measures of the three angles of a triangle is 180°. If the measures of two angles of a triangle are given, the measure of the third angle can be found by subtracting the sum of the measures of the two known angles from 180°.

Example: If m∠A = 40° and m∠B = 60°, then

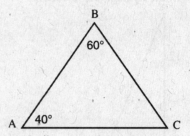

$$m\angle C = 180 - (m\angle A + m\angle B)$$
$$= 180° - (40° + 60°)$$
$$= 180° - (100°)$$
$$= 80°$$

An exterior angle of a triangle is formed by a side of a triangle and by the extension of another side of the triangle.

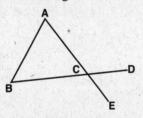

∠ACD is an exterior angle of △ABC.

∠BCE is also an exterior angle of △ABC.

Every triangle has 6 exterior angles.

- An exterior angle of a triangle is greater than either of the remote interior angles. Angles A and B are the remote interior angles for the exterior angle ∠ACD.

- An exterior angle of a triangle equals the sum of the remote interior angles (m∠ACD = m∠A + m∠B).

- m∠ACD + m∠ACB = 180°.

The total degree measure of a circle is 360°.

- A **central angle** of a circle is an angle whose vertex is the center of the circle. If a central angle represents $\frac{1}{n}$ of a circle, the measure of the central angle is $\frac{1}{n} \times 360°$.

- Angle ∠AOB is a central angle in the circle below.

- A **minor arc** of a circle consists of two points A and B, where the sides of a central angle intersect the circle, plus all points of the circle that lie in the interior of the central angle.

  The minor arc $\overparen{AB}$ is indicated in the given circle. A minor arc measures less than 180°.

- A **major arc** of a circle consists of points A and B and all points on the circle that lie in the exterior of the central angle. A major arc measures greater than 180° and less than 360°.

  The major arc $\overparen{AB}$ is indicated in the circle below.

- An **inscribed angle** of a circle is an angle whose vertex is on the circle and whose rays intersect the circle in two points different from the vertex. The measure of an inscribed angle equals one-half the measure of its intercepted arc.

  ∠ACB is an inscribed angle of the given circle. The measure of ∠ACB is one half the measure of the central angle, ∠AOB.

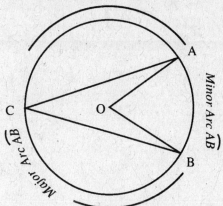

Answer Sheet

Test 1

1. Ⓐ Ⓑ Ⓒ Ⓓ	5. Ⓐ Ⓑ Ⓒ Ⓓ	9. Ⓐ Ⓑ Ⓒ Ⓓ	13. Ⓐ Ⓑ Ⓒ Ⓓ	17. Ⓐ Ⓑ Ⓒ Ⓓ
2. Ⓐ Ⓑ Ⓒ Ⓓ	6. Ⓐ Ⓑ Ⓒ Ⓓ	10. Ⓐ Ⓑ Ⓒ Ⓓ	14. Ⓐ Ⓑ Ⓒ Ⓓ	18. Ⓐ Ⓑ Ⓒ Ⓓ
3. Ⓐ Ⓑ Ⓒ Ⓓ	7. Ⓐ Ⓑ Ⓒ Ⓓ	11. Ⓐ Ⓑ Ⓒ Ⓓ	15. Ⓐ Ⓑ Ⓒ Ⓓ	19. Ⓐ Ⓑ Ⓒ Ⓓ
4. Ⓐ Ⓑ Ⓒ Ⓓ	8. Ⓐ Ⓑ Ⓒ Ⓓ	12. Ⓐ Ⓑ Ⓒ Ⓓ	16. Ⓐ Ⓑ Ⓒ Ⓓ	20. Ⓐ Ⓑ Ⓒ Ⓓ

Test 2

1. Ⓐ Ⓑ Ⓒ Ⓓ	5. Ⓐ Ⓑ Ⓒ Ⓓ	9. Ⓐ Ⓑ Ⓒ Ⓓ	13. Ⓐ Ⓑ Ⓒ Ⓓ	17. Ⓐ Ⓑ Ⓒ Ⓓ
2. Ⓐ Ⓑ Ⓒ Ⓓ	6. Ⓐ Ⓑ Ⓒ Ⓓ	10. Ⓐ Ⓑ Ⓒ Ⓓ	14. Ⓐ Ⓑ Ⓒ Ⓓ	18. Ⓐ Ⓑ Ⓒ Ⓓ
3. Ⓐ Ⓑ Ⓒ Ⓓ	7. Ⓐ Ⓑ Ⓒ Ⓓ	11. Ⓐ Ⓑ Ⓒ Ⓓ	15. Ⓐ Ⓑ Ⓒ Ⓓ	19. Ⓐ Ⓑ Ⓒ Ⓓ
4. Ⓐ Ⓑ Ⓒ Ⓓ	8. Ⓐ Ⓑ Ⓒ Ⓓ	12. Ⓐ Ⓑ Ⓒ Ⓓ	16. Ⓐ Ⓑ Ⓒ Ⓓ	20. Ⓐ Ⓑ Ⓒ Ⓓ

Test 3

1. Ⓐ Ⓑ Ⓒ Ⓓ	5. Ⓐ Ⓑ Ⓒ Ⓓ	9. Ⓐ Ⓑ Ⓒ Ⓓ	13. Ⓐ Ⓑ Ⓒ Ⓓ	17. Ⓐ Ⓑ Ⓒ Ⓓ
2. Ⓐ Ⓑ Ⓒ Ⓓ	6. Ⓐ Ⓑ Ⓒ Ⓓ	10. Ⓐ Ⓑ Ⓒ Ⓓ	14. Ⓐ Ⓑ Ⓒ Ⓓ	18. Ⓐ Ⓑ Ⓒ Ⓓ
3. Ⓐ Ⓑ Ⓒ Ⓓ	7. Ⓐ Ⓑ Ⓒ Ⓓ	11. Ⓐ Ⓑ Ⓒ Ⓓ	15. Ⓐ Ⓑ Ⓒ Ⓓ	19. Ⓐ Ⓑ Ⓒ Ⓓ
4. Ⓐ Ⓑ Ⓒ Ⓓ	8. Ⓐ Ⓑ Ⓒ Ⓓ	12. Ⓐ Ⓑ Ⓒ Ⓓ	16. Ⓐ Ⓑ Ⓒ Ⓓ	20. Ⓐ Ⓑ Ⓒ Ⓓ

Test 4

1. Ⓐ Ⓑ Ⓒ Ⓓ	8. Ⓐ Ⓑ Ⓒ Ⓓ	14. Ⓐ Ⓑ Ⓒ Ⓓ	20. Ⓐ Ⓑ Ⓒ Ⓓ	26. Ⓐ Ⓑ Ⓒ Ⓓ
2. Ⓐ Ⓑ Ⓒ Ⓓ	9. Ⓐ Ⓑ Ⓒ Ⓓ	15. Ⓐ Ⓑ Ⓒ Ⓓ	21. Ⓐ Ⓑ Ⓒ Ⓓ	27. Ⓐ Ⓑ Ⓒ Ⓓ
3. Ⓐ Ⓑ Ⓒ Ⓓ	10. Ⓐ Ⓑ Ⓒ Ⓓ	16. Ⓐ Ⓑ Ⓒ Ⓓ	22. Ⓐ Ⓑ Ⓒ Ⓓ	28. Ⓐ Ⓑ Ⓒ Ⓓ
4. Ⓐ Ⓑ Ⓒ Ⓓ	11. Ⓐ Ⓑ Ⓒ Ⓓ	17. Ⓐ Ⓑ Ⓒ Ⓓ	23. Ⓐ Ⓑ Ⓒ Ⓓ	29. Ⓐ Ⓑ Ⓒ Ⓓ
5. Ⓐ Ⓑ Ⓒ Ⓓ	12. Ⓐ Ⓑ Ⓒ Ⓓ	18. Ⓐ Ⓑ Ⓒ Ⓓ	24. Ⓐ Ⓑ Ⓒ Ⓓ	30. Ⓐ Ⓑ Ⓒ Ⓓ
6. Ⓐ Ⓑ Ⓒ Ⓓ	13. Ⓐ Ⓑ Ⓒ Ⓓ	19. Ⓐ Ⓑ Ⓒ Ⓓ	25. Ⓐ Ⓑ Ⓒ Ⓓ	31. Ⓐ Ⓑ Ⓒ Ⓓ
7. Ⓐ Ⓑ Ⓒ Ⓓ				

answer sheet

Quantitative Comparisons Test 5

1. Ⓐ Ⓑ Ⓒ Ⓓ   7. Ⓐ Ⓑ Ⓒ Ⓓ   13. Ⓐ Ⓑ Ⓒ Ⓓ   19. Ⓐ Ⓑ Ⓒ Ⓓ   24. Ⓐ Ⓑ Ⓒ Ⓓ

2. Ⓐ Ⓑ Ⓒ Ⓓ   8. Ⓐ Ⓑ Ⓒ Ⓓ   14. Ⓐ Ⓑ Ⓒ Ⓓ   20. Ⓐ Ⓑ Ⓒ Ⓓ   25. Ⓐ Ⓑ Ⓒ Ⓓ

3. Ⓐ Ⓑ Ⓒ Ⓓ   9. Ⓐ Ⓑ Ⓒ Ⓓ   15. Ⓐ Ⓑ Ⓒ Ⓓ   21. Ⓐ Ⓑ Ⓒ Ⓓ   26. Ⓐ Ⓑ Ⓒ Ⓓ

4. Ⓐ Ⓑ Ⓒ Ⓓ   10. Ⓐ Ⓑ Ⓒ Ⓓ   16. Ⓐ Ⓑ Ⓒ Ⓓ   22. Ⓐ Ⓑ Ⓒ Ⓓ   27. Ⓐ Ⓑ Ⓒ Ⓓ

5. Ⓐ Ⓑ Ⓒ Ⓓ   11. Ⓐ Ⓑ Ⓒ Ⓓ   17. Ⓐ Ⓑ Ⓒ Ⓓ   23. Ⓐ Ⓑ Ⓒ Ⓓ   28. Ⓐ Ⓑ Ⓒ Ⓓ

6. Ⓐ Ⓑ Ⓒ Ⓓ   12. Ⓐ Ⓑ Ⓒ Ⓓ   18. Ⓐ Ⓑ Ⓒ Ⓓ

Quantitative Comparisons Test 6

1. Ⓐ Ⓑ Ⓒ Ⓓ   4. Ⓐ Ⓑ Ⓒ Ⓓ   7. Ⓐ Ⓑ Ⓒ Ⓓ   10. Ⓐ Ⓑ Ⓒ Ⓓ

2. Ⓐ Ⓑ Ⓒ Ⓓ   5. Ⓐ Ⓑ Ⓒ Ⓓ   8. Ⓐ Ⓑ Ⓒ Ⓓ   11. Ⓐ Ⓑ Ⓒ Ⓓ

3. Ⓐ Ⓑ Ⓒ Ⓓ   6. Ⓐ Ⓑ Ⓒ Ⓓ   9. Ⓐ Ⓑ Ⓒ Ⓓ   12. Ⓐ Ⓑ Ⓒ Ⓓ

TEST 1

20 Questions • 15 Minutes

Directions: Each problem on this test requires logical reasoning and thinking, besides simple computations, to find the solution. Read each problem carefully and choose the correct answer from the four choices that follow. Fill in the corresponding space on your answer sheet.

1. Find the interest on $25,800 for 144 days at 6 percent per annum. Base your calculations on a 360-day year.
   - (A) $619.20
   - (B) $619.02
   - (C) $691.02
   - (D) $691.20

2. Arthur can shovel snow from a sidewalk in 60 minutes and Jack can do it in 30 minutes. How many minutes will it take them to do the job together?
   - (A) 90
   - (B) 15
   - (C) 30
   - (D) 20

3. The visitors' section of a courtroom seats 105 people. The court is in session 6 hours per day. On one particular day, 485 people visited the court and were given seats. What is the average length of time spent by each visitor in the court? Assume that as soon as a person leaves his seat it is immediately filled and that at no time during the day is one of the 105 seats vacant. Express your answer in hours and minutes.
   - (A) 1 hour 20 minutes
   - (B) 1 hour 18 minutes
   - (C) 1 hour 30 minutes
   - (D) 2 hours

4. If copy paper costs $14.50 per ream and a 5 percent discount is allowed for cash, how many reams can be purchased for $690 cash? Do not round off cents in your calculations.
   - (A) 49 reams
   - (B) 60 reams
   - (C) 50 reams
   - (D) 53 reams

5. How many hours are there between 8:30 a.m. today and 3:15 a.m. tomorrow?
   - (A) $17\frac{3}{4}$ hours
   - (B) $18\frac{3}{4}$ hours
   - (C) $18\frac{2}{3}$ hours
   - (D) $18\frac{1}{2}$ hours

6. How many days are there from September 19 to December 25 (*inclusive*)?
   - (A) 98 days
   - (B) 96 days
   - (C) 89 days
   - (D) 90 days

7. A clerk is requested to file 800 cards. If he can file cards at the rate of 80 cards per hour, what is the number of cards remaining to be filed after 7 hours of work?
   - (A) 40
   - (B) 240
   - (C) 140
   - (D) 260

GO ON TO THE NEXT PAGE

8. If your monthly electricity bill increases from $80 to $90, the percentage of increase is, most nearly,

(A) 10 percent.

(B) $11\frac{1}{9}$ percent.

(C) $12\frac{1}{2}$ percent.

(D) $14\frac{1}{7}$ percent.

9. Fifteen nurses who work the morning shift at Get Well Hospital are responsible for 135 patients. The average number of patients served by each nurse is

(A) 120.

(B) 10.

(C) 9.

(D) 140.

10. If a nursing exam contained 80 questions and you answered 72 of them correctly, what percent of the questions did you answer correctly?

(A) 90 percent

(B) 72 percent

(C) 8 percent

(D) 28 percent

11. If a patient is required to get 45 minutes of exercise each day, how many hours of exercise does he get in a week?

(A) 315 hours

(B) 5.25 hours

(C) 52 hours

(D) 6.4 hours

12. If a hospital has 120 nurses on duty during the afternoon shift and one half as many on duty for the night shift, what is the total number of nurses on duty for the two shifts?

(A) 60

(B) 180

(C) 90

(D) 120.5

13. If an inspector issued 182 summonses in the course of 7 hours, his hourly average of summonses issued was

(A) 23 summonses.

(B) 26 summonses.

(C) 25 summonses.

(D) 28 summonses.

14. Last week, 23 of the 76 patients admitted to Emergency Hospital had been in accidents. How many of the admitted patients had not been in accidents?

(A) 23

(B) 99

(C) 53

(D) 76

15. A truck going at a rate of 40 miles per hour will reach a town 80 miles away in how many hours?

(A) 1 hour

(B) 3 hours

(C) 2 hours

(D) 4 hours

16. If a barrel has a capacity of 100 gallons, how many gallons will it contain when it is two-fifths full?

(A) 20 gallons

(B) 60 gallons

(C) 40 gallons

(D) 80 gallons

17. If a monthly salary of $3,000 is subject to a 20 percent tax, the net salary is

(A) $2,000.

(B) $2,400.

(C) $2,500.

(D) $2,600.

18. If $1,000 is the cost of repairing 100 square yards of pavement, the cost of repairing 1 square yard is
    (A) $10.
    (B) $150.
    (C) $100.
    (D) $300.

19. If an employee's base pay is $3,000 per month, and it is increased by a monthly bonus of $350 and a seniority increment of $250 this month, her total salary for the month is
    (A) $3,600.
    (B) $3,500.
    (C) $3,000.
    (D) $3,700.

20. If an annual salary of $21,600 is increased by a bonus of $7,200 and by a service increment of $1,200, the total pay rate is
    (A) $29,600.
    (B) $39,600.
    (C) $26,900.
    (D) $30,000.

STOP

IF YOU FINISH BEFORE TIME IS CALLED, YOU MAY CHECK YOUR WORK ON THIS SECTION ONLY. DO NOT TURN TO ANY OTHER SECTION IN THE TEST.

TEST 2

20 Questions • 15 Minutes

Directions: Each problem on this test requires logical reasoning and thinking, besides simple computations, to find the solution. Read each problem carefully and choose the correct answer from the four choices that follow. Fill in the corresponding space on your answer sheet.

1. An emergency medical technician was standing 40 feet behind his vehicle when a second emergency medical vehicle arrived and parked 90 feet from the first vehicle. If the emergency medical technician is standing between the two vehicles, how much closer is he to the first vehicle than to the second?

   (A) 30 feet
   (B) 50 feet
   (C) 10 feet
   (D) 70 feet

2. If an IV bag has a capacity of 1,260 milliliters, how many milliliters does it contain when it's two-thirds full?

   (A) 809 ml.
   (B) 750 ml.
   (C) 630 ml.
   (D) 840 ml.

3. If an employee's salary is $2,500 a month and there are 23 working days in the month, he earns approximately how much for each day he works that month?

   (A) $108.70
   (B) $150.00
   (C) $112.50
   (D) $186.70

4. A nursing home assistant earns $360.00 a week and has deductions of $18.00 for her retirement fund, $15.00 for medical insurance, $21.00 for social security, and $72.00 for withholding taxes. How much is her take home pay?

   (A) $488.00
   (B) $296.00
   (C) $234.00
   (D) $288.00

5. A company uses 40 forty-one-cent stamps, 25 twenty-cent stamps, and 320 sixty-nine-cent stamps each day. The total cost of stamps used by the company in a five-day period is

   (A) $1,211.00.
   (B) $242.20.
   (C) $24,200.00.
   (D) $121,100.00.

6. A city department issued 12,000 applications in 2007. The number of applications that the department issued in 2005 was 25 percent greater than the number it issued in 2007. If the department issued 10 percent fewer applications in 2003 than it did in 2005, the number it issued in 2003 was

   (A) 16,500.
   (B) 13,500.
   (C) 9,900.
   (D) 8,100.

7. A secretary can add 40 columns of figures in an hour by using a calculator and 20 columns of figures an hour without using a calculator. The total number of hours it would take him to add 200 columns if he does three fifths of the work by machine and the rest without the machine is

(A) 6.

(B) 7.

(C) 8.

(D) 9.

8. In 2005, a medical office bought 500 dozen rubber gloves at a price of $2.60 per dozen. In 2008, 25 percent fewer gloves were bought than in 2005, but the price per dozen was 20 percent higher than the price in 2005. The total cost of the gloves bought in 2008 was

(A) $1,560.00.

(B) $1,170.00.

(C) $975.00.

(D) $1,040.00.

9. A nurse is assigned to check the accuracy of the entries on 490 forms. He checks 40 forms per hour. After working 1 hour on this task, he is joined by another nurse, who checks these forms at the rate of 35 per hour. The total number of hours required to do the entire assignment is

(A) 5.

(B) 6.

(C) 7.

(D) 8.

10. Assume there is a total of 420 employees in a medical care building. Thirty percent of the employees are doctors and one seventh are nurses. The difference between the number of nurses and the doctors is

(A) 60.

(B) 66.

(C) 186.

(D) 360.

11. Assume that a copying machine produces copies of a bulletin at a cost of 12 cents per copy. The machine produces 120 copies of the bulletin per minute. If the cost of producing a certain number of copies was $36, how many minutes did it take the machine to produce this number of copies?

(A) 10 minutes

(B) 6 minutes

(C) 2.5 minutes

(D) 1.2 minutes

12. The average number of medical records filed per day by a filing clerk during a five-day week was 720. She filed 610 records the first day, 720 records the second day, 740 records the third day, and 755 records the fourth day. The number of records she filed the fifth day was

(A) 748.

(B) 165.

(C) 775.

(D) 565.

13. A city department employs 1,400 people, of whom 35 percent are clerks and one eighth are stenographers. The number of employees in the department who are neither clerks nor stenographers is

(A) 640.

(B) 665.

(C) 735.

(D) 750.

14. Two nurses were assigned to take blood pressure readings at a health fair. They took the blood pressure of 190 people. If Nurse A took 40 more blood pressures than Nurse B, then the number of blood pressures taken by Nurse A was

(A) 75.

(B) 110.

(C) 115.

(D) 150.

GO ON TO THE NEXT PAGE

15. A stock clerk had on hand the following items:

500 pads, worth $0.04 each

130 pencils, worth $0.03 each

50 dozen rubber bands, worth $0.02 a dozen

If, from this stock, he issued 125 pads, 45 pencils, and 48 rubber bands, the value of the remaining stock would be

(A) $6.43.
(B) $8.95.
(C) $17.63.
(D) $18.47.

16. Joe can paint a fence in 3 hours and his friend can paint the fence in 4 hours. How long will it take them to do the job if they work together?

(A) 7 hours
(B) $\frac{15}{7}$ hours
(C) $1\frac{5}{7}$ hours
(D) 2 hours

17. A department head hired a total of 60 temporary employees to handle a seasonal increase in the department's workload.

The following lists the number of temporary employees hired, their rates of pay, and the duration of their employment:

One third of the total were hired as clerks, each at the rate of $9,750 per year, for two months.

Thirty percent of the total were hired as office machine operators, each at the rate of $11,500 per year, for four months.

Twenty-two stenographers were hired, each at the rate of $10,200 per year, for three months.

The total amount paid to these temporary employees was approximately

(A) $178,000.
(B) $157,600.
(C) $52,200.
(D) $48,500.

18. Assume that there are 2,300 employees in a city agency. Also assume that 5 percent of these employees are accountants; that 80 percent of the accountants have college degrees; and that one half of the accountants who have college degrees have five years of experience. Then the number of employees in the agency who are accountants with college degrees and five years of experience is

(A) 46.
(B) 51.
(C) 460.
(D) 920.

19. If a monthly salary of $3,000 is subject to a $425 tax deduction, the net salary is

(A) $2,557.00.
(B) $2,755.00.
(C) $2,575.00.
(D) $2,555.00.

20. A sanitation worker who reports 45 minutes early for 8:00 a.m. duty will report at

(A) 7:00 a.m.
(B) 7:30 a.m.
(C) 6:15 a.m.
(D) 7:15 a.m.

STOP

IF YOU FINISH BEFORE TIME IS CALLED, YOU MAY CHECK YOUR WORK ON THIS SECTION ONLY. DO NOT TURN TO ANY OTHER SECTION IN THE TEST.

TEST 3

20 Questions • 15 Minutes

> **Directions:** Each problem on this test requires logical reasoning and thinking, besides simple computations, to find the solution. Read each problem carefully and choose the correct answer from the four choices that follow. Fill in the corresponding space on your answer sheet.

1. If the average cost of sweeping a square foot of a small town's street is $0.75, the cost of sweeping 100 square feet is
   - **(A)** $7.50.
   - **(B)** $750.
   - **(C)** $75.
   - **(D)** $70.

2. After her car broke down on the way to a conference, a nurse had the car towed home 90 miles away. If the car was towed at a rate of 36 miles per hour, how many hours did it take to tow her car home?
   - **(A)** 0.4 hours
   - **(B)** 54 hours
   - **(C)** 2.5 hours
   - **(D)** 25 hours

3. A man is standing between a bank and a drugstore. He is 60 feet away from the bank and the drugstore is 100 feet away from the bank. How many feet nearer is the man to the bank than the drugstore is to the bank?
   - **(A)** 60 feet
   - **(B)** 40 feet
   - **(C)** 50 feet
   - **(D)** 20 feet

4. A clerk divided his 35-hour work week as follows:

   One fifth of his time in sorting mail; one half of his time in filing letters; and one seventh of his time in reception work.

   The rest of his time was devoted to messenger work. The percentage of time spent on messenger work by the clerk during the week was nearly
   - **(A)** 6 percent.
   - **(B)** 10 percent.
   - **(C)** 14 percent.
   - **(D)** 16 percent.

5. A city department has a computer unit and rents five computers at a yearly rental of $1,400 per machine. In addition, the cost to the department for the maintenance and repair of each of these machines is $100 per year. Five computer operators, each receiving an annual salary of $30,000, and a supervisor, who receives $38,000 a year, have been assigned to the unit. This unit performs the work previously performed by 10 employees whose combined salary was $324,000 per year. On the basis of these facts, the savings that will result from the operation of this unit for five years will be nearly
   - **(A)** $500,000.
   - **(B)** $947,500.
   - **(C)** $640,000.
   - **(D)** $950,000.

6. Joe can do a certain job in eight days. After working alone for four days, he is joined by Mary, and together they finish the work in two more days. How long would it take Mary alone?
   - **(A)** 5 days
   - **(B)** 6 days
   - **(C)** 7 days
   - **(D)** 8 days

GO ON TO THE NEXT PAGE

7. Eighty dozen pairs of rubber gloves were purchased for a medical facility. If the gloves are used at a rate of 32 pairs per day, what is the maximum number of days the gloves will last?

(A) Two and a half days

(B) Forty-eight days

(C) Thirty days

(D) 360 days

8. At a certain health-care facility, the average cost of providing care for 3 patients for five days is $7,200.00. What is the average cost of providing care for 24 patients for five days?

(A) $43,200.00

(B) $36,000.00

(C) $34,560.00

(D) $57,600.00

9. Typist A can do a job in 3 hours. Typist B can do the same job in 5 hours. How long would it take both, working together, to do the job?

(A) 5 hours

(B) $3\frac{1}{2}$ hours

(C) $1\frac{7}{8}$ hours

(D) $1\frac{5}{8}$ hours

10. After gaining 50 percent of his original capital, he had capital of $18,000. Find the original capital.

(A) $12,200.00

(B) $13,100.00

(C) $12,000.00

(D) $12,025.00

11. To work off 60 calories, Brenda needs to walk on the treadmill for 15 minutes. How long will it take her to work off 100 calories?

(A) 25 minutes

(B) 55 minutes

(C) 40 minutes

(D) 45 minutes

12. A student worked thirty days at a part-time job. He paid two fifths of his earnings for room and board and had $81 left. What was his daily wage?

(A) $4.50

(B) $5.00

(C) $5.50

(D) $6.25

13. A dealer bought motorcycles for $4,000. He sold them for $6,200, making $50 on each motorcycle. How many motorcycles were there?

(A) 40

(B) 38

(C) 43

(D) 44

14. An organization had one fourth of its capital invested in goods. Two-thirds of the remaining capital was invested in land. The rest was cash in the amount of $1,224. What was the capital of the firm?

(A) $4,986.00

(B) $4,698.00

(C) $4,896.00

(D) $4,869.00

15. A and B together earn $2,100. If B is paid one fourth more than A, how many dollars should B receive?

(A) $1,166.66

(B) $1,162.66

(C) $1,617.66

(D) $1,167.66

16. If a boat is purchased for $21,500 and sold for $23,650, what is the percentage of gain?

(A) 8 percent

(B) 15 percent

(C) 20 percent

(D) 10 percent

17. A person owned five sixths of a piece of property and sold three fourths of her share for $1,800. What was the value of the property?

(A) $2,808.00

(B) $2,880.00

(C) $2,088.00

(D) $2,880.80

18. A lot costing $21,250 leases for $1,900 per year. The taxes and other expenses are $300 per year. Find the percentage of net income on the investment.

(A) $7\frac{1}{2}$ percent

(B) 6 percent

(C) 4 percent

(D) 10 percent

19. B owned 75 shares of stock in a building association worth $50 each. The association declared a dividend of 8 percent, payable in stock. How many shares did he own then?

(A) 81 shares

(B) 80 shares

(C) 90 shares

(D) 85 shares

20. It requires 4 men three days to take an inventory; the weekly salary of each is as follows:

A—$250, B—$130, C—$120, D—$90.

Calculate the cost of taking the inventory, assuming that there are five full working days in a week.

(A) $119.00

(B) $196.00

(C) $354.00

(D) $588.00

STOP

IF YOU FINISH BEFORE TIME IS CALLED, YOU MAY CHECK YOUR WORK ON THIS SECTION ONLY. DO NOT TURN TO ANY OTHER SECTION IN THE TEST.

TEST 4

31 Questions • 22 Minutes

Directions: Each problem on this test requires logical reasoning and thinking, besides simple computations, to find the solution. Read each problem carefully and choose the correct answer from the four choices that follow. Fill in the corresponding space on your answer sheet.

1. In simplest form, $-11 - (-2)$ is
   (A) 7
   (B) 9
   (C) -11
   (D) -9

2. Find the average of 6.47, 5.89, 3.42, 0.65, and 7.09.
   (A) 5.812
   (B) 4.704
   (C) 3.920
   (D) 4.705

3. $\dfrac{456.3}{0.89}$ equals
   (A) $513\dfrac{13}{89}$
   (B) 512.70
   (C) 513.89
   (D) $512\dfrac{59}{89}$

4. Add 5 hours 13 minutes; 3 hours 49 minutes; and 24 minutes. The sum is
   (A) 9 hours 26 minutes.
   (B) 8 hours 16 minutes.
   (C) 9 hours 76 minutes.
   (D) 8 hours 6 minutes.

5. Two numbers are in the ratio of 18:47. If the smaller number is 126, the larger number is
   (A) 376.
   (B) 144.
   (C) 235.
   (D) 329.

6. Change 0.3125 to a fraction.
   (A) $\dfrac{3}{64}$
   (B) $\dfrac{1}{16}$
   (C) $\dfrac{1}{64}$
   (D) $\dfrac{5}{16}$

7. Divide $\dfrac{7}{8}$ by $\dfrac{7}{8}$.
   (A) 1
   (B) 0
   (C) $\dfrac{7}{8}$
   (D) $\dfrac{49}{64}$

8. In the series 5, 8, 13, 20, the next number should be
   (A) 23.
   (B) 26.
   (C) 29.
   (D) 32.

9. What is the interest on $300 at 6 percent for ten days? (Assume year = 360 days.)
   (A) $0.50
   (B) $1.50
   (C) $2.50
   (D) $5.50

10. If the scale on a map indicates that 1 and one-half inches equal 500 miles, then 5 inches on the map will represent approximately

(A) 1,800 miles.

(B) 1,700 miles.

(C) 1,300 miles.

(D) 700 miles.

11. $\frac{1}{2}$ percent equals

(A) 0.002.

(B) 0.020.

(C) 0.005.

(D) 0.050.

12. If 20 percent of an employee's bonus was $260.00, what was her entire bonus?

(A) $2,300

(B) $2,600

(C) $1,600

(D) $1,300

13. If a kilogram equals about 35 ounces, the number of grams in 1 ounce is approximately

(A) 29.

(B) 30.

(C) 31.

(D) 32.

14. An IV pump delivers medication at a constant rate of 24 milligrams per hour. How long does it take to deliver 90 milligrams?

(A) 3 hours 15 minutes

(B) 3 hours 45 minutes

(C) 3 hours 75 minutes

(D) 4 hours 15 minutes

15. If sound travels at the rate of 1,100 feet per second, in one-half minute it will travel about

(A) 6 miles.

(B) 8 miles.

(C) 10 miles.

(D) 3 miles.

16. If a kilometer is about five eighths of a mile, 2 miles is about

(A) 1.6 kilometers.

(B) 3.2 kilometers.

(C) 2.4 kilometers.

(D) 3.75 kilometers.

17. A lecture hall that is 25 feet wide and 75 feet long has a perimeter equal to

(A) 1,750 feet.

(B) 200 yards.

(C) $66\frac{2}{3}$ yards.

(D) 1,875 feet.

18. After deducting a discount of $16\frac{2}{3}$ percent, the price of a blouse was $35. The list price was

(A) $37.50.

(B) $38.

(C) $41.75.

(D) $42.

19. The number of decimal places in the product of 0.4266 and 0.3333 is

(A) 8.

(B) 4.

(C) 14.

(D) None of the above.

20. What is the cost of 5,500 bandages at $50 per thousand?

(A) $385

(B) $550

(C) $275

(D) $285

21. 572 divided by 0.52 is

(A) 1,100.

(B) 110.

(C) 11.10.

(D) 11,000.

GO ON TO THE NEXT PAGE

22. 200 percent of 800 equals
   (A) 2,500.
   (B) 16.
   (C) 1,600.
   (D) 4.

23. A seventh-grade baseball team won ten games and lost five. Their average is
   (A) 0.667.
   (B) 0.500.
   (C) 0.333.
   (D) 0.200.

24. The number of cubic feet of soil needed for a flower box 3 feet long, 8 inches wide, and 1 foot deep is
   (A) 24.
   (B) 12.
   (C) $4\frac{2}{3}$.
   (D) 2.

25. At $1,250 per hundred, 228 watches will cost
   (A) $2,850.
   (B) $36,000.
   (C) $2,880.
   (D) $360.

26. The area of the shaded portion of the rectangle below is

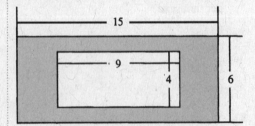

   (A) 54 square inches.
   (B) 90 square inches.
   (C) 45 square inches.
   (D) 36 square inches.

27. On February 12, 1989, the age of a boy who was born on March 15, 1979, was
   (A) 10 years, 10 months, and 3 days.
   (B) 9 years, 9 months, and 27 days.
   (C) 10 years, 1 month, and 3 days.
   (D) 9 years, 10 months, and 27 days.

QUESTIONS 28–31 ARE BASED ON THE FOLLOWING GRAPH.

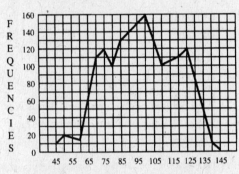

INTELLIGENCE QUOTIENTS (IQs)

28. The number of pupils having the highest IQ is about
   (A) 5.
   (B) 160.
   (C) 145.
   (D) 20.

29. The number of pupils having an IQ of 75 is about
   (A) 130.
   (B) 100.
   (C) 120.
   (D) 110.

30. The number of pupils having an IQ of 80 is identical to the number of pupils having an IQ of
   (A) 100.
   (B) 68.
   (C) 110.
   (D) 128.

31. The IQ that has the greatest frequency is
   (A) 100.
   (B) 95.
   (C) 105.
   (D) 160.

STOP

IF YOU FINISH BEFORE TIME IS CALLED, YOU MAY CHECK
YOUR WORK ON THIS SECTION ONLY. DO NOT TURN TO ANY
OTHER SECTION IN THE TEST.

QUANTITATIVE COMPARISONS TEST 5

28 Questions • 35 Minutes

Common Information: In each question, information concerning one or both of the quantities to be compared is given in the ITEM column. A symbol that appears in any column represents the same thing in Column A as it does in Column B.

Figures: Assume that the position of points, angles, regions, and so forth, are in the order shown; that the lines shown as straight are indeed straight; that figures lie in a plane unless otherwise indicated. Figures accompanying questions are intended to provide information you can use in answering the questions. However, unless a note states that a figure is drawn to scale, you should solve the problems by using your knowledge of mathematics, and NOT by estimating sizes by sight or by measurement.

Directions: For each of the following questions, two quantities are given: one in Column A and one in Column B. Compare the two quantities and mark your answer sheet with the correct lettered conclusion. These are your options:

(A) if the quantity in Column A is the greater;
(B) if the quantity in Column B is the greater;
(C) if the two quantities are equal;
(D) if the relationship cannot be determined from the information given.

Column A	Column B		Column A	Column B

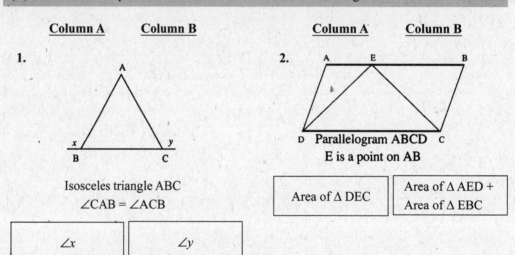

1.

Isosceles triangle ABC
∠CAB = ∠ACB

∠x	∠y

2.

Parallelogram ABCD
E is a point on AB

| Area of △ DEC | Area of △ AED +
Area of △ EBC |
|---|---|

SUMMARY DIRECTIONS

<u>Select:</u>   **(A)**   if Column A is greater;

           (B)   if Column B is greater;

           (C)   if the two columns are equal;

           (D)   if the relationship cannot be determined from the information given.

Column A	**Column B**		**Column A**	**Column B**

3. $x = -1$

$x^3 + x^2 - x + 1$	$x^3 - x^2 + x - 1$

6. x is a given number.

Area of a circle radius $= x^3$	Area of a circle radius $= 3x$

4.

The edge of a cube whose volume is 27	The edge of a cube whose total surface area is 54

7.

$\left(\dfrac{1}{4}\right)^{-2}$	4^2

5.

$\dfrac{\frac{1}{2} + \frac{1}{3}}{\frac{2}{3}}$	$\dfrac{\frac{2}{3}}{\frac{1}{2} + \frac{1}{3}}$

8.

0.02	$\sqrt{0.02}$

GO ON TO THE NEXT PAGE

SUMMARY DIRECTIONS
Select: (A) if Column A is greater;
(B) if Column B is greater;
(C) if the two columns are equal;
(D) if the relationship cannot be determined from the information given.

Column A	Column B		Column A	Column B

9.

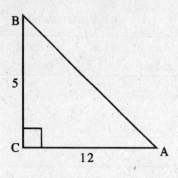

Right △ABC

(AB)²	(AC)² + 5(CB)

10.

Area of circle with radius 7	Area of equilateral triangle with side 14

11.

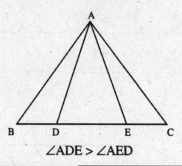

∠ADE > ∠AED

∠B	∠C

12.

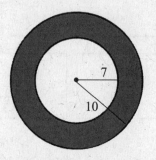

Area of shaded portion	Area of small circle

SUMMARY DIRECTIONS

Select: **(A)** if Column A is greater;

(B) if Column B is greater;

(C) if the two columns are equal;

(D) if the relationship cannot be determined from the information given.

<u>Column A</u>	<u>Column B</u>		<u>Column A</u>	<u>Column B</u>

13.

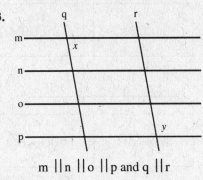

$m \parallel n \parallel o \parallel p$ and $q \parallel r$

$\angle x$	$\angle y$

15. $t < 0 < r$

t^2	r

14. $a < 0 < b$

a^2	$\dfrac{b}{2}$

GO ON TO THE NEXT PAGE

SUMMARY DIRECTIONS
Select: **(A)**   if Column A is greater;
(B)   if Column B is greater;
(C)   if the two columns are equal;
(D)   if the relationship cannot be determined from the information given.

DIAGRAM FOR PROBLEMS 16–20

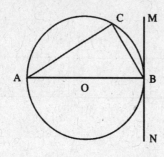

MN tangent to circle O at point B and ∠A = 30°

Column A	**Column B**
19. m∠CBA	m∠CBM

Column A	**Column B**
20. $\overline{AO} + \overline{AC}$	$\overline{BO} + \overline{BC}$

Column A	**Column B**
16. m∠ACB	m∠NBO

| **17.** $\overset{\frown}{CB}$ | $\overset{\frown}{AC}$ |

| **18.** m∠CBM | m∠CAB |

SUMMARY DIRECTIONS	
Select:	**(A)** if Column A is greater;
	(B) if Column B is greater;
	(C) if the two columns are equal;
	(D) if the relationship cannot be determined from the information given.

DIAGRAM FOR PROBLEMS 21–25

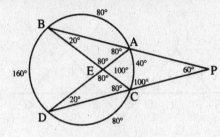

$$\overline{AB} = \overline{CD}$$

$$\overparen{BD} = 160°$$

$$\overparen{AC} = 40°$$

	Column A	Column B
24.	m∠BCP	m∠AEC + m∠ADC

	Column A	Column B
25.	$\overparen{DC} + \overparen{AC}$	$\overparen{BD}$

	Column A	Column B
21.	m∠APC	m∠ABC

22.	m∠BED	m∠BEA

23.	m∠BAD	m∠DCB

GO ON TO THE NEXT PAGE

SUMMARY DIRECTIONS
Select: **(A)**   if Column A is greater;
(B)   if Column B is greater;
(C)   if the two columns are equal;
(D)   if the relationship cannot be determined from the information given.

Column A	Column B
26. 75% of $\dfrac{3}{4}$	0.09×6

Column A	Column B
27. 4% of 0.003	3% of 0.004

Column A	Column B

28.

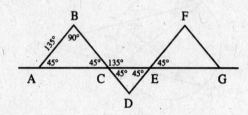

Intersecting straight lines; $AB \perp CB$, $CD = ED$

$\angle BCA$	$\angle FEG$

STOP

IF YOU FINISH BEFORE TIME IS CALLED, YOU MAY CHECK YOUR WORK ON THIS SECTION ONLY. DO NOT TURN TO ANY OTHER SECTION IN THE TEST.

QUANTITATIVE COMPARISONS TEST 6

12 Questions • 15 Minutes

Common Information: In each question, information concerning one or both of the quantities to be compared is given in the ITEM column. A symbol that appears in any column represents the same thing in Column A as it does in Column B.

Figures: Assume that the position of points, angles, regions, and so forth, are in the order shown; that the lines shown as straight are indeed straight; that figures lie in a plane unless otherwise indicated. Figures accompanying questions are intended to provide information you can use in answering the questions. However, unless a note states that a figure is drawn to scale, you should solve the problems by using your knowledge of mathematics, and NOT by estimating sizes by sight or by measurement.

Directions: For each of the following questions, two quantities are given: one in Column A and one in Column B. Compare the two quantities and mark your answer sheet with the correct lettered conclusion. These are your options:

(A) if the quantity in Column A is the greater;
(B) if the quantity in Column B is the greater;
(C) if the two quantities are equal;
(D) if the relationship cannot be determined from the information given.

Column A	Column B		Column A	Column B

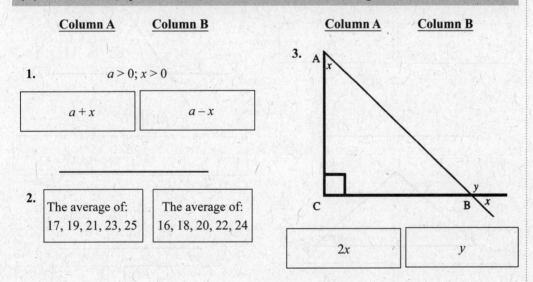

1. $a > 0; x > 0$

$a + x$	$a - x$

3.

2.

The average of:	The average of:
17, 19, 21, 23, 25	16, 18, 20, 22, 24

$2x$	y

GO ON TO THE NEXT PAGE ➤

SUMMARY DIRECTIONS

Select: (A)   if Column A is greater;
        (B)   if Column B is greater;
        (C)   if the two columns are equal;
        (D)   if the relationship cannot be determined from the information given.

Column A	**Column B**		**Column A**	**Column B**

4. $0 < a < 12;\ 0 < b < 10$

a	b

7. $\dfrac{a}{9} = b^2$

a	b

8.

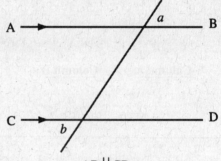

AB $\parallel$ CD

a	b

---

5. $4a - 4b = 20$

a	b

6.

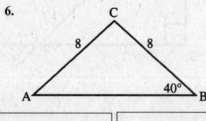

$\angle$A	$\angle$B

9.

$3 + 24(3 - 2)$	$27 + 5(0)(5)$

SUMMARY DIRECTIONS

Select: (A) if Column A is greater;

(B) if Column B is greater;

(C) if the two columns are equal;

(D) if the relationship cannot be determined from the information given.

Column A	Column B		Column A	Column B

10.

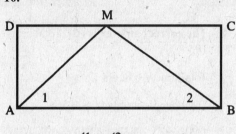

$\angle 1 > \angle 2$

$\overline{AM}$	$\overline{BM}$

12.

$\left(\dfrac{2}{3}\right)^2 (3)^3$	$(3)^2 \left(\dfrac{2}{3}\right)^3$

11.

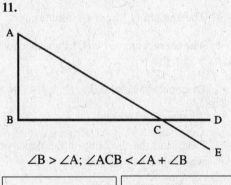

$\angle B > \angle A;\ \angle ACB < \angle A + \angle B$

$\angle A + \angle B$	$\angle ACD$

STOP

IF YOU FINISH BEFORE TIME IS CALLED, YOU MAY CHECK YOUR WORK ON THIS SECTION ONLY. DO NOT TURN TO ANY OTHER SECTION IN THE TEST.

ANSWER KEY AND EXPLANATIONS

Test 1

1. A	5. B	9. C	13. B	17. B
2. D	6. A	10. A	14. C	18. A
3. B	7. B	11. B	15. C	19. A
4. C	8. C	12. B	16. C	20. D

1. **The correct answer is (A).**

   Interest = Principal × Rate × Time
   Note: 6% = 0.06

   144 days = $\frac{144}{360}$ year

   $I = P \times R \times T$

   $= \$25,800 \times 0.06 \times \frac{144}{360}$

   $= \frac{\$222,912}{360}$

   $= \$619.20$

2. **The correct answer is (D).** Let n = number of minutes in which they can do the job together. Arthur can do $\frac{1}{60}$ of the job in 1 minute, so in n minutes he can do $\frac{n}{60}$ of the job. Jack can do $\frac{1}{30}$ of the job in 1 minute and $\frac{n}{30}$ of the job in n minutes.

   Together, in n minutes they can do the complete job.

   $\frac{n}{60} + \frac{n}{30} = 1$

   $n + 2n = 60$ (multiplying both sides by 60, the lowest common denominator)

   $3n = 60$ (combine like terms)

   $n = 20$ (divide by 3)

   They can do the job together in 20 minutes.

3. **The correct answer is (B).** Total seats = 105

   Total time = 6 hours

   Total people involved = 485

   105 seats × 6 hours = 630 seating hours

   To find the average seating time, divide

   630 ÷ 485 = 1.3 hours

   Now change the 0.3 hours to minutes

   (1 hour = 60 minutes)

   .30 hour $\times \frac{60 \text{ minutes}}{1 \text{ hour}} = 18$ minutes

   The amount is 1 hour 18 minutes.

4. **The correct answer is (C).** Paper per ream = \$14.50

   Discount = 5%, or 0.05

   Total cash = \$690.00

   First, find the discount on the paper per ream when paying cash.

   \$14.50 × 0.05 = \$0.725

   Our price per ream is \$14.50 – \$0.725 = \$13.775.

   Given \$690 to spend, divide to find how much paper can be purchased.

   \$690.00 ÷ \$13.775/ream = 50

   50 reams for \$688.75

5. **The correct answer is (B).** Use simple logic on this problem.

From	To	
8:30 a.m. →	8:30 p.m. =	12 hours
8:30 p.m. →	3:30 a.m. =	7 hours

Total = 19 hours,

but this is 15 minutes too much.

Note: Change one of the hours to minutes (1 hour = 60 minutes).

$$45 \text{ minutes} = \frac{45}{60} \text{ hours, or } \frac{3}{4} \text{ hours}$$

$$\begin{array}{r} 18 \text{ hours } 60 \text{ minutes} \\ -15 \text{ minutes} \\ \hline 18 \text{ hours } 45 \text{ minutes} \end{array}$$

$18\frac{3}{4}$ is the total number of hours.

6. **The correct answer is (A).** Again, use logic.

Month	Number of days/month	
September	from 19 to 30	12 days
October	31 days	31 days
November	30 days	30 days
December	from 1 to 25	25 days
		98 days

Note: Remember that September 19 and December 25 are included.

Total = 98 days inclusive

7. **The correct answer is (B).**

Total to be filed = 800 cards

Rate cards can be filed = 80 cards per hour

How many cards were filed in the first 7 hours?

$7 \times 80 = 560$ cards were filed

Subtract to find the remaining cards to be filed.

$800 - 560 = 240$

240 cards remain unfiled

8. **The correct answer is (C).** From \$80 to \$90, there is a \$10 increase; the percentage of increase is found by dividing the amount of increase by the original amount:

$$10 \div 80 = 0.125, \text{ or } 12\frac{1}{2}\%$$

Note: $0.125 = 12.5\%$, or $12\frac{1}{2}\%$

Percentage of increase = $12\frac{1}{2}\%$

9. **The correct answer is (C).** To find the *average* number of patients served by each nurse, divide 135 patients by 15 nurses to get 9 patients per nurse.

10. **The correct answer is (A).** To find the percent of correct answers on the test, divide the number of correct answers by the total number of items on the test.

$$\frac{72}{80} = .90$$

Change .90 to a percent.

$.90 = 90\%$

90% of the test items were correct.

11. **The correct answer is (B).** To find the number of hours of exercise the patient gets in a week, multiply

45 min. × 7 days = 315 minutes

Convert the minutes to hours by dividing by 60, since there are 60 minutes in an hour.

$$\frac{315}{60} = 5.25 \text{ hours per week}$$

12. **The correct answer is (B).** To find the number of nurses on duty for the two shifts, determine the total number of nurses who worked on the night shift by finding one half of the number who worked the afternoon shift.

$$120 \times \frac{1}{2} = 60$$

Add the number who worked the afternoon shift to the number who worked the night shift.

answers practice test 3

$120 + 60 = 180$

180 nurses worked on the two shifts.

13. **The correct answer is (B).** Total summonses in 7 hours = 182

To find the *average* number of summonses per hour, divide:

182 summonses $\div$ 7 hours = 26

Average = 26 summonses/hour

14. **The correct answer is (C).** To find the number of admitted patients who weren't in accidents, subtract the number of patients who were in accidents from the total number of patients.

$76 - 23 = 53$

53 of the admitted patients had not been in accidents.

15. **The correct answer is (C).** If it takes one truck 1 hour to go 40 miles, it will take 2 hours to go 80 miles.

$$2 \text{ hours } \times 40\frac{\text{miles}}{\text{hours}} = 80 \text{ miles}$$

16. **The correct answer is (C).** If the total capacity is 100 gallons, then

$$\frac{2}{5} \text{ of } 100 = \frac{2}{5} \times 100$$
$$= \frac{200}{5}$$
$$= 40 \text{ gallons}$$

17. **The correct answer is (B).** Total salary = $3,000

Tax = 20%, or .20

Find the amount of 20% tax by multiplying:
$3,000 \times .20 = $600

Subtract the tax from the salary to find the net:

$$\$3,000 - \$600 = \$2,400$$
$$2,400 = \text{net pay}$$

18. **The correct answer is (A).**

Total cost = $1,000

Total square yards = 100

Find the cost per square yard by dividing:

$1,000 $\div$ 100 square yards = $10

$10/square yard

19. **The correct answer is (A).**

Base pay	$3,000
Bonus	+ 350
Serv. Increment	+ 250
Total pay	$3,600

20. **The correct answer is (D).**

Annual salary	$21,600
Bonus	+ 7,200
Increment	+ 1,200
Total pay	$30,000

Test 2

1. C	5. A	9. C	13. C	17. B
2. D	6. B	10. B	14. C	18. A
3. A	7. B	11. C	15. D	19. C
4. C	8. B	12. C	16. C	20. D

1.   The correct answer is (C).

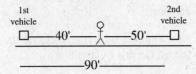

The second vehicle is 90 feet – 40 feet = 50 feet from the emergency medical technician (EMT). The first vehicle is 40 feet from the EMT. The first vehicle is 50 feet – 40 feet = 10 feet closer than the second vehicle.

2.   The correct answer is (D). To find the number of milliliters the IV bag has when it's two-thirds full, multiply 1,260 milliliters $\times \frac{2}{3} = 840$ milliliters

There are 840 milliliters in the IV bag when it's two-thirds full.

3.   The correct answer is (A).

Salary per month = $2,500

Days worked = 23

To find the earnings per day, divide:

$$\frac{\$2,500}{month} \div \frac{23\ days}{month} = \frac{\$108.70}{days}$$

or

$$\frac{\$2,500}{month} \div \frac{23\ days}{month}$$

$$= \frac{\$2,500}{\cancel{month}} \times \frac{\cancel{month}}{23\ days}$$

$$= \frac{\$2,500}{23\ days} = \frac{\$108.70}{day}$$

4.   The correct answer is (C). To find the take-home pay of the nursing home assistant, subtract the total amount of her deductions from her weekly salary.

Total deductions	= $18,00 + $15.00 + $21.00
	+$72.00 = $126.00
Weekly salary	= 360.00
Salary – deductions	= $360.00 – $126.00
	= $234.00
Take-home pay	= $234.00

5.   The correct answer is (A).

Stamps per day	Cost per day
$\frac{40}{day} \times \$0.41$	= 16.40
$\frac{25}{day} \times \$0.20$	= 5.00
$\frac{320}{day} \times \$0.69$	= 220.80
Total cost/day	$242.20

For five days, 5 × $242.20 = $1,211.00

Total cost = $1,211.00

6.   The correct answer is (B). Number of applications issued in 2007 = 12,000

In 2005, 25 percent more were issued, or 0.25 × 12,000 = 3,000 more in 2005.

So there were 3,000 + 12,000 = 15,000 issued in 2005.

In 2003, 10 percent fewer were issued than in 2005, or 0.10 × 15,000 = 1,500 fewer were issued in 2003.

The number issued in 2003 is

$15,000 - 1,500 = 13,500$.

7. **The correct answer is (B).** If three fifths of the 200 are done by calculator, then:

$$\frac{3}{5} \times 200 = \frac{600}{5} = 120$$

columns will be done by the machine. To find the number done by hand, subtract:

$200 - 120 = 80$ will be done by hand

To find the time it takes to do the 120 columns by machine and the 80 columns by hand, divide:

120 columns ÷ 40 columns per hour = 3 hours

80 columns ÷ 20 columns per hour = 4 hours

Total time = 7 hours

8. **The correct answer is (B).** To find the total cost of the rubber gloves bought in 2008, first determine the amount of the 20% increase for a dozen gloves in 2008.

$.20 \times \$2.60 = 0.52$

Add the cost in 2005 to the amount of the increase to get the cost of the gloves in 2008.

$\$2.60 + 0.52 = \$3.12$

In 2008, a dozen gloves cost $3.12.

The number of gloves purchased in 2008 was 25 percent less than the number purchased in 2005.

To find how many dozens of gloves were purchased in 2008, find 25 percent of 500 dozen and subtract the result from 500 dozen.

500 dozen $- .25 \times 500$ dozen
= 500 dozen $- 125$ dozen = 375 dozen

375 dozen gloves were purchased in 2008.

Multiply the price per dozen $3.12 × 375 dozen = $1,170.00.

The total cost of the gloves bought in 2008 was $1,170.00.

9. **The correct answer is (C).** During the first hour, 40 forms were checked, leaving 450 to be checked:

$490 - 40 = 450$

The two nurses working together can check 75 forms.

Now find the time it takes to do the 450 forms. Do this by dividing:

450 forms ÷ 75 forms/hour = 6 hours

It takes 6 hours to do the 450 and 1 hour for the first 40 forms:

6 hours + 1 hour = 7 hours to do the job

A total of 7 hours is needed.

10. **The correct answer is (B).** Total employed = 420

If 30 percent are nurses,

$420 \times 0.30 = 126$ nurses

$\frac{1}{7}$ are doctors:

$420 \times \frac{1}{7} = 60$ doctors

The difference is $126 - 60 = 66$.

11. **The correct answer is (C).** Cost = $0.12 per copy

Time = 120 copies per minute

To find the number of copies produced, divide:

$36 ÷ \$0.12 = 300$ copies

To find the number of minutes, divide:

300 copies ÷ 120 copies/minute = 2.5 minutes

12. **The correct answer is (C).** If the average number of medical records filed for five days was 720, then 5 days × 720 records/day = 3,600 records for the five-day period.

For four days:

610 + 720 + 740 + 755 = 2,825 medical records were filed

Subtract:

3,600 − 2,825 = 775 need to be filed the fifth day to get an average of 720 for the five-day period

13. **The correct answer is (C).** Total employees = 1,400

35% clerks = 1,400 × .35 = 490 clerks

$\frac{1}{8}$ stenos = 1,400 × $\frac{1}{8}$ = 175 stenos

Together (490 + 175 = 665), there are 665 clerks and stenographers. To find how many employees are neither, subtract:

1,400 − 665 = 735

Answer = 735 other employees

14. **The correct answer is (C).** If Nurse A takes 40 more blood pressure readings than Nurse B, let x represent the number of blood pressure readings taken by Nurse B. Then $x + 40 =$ the number of blood pressure readings taken by Nurse A. Add the number taken by Nurse A to the number taken by Nurse B to get the total number of blood pressure readings taken.

$$x + x + 40 = 190$$
$$2x + 40 = 190$$
$$2x = 150$$

$x = 75$, the number of blood pressure readings taken by Nurse B

$x + 40 = 75 + 40 = 115$, the number of blood pressure readings taken by Nurse A

15. **The correct answer is (D).** Stock on hand and cost per item:

		Cost
500 pads × $0.04/pad	=	$20.00
130 pencils × $0.03/pencil	=	$3.90
50 dozen rubber bands × $0.02/dozen	=	$1.00
value of stock on hand	=	$24.90

If we issue the items below,

125 pads × $0.04	=	$5.00
45 pencils × $0.03	=	$1.35
48 rubber bands or 4 dozen × $0.02	=	**$0.08**
		$6.43

To find the value of the remaining stock, subtract:

$24.90 − $6.43 = $18.47

Value = $18.47

16. **The correct answer is (C).** Let t be the amount of time for both to do the job. If Joe does $\frac{t}{3}$ part of the job, and his friend does $\frac{t}{4}$ part of the job, then $\frac{t}{3} + \frac{t}{4} = 1$ (the whole job).

$4t + 3t = 12$ (multiply lowest common denominator by 12)

$7t = 12$ (combine like terms)

$t = \frac{12}{7}$ (divide by 7)

$t = 1\frac{5}{7}$ hours

17. **The correct answer is (B).** Total employees = 60

$\frac{1}{3} × 60 = 20$ clerks

30% × 60, or .30 × 60 = 18 office machine operators (OMOs)

60 − 38 = 22 stenos

To find their *rate per month,* divide their monthly salaries by 12, because there are 12 months in a year:

clerks: $\dfrac{\$9,750}{12} = \$812.50$ per month

OMOs: $\dfrac{\$11,500}{12} = \$958.33$ per month

stenos: $\dfrac{\$10,200}{12} = \$850.00$ per month

Now find the salary for all employees for the time they worked:

If 20 clerks worked two months, total pay equals:

$20 \times 2 \times \$812.50 = \$32,500.00$

If 18 OMOs worked four months, total pay equals:

$18 \times 4 \times \$958.33 = \$68,999.76$

If 22 stenos worked three months, total pay equals:

$22 \times 3 \times \$850.00 = \$56,100.00$

Total salaries = $\$68,999.76 + \$32,500.00 + \$56,100.00 = \$157,599.76$. This amount can be rounded off to $157,600.00.

18. **The correct answer is (A).** 5 percent of 2,300 are accountants:

$0.05 \times 2,300 = 115$

80 percent of the 115 accountants have college degrees:

$0.80 \times 115 = 92$

One half of the 92 have five years of experience:

$\dfrac{1}{2} \times 92 = 46$

46 employees have all three qualifications.

19. **The correct answer is (C).** $3,000 is subject to $425 tax. The net can be found by subtracting:

$\$3,000 - \$425 = \$2,575$

20. **The correct answer is (D).** A sanitation worker who reports 45 minutes early for 8:00 a.m. duty reports

7 hours 60 minutes
    − 45 minutes
————————
7 hours 15 minutes

Note: 1 hour = 60 minutes

8 hours = 7 hours 60 minutes

This worker reports at 7:15 a.m.

Test 3

1. C	5. C	9. C	13. D	17. B
2. C	6. D	10. C	14. C	18. A
3. B	7. C	11. A	15. A	19. A
4. D	8. D	12. A	16. D	20. C

1. **The correct answer is (C).** If it costs $0.75 to sweep 1 square foot, to find the cost for 100 square feet, multiply 100 square feet × 0.75 square foot = $75.

   Total cost = $75

2. **The correct answer is (C).** To determine how many hours it will take to tow the car 90 miles at a rate of 36 mph, divide

   $$90 \div 36 = 2.5$$

   It will take 2.5 hours = $2\frac{1}{2}$ hours to tow the car 90 miles.

3. **The correct answer is (B).** To determine how many feet nearer the man is to the bank than the drugstore is to the bank, use the following diagram:

   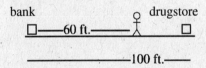

   The total distance from the bank to the drugstore is 100 feet. Subtract to find the distance from the man to the drugstore.

   100 feet − 60 feet = 40 feet

   The man is 40 feet nearer to the bank than the drug store is to the bank.

4. **The correct answer is (D).** A clerk works 35 hours per week. $\frac{1}{5}$ of his time is used to sort mail:

   $$\frac{1}{5} \times 35 = 7 \text{ hours}$$

$\frac{1}{2}$ of his time is used to file letters:

$$\frac{1}{2} \times 35 = 17\frac{1}{2} \text{ hours}$$

$\frac{1}{7}$ of his time is used for reception work:

$$\frac{1}{7} \times 35 = 5 \text{ hours}$$

Total = $29\frac{1}{2}$ hours

$29\frac{1}{2}$ hours were used for the above. To find the time left for messenger work, subtract

$$35 - 29\frac{1}{2} = 5\frac{1}{2} \text{ hours}$$

Now to find what percentage of 35 is $5\frac{1}{2}$, divide:

$$5.5 \div 35 = 0.16 \text{ or } 16\%$$

Note: $5\frac{1}{2} = 5.5$

16% remains for messenger work.

5. **The correct answer is (C).**

   Item

5 computers $1,400/year	5 × 1,400	$7,000
Maintenance, repairs $100/computer	5 × 100	$500
5 operators' annual salaries $30,000	5 × $30,000	$150,000
Supervisor's annual salary $38,000	1 × $38,000	$38,000
Total cost		$195,500

   If 10 employees were paid a total of $324,000, find the savings by subtracting:

   $324,000 − $195,500 = $128,500 one year's savings

   To find the savings for five years, multiply:

   $128,500 × 5 = $642,500

   This amount *rounds off* to (or, is nearest to) $640,000.

6. **The correct answer is (D).** If Joe can do the job alone in eight days, then he can do $\frac{1}{8}$ in one

   day and $\frac{6}{8}$, or $\frac{3}{4}$, in six days.

   Let *n* be the number of days it would take Mary to do the job alone. Then:

   $\frac{1}{n}$ is the part of the job she can do in one day,

   and $\frac{2}{n}$ is the part of the job she can do in the two

   days she works with Joe.

   Now, the sum of parts done by Joe and Mary equals one whole job:

   $$\frac{3}{4} + \frac{2}{n} = 1$$

   $3n + 8 = 4n$ (multiply by the lowest common
   denominator, 4*n*)

   $8 = 4n - 3n$ (subtract 3*n* from both sides of the
   equation)

   $8 = n$ (subtract like terms)

   $n = 8$

   Mary alone could do the job in eight days.

7. **The correct answer is (C).**

Eighty dozen = $80 \times 12 = 960$

960 pairs of gloves were purchased.

To find the maximum number of days the gloves will last, divide $960 \div 32 = 30$

If the gloves are being used at a rate of 32 pairs per day, they will last thirty days.

8. **The correct answer is (D).** To determine the cost of caring for 24 patients for five days, find the cost of caring for 1 patient by dividing.

$\$7,200.00 \div 3 = \$2,400.00$

To get the cost for caring for 24 patients, multiply

$24 \times \$2,400.00 = \$57,600.00$

The cost for caring for 24 patients is $57,600.00.

9. **The correct answer is (C).** A can do one third of the job in 1 hour. B can do one fifth of the job in 1 hour. Together they can do $\frac{1}{3} + \frac{1}{5}$ of the job in 1 hour. Let t be the time it takes for both to do the job. Together, they can do $\frac{1}{t}$ of the job in 1 hour. Thus:

$$\frac{1}{3} + \frac{1}{5} = \frac{1}{t}$$

$5t + 3t = 15$ (multiply by the lowest common denominator, $15t$ or $3 \times 5 \times t$)

$8t = 15$ (add like terms)

$t = \frac{15}{8}$ (divide both sides by 8 hours)

$t = 1\frac{7}{8}$

10. **The correct answer is (C).** Let x be the unknown original capital and $0.50x$ be 50 percent of the unknown capital.

$x + .50x = \$18,000$

$1.50x = \$18,000$ (add like terms)

$\frac{150x}{1.50} = \frac{\$18,000}{1.50}$ (divide both sides by 1.50)

$x = \$12,000$

$12,000 is the original amount of the capital.

11. **The correct answer is (A).** Let x represent the amount of time it takes to work off 100 calories.

The ratio of the amount of time it takes to work off 60 calories equals the ratio of the amount of time it takes to work off 100 calories:

$$\frac{15 \text{ minutes}}{60 \text{ calories}} = \frac{x \text{ minutes}}{100 \text{ calories}}$$

$60x = 15 \times 100$

$60x = 1,500$

$x = 25$ minutes

It will take 25 minutes on the treadmill to work off 100 calories.

12. **The correct answer is (A).** If two fifths of his salary was used, then three fifths was left; three fifths of his salary is $81. Now, since his salary is unknown, let x represent it:

$\frac{3}{5} \times x = \$81$

$x = \$81 \div \frac{3}{5}$ (divide both sides by $\frac{3}{5}$)

$x = \$81 \times \frac{5}{3}$ (invert and multiply)

$x = \$135$

His salary is $135 for 30 days of work. To find the *daily wage,* divide the salary by 30:

$\$135 \div 30$ days $= \$4.50$/day

Daily wage $= \$4.50$

13. **The correct answer is (D).** To find the number of motorcycles purchased, first subtract his original purchase price from the selling price:

$\$6,200 - \$4,000 = \$2,200$ profit

Since the profit was $2,200, and the profit on each motorcycle was $50, the number of motorcycles sold is:

$\$2,200$ profit $\div \$50$ profit/motorcycle $= 44$ motorcycles sold

14. **The correct answer is (C).** $\frac{1}{4}$ in *goods*

(given)

$\frac{2}{3} \times \frac{3}{4} = \frac{1}{2}$ in *land* (because $\frac{3}{4}$ is the re-

mainder after the goods are invested), $\frac{1}{4}$

is left in *cash*, because if $\frac{1}{4}$ is in goods,

and $\frac{1}{2}$ is in land, then $\frac{3}{4}$ is invested, leav-

ing $\frac{1}{4}$ for cash.

If $\frac{1}{4}$, which is the cash, is valued at $1,224,

To find total capital, multiply $1,224 × 4.

Total capital = $4,896

15. **The correct answer is (A).** Let *A* equal the amount A earned, and *B* equal the amount B earned.

Together, they earned $A + B = \$2,100$.

If B is paid $\frac{1}{4}$ more than A, then A's sal-

ary plus $\frac{1}{4}$ of A's salary is equal to B's

salary.

Express this as follows:

$$A + B = \$2,100$$

$$B = A + \frac{1}{4}A$$

$$B = 1\frac{1}{4}$$

$$A + 1\frac{1}{4}A = 2,100$$

$$2\frac{1}{4}A = 2,100$$

$$A = 933\frac{1}{3}$$

A earns $933.33

B earns $933.33 \times 1\frac{1}{4} = 1,166\frac{2}{3}$

B earns $1,166.66

16. **The correct answer is (D).** The boat costs $21,500 and was sold for $23,650. Subtract:

$$\$23,650 - \$21,500 = \$2,150$$

$2,150 was gained. To find the percentage gained, divide the amount gained by the original amount:

$$\$2,150 \div \$21,500 = 0.10, \text{ or } 10\%$$

Percentage gained = 10%

17. **The correct answer is (B).** $\frac{5}{6} \div \frac{3}{4} = \frac{5}{8}$ of

the property costs $1,800

Then, letting *y* represent the value of the property,

$$\frac{5}{8} \times y = \$1,800$$

$$y = \$1,800 \div \frac{5}{8} \left(\text{divide both sides by } \frac{5}{8} \right)$$

$$y = \$1,800 \times \frac{8}{5} \text{ (invert and multiply)}$$

Therefore, $2,880 is the price of the property.

18. **The correct answer is (A).** A lot costs $21,250.

$1,900	is received for lease
− 300	is deducted for expenses
$1,600	is net income

To find what percentage $1,600 is of the cost of the lot, divide:

$$1,600 \div 21,250 = 0.075, \text{ or } 7\frac{1}{2}\%$$

$7\frac{1}{2}\% = $ percentage of cost

19. The correct answer is (A). Total shares currently owned = 75

Values per share = $50

To find the value of the stock, multiply

$75 \times \$50 = \$3,750$

To find 8%, multiply the stock value by 0.08

$\$3,750 \times 0.08 = \$300$ (dividend)

Given $300, divide by $50 to see how many additional shares of stock can be purchased:

$\$300 \div 50 = 6$ shares

Therefore, he now owns $75 + 6 = 81$ shares.

20. The correct answer is (C). First, find the salary each man is paid for 1 day. To do so, divide their salaries by 5 days:

		salary/day	salary/ 3 days
A	$\dfrac{\$250}{5} =$	$\$50.00 \times 3 =$	$\$150$
B	$\dfrac{\$130}{5} =$	$\$26.00 \times 3 =$	$\$78$
C	$\dfrac{\$120}{5} =$	$\$24.00 \times 3 =$	$\$72$
D	$\dfrac{\$90}{5} =$	$\$18.00 \times 3 =$	$\$54$

Total salaries for 3 days = $354

Test 4

1. D	8. C	15. A	21. A	27. D
2. B	9. A	16. B	22. C	28. A
3. B	10. B	17. C	23. A	29. C
4. A	11. C	18. D	24. D	30. C
5. D	12. D	19. A	25. A	31. A
6. D	13. A	20. C	26. A	
7. A	14. B			

1. The correct answer is (D).

$-11 - (-2)$
$= -11 + 2$
$= -9$

2. The correct answer is (B). $6.47 + 5.89 + 3.42 + .65 + 7.09 = 23.52$

To find the average, divide the sum by 5 (the number of terms involved)

$23.52 \div 5 = 4.704$

Average = 4.704

3. **The correct answer is (B).**

$$512.69\frac{59}{89}$$

$$.89\overline{)456.30.00}$$
$$\underline{445}$$
$$113$$
$$\underline{89}$$
$$240$$
$$\underline{178}$$
$$620$$
$$\underline{534}$$
$$860$$
$$\underline{801}$$
$$59 \text{ remainder}$$

$512.69\frac{59}{89}$ rounds off to 512.70.

4. **The correct answer is (A).**

$$
\begin{array}{l}
5 \text{ hours } 13 \text{ minutes} \\
3 \text{ hours } 49 \text{ minutes} \\
+ \qquad\qquad 24 \text{ minutes} \\
\hline
8 \text{ hours } 86 \text{ minutes}
\end{array}
$$

Since there are 60 minutes in 1 hour, then 86 minutes = 60 minutes + 26 minutes or 1 hour and 26 minutes.

So, 8 hours and 86 minutes = 9 hours and 26 minutes.

5. **The correct answer is (D).** $\dfrac{18}{47} = \dfrac{126}{x}$

$18x = 47(126)$ (cross-multiply)
$18x = 5,922$
$x = 329$ (divide by 18)

6. **The correct answer is (D).**
$0.3125 = \dfrac{3,125}{10,000} = \dfrac{5}{16}$

7. **The correct answer is (A).** $\dfrac{7}{8} \div \dfrac{7}{8}$

$= \dfrac{7}{8} \times \dfrac{8}{7}$ (invert the second term
and multiply)

$= 1$

8. **The correct answer is (C).** 5, 8, 13, 20. To each number, add the next odd number to determine the next number in the series.

Series		Odd Number	
5	+	3	= 8
8	+	5	= 13
13	+	7	= 20
20	+	9	= 29

29 will be the next number.

9. **The correct answer is (A).** *Interest = Principal × Rate × Time*

$= \$300 \times 0.06 \times \dfrac{10}{360}$

$= \dfrac{\$180}{360} = \dfrac{\$1}{2}$

$= \$.50$

10. **The correct answer is (B).** First, find the number of $1\frac{1}{2}$ inch units there are in 5 inches. Do this by dividing:

$5 \div 1\frac{1}{2}$

$= 5 \div \dfrac{3}{2}$ $\left(\text{change } 1\frac{1}{2} \text{ to } \dfrac{3}{2}\right)$

$= 5 \times \dfrac{2}{3}$ (invert and multiply)

$= \dfrac{10}{3}$

Now find the total miles by multiplying:

$500 \times \dfrac{10}{3} = 1,666.67$

Five inches represents approximately 1,700 miles.

11. **The correct answer is (C).** $\dfrac{1}{2}\% = 0.5\%$,

or $\dfrac{0.5}{100} = 0.005$

12. **The correct answer is (D).** $260 is 20% of the bonus. Write this in equation form. Let the bonus be x.

$$\$260 = .20x$$
$$\frac{260}{.20} = \frac{.20x}{.20} \quad \text{(divide by 0.20)}$$
$$\$1,300 = x$$

Her entire bonus was $1,300.

13. **The correct answer is (A).** 1 kilogram = 35 ounces

Find how many grams there are in 1 ounce.

Note: 1 kilogram = 1,000 grams

$$1,000 \text{ grams} = 35 \text{ ounces}$$

$$1 \text{ ounce} \times \frac{1,000 \text{ grams}}{35 \text{ ounces}} = \frac{1,000 \text{ grams}}{35}$$
$$= 28.6, \text{ or } 29 \text{ grams}$$
$$\text{in 1 ounce}$$

14. **The correct answer is (B).** To find the amount of time it takes to deliver the 90 milligrams at a rate of 24 milligrams per hour, divide

amount of time = 90 milligrams ÷

24 milligrams per hour = 3.75 hours

3.75 hours = $3\frac{3}{4}$ hours =

3 hours and 45 minutes

15. **The correct answer is (A).** First, find the number of seconds there are in one-half minute:

$$\frac{1}{2} \times 60 \text{ sec/min} = 30 \text{ seconds}$$

Since sound travels 1,100 feet per second, it will travel:

30 sec. × 1,100 ft. = 33,000 ft.

Change the 33,000 feet to miles (1 mile = 5,280 feet)

$$33,000 \text{ feet} \times \frac{1 \text{ mile}}{5,280 \text{ feet}} = \frac{33,000}{5280}$$
$$= 6.25$$

Round off: 6.25 miles = about 6 miles

16. **The correct answer is (B).** 1 kilometer = $\frac{5}{8}$ mile

x kilometer = 2 miles

$$\frac{1 \text{ kilometer}}{\frac{5}{8} \text{ mile}} = \frac{x}{2}$$
$$\frac{5}{8}x = 2$$
$$5x = 16$$
$$x = 3.2$$

2 miles = about 3.2 kilometers

17. **The correct answer is (C).** Perimeter of a rectangle (the hall is shaped like a rectangle) is:

$$Perimeter = 2 \, length + 2 \, width$$
$$= 2(75) + 2(25)$$
$$= 150 + 50$$
$$= 200 \text{ feet}$$

The perimeter is 200 feet.

Now change 200 feet to yards (3 feet = 1 yard).

$$200 \text{ feet} \times \frac{1 \text{ yard}}{3 \text{ feet}} = 66\frac{2}{3} \text{ yards}$$

18. **The correct answer is (D).** Let the price of a blouse be x. Then:

$$x - 16\frac{2}{3}\% = 35$$

$$\frac{2}{3} = 0.67, \text{ so } 16.6770\% = 0.1667$$

$$x - 0.1667x = \$35 \text{ (change the percent to a decimal)}$$

$$0.8333x = \$35 \text{ (combine like terms)}$$

$$x = \$42 \text{ (divide by 0.8333)}$$

The list price was $42.

19. **The correct answer is (A).** To find the number of decimal places in the product of two numbers, find the sum of the number of digits to the right of the decimal of each number.

0.4266 has 4 digits to the right.
0.3333 has 4 digits to the right.

There should be 8 digits in the product.

20. **The correct answer is (C).** 5.5 thousand × $50 thousand = $275

21. **The correct answer is (A).**

$$\begin{array}{r} 1100. \\ .52\overline{)572.00.} \\ \underline{52} \\ 52 \\ \underline{52} \\ 52 \\ \underline{52} \\ 0 \end{array}$$

Answer: 1,100

22. **The correct answer is (C).** 200 percent of 800

$$2.00 \times 800 = 1,600$$

23. **The correct answer is (A).** The total games played was 15. To find their average, divide games won by total played:

$$10 \div 15 = 0.667$$

Their average is 0.667.

24. **The correct answer is (D).** To find the soil needed, first change the 8 inches to feet, so all units will be the same.

$$8 \text{ inches} \times \frac{1 \text{ foot}}{12 \text{ inches}} = 0.67 \text{ feet}$$

Now multiply all units.

$$3 \text{ feet} \times 0.67 \text{ feet} \times 1 \text{ foot} = 2 \text{ cubic feet}$$

2 cubic feet of soil will be needed to fill the box.

25. **The correct answer is (A).** Find the price for one watch by dividing:

$$\$1,250 \text{ (per hundred)} \div 100 = \$12.50 \text{ (price of one watch)}$$

To find the cost of 228, multiply the number of watches by the price per watch.

$$228 \text{ watches} \times \$12.50 \text{ per watch} = \$2,850$$

The cost of the watches will be $2,850.

26. **The correct answer is (A).** Find the area of the small rectangle and subtract its area from the large rectangle to determine the shaded area.

Large rectangle

$$\begin{aligned} A &= length \times width \\ &= 6 \times 15 \\ &= 90 \text{ square inches} \end{aligned}$$

Small rectangle

$$\begin{aligned} A &= length \times width \\ &= 4 \times 9 \\ &= 36 \text{ square inches} \end{aligned}$$

$$90 - 36 = 54 \text{ square inches}$$

The area of the shaded area is 54 square inches.

27. **The correct answer is (D).**

From	To	Time
March 15, 1979	March 15, 1988	9 years
March 15, 1988	Jan. 15, 1989	10 months
Jan. 15, 1989	Feb. 12, 1989	27 days

His age will be 9 years, 10 months, 27 days.

28. **The correct answer is (A).** On the chart, each line represents 10 units. The highest IQ is about halfway on the first line, which is half of 10.

So, the answer is 5.

29. **The correct answer is (C).** Locate 75 on the base and trace it to the horizontal intersection.

30. **The correct answer is (C).** There are 100 students with an IQ of 80. Looking across the chart we see that there are also 100 students with an IQ of 110.

31. **The correct answer is (A).** The highest point on the graph points to an IQ of 100.

Quantitative Comparisons Test 5

1. D		7. C		13. D		19. A		24. B	
2. C		8. B		14. D		20. A		25. B	
3. A		9. C		15. D		21. A		26. A	
4. C		10. A		16. C		22. A		27. C	
5. A		11. D		17. B		23. C		28. C	
6. D		12. A		18. C					

1. **The correct answer is (D).** The value of $\angle x$ or $\angle y$ cannot be determined unless the measure of at least one angle is known.

2. **The correct answer is (C).**

   Area of $\triangle DEC = \frac{1}{2}$ base $\times$ height

   Area of parallelogram = base $\times$ height

   Area of $\triangle ADE + \triangle EBC =$ (area of the whole parallelogram – area of $\triangle DEC$)

   $= \left($base $\times$ height $- \frac{1}{2}$ base $\times$ height$\right)$

   $= \frac{1}{2}$ base $\times$ height

3. **The correct answer is (A).**

   $$x^3 + x^2 - x + 1 = (-1)^3 + (-1)^2 - (-1) + 1$$
   $$= -1 + 1 + 1 + 1$$
   $$= 2$$
   $$x^3 - x^2 + x - 1 = (-1)^3 - (-1)^2 + (-1) - 1$$
   $$= -1 - 1 - 1 - 1$$
   $$= -4$$

4. **The correct answer is (C).** A cube has six surfaces; each one's area is e^2:

   $$e^3 = 27$$
   $$e = 3$$
   $$6e^2 = 54$$
   $$e^2 = 9$$
   $$e = 3$$

5. **The correct answer is (A).**

   $$\frac{\frac{1}{2} + \frac{1}{3}}{\frac{2}{3}} = \frac{\frac{3}{6} + \frac{2}{6}}{\frac{4}{6}} = \frac{\frac{5}{6}}{\frac{4}{6}} = \frac{5}{6} \times \frac{6}{4} = \frac{5}{4}$$

   $$\frac{\frac{2}{3}}{\frac{1}{2} + \frac{1}{3}} = \frac{\frac{4}{6}}{\frac{3}{6} + \frac{2}{6}} = \frac{\frac{4}{6}}{\frac{5}{6}} = \frac{4}{6} \times \frac{6}{5} = \frac{4}{5}$$

   $$\frac{5}{4} = \frac{5}{4} \times \frac{5}{5} = \frac{25}{20}$$

   $$\frac{4}{5} = \frac{4}{5} \times \frac{4}{4} = \frac{16}{20}$$

   $$\frac{25}{20} > \frac{16}{20}$$

6. **The correct answer is (D).** Area of circle with radius x^3:

   $$A = \pi r^2 = \pi(x^3)^2 = \pi x^6$$
   $$= 3.14x^6$$

   Area of circle radius $3x$:

   $$A = \pi r^2 = \pi(3x)^2 = \pi(9x^2) = 3.14(9x^2)$$
   $$= 28.26x^2$$

   We cannot know whether $3.14x^6$ or $28.26x^2$ is larger unless we know the value of x.

   $$\left(\frac{1}{4}\right)^{-2} = \frac{1}{\left(\frac{1}{4}\right)^2} \quad \text{(Note that } 4^2 = 16.\text{)}$$

7. **The correct answer is (C).**

$$= \frac{1}{\frac{1}{16}}$$
$$= 16$$

8. **The correct answer is (B).**

$$\sqrt{0.02} = .1414$$
$$0.02 < .1414$$

9. **The correct answer is (C).** By the Pythagorean theorem, $(AB)^2 = (AC)^2 + (BC)^2$

However, $(BC)^2 = 5^2 = 25$ and $5CB = 5 \times 5 = 25$

Therefore, $(BC)^2 = 5CB$

$(AB)^2 = (AC)^2 + 5CB$ [substituting $5CB$ for $(BC)^2$ in the Pythagorean theorem]

10. **The correct answer is (A).** Area of circle with radius

$$A = \pi r^2 = 3.14 \times 7^2$$
$$= 3.14 \times 49 = 153.86$$
Note : $\pi \approx 3.14$

Area of equilateral Δ with side of 14:

A line from one vertex to the mid-point of the opposite side is perpendicular to the opposite side. It is, therefore, the height of the triangle.

Let the length of this line be h. Then, by the Pythagorean theorem, $7^2 + h^2 = 14^2$.

$$h^2 = 14^2 - 7^2 = 147$$
$$h^2 = 3 \times 7 \times 7$$
$$h = 7\sqrt{3}$$

$$\text{Area of } \Delta = \frac{1}{2} \text{ base} \times \text{height}$$
$$= \frac{1}{2}(14)(7\sqrt{3}) \quad Note : \sqrt{3} \approx 1.732$$
$$\text{Area of } \Delta = (7)7\sqrt{3}$$
$$= 49\sqrt{3}$$
$$= 49 \times 1.732 = 84.87$$
$$153.86 > 84.87$$

Thus, the area of the circle is greater than the area of the triangle.

11. **The correct answer is (D).** Not enough information is given to determine the values of the angles.

12. **The correct answer is (A).** (Area of shaded portion) = (Area of larger circle) – (Area of smaller circle)

$$\text{Area of larger circle} = \pi r^2 \quad = \pi \times 10^2$$
$$= 3.14 \times 10^2$$
$$= 3.14 \times 100$$
$$= 314$$
$$\text{Area of smaller circle} = \pi r^2 \quad = \pi \times 7^2$$
$$= 3.14 \times 7^2$$
$$= 3.14 \times 49$$
$$= 153.86$$
$$\text{Area of shaded region} = 314 - 153.86 = 160.14$$
$$160.14 > 153.86$$

13. **The correct answer is (D).**

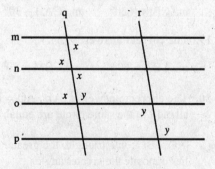

All that can be determined is that x and y are supplementary.

14. **The correct answer is (D).** There is insufficient information to determine an answer.

15. **The correct answer is (D).** There is insufficient information to determine an answer.

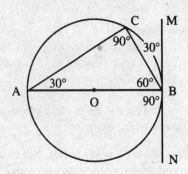

16. **The correct answer is (C).** m∠ACB = 90°

    m∠NBO = 90°

    A tangent to a circle is perpendicular to the radius of the circle at their point of contact. An inscribed angle is equal to one half its intercepted arc. Therefore, m∠ACB = 90°.

17. **The correct answer is (B).**

    $\overarc{AC} = 120°$ $\overarc{CB} = 60°$

    An inscribed angle is equal to one half its intercepted arc.

18. **The correct answer is (C).**

    m∠CBM = 30°   m∠CAB = 30°

19. **The correct answer is (A).**

    m∠CBA = 60°   m∠CBM = 30°

20. **The correct answer is (A).** $\overline{AO} = \overline{BO}$; all radii in the same circle are equal.

    $\overline{AC} > \overline{BC}$; in a triangle, the greater side lies opposite the greater angle.

    $\overline{AO} + \overline{AC} > \overline{BO} + \overline{BC}$

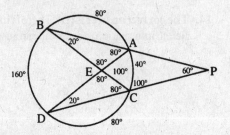

21. **The correct answer is (A).**

    m∠APC = 60°   m∠ABC = 20°

22. **The correct answer is (A).**

    m∠BED = 100°   m∠BEA = 80°

23. **The correct answer is (C).**

    m∠BAD = 80°   m∠DCB = 80°

24. **The correct answer is (B).**

    m∠BCP = 100°

    m∠AEC + m∠ADC = 100° + 20° = 120°

25. **The correct answer is (B).**

    $\overarc{DC} + \overarc{AC} = 80° + 40° = 120°$

    $\overarc{BD} = 160°$

26. **The correct answer is (A).**

    75% of $\frac{3}{4}$ = .75 × .75   .09 × 6 = .54

    = .5625

27. **The correct answer is (C).**

    4% of 0.003 = 0.04 × .003

    = 0.00012

    3% of 0.004 = 0.03 × 0.004

    = 0.00012

28. **The correct answer is (C).**

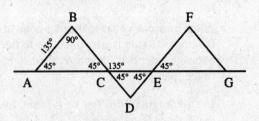

    ∠BCA = 45°   ∠FEG = 45°

Quantative Comparisons Test 6

1. A	4. D	7. D	9. C	11. C
2. A	5. A	8. C	10. B	12. A
3. B	6. C			

1. **The correct answer is (A).** The statement $a > 0$ and $x > 0$ implies both a and x are positive. The sum of two positive numbers is always greater than their difference.

2. **The correct answer is (A).** The averages of Column A and Column B are 21 and 20, respectively.

3. **The correct answer is (B).** $\angle ABC = x$ (vertical angles are equal). Since $\angle C = 90°$, $\angle A + \angle ABC = 90°$ (180° in a triangle). Therefore, $2x = 90°$, and $x = 45°$. $\angle ABC$ and $\angle y$ are supplementary; hence, $y = 135°$. Therefore, $y > 2x$.

4. **The correct answer is (D).** This is impossible to determine because a could be any number between 0 and 12 and b, any number between 0 and 10.

5. **The correct answer is (A).** $4a - 4b = 20$

$$a - b = 5$$
$$a - 5 = b$$

For all values of a and b, $a > b$.

6. **The correct answer is (C).** Angles opposite equal sides of a triangle are equal.

7. **The correct answer is (D).** This is impossible to determine because b could be positive or negative.

8. **The correct answer is (C).** If two parallel lines are cut by a transversal, the alternate exterior angles are equal.

9. **The correct answer is (C).** Column A and Column B both equal 27.

10. **The correct answer is (B).** The greater side lies opposite the greater angle.

11. **The correct answer is (C).** The exterior angle of a triangle is equal to the two interior nonadjacent angles.

12. **The correct answer is (A).** The value of Column A is 12, and the value of Column B is $2\frac{2}{3}$. Therefore, A > B.

Final Mathematics Examination Answer Sheet

Part 1: General Mathematics

1. Ⓐ Ⓑ Ⓒ Ⓓ	10. Ⓐ Ⓑ Ⓒ Ⓓ	19. Ⓐ Ⓑ Ⓒ Ⓓ	27. Ⓐ Ⓑ Ⓒ Ⓓ	35. Ⓐ Ⓑ Ⓒ Ⓓ
2. Ⓐ Ⓑ Ⓒ Ⓓ	11. Ⓐ Ⓑ Ⓒ Ⓓ	20. Ⓐ Ⓑ Ⓒ Ⓓ	28. Ⓐ Ⓑ Ⓒ Ⓓ	36. Ⓐ Ⓑ Ⓒ Ⓓ
3. Ⓐ Ⓑ Ⓒ Ⓓ	12. Ⓐ Ⓑ Ⓒ Ⓓ	21. Ⓐ Ⓑ Ⓒ Ⓓ	29. Ⓐ Ⓑ Ⓒ Ⓓ	37. Ⓐ Ⓑ Ⓒ Ⓓ
4. Ⓐ Ⓑ Ⓒ Ⓓ	13. Ⓐ Ⓑ Ⓒ Ⓓ	22. Ⓐ Ⓑ Ⓒ Ⓓ	30. Ⓐ Ⓑ Ⓒ Ⓓ	38. Ⓐ Ⓑ Ⓒ Ⓓ
5. Ⓐ Ⓑ Ⓒ Ⓓ	14. Ⓐ Ⓑ Ⓒ Ⓓ	23. Ⓐ Ⓑ Ⓒ Ⓓ	31. Ⓐ Ⓑ Ⓒ Ⓓ	39. Ⓐ Ⓑ Ⓒ Ⓓ
6. Ⓐ Ⓑ Ⓒ Ⓓ	15. Ⓐ Ⓑ Ⓒ Ⓓ	24. Ⓐ Ⓑ Ⓒ Ⓓ	32. Ⓐ Ⓑ Ⓒ Ⓓ	40. Ⓐ Ⓑ Ⓒ Ⓓ
7. Ⓐ Ⓑ Ⓒ Ⓓ	16. Ⓐ Ⓑ Ⓒ Ⓓ	25. Ⓐ Ⓑ Ⓒ Ⓓ	33. Ⓐ Ⓑ Ⓒ Ⓓ	41. Ⓐ Ⓑ Ⓒ Ⓓ
8. Ⓐ Ⓑ Ⓒ Ⓓ	17. Ⓐ Ⓑ Ⓒ Ⓓ	26. Ⓐ Ⓑ Ⓒ Ⓓ	34. Ⓐ Ⓑ Ⓒ Ⓓ	42. Ⓐ Ⓑ Ⓒ Ⓓ
9. Ⓐ Ⓑ Ⓒ Ⓓ	18. Ⓐ Ⓑ Ⓒ Ⓓ			

Part 2: Quantitative Comparisons

1. Ⓐ Ⓑ Ⓒ Ⓓ	4. Ⓐ Ⓑ Ⓒ Ⓓ	7. Ⓐ Ⓑ Ⓒ Ⓓ	10. Ⓐ Ⓑ Ⓒ Ⓓ
2. Ⓐ Ⓑ Ⓒ Ⓓ	5. Ⓐ Ⓑ Ⓒ Ⓓ	8. Ⓐ Ⓑ Ⓒ Ⓓ	11. Ⓐ Ⓑ Ⓒ Ⓓ
3. Ⓐ Ⓑ Ⓒ Ⓓ	6. Ⓐ Ⓑ Ⓒ Ⓓ	9. Ⓐ Ⓑ Ⓒ Ⓓ	12. Ⓐ Ⓑ Ⓒ Ⓓ

answer sheet

FINAL MATHEMATICS EXAMINATION

Part 1: General Mathematics

42 Questions • 40 Minutes

Directions: Each problem on this test requires logical reasoning and thinking, besides simple computations, to find the solution. Read each problem carefully and choose the correct answer from the four choices that follow. Fill in the corresponding space on your answer sheet.

1. Jane Doe borrowed $225,000 for five years at $13\frac{1}{2}$ percent. The annual interest charge was
   - (A) $1,667.
   - (B) $6,000.
   - (C) $30,375.
   - (D) $39,375.

2. A junior salesman gets a commission of 14 percent on his sales. If he wants his commission to amount to $140, he will have to sell merchandise totaling
   - (A) $1,960.
   - (B) $10.
   - (C) $1,000.
   - (D) $100.

3. On a list price of $200, the difference between a single discount of 25 percent and successive discounts of 20 percent and 5 percent is
   - (A) $0.
   - (B) $48.
   - (C) $8.
   - (D) $2.

4. *A* worked five days on overhauling an old car. *B* worked four days more to finish the job. After the sale of the car, the net profit was $243. They wanted to divide the profit on the basis of the time spent by each. *A*'s share of the profit was
   - (A) $108.
   - (B) $135.
   - (C) $127.
   - (D) $143.

5. If cloth costs $42\frac{1}{2}$ cents per yard, how many yards can be purchased for $76.50?
   - (A) 220
   - (B) 180
   - (C) 190
   - (D) 230

6. A fashionable dress shop offers a 20 percent discount on selected items. For a dress marked at $280, what is the discount price?
   - (A) $224.00
   - (B) $232.00
   - (C) $248.00
   - (D) $261.00

7. If *A* takes six days to do a task and *B* takes three days to do the same task, working together they should do the same task in
   - (A) $2\frac{2}{3}$ days.
   - (B) 2 days.
   - (C) $2\frac{1}{3}$ days.
   - (D) $2\frac{1}{2}$ days.

8. The area of a mirror 40 inches long and 20 inches wide is approximately
   - (A) 8.5 square feet.
   - (B) 5.5 square feet.
   - (C) 8.0 square feet.
   - (D) 2.5 square feet.

9. $\frac{2}{3}$ plus $\frac{1}{8}$ equals

(A) $\frac{37}{72}$

(B) $\frac{82}{72}$

(C) $\frac{3}{11}$

(D) $\frac{19}{24}$

10. A student has received two grades of 90 and two grades of 80 in an English course. Assuming the grades are weighted equally, what is the student's average for the course?

(A) 90
(B) 87
(C) 85
(D) 84

11. If a man has only quarters and dimes totaling $2.00, the number of quarters CANNOT be

(A) 2.
(B) 4.
(C) 6.
(D) 3.

12. The number that increased by one sixth of itself yields 182 is

(A) 156.
(B) 176.
(C) 148.
(D) 160.

13. $0.16\frac{3}{4}$ written as a percent is

(A) $16\frac{3}{4}$ percent.

(B) $16.\frac{3}{4}$ percent.

(C) $0.016\frac{3}{4}$ percent.

(D) $0.0016\frac{3}{4}$ percent.

14. If 4 ounces of protein provide 448 calories, how much protein is needed to provide 392 calories?

(A) 2.8 ounces
(B) 3.5 ounces
(C) 4.57 ounces
(D) 56 ounces

15. $1,296.53 minus $264.87 is

(A) $1,232.76.
(B) $1,032.76.
(C) $1,031.66.
(D) $1,132.53.

16. $12\frac{1}{2}$ minus $6\frac{1}{4}$ is

(A) $5\frac{3}{4}$.

(B) $6\frac{1}{4}$.

(C) $6\frac{1}{2}$.

(D) $5\frac{1}{4}$.

17. Men's handkerchiefs cost $1.29 for three. The cost per dozen handkerchiefs is

(A) $7.74.
(B) $3.87.
(C) $14.48.
(D) $5.16.

18. Add: $\frac{1}{4}, \frac{7}{12}, \frac{3}{8}, \frac{1}{2}$, and $\frac{5}{6}$:

(A) $2\frac{1}{2}$

(B) $2\frac{13}{24}$

(C) $2\frac{3}{4}$

(D) $2\frac{15}{24}$

19. A floor is 25 feet wide by 36 feet long. To cover this floor with carpet will require
    (A) 100 square yards.
    (B) 300 square yards.
    (C) 900 square yards.
    (D) 25 square yards.

20. 72 divided by 0.0009 is
    (A) 0.125.
    (B) 800.
    (C) 80,000.
    (D) 80.

21. 345 safety pins at $4.15 per hundred will cost
    (A) $0.1432.
    (B) $1.4320.
    (C) $14.32.
    (D) $143.20.

22. The number that decreased by one fifth of itself yields 132 is
    (A) 165.
    (B) 198.
    (C) 98.
    (D) 88.

23. 285 is 5 percent of
    (A) 1,700.
    (B) 7,350.
    (C) 1,750.
    (D) 5,700.

24. A store sold jackets for $65 each. The jackets cost the store $50 each. The percentage of increase of selling price over cost is
    (A) 40 percent.
    (B) $33\frac{1}{2}$ percent.
    (C) $33\frac{1}{3}$ percent.
    (D) 30 percent.

25. The denominator of a fraction is 20 more than the numerator. What is the numerator if the fraction is equivalent to $\frac{3}{5}$?
    (A) 12
    (B) 30
    (C) –50
    (D) 10

26. Which statement below is true about the inequality of $2 < x \le 7$?
    (A) $x < 2$
    (B) $x = 2$
    (C) x is greater than 7
    (D) $x > 2$

27. $\frac{x}{5} - 4 = 11$. Find the value of x.
    (A) 75
    (B) 3
    (C) 35
    (D) 59

28. A punch recipe for a half gallon (64 ounces) of punch requires one pint (16 ounces) of grape juice. How many quarts (1 quart = 32 ounces) of grape juice are required for $2\frac{1}{2}$ gallons of the punch?
    (A) 5 quarts
    (B) 10 quarts
    (C) $1\frac{1}{4}$ quarts
    (D) $2\frac{1}{2}$ quarts

29. Mrs. Bowler got up at 7:00 a.m. last Wednesday morning and went to bed at 11:00 p.m. Wednesday night. During the time that she was up, she spent $\frac{1}{2}$ of her time at work, $\frac{1}{8}$ of her time bowling with friends, and $\frac{1}{4}$ of her time with her family. How much time did she have left for other activities?
    (A) 2 hours
    (B) 4 hours
    (C) 1 hour
    (D) 8 hours

30. If 24 percent of the students who enrolled in an algebra class of 50 students dropped the course before the semester ended, how many students remained in the class?
    (A) 27
    (B) 76
    (C) 12
    (D) 38

31. How many $\frac{3}{4}$–gram tablets are needed for a dosage of $4\frac{1}{2}$ grams?
    (A) 3.75
    (B) 1.5
    (C) 6
    (D) 3

32. $3.6 - 1.2(0.8 - 0.3) + 8 \div 0.4 =$
    (A) 23
    (B) 20.5
    (C) 50
    (D) 3.2

33. Find 0.2 percent of 400.
    (A) 80
    (B) 800
    (C) 0.8
    (D) 2,000

34. An 8-ounce bottle of fruit juice provides 200 calories. What percent of the 200 calories is provided by 3 ounces of the fruit juice?
    (A) 12.5 percent
    (B) 22.5 percent
    (C) 37.5 percent
    (D) 75 percent

35. Find the length of the hypotenuse in the triangle below.

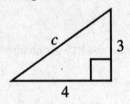

    (A) 7
    (B) 5
    (C) 25
    (D) 6

36. What is the width of a rectangle with an area of 63 square feet and a length of 9 feet?
    (A) 22.5 feet
    (B) 7 feet
    (C) 567 feet
    (D) 144 feet

37. If the triangles below are similar, find the length of side x.

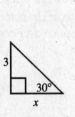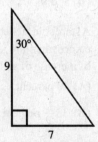

    (A) 21 inches
    (B) 11 inches
    (C) 13 inches
    (D) $3\frac{6}{7}$ inches

38. If two lines are parallel, which of the following statements is true?

    (A) The two lines have equal slopes.

    (B) The two lines have one point in common.

    (C) The product of the slopes of the lines is −1.

    (D) The two lines form right angles.

39. If the area of a square is 144 m², what is the length of a side of the square?

    (A) 12m

    (B) 12m²

    (C) 72m

    (D) 72m²

40. Find the area of the figure below.

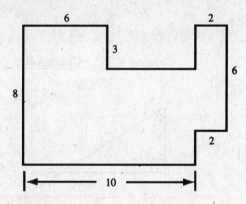

    (A) 40m

    (B) 46m

    (C) 80m²

    (D) 96m²

41. Consider the circle with central angles shown below:

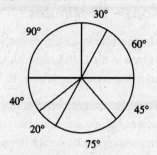

What percent of the circle does the central angle of 60° represent? (Give answer to the nearest degree.)

    (A) 6 percent

    (B) 60 percent

    (C) 17 percent

    (D) 25 percent

42. If $\frac{1}{12}$ of a family's weekly budget is spent on entertainment and $\frac{1}{8}$ of the budget is spent on gasoline, which central angle represents the total spent on entertainment and gasoline?

    (A) 20

    (B) 45

    (C) 90

    (D) 75

Part 2: Quantitative Comparisons

12 Questions • 20 Minutes

Common Information: In each question, information concerning one or both of the quantities to be compared is given in the ITEM column. A symbol that appears in any column represents the same thing in column A as it does in column B.

Figures: Assume that the position of points, angles, regions, and so forth, are in the order shown; that the lines shown as straight are indeed straight; that figures lie in a plane unless otherwise indicated. Figures accompanying questions are intended to provide information you can use in answering the questions. However, unless a note states that a figure is drawn to scale, you should solve the problems by using your knowledge of mathematics, and NOT by estimating sizes by sight or by measurement.

Directions: For each of the following questions, two quantities are given: one in Column A and one in Column B. Compare the two quantities and mark your answer sheet with the correct lettered conclusion. These are your options:

(A) if the quantity in Column A is the greater;
(B) if the quantity in Column B is the greater;
(C) if the two quantities are equal;
(D) if the relationship cannot be determined from the information given.

Column A	Column B		Column A	Column B

1. $n < 0; a < 0$

$n + a$	$n - a$

3.

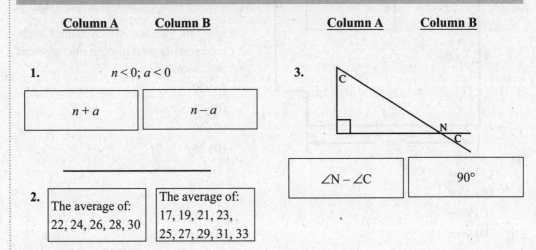

$\angle N - \angle C$	$90°$

2.

The average of: 22, 24, 26, 28, 30	The average of: 17, 19, 21, 23, 25, 27, 29, 31, 33

SUMMARY DIRECTIONS

Select: **(A)**   if Column A is greater;

        (B)   if Column B is greater;

        (C)   if the two columns are equal;

        (D)   if the relationship cannot be determined from the information given.

| Column A | Column B | | Column A | Column B |

4. $0 < y < 5; 0 < n < 7$

| y | n |

8.

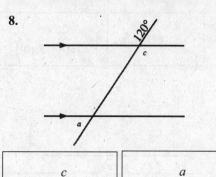

| c | a |

5. $5n - 5a = 25$

| n | a |

9.

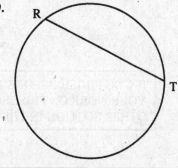

6.   In isosceles $\triangle NCY$:

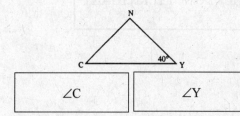

| $\angle C$ | $\angle Y$ |

| $\overarc{RT}$ | $\overline{RT}$ |

7. $\dfrac{m}{2} = c^2$

| m | c |

GO ON TO THE NEXT PAGE →

SUMMARY DIRECTIONS

Select: **(A)**   if Column A is greater;

 (B)   if Column B is greater;

 (C)   if the two columns are equal;

 (D)   if the relationship cannot be determined from the information given.

Column A	Column B		Column A	Column B

10.

$$5 + 16(3 - 2)$$

$$21 + 5 - [3(4 - 3)(0)]$$

12.

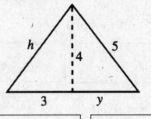

h	y

11.

$$8[2x - 3 (4x - 6) - 9]$$

$$6[3x - 2 (6x - 3) + 2]$$

STOP

IF YOU FINISH BEFORE TIME IS CALLED, YOU MAY CHECK YOUR WORK ON THIS SECTION ONLY. DO NOT TURN TO ANY OTHER SECTION IN THE TEST.

ANSWER KEY AND EXPLANATIONS

Final Mathematics Examination

Part 1: General Mathematics

1. C	10. C	19. A	27. A	35. B
2. C	11. D	20. C	28. D	36. B
3. D	12. A	21. C	29. A	37. D
4. B	13. A	22. A	30. D	38. A
5. B	14. B	23. D	31. C	39. A
6. A	15. C	24. D	32. A	40. C
7. B	16. B	25. B	33. C	41. C
8. B	17. D	26. D	34. C	42. D
9. D	18. B			

1. **The correct answer is (C).**
$I = P \times R \times T$

$= \$225,000 \times 0.135 \times 1 \text{ year}$

$= \$30,375$

2. **The correct answer is (C).** 14% of $x =$ $140 (Let x be the total sales.)

$0.14 \times x = \$140$

$x = 1,000$ (divide by 0.14)

3. **The correct answer is (D).**

25% of $200 = 0.25 \times \$200 = \$50$

Next, find the 20% discount on $200:

$0.20 \times \$200 = \$40$

The list price is $200 – $40 = $160

Now take 5% of $160:

$0.05 \times \$160 = \$8$

The discount is $48 when taken at 20% and 5% successively.

$50 – $48 = $2

4. **The correct answer is (B).** The job took nine days to complete.

A worked five days: he completed $\frac{5}{9}$ of the work.

B worked four days: he completed $\frac{4}{9}$ of the work.

If the net profit was $243, then A received

$\frac{5}{9} \times \$243 = \$135$

5. **The correct answer is (B).**
$\$76.50 \div 42\frac{1}{2} ¢/\text{yard}$

$\left(42\frac{1}{2}¢ = \$0.425\right)$

$= \$76.50 \div \$0.425 / \text{yard}$

$= 180 \text{ yards}$

6. **The correct answer is (A).**

Discount = 20%

Sale price = 80%

$0.80 \times \$280.00 = \$224.00$

7. **The correct answer is (B).** $\frac{n}{6} + \frac{n}{3} = 1$

$n + 2n = 6$ (multiply by 6)

$3n = 6$ (combine like terms)

$n = 2$ (divide by 3)

8. **The correct answer is (B).** Area of a rectangle is

$A = length \times width$

$= 40 \text{ inches} \times 20 \text{ inches}$

$= 800 \text{ square inches}$

Note: 1 square foot = 144 square inches

$\frac{800 \text{ square inches}}{144 \text{ square inches}} = 5.5 \text{ square feet}$

9. **The correct answer is (D).**

$\frac{2}{3} \times \frac{8}{8} = \frac{16}{24}$ (lowest common denominator is 24)

$+\frac{1}{8} \times \frac{3}{3} = \frac{3}{24}$

$= \frac{19}{24}$

10. **The correct answer is (C).** To arrive at the average, add all numbers and divide by total number of grades.

80
80
90
$+90$
$340 \div 4 = 85$

11. **The correct answer is (D).** The number of quarters must be even; otherwise, adding dimes will not give $2.00 *exactly*. So the answer cannot be 3, choice (D).

$3 \times 25¢ = 75¢$ or 0.75

$2.00 - 0.75 = 1.25$

$1.25 cannot be changed to all dimes.

12. **The correct answer is (A).** Let the *number* be x. A *number* increased by $\frac{1}{6}$ of itself is 182. To put this in equation form:

$x + \frac{1}{6} = 182$

$6x + x = 1,092$ (multiple each term by 6)

$7x = 1,092$ (combine like terms)

$x = 156$ (divide by 7)

13. **The correct answer is (A).**

$0.16\frac{3}{4} = 16\frac{3}{4} \text{ percent}$

When changing decimals to percents, move the decimal to the right two places.

14. **The correct answer is (B).** Let p represent the amount of protein needed for 392 calories. Use a proportion

$\frac{4 \text{ ounces}}{448 \text{ calories}} = \frac{p \text{ ounces}}{392 \text{ calories}}$

$448p = 4 \times 392$

$448p = 1,568$

$p = 3.5 \text{ ounces of protein}$

3.5 ounces of protein are needed for 392 calories.

15. **The correct answer is (C).**

$1,296.53$
$\underline{-246.87}$
$1,031.66$

16. **The correct answer is (B).**

$12\frac{1}{2} = 12\frac{2}{4}$

$\underline{-6\frac{1}{4} = -6\frac{1}{4}}$

$6\frac{1}{4}$

Note $: \frac{1}{2} \times \frac{2}{2} = \frac{2}{4}$

17. **The correct answer is (D).** Price per dozen can be found by multiplying the $1.29 by 4. (There are 4 groups of 3 in a dozen.)

$$\$1.29 \times 4 = \$5.16$$

18. **The correct answer is (B).**

$$\frac{1}{4} + \frac{7}{12} + \frac{3}{8} + \frac{1}{2} + \frac{5}{6} = \frac{6}{24} + \frac{14}{24} + \frac{9}{24} + \frac{12}{24} + \frac{20}{24}$$

Note: The lowest common denominator is 24. Each fraction needs to be rewritten to an equivalent fraction, so the denominator will be 24.

$$\frac{6 + 14 + 9 + 12 + 20}{24} = \frac{61}{24}$$

Divide:

$$24\overline{)61} = 2\frac{13}{24}$$
$$\underline{48}$$
$$13$$

19. **The correct answer is (A).** 25 feet × 36 feet = 900 square feet

Now change 900 square feet to square yards.

Note: 9 square feet = 1 square yard

$$900 \text{ square feet} \times \frac{1 \text{ square yard}}{9 \text{ square feet}}$$
$$= 100 \text{ square yards}$$

20. **The correct answer is (C).**

$$0.0009\overline{)72.0000}, \text{ or } 80,000$$
$$80000.$$

21. **The correct answer is (C).** One safety pin costs:

$$\$4.15 \div 100 = \$.0415$$

So 345 safety pins cost:

$$345 \times 0.0415 = \$14.32$$

22. **The correct answer is (A).** A number, x, that decreased by $\frac{1}{5}$ of itself equals 132, can be expressed as:

$$x - \frac{1x}{5} = 132$$
$$5x - x = 660 \quad \text{(multiply each term by 5)}$$
$$4x = 660 \quad \text{(combine like terms)}$$
$$x = 165 \quad \text{(divide by 4)}$$

23. **The correct answer is (D).** $285 = 0.05y$ (y is the unknown value)

$$5,700 = y \text{ (divide by 0.05)}$$

24. **The correct answer is (D).** $65 − $50 = $15 is the increase, but to find the percentage of increase, we divide the increase by the original amount:

$$\$15 \div \$50 = 0.30, \text{ or } 30\%$$

25. **The correct answer is (B).** Let x represent the numerator of the fraction, then the denominator will be $x + 20$.

Since the fraction is equivalent to $\frac{3}{5}$, we get

$$\frac{x}{x + 20} = \frac{3}{5}$$
$$5x = 3(x + 20)$$
$$5x = 3x + 60$$
$$2x = 60$$
$$x = 30$$

26. **The correct answer is (D).** $2 < x \leq 7$ means that x is greater than 2 and it is less than or equal to 7.

27. **The correct answer is (A).**

$$\frac{x}{5} - 4 = 11$$
$$\frac{x}{5} - 4 + 4 = 11 + 4$$
$$\frac{x}{5} = 15$$
$$5 \times \frac{x}{5} = 5 \times 15$$
$$x = 75$$

28. **The correct answer is (D).** Note that one gallon of punch contains 128 ounces (one-half gallon contains 64 ounces; hence, $2\frac{1}{2}$ gallons equals 320 ounces). A direct proportion can be used to solve the problem.

Let x = the number of ounces of grape juice needed.

$$\frac{16 \text{ ounces grape}}{64 \text{ ounces punch}} = \frac{x}{320 \text{ ounces punch}}$$

$$\frac{1}{4} = \frac{x}{320}$$

$$4x = 320$$

$$x = 80 \text{ ounces grape juice}$$

Since the answer is to be given in quarts, change 80 ounces to quarts by dividing 80 by 32. (There are 32 ounces in a quart.)

$80 \div 32 = 2.5$; thus, 2.5, or $2\frac{1}{2}$ quarts of grape juice are needed to make $2\frac{1}{2}$ gallons of punch.

29. **The correct answer is (A).** There are 16 hours from 7:00 a.m. until 11:00 p.m. Hence, Mrs. Bowler was up 16 hours.

Let x = the time Mrs. Bowler had left for other activities, then

$$\frac{1}{2}(16) + \frac{1}{8}(16) + \frac{1}{4}(16) + x = 16$$

$$8 + 2 + 4 + x = 16$$

$$14 + x = 16$$

$$x = 2$$

30. **The correct answer is (D).** 24 percent of the 50 students dropped the class.

24 percent of 50 = $0.24 \times 50 = 12$

Since 12 students dropped, $50 - 12$, or 38 students remained in the class.

31. **The correct answer is (C).** Divide $4\frac{1}{2}$ by $\frac{3}{4}$. (First change $4\frac{1}{2}$ to $\frac{9}{2}$.)

$$4\frac{1}{2} \div \frac{3}{4} = \frac{9}{2} \times \frac{4}{3} = \frac{36}{6} = 6$$

32. **The correct answer is (A).**
$$3.6 - 1.2(0.8 - 0.3) + 8 \div 0.4$$
$$= 3.6 - 1.2(0.5) + 8 \div 4$$
$$= 3.6 - 0.6 + 8 \div 0.4$$
$$= 3.6 - 0.6 + 20$$
$$= 3 + 20$$
$$= 23$$

(*Note:* Operations must be performed in the correct order. (Parentheses first, then multiplication and division before addition and subtraction.)

33. **The correct answer is (C).** Change 0.2 percent to a decimal and multiply 0.2 percent by 400.

$0.002 \times 400 = 0.800$, or 0.8

34. **The correct answer is (C).** Find the number of calories provided by 3 ounces of fruit juice.

$$\frac{8}{200} = \frac{3}{c}$$

$$8c = 600$$

$$c = 75$$

75 calories are provided by 3 ounces of fruit juice.

Now determine what percent 75 is of 200.

n% of 200 = 75

$$200n = 75$$

$$n = .375 = 37.5\%$$

Three ounces of the fruit juice provide 37.5% of the calories in the 8 ounces.

35. The correct answer is (B). Use the Pythagorean theorem.

$$c^2 = a^2 + b^2$$
$$c^2 = 3^2 + 4^2$$
$$c^2 = 9 + 16$$
$$c^2 = 25$$
$$c = \sqrt{25}$$
$$c = 5$$

36. The correct answer is (B). The formula for the area of a rectangle is $A = LW$. We know the area of the rectangle is 63 and the length is 9 feet. Thus,

$$63 \text{ square feet} = 9W \text{ feet}$$
$$\frac{63 \text{ square feet}}{9 \text{ feet}} = \frac{9W \text{ feet}}{9 \text{ feet}}$$
$$7 \text{ feet} = W$$

37. The correct answer is (D). The corresponding sides of similar triangles are proportional. Therefore,

$$\frac{3}{7} = \frac{x}{9}$$
$$7x = 27$$
$$x = 3\frac{6}{7}$$

38. The correct answer is (A). Parallel lines have equal slopes; they do not intersect.

39. The correct answer is (A). The area of a square is found by squaring a side of the square.

If $A = 144\text{m}^2$

$144\text{m}^2 = s^2$ where s is a side of the square

$$\sqrt{144\text{m}^2} = s$$
$$12\text{m} = s$$

40. The correct answer is (C). Divide the figure into nonoverlapping rectangles. Find the area of each rectangle. Add the areas of the rectangles to get the total area of the figure.

$A = 48\text{m}^2 + 20\text{m}^2 + 12\text{m}^2 = 80\text{m}^2$

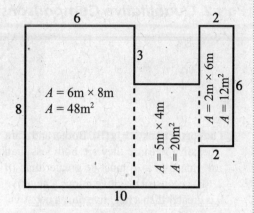

41. The correct answer is (C). The entire circle contains 360°. The central angle of 60° represents $\frac{60}{360} = \frac{1}{6}$.

Change $\frac{1}{6}$ to a percent by dividing the denominator into the numerator. Thus, $\frac{1}{6} = 16\frac{2}{3}\%$. We get 17 when we express $16\frac{2}{3}$ to the nearest whole percent.

42. The correct answer is (D). The weekly budget is represented by the entire circle; $\frac{1}{12}$ of the circle represents $\frac{1}{12} \times 360 = 30°$, which is the measure of the central angle for the amount spent on entertainment. $\frac{1}{8}$ of the circle represents $\frac{1}{8} \times 360 = 45°$, which is the measure of the central angle for the amount spent on gasoline. A central angle that represents the total spent on entertainment and gasoline is $30° + 45° = 75°$. (Alternatively, $\frac{1}{8} + \frac{1}{12} = \frac{5}{24}$ and $\frac{5}{24} \times 360° = 75°$.)

Part 2: Quantitative Comparisons

1. B	4. D	7. D	9. A	11. D
2. A	5. A	8. A	10. B	12. A
3. C	6. D			

1. **The correct answer is (B).** Both n and a are negative because they are both less than 0. Hence $(n - a)$ must be greater than $(n + a)$ because a negative minus a negative is greater than a negative plus a negative.

   $-a > +a$ ($-a$ = positive, $+a$ = negative)

   $n - a > n + a$ (adding n to both sides)

2. **The correct answer is (A).** The average of Column A is 26, while the average of Column B is 25.

3. **The correct answer is (C).**

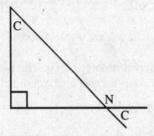

   $\angle N = \angle C + 90°$ An exterior angle is equal to the sum of the interior remote angles.

   $\angle N - \angle C = 90°$ When equals are subtracted from equals, the differences are equal.

4. **The correct answer is (D).** It is impossible to determine because y could be any number from 0 to 5 and n any number from 0 to 7.

5. **The correct answer is (A).** $5n - 5a = 25$

   $n - a = 5$ (equals divided by equals are equals)

   $n = a + 5$ (equals plus equals are equal)

   n is 5 greater than a.

6. **The correct answer is (D).** An isosceles triangle has two equal angles, but from the information given, it is impossible to determine which two angles are actually equal.

7. **The correct answer is (D).** There is insufficient information to determine whether m or c is the greater. By substituting numbers for m and c, we see that either quantity could be greater—for example

   (1) $m = 2$, $c = 1$;

   (2) $m = \frac{1}{8}$, $c = \frac{1}{4}$.

8. **The correct answer is (A).**

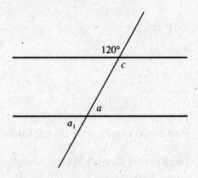

   $\angle c = 120°$ and $\angle a = \angle a_1$ since all vertical angles are equal.

   $\angle c + \angle a_1 = 180°$ since the two interior angles on the same side of a transversal are supplementary.

   $\angle a_1 = 60°$

   $\angle a = 60° < \angle c = 120°$

9. **The correct answer is (A).** The shortest distance between two points is a straight line. Therefore, the chord, a straight line, must be shorter than the arc.

10. **The correct answer is (B).**

$$5 + 16(3 - 2) = 5 + 16(1)$$
$$= 5 + 16$$
$$= 21$$

$$21 + 5 - [3(4 - 3)(0)] = 21 + 5 - 0$$
$$= 26$$

11. **The correct answer is (D).** Since the value of x cannot be determined, the values of Columns A and B remain unknown.

12. **The correct answer is (A).** It can be readily seen that the figure consists of two 3-4-5 right triangles. Therefore, $h = 5$ and $y = 3$.

Science

OVERVIEW

- **Characteristics of organisms**
- **Basic principles of life sciences**
- **Anatomy and physiology**
- **Humans and their environment**
- **Science Glossary**

Unit 3 provides a review of important life science and physical science information to help you prepare for the registered nursing school entrance exam. The unit includes relevant concepts and principles related to general biology, anatomy and physiology, nutrition, chemistry, and physics as well as practice tests that simulate the testing experience. Emphasis is on the descriptions of the activities and characteristics of life with respect to humans.

CHARACTERISTICS OF ORGANISMS

The modern classification of organisms divides all living species into one of six kingdoms. There is some debate as to how many kingdoms there are, and some taxonomists classify species into only five kingdoms, but in the United States, it is currently accepted practice to classify species into six kingdoms.

1. **Monera:** The kingdom Monera consists of prokaryotic organisms. Prokaryotes are cells that do not have a nucleus or any membrane-bound organelles. All monerans are single-cell organisms that reproduce asexually. Monerans can live in colonies, as is the case with bacteria and cyanobacteria. These organisms can be autotrophs (self-feeders) or decomposers that feed off dead matter (saprotrophic).

2. **Archaeabacteria:** The kingdom Archaeabacteria also consists of single-celled prokaryotes. These organisms are bacteria that can live under very extreme conditions such as extreme temperatures, acidity, alkalinity, or salinity. Some archaeabacteria can live under extremely low oxygen conditions.

3. **Protista:** The kingdom Protista consists of unicellular and multicellular eukaryotic organisms. Eukaryotic cells are those with a nucleus and compartmentalized, membrane-bound organelles. There are three informal groups of Protista: protozoa (amoeba, flagellates,

ciliates), algae, and slime and water molds. Organisms in the kingdom Protista can be autotrophs, saprotrophs, or heterotrophs.

4. **Fungi:** Members of the kingdom Fungi are unicellular or multicellular heterotrophs. This kingdom includes mushrooms, yeasts, and molds. Multicellular fungi are composed of a mass of slender filaments called mycelium, and yeasts are a type of unicellular fungi. Fungi do not perform photosynthesis because they lack chlorophyll. Some fungi are parasitic and pathogenic. Fungi are generally saprotrophic.

5. **Plantae:** Members of the kingdom Plantae are eukaryotic, multicellular organisms that consist of a cell wall made of cellulose. The kingdom Plantae includes flowering plants, conifers, ferns, and mosses. They are all photosynthetic green plants that contain chlorophyll. These species are autotrophs and nonmotile. Plants are the primary producers for all living land organisms, and they are an essential source of oxygen on Earth.

6. **Animalia:** The kingdom Animalia consists of eukaryotic multicellular heterotrophs. Heterotrophs are consumers that must ingest food as an energy source. They can be herbivores, carnivores, or omnivores. Species belonging to the kingdom Animalia include all vertebrates and invertebrates. These species commonly exhibit tissue differentiation and complex organ systems, and they are motile. Species included in the kingdom Animalia are sometimes parasitic organisms.

Regardless of the kingdom into which a species is classified, all living organisms share certain common characteristics. These characteristics are sometimes used to describe life. In particular all living organisms are composed of cells; respond to stimuli (external or internal), reproduce, exhibit growth and development, obtain and metabolize food as an energy source, possess nucleic acids, and are able to adapt to their environments.

Organisms can be interdependent. Two species can exist in an indirect relationship in which they adapt to occupy the same habitat without interacting with each other. Other species can exist in a direct relationship in which one or both species benefit from the relationship (symbiosis), or one species is threatened by the other (predation). In addition, organisms can have an effect on their environment, or an environment may have an effect on the organisms that live within it.

BASIC PRINCIPLES OF LIFE SCIENCES

All substances, either inorganic or organic, are composed of matter. Matter obeys certain physical and chemical laws. These laws are the foundation of all the life sciences.

The Cell

All living organisms are composed of cells. Cells are the basic unit of life. There are two types of cells that define an organism: prokaryotic and eukaryotic. Prokaryotic cells are cells that lack a nuclear membrane and defined organelles. These cells make up organisms such as bacteria and archaea. Eukaryotic cells are more complex. DNA in eukaryotic cells is contained within a nuclear membrane, separating it from the cytoplasm. Within the cytoplasm are clearly defined membrane-bound organelles. Some types of eukaryotic cell, such as red blood cells, lack a clearly defined nucleus when they are fully mature. Immature red blood cells have a nucleus, but lose it for functional reasons when they are fully developed. All vertebrates, including humans, are composed of eukaryotic cells.

NOTE

The science part of the Registered Nursing Exam tests knowledge of concepts rather than critical thinking ability.

There are several differences between plant and animal cells. Organelles that are found in animal cells, but not in plant cells, include lysosomes, centrioles, and flagella (although these are found in some plant sperm cells). Organelles that are found in plant cells, but not in animal cells, include chloroplasts, central vacuole and tonoplasts, cell wall, and plasmodesmata.

Cell Division

All eukaryotic cells divide in order to reproduce themselves. Typical nonsex cells divide through the process of mitosis. Mitosis is the division of the cell's nuclear material, and it is divided into five stages: prophase, prometaphase, metaphase, anaphase, and telophase. DNA replicates in a cell during the cell cycle phase known as interphase. Interphase occurs before the process of mitosis. Mitosis conserves numbers of chromosomes equally, allocating replicated chromosomes to each of the new daughter nuclei. One round of mitosis of a diploid cell (two copies of each chromosome) produces two new daughter cells that are also diploid. In some cases, mitosis may occur without cell division, resulting in a multinucleate cell.

Sex cells in eukaryotic organisms undergo a variation of cell division called meiosis. Meiosis results in four nonidentical daughter cells that each have only one set of chromosomes. Meiosis occurs only in the gonads (ovaries and testes). Cells that undergo meiosis are called gametes and include ovum and sperm cells.

Cellular Organelles

Cellular functions are accomplished by one or more parts, or organelles, in each cell.

- **Cell membrane:** The cell, or plasma, membrane is a phospholipid bilayer impregnated with proteins. It is differentially permeable and functions in regulating the passage of materials into and out of the cell. Mechanisms by which material can pass through the plasma membrane include osmosis, diffusion, and active transport. Cells constantly interact with their environment through osmosis and diffusion. Diffusion is the passive movement of a substance from an area of higher concentration to an area of lower concentration. Osmosis is another mechanism of passive transport in which a solvent (usually water) will travel from an area of higher concentration to an area of lower concentration. Mechanisms of active transport include a sodium-potassium ion pump, endocytosis, phagocytosis, pinocytosis, and exocytosis. The outside surface of the plasma membrane of animal cells is covered with tiny microvilli, projections that increase the surface area of the cell.

- **Cell wall:** The cell wall is the outer layer of plant cells that maintains the cell's shape and protects the cell from mechanical and physical damage. The cell wall is composed of cellulose, other polysaccharides, and proteins.

- **Central vacuole:** The central vacuole is an organelle found in plant cells, but not in animal cells. It functions include storage, the breakdown of waste products, and the hydrolysis of macromolecules. The enlargement of the central vacuole is a major mechanism in plant growth.

- **Centrosome:** The centrosome is the region of the cell where microtubules initiate. Each animal cell contains a pair of centrioles within the centrosome. Centrioles are tiny, barrel-shaped organelles with an as yet unknown function. Centrioles are not completely understood. It is known that they provide a framework for functional structure construction, such as centrosomes and cilia.

- **Contractile vacuole:** Contractile vacuoles are membranous sacs that maintain a proper concentration of water inside the cell. They function to drain excess water from the cytoplasm and remove it from the cell. Contractile vacuoles are found in many protists and some animal cells.

- **Cytoskeleton:** The cytoskeleton reinforces and maintains a cell's shape. It also functions in cell movement. The components of the cytoskeleton are microfilaments, intermediate filaments, and microtubules.

- **Endoplasmic reticulum:** The endoplasmic reticulum, ER, is a network of membranous sacs and tubules. The ER is active in membrane synthesis and functions as an intracellular transport system for many proteins and substances. The ER extends throughout the cytoplasm.
  There are two types of endoplasmic reticulum: the rough ER and the smooth ER. The rough ER is studded with ribosomes that produce many secretory proteins in the cell. The rough ER is also involved in membrane synthesis. The smooth ER is involved in processes including the synthesis of lipids, cellular metabolism of carbohydrates, and the detoxification of drugs and poisons.

- **Flagella/Cilia:** Flagella and cilia are slender projections from the cell that function to aid in cell movement. Flagella are longer than cilia and are composed of membrane-enclosed microtubules. Cilia are small hair-like structures that also have an internal arrangement of microtubules.

- **Golgi apparatus:** The Golgi apparatus functions in the synthesis, modification, sorting, and secretion of cell products. Products of the ER are modified and stored in the Golgi and then sent to other destinations. The Golgi apparatus consists of flattened membranous sacs called cisternae. Responsible for carbohydrate synthesis, phosphorylation of proteins and synthesis of other non-protein macro molecules.

- **Lysosome:** The lysosomes are digestive organelles in which macromolecules are hydrolyzed. In addition, phagocytic vacuoles, also called food vacuoles, are membranous sacs used by some types of cells to engulf and digest food material. Other vacuoles called autophagatic vacuoles function to engulf, digest, and recycle worn-out cytoplasmic organelles.

- **Mitochondria:** Mitochondria are important organelles in the cell in which cellular respiration occurs. Macromolecules such as carbohydrates, fats, and proteins are oxidized, resulting in the release of ATP, a form of usable energy that all cells require.

- **Nucleus:** The nucleus is the genetic control center of the cell. The cell nucleus is enclosed within a porous double membrane called the nuclear envelope. The nucleus contains all the genetic material of the cell (DNA). DNA and protein form structures called chromatin, which are visible as individual chromosomes in a dividing cell. The nucleolus is a nonmembraneous organelle within the nucleus that is involved in the production of ribosomal RNA (rRNA) and ribosomes. Transcription, the biosynthesis of RNA from a DNA template, occurs within the cell's nucleus. The messenger RNA, mRNA, then moves to the ribosomes in the cytosol where the mRNA acts as a template for protein synthesis in the process of translation.

- **Peroxisome:** A peroxisome is an organelle with specialized metabolic functions that produce hydrogen peroxide.

- **Plasmodesmata (plasmodesma, singular):** Plasmodesmata are also only found in plant cells. They are the channels through cell walls that connect the cytoplasm of adjacent cells.

- **Plastid:** Plastids are only found in plant cells. There are two different types of plastids, and they vary in function. Chloroplasts are green organelles in which photosynthesis takes place. They are what give plants their green color. Chloroplasts convert the energy from sunlight into chemical energy, which is stored in a plant cell in the form of glucose. Chromoplasts and leucoplasts function in storage and other processes such as starch collection.

- **Ribosomes:** Ribosomes are small nonmembranous organelles that synthesize proteins from mRNA. They may be found free in the cytoplasm or bound to endoplasmic reticulum.

Cells are grouped together to form tissues. Well-developed tissues are specialized for certain functions. Furthermore, different tissues work together to form organs and organs are grouped together by function to form a system. Throughout the body, organ systems have highly specialized functions, but in many cases the function of one system is dependent on the function of one or more other systems. Most organisms, from the round and segmented worm to vertebrates, are characterized by the organization of their systems.

The Cell Cycle

Cell growth occurs in a regular pattern called the cell cycle. The cell cycle is divided into several phases: the mitotic (M) phase and the interphase, which is divided into the following phases: G1, S, and G2.

1. **M phase:** Mitosis occurs during the M phase of the cell cycle. Mitosis is the division of the cell nucleus followed immediately by division of the cytoplasm in a process known as cytokinesis. There are five phases of mitosis that are involved in division of the nucleus. Chromatin fibers become denser during prophase. The nuclear envelope fragments and microtubules that form spindles invade the nuclear area during prometaphase. Metaphase is the longest phase of mitosis in which the chromosomes line up along the center of the cell, midway between the poles of the mitotic spindle. Anaphase is the shortest phase of mitosis during which the chromatid pairs separate and each chromosome moves to opposite poles of the cell. During telophase, two daughter cells begin to form, two nuclear envelopes form, and the original nucleus is now divided into two. The cytoplasm divides during cytokinesis, and the result is two new cells.

2. **G1 and G2 phase:** The cell grows during both the G1 and the G2 portions of interphase. The G1 phase is known as the first "gap," and the G2 phase is called the second "gap."

3. **S phase:** The S phase, or the synthesis phase, is the phase in which the DNA of the cell is replicated resulting in duplication of each chromosome.

Reproduction

All living organisms undergo either sexual or asexual reproduction. Reproduction maintains the continuity of a species or population.

Asexual Reproduction

Asexual reproduction occurs through mitosis and does not involve a union of reproductive cells (gametes). There are several mechanisms of asexual reproduction.

- **Sporulation:** Sporulation is a process that involves the production of asexual reproductive cells called spores. These spores develop into mature individuals that are identical.

- **Binary fission:** Binary fission involves the division of an organism (usually a unicellular organism) into two organisms. In the case of unicellular eukaryotes, binary fission usually involves mitosis.

- **Multiple fission or fragmentation:** Fragmentation is seen in organisms such as filamentous algae. It involves the breaking of an organism into smaller units. Each of these fragments can then develop into an identical species.

- **Budding:** Budding involves the production of an outgrowth or miniature organism that eventually breaks away from the parent, forming a new identical individual.

Sexual Reproduction

Sexual reproduction involves the process of meiosis followed by fertilization. Thus, there is a union between the nuclei of a male and female reproductive cell. Sexual reproduction allows for variation between parents and offspring, whereas asexual reproduction produces offspring that are identical to the parent. There are three general mechanisms of sexual reproduction.

1. **Isogamy:** Isogamy is a mechanism of sexual reproduction involving the fusion of gametes of identical size and structure. This type of reproduction is most common in lower plant species.

2. **Heterogamy:** Heterogamy is a mechanism of sexual reproduction involving the fusion of gametes that differ in size and/or structure. Ansiogamy is a type of heterogamy that involves motile gametes that differ only in size. Oogamy is a type of heterogamy that involves gametes that differ in size and structure.

   Human sexual reproduction is a form of oogamy. The spermatozoa produced by males differs in size and structure from the ovum produced by females. In humans and most other mammals, gametes are produced in gonads or sex organs. The male gonads are the testes, and the female gonads are the ovaries. Gonads in humans and other higher-order animal species also have an endocrine function. Gonads produce hormones that function in the development of secondary sex characteristics and reproductive cycles (female menstruation cycle).

3. **Conjugation:** Conjugation is a mechanism of sexual reproduction that involves the temporary union of cells to allow for the exchange or transmission of DNA or nuclei.

Meiosis

The production of gametes (sex cells) or spores involves the process of meiosis. Gametes are haploid cells, meaning that they have half the number of chromosomes of a zygote, or fertilized ovum. Meiosis has several stages that occur in two rounds (meiosis I and meiosis II). Round 1 consists of interphase, prophase, prometaphase, metaphase I, anaphase I, and telophase I. Round 2 consists of interphase II, metaphase II, anaphase II, telophase II, and cytokinesis. During the first round (interphase through telophase I), two diploid cells are formed. The cell undergoes DNA replication during interphase, just as it would in the process of mitosis. During the second round (interphase II through cytokinesis), four haploid cells are formed. The process of meiosis is similar to mitosis, except that a single replication of chromosomes is followed by two consecutive cell divisions (meiosis I and meiosis II).

Once the two gametes, such as a sperm and an ovum, are united, the zygote forms, and there is a diploid number of chromosomes. This process is called fertilization. The zygote typically develops mitotically into an embryo, thus the developing embryo has cells that contain a diploid number of chromosomes (except for any developing gametes). Because of meiosis and the union of two gametes (syngamy), the individual developing from the zygote receives half of its chromosomes (DNA) from each parent. In this way, the number of chromosomes in a species remains constant.

Growth and Development

The growth and development of an organism allows for the characteristic size range of a species to be maintained. Also, through the development and growth of offspring, differentiation of tissue and organs is accomplished. In a multicellular organism, growth most often involves an increase in the number of cells. It may also occur through an increase in the size of the cells or an increase in both the number and size of the cells.

Embryogenesis is the process by which an embryo forms and develops, eventually becoming a fetus. In higher-order animals such as humans, the basic pattern of development is as follows:

1. **Cleavage:** The zygote undergoes cleavage that results in the formation of a cluster of cells called morula.

2. **Blastocyst or Blastula:** The morula develops into a blastula or blastocyst. The blastocyst is a hollow ball of cells with a cavity known as a blastocoel.

3. **Gastrula:** The blastocyst develops into a two-layered gastrula. The gastrula has a cavity known as a gastrocoel or archenteron. The outer, or germ, layer of the gastrula is called the ectoderm, and the inner layer is called the endoderm. A third germ layer called the mesoderm develops between the ectoderm and the endoderm.

    Each of these three germ layers gives rise to specific tissues and body structures. The nervous system, including some sensory organs such as the eyes and the outer skin, develops from the ectoderm layer. The musculoskeletal system, muscles of the viscera, mesenteries, and the circulatory system develop from the mesoderm. The lungs, liver, pancreas, thyroid, parathyroid, thymus glands, and the lining of the digestive tract all develop from the endoderm layer.

In addition to these three primary germ layers, some animals develop extraembryonic membranes. There are four basic extraembryonic membranes: the yolk sac, amnion, chorion, and allantois. The yolk sac provides nutrition to the embryo. The amnion forms a fluid-like sac filled with amniotic fluid that protects the developing embryo. Allantois is the membrane involved in gas exchange to and from the developing embryo. The outermost fetal membrane, the chorion, is formed from the secretion of ectoderm.

The complete development of a human takes about 38 weeks. During the first two months, the developing baby is referred to as an embryo. From the third month until the ninth month, the baby is then referred to as a fetus.

Nutrition

The nutritional processes of ingesting and utilizing food as an energy source are exhibited by all organisms. Food is defined "as any substance that can be used by an organism as an energy source that helps to promote growth and maintenance of the body."

Most food sources ingested by humans are organic (carbon-based substances). The process of converting inorganic materials into an organic food source is carried out in plants through the process of photosynthesis. Sunlight provides energy for the process of photosynthesis, and green plants have chloroplasts that are the major site of photosynthesis. Chloroplasts are found mainly in the mesophyll, the tissue in the interior of the leaf. Light energy absorbed by chlorophyll drives the synthesis of inorganic compounds into organic molecules. During photosynthesis, light energy drives a reaction between carbon dioxide and water in the leaf tissue. The resulting products are the sugar glucose, $C_6H_{12}O_6$, and oxygen. Carbon dioxide enters the leaf and oxygen exits the leaf through microscopic pores called stomata. All organisms (with the exception of some algae and prokaryotes) depend either directly or indirectly on photosynthesis for food.

Organisms such as green plants that are able to manufacture food and energy within their body from inorganic materials in the environment are called autotrophs. Organisms that receive an organic food source from their environment are called heterotrophs. There are three different types of heterotrophs.

1. **Saprotrophs:** Saprotrophs digest food internally and absorb the digested food into the body. Most bacteria and fungi are saprotrophs.

2. **Parasites:** Parasites are dependent on a host for survival and are harmful to the host on or in which they live.

3. **Phagotrophs**: Humans and most animals are phagotrophs. Phagotrophs ingest solid food into a digestive cavity. The digestive cavity may be as simple as a food vacuole in primitive organisms. Other simple organisms such as coelenterates and flatworms have a gastrovascular cavity with a mouth opening at one end. More complex organisms such as humans and other animals have a complete digestive tract. The human digestive system has a mouth opening for ingesting food and an anal opening for expelling food waste.

Food that has been ingested by an organism must be changed into a usable and absorbable state. The digestive system alters ingested food so that the body can absorb the necessary nutrients. The undigested and nutritionally expended food remains are expelled as waste. In humans and most animals, this occurs in the digestive tract. In lower organisms, this will occur in the food vacuole or gastrovascular cavity.

Once food has been digested, nutrients and molecules from the food are distributed to cells throughout the body. In humans, it is the circulatory system that distributes food products to the cells. Within the cells, the process of metabolism converts these molecules obtained from food into energy for the cell.

There are three classes of organic macromolecules found in foods that are essential to life: proteins, carbohydrates, and lipids.

1. **Proteins:** Proteins are made up of long chains of amino acids. Twenty different types of amino acids form long polypeptide chains that can be folded into a three-dimensional structure. The final folded structure is a protein. Structural proteins are made up of long filaments (collagen). Structural proteins are found in hair, skin, and connective tissue. Globular proteins are larger proteins such as hemoglobin, enzymes, and antibodies. Most proteins are globular.

2. **Carbohydrates:** Carbohydrates consist of carbon, hydrogen, and oxygen atoms. All sugars are carbohydrates. A sugar molecule is called a saccharide. A saccharide can contain one, two, or many sugar molecules. Monosaccharides are simple sugars such as glucose and fructose. Disaccharides contain two sugars. These include sucrose, lactose, and maltose. Polysaccharides have many sugars. Examples of polysaccharides include glycogen (the form in which animals store glucose), starch (the form in which plants store glucose), and cellulose (a structural polysaccharide that forms cell walls in plants.)

    Saccharides serve as an energy source for cells. This energy can be used immediately or stored as glycogen for later use.

3. **Lipids:** Lipids are organic compounds that, like carbohydrates, contain carbon, hydrogen, and oxygen. Lipids are important for maintaining the structure of cell membranes, and they are a source of insulation and a means of storing energy in the body. Lipids include fats, oils, waxes, phospholipids, and steroids. A fat molecule contains one glycerol molecule and three fatty acid chains; thus, the term *triglyceride* is also used to refer to fats. The human body stores both health beneficial lipids called high-density lipids, or HDLs, and health harmful lipids called low-density lipids, or LDLs. Too many lipids can lead to clogged arteries, which cause coronary diseases such as arteriosclerosis and atherosclerosis. These conditions can lead to heart attacks and stroke. Both LDL and HDL are referred to as cholesterols. Cholesterol is a unique organic lipid made up of hydrocarbon rings. It is a lipid that is necessary to build and maintain cell membranes and gives the cell an elastic quality. Cholesterol also functions to produce steroid hormones in the body.

Metabolism

Metabolism occurs in cells and is the sum of the chemical reactions that take place within a cell. Macromolecules such as carbohydrates, lipids, and proteins are metabolized in the cell to provide energy for cell maintenance and function. When a cell needs energy, it uses a molecule called adenosine triphosphate, or ATP, and breaks it down to release energy. In cells, the process of cellular respiration breaks down chemicals into usable energy. Cellular respiration occurs in a series of small reaction steps designed to maximize the production of energy. The steps of cellular respiration in human and animal cells are glycolysis, the Krebs cycle (or citric acid cycle), and oxidative phosphorylation. Respiration breaks down fuel in the form of glucose and generates ATP, the usable form of energy in the cell.

- **Glycolysis:** Glycolysis takes place in the cytosol in the absence of oxygen and involves the splitting of a glucose molecule (through the process of oxidation) into two molecules of pyruvate (the ionized form of pyruvic acid). The initial glycolysis reaction involves the breakdown of two ATP molecules into ADP. However, the overall glycolysis reaction produces four ATP molecules, so there is a net gain of two ATP molecules in the overall reaction. The overall reaction also produces two NADH molecules, also a form of usable energy in the cell. Therefore, the overall

TIP

Remember that the Krebs cycle is also called the citric acid cycle. You might find either term on the exam.

yield of one round of glycolysis in which glucose is oxidized in the cell is two pyruvate, two ATP, and two NADH molecules. No CO2 is released during glycolysis because the reaction takes place in the absence of oxygen.

- **Krebs Cycle:** After the completion of glycolysis, pyruvate is transported to the mitochondria. In the mitochondria, each pyruvate is first converted into acetyl coenzyme A. Pyruvate's COOH group is removed, and CO2 is released from the reaction. The remaining fragment of pyruvate is oxidized and several more reaction steps take place involving NAD^+ and coenzyme A, resulting in acetyl coA. During the Krebs cycle, eight (8) reaction steps are catalyzed by different enzymes. The result is the release of two (2) ATP molecules, six (6) NADH molecules, and two (2) FADH molecules, all of which provide usable energy to the cell.

The Krebs Cycle (Citric Acid Cycle)

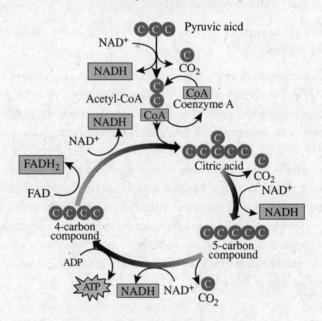

- **Oxidative phosphorylation:** The process of oxidative phosphorylation is comprised of two stages: electron transport and chemiosmosis. The electron transport chain is a collection of molecules embedded in the inner membrane of the mitochondrion. Most components of the electron transport chain are protein complexes. Electron transport through these complexes creates an H+ ion gradient across the cell membrane. The two sources of H+ for the electron transport chain are NADH and FADH2. No ATP is made during this process, but the purpose of the electron transport chain is so the mitochondrion couples the electron transport with the process of chemiosmosis. Oxygen is the final electron acceptor of the electron transport chain. The energy stored in the H+ gradient across the membrane couples the redox reaction of the chain to ATP synthesis. Protons (H+) from the electron transport chain flow through the membrane by way of a large enzyme complex called ATP synthase. There are three (3) catalytic sites in the enzyme complex that join ADP with inorganic phosphate to form ATP. Oxidative phosphorylation results in the production of thirty-two (32) to thirty-four (34) ATP molecules.

The total yield of ATP molecules during cellular respiration is thirty-six to thirty-eight ATP molecules. Cellular respiration is a remarkably efficient process in its energy conversion.

During the metabolism process of cellular respiration, aerobic oxidation requires free molecular oxygen. Oxygen is made available to the cells by means of the human respiratory system or, in other animals, by the respiratory organs. Oxygen is inhaled and absorbed from the air into the lungs. It is transported throughout the body by the circulatory system. In humans, oxygen is transported through the blood by hemoglobin and red blood cells. Once glucose is oxidized, CO_2 is produced. The resulting CO_2 is removed from cells by the circulatory system and is expelled from the body through expiration of air from the lungs (respiratory system). Liquid waste formed as a result of metabolism is collected, concentrated, and eliminated through the excretory (urinary) system.

When food is ingested, the production of other necessary compounds such as proteins and secretory products also occurs in the cell. Any solid indigestible waste from food is eliminated from the digestive system through the excretory system.

Enzymes

All cellular functions depend on specific proteins, and in particular, they depend upon enzymes. Enzymes are highly specialized proteins that serve as biological catalysts to help speed up certain biological reactions. Enzymes are able to change the rate of a chemical reaction without themselves being changed or consumed during the reaction. A substrate is a particular substance acted upon by an enzyme. A substrate fits into a region of the enzyme called the active site, which is typically a pocket or groove on the enzyme's surface. Enzymes are specific because their active sites will only fit a specific substrate molecule. Once the substrate "fits" into the enzyme's active site, the reaction is catalyzed and product is formed. The enzyme releases the product and emerges unchanged from the reaction, so it can bind another of the same type of substrate molecule.

Nucleic Acids

Nucleic acids are macromolecules found in every cell. There are two types of nucleic acids: DNA and RNA. All living organisms possess one or both types of nucleic acids. DNA, or deoxyribonucleic acid, functions as the source of genetic information for an individual. DNA exists as two long chains of individual molecules called nucleotides. The long strands of DNA nucleotides are twisted into a double helix structure in which one nucleotide forms a base pair with another. These base pairs are held together by hydrogen bonds. Each nucleotide consists of a sugar called deoxyribose, a phosphate group, and a purine or pyrimidine base. There are two purine bases, guanine and adenine, and two pyrimidine bases, cytosine and thymine. The purine guanine, G, only forms base pairs with the pyrimidine cytosine, C, and the purine adenine, A, only forms base pairs with the pyrimidine thymine, T. All eukaryotic cells contain DNA within their nucleus, and prokaryotic cells contain DNA attached to the inside of the cell membrane.

DNA can function is several processes, including cellular metabolism, reproduction (heredity), and the production of another nucleic acid called RNA (ribonucleic acid). RNA is synthesized from a DNA template during the process of transcription. RNA is also composed of nucleotides. However, RNA exists mostly as a single strand of nucleotide molecules, and it is generally smaller in size than DNA. The nucleotides of RNA are slightly different than those of DNA in that the pyrimidine base uracil replaces thymine. Uracil pairs with adenine. Guanine pairs with cytosine.

There are three types of RNA, all of which play a role in protein synthesis. Messenger RNA, or mRNA, is the template for amino acid synthesis. These amino acid chains, or polypeptide chains,

TIP

If you aren't sure of an answer, use the process of elimination to rule out answers that you know are wrong.

synthesized by an mRNA template, are modified and folded into a protein structure. The information in the mRNA that leads to the synthesis of a protein comes from the original DNA template that was transcribed into RNA. The segments of DNA that code for specific proteins are called genes.

Transfer RNA, or tRNA, matches each specific amino acid to its codon on an mRNA strand. The codon is a three-nucleotide sequence that is specific for only one of the twenty-six amino acids. Thus, tRNA molecules are able to pick up a specific amino acid and deliver it to a specific amino acid codon. This ensures that all amino acids are placed in the correct sequence for a particular protein.

A third type of RNA, ribosomal RNA, or rRNA, is the key component of ribosomes. Ribosomes are present in the cytoplasm of the cell and are the site of protein synthesis.

Heredity

Heredity is defined as the transmission of traits from one generation to the next. The transmission of these traits can be explained in terms of several concepts, including gene theory, Mendel's law, gene theory, meiosis, and chromosomes.

Gene Theory

Gregor Mendel deduced the fundamental principles of modern genetics by breeding garden peas. The pea plants he studied produced a large number of offspring and came in many distinguishable varieties. A heritable feature that varies among individuals in a population is called a character, and each variable of a character is called a trait. Mendel was able to strictly control the breeding of the pea plants and worked with his plants until he had true breeding varieties that produced offspring identical to the parent. Mendel was then able to create hybrid offspring by mating two different true-breeds of a pea plant variety. The cross fertilization of two species is called hybridization, or a cross.

Mendel's Laws

Mendel performed many experiments in which he tracked the inheritance patterns of specific traits in plants. The results of his experiments led him to formulate several ideas about inheritance.

- **The law of segregation:** Mendel's law of segregation, based on his observations during his studies of inheritance patterns of plants, states that for a specific inheritable trait, there are two alleles (versions of the same gene) that separate during gamete formation and end up in two separate gametes during meiosis. For each trait, an individual inherits one allele from each parent. An individual with two identical alleles for a gene is said to be homozygous for that allele, and an individual with two different alleles for a gene is said to be heterozygous for that gene. If the two alleles for one gene are different, one allele determines the physical trait expressed by the gene and is called the dominant allele. The other allele has no noticeable effect on the appearance of the individual and is called the recessive allele.

- **The law of independent assortment:** Mendel's law of independent assortment states that each pair of alleles for a specific gene segregates independently of the alleles for a different gene. This law was revealed by the tracking of two traits at one time.

Punnett Squares

Since Mendel's laws of segregation and independent assortment reflect the rules of probability, the distribution of hereditary traits among offspring can be predicted using a tool called the Punnett square. In order to construct a Punnett square, the genotypes of each parent must be known. The genotype of an individual identifies each allele for a specific gene. Individuals can either be homozygous for the dominant trait, homozygous for the recessive trait, or heterozygous for both traits. The Punnett square predicts the percentage of each type of offspring based on the genotypes of the parents. For example, if two heterozygous individuals mate, 50% of the offspring will be heterozygous, 25% will be homozygous for the dominant trait, and 25% will be homozygous for the recessive trait.

	PATERNAL	
MATERNAL	**A**	**a**
A	AA	Aa
a	Aa	aa

AA = 25% heterozygous (two dominates)
Aa = 50% heterozygous (one dominate and one recessive)
aa = 25% homozygous (two recessives)

Meiosis and Chromosomes

During meiosis, four haploid gamete cells are produced. Each of these cells contains one copy of each gene packaged into chromosomes. When two gametes are joined during fertilization, the offspring receives one copy of each allele from each of its parents. In this way, a population experiences genetic variation during sexual reproduction that is not seen in asexual reproduction.

DNA in most species is divided into separate segments and packaged into chromosomes. Genes occupy specific loci, or positions, on a chromosome, and it is the chromosomes that undergo segregation and independent assortment. Therefore, it is the behavior of chromosomes during meiosis and fertilization that account for inheritance patterns.

Many species have a pair of sex chromosomes, designated by the symbols X and Y. These sex chromosomes are responsible for determining the sex of an individual. In humans, individuals with one X chromosome and one Y chromosome are male and those with two X chromosomes are female. All ova contain a single copy of the X chromosome, and sperm can contain either an X or a Y chromosome. Thus, the sex of an individual is determined by whether the sperm that fertilizes the ovum is carrying an X or a Y chromosome.

ANATOMY AND PHYSIOLOGY

Essential life functions are carried out through biological systems that work together to maintain an organism. These biological systems include the nervous system, the respiratory system, the circulatory system, the digestive system, the excretory system, the endocrine system, and the musculoskeletal system.

The Nervous System

All living organisms exhibit a response to both external and internal stimuli. A response to a stimulus involves the reception of the stimulus (sensory input), transmission of an impulse (integration), and a reaction to a stimulus (motor output).

Response

In higher animals such as humans, well-developed sensory organs are involved in the reception of a stimulus. External sensory organs include the skin, eyes, ears, and nose. More primitive sense organs can be seen in some species, and other animals have well-developed sensory organs. Single-cell organisms such as *Euglena* have a primitive sensory organ called an eyespot.

Internal sensory information such as blood pressure, blood CO_2 level, muscle tension, and pain are received by internal sensory neurons.

Transmission

The transmission of sensory input from the sensory organ to the central nervous system (brain) involves nerves or nerve fibers. Humans and many other animals have a complex nervous system consisting of the peripheral nervous system (throughout the body) and the central nervous system (the brain and the spinal cord).

The transmission of nerve impulses is electrical in nature and involves a difference in the concentration of certain ions, in particular sodium (Na^+) and potassium (K^+). The difference in concentration forms a gradient along the nerve fibers. The electrical potential difference generated by the ion gradient between the inside of a nerve cell (neuron) and the outside is called the membrane potential. A neuron that is not transmitting a signal is at its resting membrane potential. The threshold potential in a neuron that is transmitting a signal is called an action potential.

Nerve impulses, or electrical signals, are transmitted from one neuron to another across a tiny gap between the cells called a synapse. Most synapses are chemical synapses, which involve the release of chemicals called neurotransmitters by the presynaptic neuron (the neuron that is transmitting the nerve impulse). Presynaptic neurons synthesize neurotransmitters and package them into synaptic vesicles. The vesicles are stored in the neuron's synaptic terminals. The release of a neurotransmitter into the synaptic space between two neurons either stimulates or blocks the generation of a nerve impulse in the postsynaptic neuron (the neuron that is receiving the nerve impulse). This mechanism allows the synapse to function as a point of control in a neural pathway.

Reaction

A reaction to a stimulus may involve a change in position, movement, or secretory activity. Several biological systems may be involved in the motor output, or reaction, to stimuli. These systems include the skeletal and muscular systems, the endocrine system, and the digestive system. Other systems more indirectly involved in the reaction to stimuli are the circulatory system, the respiratory system, and the excretory system. The motor output response leaves the central nervous system through motor neurons, which communicate with effector cells such as muscle or endocrine cells.

The Respiratory System

The function of the respiratory system in humans is to exchange gases with the environment. The respiratory system supplies oxygen to blood and expels carbon dioxide from the blood. The quantity of available oxygen determines the effectiveness of respiration. In addition, oxygen consumption by the body is directly proportional to the rate of energy use and the level of physical activity of the body. Changes in oxygen consumption caused by an increase or decrease in physical activity have a temporary affect on the concentration of oxygen in the blood. Blood oxygen levels are restored to normal by a change in the respiratory rate. Metabolic processes are also affected by the level of oxygen in the blood.

The human respiratory system consists of the following parts:

- **Nasal/Oral Cavity:** The nasal cavity (nose) and the oral cavity (mouth) are the openings through which air is drawn into the body. Both cavities moisten and warm the air that enters the body. Nose hairs help to filter inspired air by trapping some particulate matter.

- **Pharynx (throat):** The pharynx forms the nose and mouth, and air passes into the pharynx. When food is not being ingested, the air passage to the pharynx remains open so air can travel to the larynx.

- **Larynx (voice box):** The larynx contains vocal cords, and as air rushes out of the larynx past the vocal cords, sound is produced.

- **Trachea (windpipe):** The trachea, or windpipe, is encircled by rings of cartilage so that it always remains open. Mucous in the trachea prevents dust and pollutants from entering the lungs.

- **Bronchi:** The trachea branches into two bronchi leading to the right and left lungs. The bronchi branch into narrower and narrower tubes called bronchioles.

- **Lungs:** Lungs are large sacs of air space and connective tissue. The lungs expand when air is taken in and contract when air is expelled.

- **Alveoli:** The alveoli are small clusters of cells in the lungs that secrete a substance that prevents the lungs from sticking together.

- **Diaphragm:** The diaphragm is a large muscle in the lower portion of the respiratory system. The diaphragm contracts to expand the chest when air is taken in and relaxes to decrease the volume of the lungs as air is expelled.

The Circulatory System

The circulatory system in humans delivers oxygen and nutrients to cells throughout the body and carries carbon dioxide to the lungs and metabolic waste to the excretory system.

Pulmonary Circulatory System

The force that causes blood to circulate throughout the body is called blood pressure. Blood pressure is created by the pumping of the heart. Blood is pumped to capillaries, where there is an exchange of materials between the blood and tissue.

The heart is a strong muscle divided into four chambers: the right atrium, the right ventricle, the left atrium, and the left ventricle. The left and right side of the heart are separated by the septum. The atria and ventricles are separated by valves. Blood flows through the heart and the body and then back to the heart in the following manner:

1. Oxygen-rich blood leaves the left ventricle and enters the aorta, which is the largest blood vessel in the body.

2. Blood travels through the aorta into the systemic circulatory system, which is made up of smaller arteries, arterioles, and capillaries.

3. The gas-and-nutrient exchange takes place between the blood and tissue through the capillary walls by the mechanisms of diffusion and osmosis. Oxygen and glucose are delivered to cells. The cells use oxygen and glucose to make ATP, which provides energy for the cell. Carbon dioxide, water, and other waste products are delivered to the blood to be carried away from the cells.

4. This oxygen-poor blood passes from capillaries to venules to veins. From the veins, blood flows to the superior or inferior vena cava, the largest veins in the body. Blood is returned to the heart through the veins by a passive mechanism of pushing from behind and a squeezing of the veins by skeletal muscles and gravity. The walls of veins do not contain muscle fibers like the walls of arteries.

5. The vena cava deliver the oxygen-poor blood to the right atrium of the heart. The blood passes through the tricuspid valve into the right ventricle.

6. The right ventricle sends the blood through the right and left pulmonary arteries to the lungs. In the lungs, the blood becomes oxygen-rich. The pulmonary arteries branch off into pulmonary capillaries. Carbon dioxide and water are exchanged for oxygen.

7. The pulmonary veins carry oxygenated blood to the left atrium of the heart. Blood passes from the left atrium through the bicuspid valve into the left ventricle.

8. The left ventricle pumps the blood back out to the body through the aorta.

The stimulation of the heart comes from within the heart muscle, but the rate of the heart beat, or muscle contractions, is modified by chemicals such as hormones and nerve transmissions from the brain. The rate and volume of blood flowing through the vessels are directly proportional to the blood pressure and is partially maintained by the closed nature of the circulatory system. Arteries are able to alter their internal diameter through the processes of constriction and dilation, and blood pressure is inversely proportional to the diameter of the arteries. It is important to remember that arteries have high pressure, muscular walls, and can regulate the rate of blood flow. Arteries do not have valves. Veins, on the other hand, have low pressure, no muscle, and are passive receivers of blood. Veins have an internal, one-way valve leading to the heart to prevent the backflow of blood.

Systemic Circulatory System

The lymphatic system consists of a network of branching vessels, lymph nodes, the tonsils and adenoids, the spleen, and the appendix. The lymphatic system returns excess body fluid to the circulatory system so that it can be expelled. The system also functions as part of the immune system.

Lymphatic vessels carry fluid called lymph. Lymph flows toward the heart. Lymphatic capillaries are permeable, so fluids can pass into and out of them, and they can pick up interstitial fluids. As lymph cycles through lymphatic organs such as the lymph nodes, it picks up and carries microbes or toxins from the site of infection in the body. An immune response is triggered when these materials are picked up by the lymph. When the body is fighting an infection, lymph nodes will fill with a large quantity of defensive cells, causing the nodes to be swollen and tender. An immune response in the lymph node is carried out by B-lymphocytes that fight off infection.

Blood Type

Blood is made in the marrow of the bone. It begins in pluripotent stem cells that mature to become one of three types of blood cells: erythrocytes (red blood cells), leukocytes (white blood cells), or platelets. Plasma is a fluid component in the blood that is similar to lymph, but contains more proteins. Red blood cells contain an iron-rich protein called hemoglobin, which binds to oxygen and carries it through the bloodstream and throughout the body. White blood cells serve to fight infection in the body. White blood cells consist of phagocytes that consume toxins, or infectious material, and lymphocytes that participate in cell defense and immunity. B-cells are a type of white blood cell that produces antibodies against foreign antigens. Helper T-cells help the B-cells and other T-cells. Killer T-cells kill off cells that have been infected with a virus. Platelets are small fragments in the blood that are important for clotting. When a body is injured, platelets rupture to release clotting factor.

There are four blood groups: A, B, AB, and O, which are based on the type of antigen found in the red blood cells. Individuals with type O blood can donate to any other type and are considered universal donors. Individuals with type AB blood can receive any type of blood and are considered universal recipients.

An individual with type A blood carries the A antigen and anti-B antibodies. These individuals may donate blood to others who have type A or type AB blood. They can receive blood from type O or type A donors. Individuals with type B blood carry the B antigen and anti-A antibodies. They may donate blood to others with type B or type AB blood. They can receive blood from others with type B and type O blood. AB blood carries both the A and the B antigen and does not make antibodies against either A or B. These individuals may donate to others with AB blood only and can receive all four types of blood. Individuals with type O blood do not have antigens for A or B and have antibodies against both A and B. They may donate to all blood types, but can receive only type O blood.

The Digestive System

The human digestive system ingests and breaks down food, absorbs nutrients, and eliminates undigested food as waste. Food is ingested into the digestive system, mixed with digestive substances such as the gastric juices of the stomach, and chemically broken down. Certain nutrients are then absorbed into the bloodstream. The rate of digestion is directly proportional to the type and quantity of food ingested.

The human digestive system includes the alimentary canal and associated organs. The alimentary canal is called the gastrointestinal (GI) tract and consists of the mouth, pharynx, esophagus, stomach, small intestine, and large intestine. The lining of the GI tract secretes mucous to lubricate the passage of food and to protect the lining of the tract from enzymes or acids. The associated organs of the

NOTE

Be sure you know the donors and recipients for the different blood types.

digestive system aid the GI tract either by providing secretions, or helping to break down food. These organs include the teeth, tongue, salivary glands, bladder, liver, and pancreas.

There are several processes that occur in the digestive system:

1. **Ingestion:** Food is taken into the body through the mouth.

2. **Propulsion:** The tongue pushes food into the pharynx and triggers a swallowing reflex. Once food enters the pharynx, it is propelled through the GI tract by peristalsis. Peristalsis involves alternating involuntary waves of constriction and relaxation that moves the food along the tract.

3. **Mechanical digestion:** Mechanical digestion involves the chewing of food, the churning and mixing of the food in the stomach, and the breaking down of food in the small intestine.

4. **Chemical digestion:** Chemical digestion takes place along the digestive tract between the mouth and the small intestine. Chemicals and enzymes break down food. Gastric juices in the stomach include stomach acids, mucous, and enzymes. Digestion of food begins in the stomach and continues in the small intestine. The liver and the pancreas aid in the digestion process that occurs in the small intestine. The liver produces bile that helps in the digestion of fats, and the pancreas produces pancreatic juice, which is a mixture of digestive enzymes and alkaline solution.

   All four types of molecules—carbohydrates, proteins, fats, and nucleic acids—are digested by enzymes in the small intestine that are specific to each type of molecule. The digestion of carbohydrates begins in the oral cavity and is completed in the small intestine. The digestion of proteins begins in the stomach and is completed in the small intestine. Pancreatic juice that is released into the small intestine contains nucleases (pancreatic ribonuclease and deoxyribonuclease) to hydrolyze ingested nucleic acids. Nucleosidases and phosphatases continue to break down the nucleic acids in the small intestine. Fats remain undigested until they reach the duodenum of the small intestine.

5. **Absorption:** The absorption of nutrients from food into the bloodstream occurs mostly in the small intestine. Some nutrients are absorbed by diffusion and others are pumped across a concentration gradient into cells. Large vessels transport nutrients from the intestine directly into the liver. The liver is involved in body metabolism by regulating the amount of glycogen it stores and the amount of glucose that is released into the bloodstream. Water is also absorbed by the large intestine and reabsorbed back into the bloodstream.

6. **Defecation:** Defecation includes ridding the body of waste material in the form of feces. This occurs through the large intestine, or colon. Waste products consist mostly of indigestible plant fibers and bacteria.

The Excretory System

The excretory, or urinary, system removes nitrogen-containing waste products from the blood and regulates the chemical composition, pH, and water balance of the blood. The key processes of the urinary system include filtration, reabsorption, secretion, and excretion. The kidneys are able to absorb wastes and excess substances from the blood selectively and pass them to urine. The kidneys then reabsorb any necessary nutrients needed by the body and return them to the blood. A huge volume of blood passes through the kidneys to extract a liquid filtrate, containing water, urea, glucose, amino acids, ions, and vitamins. The body requires many of these nutrients, and the kidneys concentrate the urea to pass in urine and return most of the water and nutrients to the bloodstream. This selective reabsorption conserves water and electrolytes in the body and balances their concentration in the blood and body tissues. The circulating volume of blood has a direct effect on kidney activity.

Urine contains urea, which accumulates from the breakdown of amino acids; uric acid, which accumulates from the breakdown of nucleic acids; and creatinine, which is a waste product from muscle metabolism. Urine is formed by filtration, reabsorption, and secretion. Urine is produced in the renal cortex of the kidneys and drains through collecting ducts and pyramids in an area called nephrons. The nephrons are the functional units of the kidneys, and the human body has millions of nephrons. Concentrated urine is formed in the collecting ducts of the kidneys and then moves from the collecting ducts into ureters and down into the bladder. The ureters connect the kidneys to the bladder, and the bladder serves as a receptacle for holding urine until it is excreted through the urethra. Urination, or micturition, is a reflex action of the body.

The Endocrine System

The endocrine system secretes chemicals called hormones that regulate biological processes such as digestion, metabolism, growth, reproduction, heart rate, and water concentration. Chemical messengers, or hormones, can be produced in one region of the body and act on target cells in another region of the body. Hormones are produced in specialized organs called endocrine glands, and these secrete hormones into the blood and tissue. This secretion is regulated by chemical and neural factors.

The major endocrine glands include the following:

- **The hypothalamus:** The hypothalamus exerts master control over the endocrine system. It receives information from nerves about internal and external body conditions and responds by sending out the appropriate neural, or endocrine, signal.

- **The pineal gland:** The pineal gland is a small pea-sized gland near the center of the brain that synthesizes and secretes melatonin. Melatonin links biorhythms with environmental light (daily and seasonal).

- **The pituitary gland:** The pituitary gland sits at the base of the hypothalamus. One lobe of the pituitary gland secretes hormones made in the hypothalamus, including oxytocin and antidiuretic hormone (ADH). The other lobe of the pituitary gland makes and secretes hormones into the bloodstream.

- **The thyroid gland:** The thyroid gland is located in the throat region, and hormones secreted from the thyroid affect almost every tissue type in the body. The thyroid produces thyroxine (T4) and triiodothryonine (T3), which stimulate and maintain metabolic processes. An excess of T3 and T4 can cause hyperthyroidism, and a deficit of these hormones can cause hypothyroidism.

- **The parathyroid gland:** There are four parathyroid glands and all are located on the surface of the thyroid. The parathyroid glands secrete calcitonin, which lowers blood calcium levels, and parathyroid hormone, which raises blood calcium levels. The action of these two hormones maintains calcium homeostasis in the body.

- **Adrenal glands:** Adrenal glands are located above the kidneys and secrete hormones in response to stress on the body. Two of the hormones secreted are epinephrine and norepinephrine; they increase blood glucose and increase metabolic activity while constricting certain blood vessels. These hormones trigger a "fight-or-flight response." Adrenal glands also secrete glucocorticoids such as cortisol, (increase blood glucose) and mineralocortoids (promote reabsorption of Na+ and excretion of K+ in the kidneys); they provide a slower, longer-lasting response to stress in the body.

- **The pancreas:** The pancreas produces two hormones that play a role in maintaining the body's energy supply. The pancreas produces insulin, which lowers blood glucose, and glucagon, which raises blood glucose.

- **The gonads:** The ovaries and testes are gonads, or sex glands, that secrete sex hormones and produce gametes (sperm and ova). The testes produce hormones called androgens (including testosterone) that support sperm formation and promote development and maintenance of male secondary sex characteristics. The ovaries produce hormones called estrogen and progesterone. Estrogen stimulates growth of the uterine lining and promotes the development and maintenance of female secondary sex characteristics. Progesterone promotes growth of the uterine lining so that it can support an embryo during pregnancy.

- **The thymus gland:** The thymus gland secretes the hormone thymosin that stimulates T-cell production for the immune system.

Hormones regulate primary metabolic processes. The mechanism by which a hormone works depends on whether the hormone is a steroid, a protein, a peptide, or an amine. If the hormone is a steroid, it can diffuse across the membrane of its target cell. It then binds to a receptor protein in the cell nucleus and activates specific genes on the DNA. If the hormone is a protein, a peptide, or an amine (all amino-acid based hormones), it binds to a receptor protein on the surface of the target cell. This receptor protein then stimulates the production of a second messenger called cyclic AMP or cAMP. The cAMP triggers various enzymes in the cell that initiate specific cellular changes or processes.

The Musculoskeletal System

The musculoskeletal system functions to generate motion and maintain posture. The skeletal system supports the body, protects certain internal organs such as the brain and lungs, and provides the framework for muscles to produce movement. The muscular system produces movement of the body and maintains posture. Bones and muscles are combined into individual systems resembling levers. This lever system consists of a muscle that provides force to the system, a joint that acts as the fulcrum, and a bone that acts like a lever. This arrangement allows for movement with a minimal expenditure of energy. A longer axis of the lever, or the bone, produces a greater extent of the movement of the body.

The skeleton is made up of bones and cartilage. Bone is a rigid and dense substance formed from connective tissue made up of collagen and calcium salts. Bones can be short, long, flat, or irregularly shaped. Bones contain nerves and blood vessels. Cartilage is found in developing embryos to a greater extent than it is found in a fully developed human. Cartilage does not contain nerves or blood vessels. Compact bone tissue is the superficial, dense surface of the bone. Spongy bone tissue is the deeper bone tissue that is honeycombed with small cavities; it is found in the midsection of the bone. Bone tissue is continually being deposited by osteoblasts and continually absorbed by osteoclasts. Bone is deposited in different regions based on the compressional load that the bone must carry. The function of bone is to support the body framework, aid in movement, protect vital organs such as the brain (skull), store fat in the form of yellow bone marrow, and store calcium and phosphate. Bones are also the site of blood cell formation.

Joints act as points of balance and are sculptured to regulate the extent or direction of the movement. All joints are classified according to how they are constructed. Fibrous joints are joined by fibrous tissue full of collagen fibers; these types of joints are immovable. Cartilaginous joints are articulating bones that are joined together by cartilage; almost all cartilaginous joints are immovable. Synovial joints are articulating bones that are separated by a fluid-containing joint cavity; these types of joints are generally free moving. The three basic movements allowed by these joints are gliding, angular motion, and rotational movements. Ligaments act to hold joints together.

A change in body position is produced by a shift in weight, which is accomplished by muscular force. The use of muscular force utilizes a large amount of energy and results in waste given off as thermal energy. The release of thermal energy during the application of muscular force helps to maintain a constant body temperature.

There are three types of muscle in the body. Skeletal muscle is attached to bones by tendons. It is a voluntary muscle that the body has conscious control over. The skeletal muscles contract to produce movement. Skeletal muscle is striated. Cardiac muscle is striated muscle that is only found in the heart. Its movement is involuntary and self-excitatory (initiates its own contraction). Smooth muscle is not striated and is found in the walls of organs such as the stomach, blood vessels, intestines, and the bladder. Smooth muscle tissue is also involuntary; that is, the body is not capable of conscious movement of smooth muscle.

The function unit of the muscle cell is the sacromere, which is composed of filaments called actin (thin filaments) and myosin (thick filaments). Muscles contract in the following manner:

1. Muscles can contract when a nerve impulse is sent to a skeletal muscle.

2. The neuron sending the impulse releases neurotransmitters onto the muscle cell.

3. The muscle depolarizes.

4. Depolarization of the muscle causes the sacroplasmic reticulum to release calcium ions.

5. The calcium ions released cause the actin and myosin filaments in the striated muscle to slide past one another. This action is explained by the sliding filament theory.

6. The sliding movement causes the muscle to contract, a motion driven by ATP. Muscle contractions cause movement of the body.

HUMANS AND THEIR ENVIRONMENT

Organisms must adapt to the environment in which they live in order to survive. Organisms may possess or develop certain traits that enable them to live or thrive in a specific environment. These adaptations, or changes, may originate in an individual and spread throughout a population, making the survival rate of that population greater. The changes that are most conducive to survival are preserved in the next generation and may eventually lead to a new species, or subspecies.

Energy in Ecosystems

Humans—like other species—form a complex relationship with their environment. Organisms in any given environment can be divided into three categories: producers, consumers, and decomposers.

1. **Producers:** Producers are organisms that are able to use energy from the sun to make complex organic molecules from simple inorganic substances, such as nitrogen and phosphorous, in their environment. Plants are producers that carry out the process of photosynthesis. All other organisms rely upon producers as a food source, either directly or indirectly.

2. **Consumers:** Consumers are organisms that either eat producers or other consumers to obtain energy. Humans are classified as consumers. In particular, humans are omnivores because they eat both producers (plants) and consumers (animals).

3. **Decomposers:** Decomposers are organisms that rely upon nonliving organic matter as a source of energy and material for growth. When an organism dies, sheds, or excretes waste, it provides a source of food for decomposers.

Biomes

The kinds and amounts of life found in each environment is dependent upon abiotic, or "nonliving," factors such as temperature, moisture (rainfall), sunlight, soil conditions, and climate. Environments with different conditions form biomes. Each biome is most dependent upon temperature and amount of precipitation. Some biomes in which humans and animals live include deserts, grasslands, savannas, Mediterranean shrublands, tropical dry forests, tropical rainforests, temperate deciduous forest, northern coniferous forests (taiga), and tundra.

Food Webs

Because only organisms that contain chlorophylls—such as plants—can make their own food, food webs exist in all environments so that all organisms can obtain energy. The energy from the sun is passed on to the producers in the environment. In turn, producers pass on the energy to primary consumers that eat the plants. A simple food chain continues to pass on energy as follows:

producer → primary consumer → secondary consumer → tertiary consumer → decomposer.

Each step in the flow of energy through an ecosystem is known as a trophic level. Because most consumers rely upon two or more types of organisms at different trophic levels for their energy, multiple food chains can overlap and intersect, forming a complex food web. Complex food webs are more stable than a simple food chain because the organisms are all dependent on more than one source of energy. The survival of humankind and other species is influenced by other species in the same environment. If one species struggles for survival or dies off, then due to the nature of a food web, many species may also struggle for an energy source.

Symbiosis

Symbiosis is a close, long-lasting physical relationship between two species. In a given environment, living organisms form an interrelated community in which many species live in close associations with one another. There are three different categories of symbiotic relationships:

1. **Mutualism:** Mutualism is a relationship between organisms that is beneficial to both species. Most symbiotic relationships are mutualistic.

2. **Commensalism:** Commensalism is a relationship between organisms in which one organism benefits from the relationship and the other is not affected.

3. **Parasitism:** Parasitism is a relationship in which one organism called the parasite lives in or on another organism called the host. The parasite derives energy and nourishment from the host, but the host is harmed by the relationship.

Conservation of Resources

The supply of natural resources in the environment is limited. Soil, wind, water, and fossil fuels are all examples of natural resources. A renewable resource can be formed or generated by natural processes and will not be used up. A nonrenewable resource is not replaced by natural processes. In relation to the human time scale, fossil fuels and mountain ranges are examples of resources that are not renewable. Humans often practice conservation in order to limit use of natural resources, so that they are preserved for future generations.

Population growth can reduce the amount of resources available to individuals in an environment. A renewable resource can be formed, generated, or replenished by natural biological, chemical, mechanical, or physical processes. Population control may be another way to ensure adequate amounts of food, energy, and other resources that humans depend upon.

Human Interaction with the Environment

Organisms within an environment may cause changes within the environment because of exploitation or overpopulation. The changes made to the environment may be to the extent that the environment then becomes suitable for a different group or species. In this way, succession occurs as the environment continues to change under the influence of different species, in turn causing other species to adapt or invade the environment. Succession is a series of recognizable and predicable changes over time that act to re-stabilize a community. When an ecosystem or environment is disturbed in some manner, either through natural disaster or overuse of land, succession can occur and new species may become better adapted to an environment than existing species.

In addition to protecting the environment, humans must also protect themselves from biological, chemical, physical, and radiological hazards. Vaccines are one way in which humans can protect themselves from certain biological hazards. Acquiring a natural immunity to viruses is another form of protection. Other biological hazards can be controlled through the use of antibiotics (to fight bacterial infections) and disinfectants. Sterilization, pasteurization, and refrigeration are all ways in which humans can keep their food supply safe from biological hazards.

Staying healthy and following safety precautions are ways in which humans can avoid biological, chemical, and physical hazards. Radiological hazards can be avoided by practicing safe laboratory and industrial methods.

SCIENCE GLOSSARY

TIP

This glossary lists terms and definitions useful to review for the registered nurse and allied health school exams.

A

absolute zero
The lowest known temperature possible, where all molecular motion nearly ceases.
Fahrenheit Scale—approximately 460°F (actual—459.67°F)
Celsius Scale— approximately 273°C (actual—273.15°C)
Kelvin Scale 0°K

absorption
The movement of water and/or dissolved substances into a cell, tissue, or organism.

acceleration
A change in the speed of an object. If the object speeds up, this is called *positive acceleration*. If the object slows down, it is called *negative acceleration*.

acid
A compound with a pH less than 7, which means that it releases hydrogen ions when dissolved in water. An acid changes blue litmus paper to red and tastes sour.

acquired immunity
Immunity that is not natural or congenital; obtained after birth.

active immunity
Immunity brought about by activity of certain cells of the body as a result of being exposed to an antigen.

active transport
An energy-requiring process by means of which materials are moved across a cell membrane.

adsorption
The gathering of molecules of a substance on a surface.

aerobe
Any organism living in the presence of and utilizing free, molecular oxygen (that is, oxygen not in chemical combination) in its oxidative processes.

alchemy
The science of transforming less valuable metals into gold or silver, and the philosophy behind this idea. The theories of the alchemists of the Middle Ages were false, but their experiments laid the foundation for modern chemistry.

alkali
A compound, when dissolved in water, with a pH greater than 7. An alkaline substance changes red litmus paper to blue, and it can combine with hydrogen ions of acids. *See* BASE.

alkaline

A substance having the properties of an ALKALI.

allantois

One of four extraembryonic membranes attached to the body of the embryo or fetus of a land-dwelling vertebrate. In humans, it is modified to form part of the placenta and umbilicus.

amino acid

An organic molecule containing an amino group (NH_2) and a carboxyl group (COOH) bonded to the same carbon atom; the "building blocks" of proteins. There are 20 amino acids that are used in metabolic processes.

amnion

The innermost of four extraembryonic membranes attached to the body of the embryo or fetus of a land-dwelling vertebrate. It forms a fluid-filled sac around the body that provides an aqueous environment (amniotic fluid) and cushions the embryo from shocks.

ampere

A measurement of electric current, abbreviated *amp*. It was named after French scientist ANDRÉ-MARIE AMPÈRE.

Ampère, André-Marie

A French scientist (1775–1836) whose work and theory laid the foundation for the André-Marie science of electrodynamics. His name lives on in the electrical measurement AMPERE.

amphipods

A crustacean group that includes sand fleas.

anaerobe

Any organism not requiring free, molecular oxygen (O_2) for its cellular oxidative processes. Some anaerobes are *obligate* and cannot survive in the presence of oxygen; others are *facultative* and can survive with or without oxygen.

anatomy

The study of the structure of living things. Usually, refers to the structure of the human body.

anemone

A sea animal (a coelenterate) that resembles the flower of the same name.

antibiotic

A substance derived from lower organisms that can be used to prevent growth of certain pathogens, thus combating infection.

antibody

A specific type of protein molecule that is manufactured in the tissues, blood, or lymph in response to the presence of viruses or foreign cells. Each variety of antibody will attach to the surface of only one type of invader, enabling it to be recognized and marked for destruction by the immune system.

antigens

Protein molecules on the surface of viruses or foreign cells that provoke the manufacture of matching antibodies, enabling invaders to be recognized as such so they can be destroyed.

apolipoprotein

(apo E) A gene that codes for a protein that facilitates the transport of cholesterol and influences human longevity.

ATP

(adenosine triphosphate) The energy-transport compound of a cell which is produced in the mitochondria.

atrium

The two anterior chamber(s) of the heart of vertebrates.

attenuated

The state of being weakened, as in the case of pathogens used to induce active immunity.

auricle

The projecting outer portion, or pinna, of the ear.

autotroph

An organism, such as a green plant, capable of manufacturing its food from inorganic environmental materials.

B

bacteria

Unicellular, microscopic, prokaryotic organisms, mostly saprotrophic or parasitic.

base

A compound, when dissolved in water, with a pH greater than 7 that can react with an acid to accept a hydrogen ion and form a salt. *See* ALKALI.

biochemistry

The study of the chemical makeup of organisms. This science is a branch of both chemistry and biology.

biology

The study of living things; a major science.

biome

A type of community recognized by certain characteristics of plants and climate, such as the plains of the Midwest United States, tropical rainforests, and arctic tundra.

bond

The force of attraction that holds 2 atoms together in a molecule. There are two major types of chemical bonds: COVALENT BONDS and IONIC BONDS.

botany

The study of plant life. Botany is a branch of BIOLOGY.

Brahe, Tycho

A Danish astronomer (1546–1601) who made a systematic study of the movement of celestial bodies. He is often referred to only as *Tycho*.

C

carbohydrate

A food substance made up of carbon, hydrogen, and oxygen.

carbon

An important chemical element that forms the basic skeleton of all ORGANIC compounds. Atoms of other elements are bonded to the carbon skeleton to form the many different varieties of organic compounds.

carbon dioxide (CO_2)

A compound made up of 1 atom of carbon (C) and 2 atoms of oxygen (O). It exists in the form of a gas and is one of the principal waste byproducts resulting from CELLULAR RESPIRATION.

carcinogen

A cancer-causing substance that may be physical, chemical, biological, or radiological.

catalyst

A chemical substance that lowers the energy necessary for a chemical reaction to take place and makes the reaction proceed more rapidly. ENZYMES act as catalysts in living organisms. Catalysts do not become part of the end-product. They can be reused many times.

celestial

An adjective referring to the sky.

cell

The basic structural and functional unit of organisms.

cellular respiration

The oxidation of glucose into carbon dioxide and water (or into other products, in the case of anaerobic respiration), leading to the release of energy.

Celsius

A system of measurement of temperature, often referred to as *centigrade*. On the Celsius scale, the freezing point for water is 0 degrees and the boiling point is 100 degrees.

centriole

A cellular organelle characteristic of animal cells, but not plant cells, that migrates to the poles during mitosis; spindle fibers and astral rays arise from it.

centromere

The portion of the chromosome that holds the chromatids together and to which spindle fibers apparently attach.

chelicerae

The claw-like head appendages on certain arthropods, such as spiders.

chemistry

The science that studies the composition and transformation of matter; a major science.

chlamydiae

Small intracellular obligate parasites closely related to the *Rickettsiae*.

chlorophylls

The green pigments of plants, produced in the presence of light and essential for photosynthesis.

chromosomes

Small cellular bodies containing tightly bound and packaged DNA that are formed during MITOSIS and MEIOSIS from loosely packaged DNA (chromatin). The hereditary determinants called GENES are carded on chromosomes.

colloid

A type of mixture intermediate between a SOLUTION and a SUSPENSION, consisting of liquid plus particles that are too small to settle out of the mixture and too large to dissolve. Colloids can exist in the form of a gel and pass through membranes either slowly or not at all.

commensalism

A symbiotic relationship in which one member is benefited, and the other member is neither benefited nor harmed.

compound

The combination of two or more elements into a single unit.

condensation

The transition of water vapor to liquid water due to a lowering of temperature.

conduction

The transfer of heat from one object or physical medium to another by direct contact.

conservation of energy

The principle that energy changes its form but cannot be created or destroyed.

conservation of matter

The principle that matter can change its form but cannot be created or destroyed.

constellation

A particular grouping of stars.

copepod

A small aquatic crustacean.

Copernicus, Nicholas

A Polish astronomer (1473–1543) who proposed the theory that the earth moves through space. It was generally believed up to that time that the earth was the immobile center of the universe.

cosmic year

The time it takes the sun to go around its galaxy.

covalent bond

A type of chemical bond created by the sharing of electrons between 2 atoms to achieve the maximum number of electrons in the outer electron orbit of each atom. Covalent bonds are the strongest type of chemical bonds.

crop rotation

An agricultural method by which crops in an area are changed each year, helping to maintain the fertility of the soil.

crustaceans

A group of aquatic animals with a hard outside covering. They are often included with MOLLUSKS in the group of "shellfish."

crystal

A form of solid in which the constituent atoms or molecules are arranged in a very regular, repeating pattern.

cytoplasm

In a prokaryotic cell, the entire contents of the cell contained within the plasma membrane. In a eukaryotic cell, the region of the cell lying within the plasma membrane but exterior to the nucleus.

D

Dalton, John

An English chemist and physicist (1766–1844) who introduced the theory that matter is composed of atoms.

Darwin, Charles

An English naturalist (1809–1883) who developed a THEORY OF EVOLUTION.

deforestation

The process by which land is cleared of forests. Excessive removal of forests for agriculture, development, mining, timber, and other human interests. If deforested areas remain barren, it can result in many negative ecological and environmental consequences, such as soil erosion and flooding.

density

Mass per unit volume, often expressed as grams per milliliter.

dictyosome

The *Golgi apparatus* of plant cells, which serves as a collecting and packaging center for secretions.

diffusion

The spontaneous movement of dissolved molecules from an area where they are in high concentration to an area where they are in lower concentration. This process requires no energy and, in living organisms, often takes place across semipermeable membranes.

distillation

The purification of a liquid substance by heating it until it vaporizes and then cooling it to cause it to condense into liquid again. Useful for separating and purifying liquids with different boiling points.

DNA

Deoxyribonucleic acid; a large, helical, double-stranded molecule in which the chromosomes code hereditary information.

dorso-ventral

An adjective referring to a back-to-front plane.

Down Syndrome

A genetic disorder of humans caused by the presence of an extra, third copy of chromosome 21. Individuals with Down Syndrome are mentally retarded and possess characteristic physical features.

E

eclipse

The obscuring of a celestial body that takes place when one celestial object moves in front of another. When the moon comes between the earth and the sun, it casts a shadow, or *umbra,* on part of the earth. This is known as a *solar* eclipse, since during this time the sun cannot be seen on that part of the earth. When the earth comes between the sun and the moon, it casts a shadow on the moon. Since the moon cannot be seen during this time, this is called a *lunar* eclipse.

Einstein, Albert

A German physicist (1879–1955) who lived the last years of his life in the United States. His theories changed the field of PHYSICS. He, more than any other scientist, was responsible for nuclear fission.

electron

A negatively charged particle in the atom that moves in an orbit around the NUCLEUS of the atom.

electronics

The study of the motion or movement of free electrons and ions to power countless communication and entertainment devices.

electrophoresis

A biochemical technique used to separate organic molecules such as PROTEINS or NUCLEIC ACIDS out of a mixture. In the most commonly used version of the technique, a sample of the mixture is placed at one end of a slab-shaped gel immersed in a buffer solution. An electric current is passed through the chamber containing the gel, and molecules travel through the gel at different distances according to their size and electrical charge. Each type of molecule accumulates in its own distinct zone or band in the gel.

element

One of more than 118 known basic substances. These substances and their combinations make up all matter, as far as is known. A pure chemical substance composed of a single type of atom, distinguished by having the same number of protons and electrons.

embryology

The study of the development of organisms from the time of conception until birth.

energy

The capacity to do work.

enthalpy

The heat content of the reactants and products in a chemical reaction.

entropy

The concept that closed systems move to a state of maximum disorder unless energy enters from the surroundings.

enzyme

An organic CATALYST; specific types of proteins produced by cells that govern or otherwise affect all biological reactions. *Exoenzymes* act outside the cells that produce them, and *endoenzymes* act within the cells that produce them. Enzymes are sensitive to the pH and temperature of their environment, and deviations from the optimal pH and temperature for an enzyme will lessen its activity. The maintenance of optimal internal environments for enzymes is a major objective of HOMEOSTASIS.

erg

A unit of work or energy.

erythrocytes

Red blood cells.

eugenics

A science that deals with the improvement of hereditary qualities of a race or breed.

eukaryote

An organism characterized by cells containing a true or visible nucleus.

evaporation

The process by which liquids change to gases.

evolution, theory of

Usually refers to Darwin's theory that changes occur in populations because natural selection favors the survival of those organisms best fitted for their environment.

exergonic reaction

Downhill reaction, whose products have less energy than the reactant.

experiment

A test to see if an idea is true or false.

F

Fahrenheit

The system of measuring temperature as generally used in the United States was developed by Gabriel Fahrenheit (1686–1736), a German scientist. On the Fahrenheit scale, 32 degrees is the freezing point of water, 212 degrees is the boiling point of water, and 98.6 degrees is the average temperature of the human body. Another widely used temperature measurement is the CELSIUS scale.

Faraday, Michael

An English physicist and chemist (1791–1867) who developed the first dynamo (electric generator) and discovered that a magnet could induce an electric current in a conductor, such as metal.

fertility

The ability to reproduce. *See* REPRODUCTION.

force

That which stops, creates, or changes the velocity of motion.

friction

The resistance created to the movement of an object when it rubs or collides with other objects.

fungi

A group of organisms, typically saprotrophic (or parasitic), many of which have a MYCELIUM. A few fungi, such as yeasts, do not have a mycelial body. *See* SAPROTROPH.

G

galaxy

A massive grouping of stars, often orbiting a central black hole. Astronomers estimate there are over 100 billion galaxies in the visible universe.

Galileo

An Italian astronomer and physicist (1564–1642) who made many contributions to science. He discovered that objects of different weights and shapes fall to the ground at the same rate of speed, attracted by GRAVITY. He was a strong believer in COPERNICUS' theory that the earth moved in space, and he was persecuted for this belief.

gene

A hereditary determinant consisting of a segment of a DNA molecule that contains the coded information necessary for assembling a specific type of protein molecule. Each gene occupies a fixed locus on a specific CHROMOSOME, enabling the transmission of hereditary determinants from one generation to the next.

genetic code

The sequence of NUCLEOTIDE bases in a molecule of DNA or RNA that, when translated by a RIBOSOME, specifies the sequence of AMINO ACIDS in a PROTEIN molecule.

genetic disorder

A metabolic disorder caused by inheritance of a damaged gene, a damaged chromosome, or an incorrect number of chromosomes. *See* DOWN SYNDROME, HEMOPHILIA, PHENYLKETONURIA, and SICKLE CELL ANEMIA.

genetics

The study of HEREDITY, or the manner in which hereditary traits are passed on from one generation to the next.

genome

The genetic makeup of an individual; the genotype.

geology

The study of the formation, structure, and history of the earth.

geriatrics

The science of the diseases of aged persons.

glycolysis

The anaerobic decomposition of a glucose into 2 molecules of pyruric acid, with the production of 2 net molecules of ATP.

Golgi
An organelle in animal and plant cells where proteins from the endoplasmic reticulum are processed, modified, and secreted.

gravitation
The tendency of objects in space to move toward each other.

gravity
A fundamental force in nature. The force of attraction between two bodies where the strength of the force is proportional to the bodies' masses and distance between them.

greenhouse effect
The warming effect of the Earth caused by an accumulation of carbon dioxide and other gases, such as methane, which are expelled from vehicles and industrial operations into the atmosphere. Heat is trapped under the layer of greenhouse gases and is attributed to causing global warming and climate change.

H

habitat
The immediate surroundings or environment in which a particular species may live.

half-life
The length of time required for the degradation to another substance of half the molecules in an amount of radioactive substance. The half-lives of radioactive ISOTOPES of elements can be used to date material containing radioactive substances. An example is the carbon-14 dating of living material.

Harvey, William
An English physician and anatomist (1578–1657) who discovered how the blood moves through the body.

heat
A measurable form of energy.

heat shock proteins
A protein that prevents the denaturation of other proteins when the temperature rises to abnormally high levels.

hemoglobin
A type of protein molecule that is bright red in color and binds reversibly to oxygen. It is carried within ERYTHROCYTES, enabling them to transport oxygen.

hemophilia
A GENETIC DISORDER caused by inheritance of a defective gene for one of the proteins that act as blood-clotting factors. The blood of affected persons fails to clot normally if an injury occurs, creating the danger that they might bleed to death from even minor wounds.

heredity
The transmission of traits from generation to generation.

homeostasis
The maintenance of internal balance by a living organism.

hormone

A chemical regulator of many bodily activities. A hormone is produced by an endocrine gland.

hydridoma

Recombinant (mixed) cells produced by the fusion of plasma cells and cancer cells.

hydrogen

The element with the smallest atom, consisting of one (1) proton and one (1) electron. It exists as a gas and is common in nature. Hydrogen is important to living organisms because it is a constituent of water and most organic compounds.

hypha

A mycelial thread; one of the "strands" making up a MYCELIUM, which is a fungus body.

hypothesis

An unproven explanation of something that has happened or might happen.

I

immunity

Resistance to a particular disease or condition. *See* ACQUIRED IMMUNITY, ACTIVE IMMUNITY, NATURAL IMMUNITY, and PASSIVE IMMUNITY.

immunization

The process of making one immune, usually by giving antigens to induce active immunity via the production of antibodies specific to that antigen.

immunoglobulins

Antibodies.

indicator

A substance whose color is sensitive to the hydrogen-ion concentration of the solution to which it is added.

inorganic

An adjective meaning "not organic" and generally applied to any atom other than carbon, or to a molecule not containing carbon. *See* ORGANIC.

insecticides

Natural or synthetic chemical compounds used to control insects.

interferon

An antiviral agent secreted by cells under attack from viruses.

interstellar

An adjective meaning "between stars."

ion

An atom or radical that has acquired a positive charge by giving up or losing electron(s), or a negative charge by gaining electron(s).

ionic bond

A type of chemical bond created by one atom giving up all electron or electrons to another atom to achieve the maximum number of electrons in the outer orbit of each atom. Ionic compounds will separate in water to yield IONS in a process called *dissociation*.

isotopes

Atoms that belong to the same chemical element, having the same number of protons and electrons, differing only in the number of neutrons and therefore atomic mass.

K

Kepler, Johannes

A German astronomer (1571–1630) who made important discoveries about the orbits of planets.

kinetic energy

Energy that is in motion. The energy of a boulder tumbling down a mountainside is an example of kinetic energy. *See* POTENTIAL ENERGY.

Koch, Robert

A German doctor (1843–1910) who studied bacteria. He and LOUIS PASTEUR are considered the founders of the science of bacteriology.

Krebs cycle

The aerobic breakdown of glucose, forming carbon dioxide, water, and ATP.

L

Lamarck, Chevalier de

A French naturalist (1744–1829) who developed a theory of evolution. *See* CHARLES DARWIN.

Lavoisier, Antoine

A French chemist (1743–1794) who made important discoveries concerning combustion, the conservation of matter, and the role of oxygen in respiration.

leukocytes

White blood cells that defend the body against bacteria, infectious diseases, and foreign bodies.

lever system

An assemblage of parts for moving weight with the least amount of applied force. A lever system consists of a rigid rod (*lever*) applied to the weight, a point of balance (*fulcrum*) for the lever, and mechanical force applied to the lever. These parts can be arranged in different ways to accommodate different amounts of weight, but a common principle of all lever systems is that the greatest amount of lifting force is achieved when the point at which the force is applied is farthest from the fulcrum.

light year

The distance light travels in one year. 9.46 trillion kilometers; 5.88 trillion miles.

Linnaeus, Carolus

A Swedish botanist (1707–1778) best known for developing a system of nomenclature for animals and plants.

lipopoly-saccharide

A polymer of simple sugars linked with fragments of lipid molecules.

litmus

An indicator used to test for pH, or hydrogen-ion concentration. Litmus is red in acid solutions and blue in basic solutions.

litmus paper

A special paper containing LITMUS, used by chemists to test for acid and alkali.

lunar

An adjective referring to the moon. A lunar eclipse is an eclipse of the moon.

lymph

A colorless fluid that has passed from the bloodstream through capillary walls into the intercellular spaces; lymph is collected by lymph ducts and returned to the bloodstream.

lysosomes

Cellular organelles that contain powerful hydrolytic enzymes.

M

mandible

The lower jaw bone of vertebrates; the mouth part of arthropods that resembles a jaw and functions in biting.

marine

An adjective meaning "of or relating to the sea."

mechanics

The study of the effects of force on moving or motionless bodies; a branch of PHYSICS.

meiosis

A type of cellular division that results in gametes (sex cells) or gametic nuclei. It consists of two divisions resulting in four daughter cells, and the number of chromosomes in each daughter is reduced by half (haploid).

membrane

A thin sheet forming a semipermeable boundary, as in (1) a thin layer of soft tissue; (2) the outer boundary of a cell (*see* PLASMA MEMBRANE); or (3) the enclosing boundary of an intracellular structure (for example, the nucleus).

Mendel, Gregor Johann

An Austrian monk and botanist (1822–1884) who made important discoveries concerning HEREDITY.

metabolism

The sum total of the cellular chemical processes that allow a cell to survive.

meteorology

A science that studies the weather and the atmosphere.

facebook.com/petersonspublishing

microscope

An instrument that produces a magnified image of an object. Light microscopes use a set of glass lenses to focus and magnify rays of light that either pass through or bounce off the object. Electron microscopes use magnetic lenses and beams of electrons to produce more sharply focused and highly magnified images than can be produced with a light microscope.

mineral

An INORGANIC substance that occurs naturally in rocks or soil. Minerals such as calcium, sodium, potassium, and zinc are used by living organisms in various metabolic processes. Calcium carbonate (limestone) is an example.

mitochondrion

The cellular organelle of EUKARYOTES in which cellular oxidation (*cellular respiration*) generates energy in the form of ATP.

mitosis

A type of cellular division that results in exact duplicates of the parent cell, as in asexual reproduction or growth. It consists of one division resulting in two daughter cells, and the number of chromosomes in each daughter is the same as in the parent (diploid).

molecule

A collection of atoms arranged in a specific manner and is the smallest unit into which a compound can be divided; yet still retain its physical and chemical properties.

mollusks

Animals of the phylum *Mollusca,* characterized by a *mantle,* a *radula,* and a *muscular foot.* Some mollusks are aquatic, like the octopus, clam, and oyster. Others are terrestrial, like the snail and slug.

mutation

A stable and abrupt change in a gene, and thus in the trait the gene determines, that is transmitted from generation to generation.

mutualism

A symbiotic relationship of mutual benefit to its partners.

mycelium

A mass of fungal threads or hyphae, composing the fungus body.

N

natural immunity

Immunity or resistance to disease with which a person is born.

nebula

An intersteller gas cloud mostly composed of ionized hydrogen and helium atoms, primarily responsible for star formation.

nephron

A functional unit of the kidney, consisting of Bowman's capsule with its glomerulus, and the associated ducts and convoluted tubules, with their capillaries.

neutron

A small particle that is part of the atom and has no electrical charge. *See* ELECTRON and PROTON.

Newton, Isaac

An English mathematician and natural philosopher (1642–1727) who made major discoveries in astronomy and PHYSICS. His most important work was his study of GRAVITATION and OPTICS.

nonpolar compound

A substance in which the electromagnetic charge of each molecule is balanced so that there is no positively or negatively charged end to the molecule. Oils and fats are examples. *See* POLAR COMPOUND and SOLUBLE.

norepinephrine

A biogenic amine derivative of tyrosine that serves as a neurotransmitter in the central nervous system and the peripheral nervous system.

nuclear

An adjective referring to the NUCLEUS of an atom or cell.

nuclear fission

The splitting of an atom in order to produce energy and different atomic weight elements.

nuclear fusion

The joining together of lightweight atoms resulting in the release of energy.

nucleic acid

DNA and RNA; the nucleic acids code and transcribe information about heredity.

nucleolus

A separate area within the NUCLEUS in which RNA is synthesized.

nucleotide

The "building unit" of NUCLEIC ACIDS, consisting of a sugar (ribose or deoxyribose), a phosphate, and a base (a purine or a pyrimidine).

nucleus

The center core of an object, as (1) the center of an atom, containing protons and neutrons; or (2) the regulatory center of a cell of an organism.

O

observatory

A specially constructed building containing one or more telescopes for observation of the heavens.

ohm

A unit for measuring electric resistance.

oncogen

Specific genes that initiate malignancies.

optics

The study of light and its effects; a branch of PHYSICS.

orbit

The path of an object or particle around a body, such as the Moon circling the Earth, and an electron around an atomic nucleus.

organ

A structure consisting of several different types of TISSUE combined into a single unit. A single organ can perform one or more major functions and is usually linked with other organs to form a *system*.

organelle

An intracellular structure that performs a major function for the cell; the cellular equivalent of an organ.

organic

Characteristic of, pertaining to, or derived from organisms; an adjective referring to living things or organisms.

organism

A living thing, such as a human, a plant, or an animal.

osmosis

The movement of water across a semipermeable membrane.

oxidation

Any chemical reaction that results in a molecule losing an electron, losing a hydrogen atom, or gaining an oxygen atom.

oxide

A compound made of oxygen and another element.

P

parasitism

A symbiotic relationship in which one organism (*parasite*) lives on and at the expense of another (*host*).

passive immunity

(usually temporary) Imparted without the person's body acting in its immunity build-up; the immunity is imparted by the administration of foreign antibodies.

Pasteur, Louis

A French chemist (1822–1895) who made major discoveries in chemistry and biology, especially in the control of many diseases. He and ROBERT KOCH were the founders of the science of bacteriology.

pasteurization

The heating of milk, or some other liquid, to a certain temperature for a definite period of time to destroy certain pathogens without changing the flavor or quality of the beverage.

PCR

Polymerase chain reaction is an *in-vitro* technique for the rapid reproduction of many copies of DNA segments.

peptide bond

A chemical bond that joins two amino acids by connecting the carboxyl group of one amino acid and the amino group of the other.

peptidoglycan

A polymer of amino acids and sugars arranged in a mesh-like structure to form bacteria cell walls.

pH

A symbol used in expression of acidity or alkalinity. It denotes the negative logarithm of the concentration of hydrogen ions in gram atoms or moles per liter.

phagotroph

An organism that feeds on other organisms, usually while they are still alive, by engulfing them to allow digestion and absorption to take place within the body.

phenylketonuria (PKU)

A GENETIC DISORDER caused by inheritance of a damaged gene for the enzyme that converts excess molecules of the AMINO ACID phenylalanine to the AMINO ACID tyrosine. High levels of phenylalanine and phenylketones, molecules intermediate between phenylalanine and tyrosine, accumulate in the blood of the affected person unless dietary intake of phenylalanine is severely restricted. Untreated PKU in infants results in severe brain damage and mental retardation.

physics

The study of matter and energy and their interactions.

phytogeographic map

A visual reference, illustration, or imagery of vegitarian and plant distribution in a given area.

Planck, Max

A German physicist (1858–1947) who did notable work in thermodynamics; the "father of quantum physics."

planet

A large body that moves around the Sun or another star, for example, the Earth.

plankton

A group of sea life—both plant and animal—that drifts with tides and currents.

plasma

The liquid portion of the blood in which proteins and other substances are dissolved. Also, a fourth state of matter, such as fire.

plasma membrane

The cell membrane; the living covering of the cell.

plasmid

Small circular DNA molecules in bacterial cells capable of self-duplication; often different genes are inserted.

plastids

Cellular organelles that are found in plant cells and may contain pigments. The types of plastids are (1) *chloroplasts,* which contain the chlorophyll and carotenoid pigments and which are green; (2) *chromoplasts,* which contain carotenoid pigments and range in color from yellow to brown; and (3) *leucoplasts,* which are colorless.

polar compound

A substance (for example, water) in which the electromagnetic charge of each molecule is unevenly distributed so that the molecule is positively charged on one end and negatively charged on the other end. *See* NONPOLAR COMPOUND and SOLUBLE.

potential energy

Energy that is available for use. The energy of a boulder balanced on a mountainside is an example of potential energy. It becomes *kinetic energy* when the boulder begins to roll.

precipitation

The settling out of particles suspended in liquid. Precipitation can be the result of a chemical reaction in which dissolved reactants form an insoluble product. Material that settles out of a suspension is a *precipitate*.

Priestley, Joseph

The English chemist (1738–1804) who discovered oxygen, though the element was named, and its importance first recognized, by ANTOINE LAVOISIER.

primeval

An adjective meaning "the first" or "early."

prokaryote

An organism characterized by cells not containing a true or definite NUCLEUS surrounded by a nuclear membrane.

protein

A complex organic compound consisting of AMINO ACIDS in polymeric form.

proton

A positively charged particle found in the nucleus of atoms.

protoplasm

An outdated term for the living substance within a cell. Current terminology divides cellular content into CYTOPLASM and *nucleoplasm* (material within the nuclear membrane).

protoplast

The entire cellular contents, surrounded by and including the cell membrane. The cell wall and/or capsule are not a part of the protoplast.

R

radical

An atom or compound that contains an unpaired electron.

radio astronomy

The study of radio waves received from outer space.

reduction

Any chemical reaction that results in a molecule gaining an electron, gaining a hydrogen atom, or losing an oxygen atom.

regeneration

The ability of an organism to regrow parts of itself after an injury.

replication

The process by which DNA duplicates itself for distribution to daughter nuclei during mitosis and/or meiosis.

reproduction

The process by which organisms create offspring of their own species.

respiration

In cells, the oxidation of food for the release of energy; in aerobes, the intake of oxygen and the release of carbon dioxide.

restriction fragment

A piece of DNA produced by breaking a large piece of DNA at specific points with restriction enzymes extracted from bacteria.

retrovirus

An RNA virus that produces new DNA from its RNA, as catalized by the enzyme reverse transcriptase. Example, human immunodeficiency virus (HIV).

RFLP

(restriction fragment length polymorphism) Differences in the lengths of RESTRICTION FRAGMENTS seen when DNA from different individuals is exposed to the same set of restriction enzymes. Using RFLPs to determine the identity of a person with DNA obtained from blood or other bodily materials is often referred to as "DNA fingerprinting." RFLPs can also be used to diagnose the presence of genetic disorders resulting from damaged genes.

ribosome

An intracellular structure consisting of RNA and protein whose function is to provide a site for the TRANSLATION phase of protein synthesis.

RNA

(ribonucleic acid) A large, helical, single-stranded molecule whose different types perform various tasks in the process of protein synthesis. Responsible for decoding the DNA sequence to construct protein chains.

S

salinity

The amount of dissolved salt in a fluid, typically referring to sodium chloride. However, other salts can be present.

salt

A substance formed when an acid is mixed with a base and composed of ionic bonds.

saprotroph

An organism feeding on dead organic matter, usually digesting the food externally and absorbing the digested material into its body such as fungi.

satellite

A man-made or natural object that orbits around a planet.

serotonin

A biogenic amine derivative of tryptophan that serves as a neurotransmitter in the central nervous system.

serum

The fluid portion of blood plasma after clotting.

sickle cell anemia

A GENETIC DISORDER caused by inheritance of a damaged gene for two of the four PROTEIN subunits of the HEMOGLOBIN molecule. The defective hemoglobin molecules stick to one another, forming clusters that distort the shape of the ERYTHROCYTES, reducing their ability to transport oxygen. Defective erythrocytes can also burst or clog capillaries.

slime mold

Large amoeboid protozoans that form spores similar to those of fungi.

solar

An adjective referring to the sun. A solar eclipse is an eclipse of the sun.

solar system

The Sun, planets, moons, asteroids, and comets.

soluble

The ability of a substance to mix completely with a liquid at the molecular level, such that no particles of any kind are visible in the mixture. The substance must be compatible with the liquid; nonpolar substances will not dissolve in polar liquids or the reverse. Dissolved substances will often be able to pass through semipermeable membranes. *See* NONPOLAR COMPOUND, POLAR COMPOUND, SOLUTE, and SOLUTION.

solute

The substance dissolved in a fluid to form a solution. *See* SOLUTION, SOLUBLE, and SOLVENT.

solution

A solution is a type of mixture formed when one substance mixes completely with a liquid at the molecular level. For example, when sugar (POLAR COMPOUND) is mixed with hot water (also a POLAR COMPOUND), the result is a solution. *See* SOLUTE, SOLVENT, and SOLUBLE.

solvent

The fluid in which a solute is dissolved to form a SOLUTION. *See* SOLUBLE.

sonic

An adjective referring to sound.

spawn

(noun) eggs of certain aquatic and marine animals, such as fish, crabs, shrimp, frogs, and turtles (verb) to lay eggs.

stimulus

Any change in the external or internal environment of a living organism. Many stimuli cause a change in the organism's activity (response). For example, if a person has not eaten for some time, the smell of the food might make his mouth water. The stimulus is the sudden presence of food (detected by smell); the response is secretion of saliva.

sublimation

The transformation of a substance from a solid directly to a gaseous state without passing through a liquid state.

substratum

A layer lying beneath the top layer (geology); the surface of a medium on which microorganisms grow (biology); a material or compound on which enzymes act (biology). Also called the *substrate*.

supersonic

Faster than the speed of sound.

suspension

A type of mixture in which large particles are mixed with a liquid and remain mixed only as long as they are agitated. The particles in a suspension will settle out if not continuously agitated. An example is the suspension of blood cells in the plasma of blood. Particles in suspension will not pass through a semipermeable membrane. *See* COLLOID and SOLUTION.

symbiosis

A relationship between two different species living together. The relationship may be PARASITISM, MUTUALISM, or COMMENSALISM.

synergism

A phenomenon in which the total is greater than the sum of the individual parameters.

T

theory

An explanation of natural events based on hypotheses and confirmed by testing.

thermodynamics

The study of heat and energy flow.

tissue

A group of similar CELLS specialized to perform a single task. When different tissues are combined, they are arranged in sequential layers. *See* ORGAN.

transcription

The formation of messenger RNA from the coded DNA.

transduction

The passage of genetic material from one bacterial cell to another by means of viral parasites called *phages*.

transformation

The passage of genetic material from one bacterium to another through the medium in which they are growing.

translation

The formation of proteins from amino acids by the use of the coded information in the messenger RNA (mRNA) and transfer (tRNA).

translocation

The movement of materials throughout a plant.

U

unicellular

An adjective meaning single-celled. *See* CELL.

universe

All things that exist and taken as a whole but generally referring to as in space.

V

valence

The number of electrons that can be accepted, given up, or shared by an atom or RADICAL. Positive valence numbers indicate electrons that can be given up to or shared with another atom or radical; negative valence numbers indicate electrons that can be accepted from another atom or radical. The positive and negative valences of reactants must balance for a chemical reaction to occur.

vapor

The gaseous phase of a substance that is usually in a liquid state. Vaporization (*evaporation*) of water or another liquid is accomplished by heating the liquid.

vascular tissue

Tissue used to transport materials in multicellular organisms. In higher animals, blood is vascular tissue; in higher plants, xylem and phloem are vascular tissues.

vector

An organism that carries and transmits pathogens from one animal to another.

velocity

The rate of motion of one object relative to another object.

Vesalius, Andreas

A Flemish anatomist (1514–1564) who studied the body. His discoveries were so important that he is often referred to as "the father of anatomy." *See* ANATOMY.

virus

An obligate intracellular parasite consisting essentially of a nucleic acid surrounded by a protein coat.

vitamin

An organic substance other than an ENZYME that is necessary for the proper maintenance of a metabolic process. A vitamin deficiency will cause metabolic dysfunction and an overall decline in health. Animals, including humans, must get their vitamins from the foods they eat.

volt

The practical unit of measurement of electric potential and electromotive force.

W

water table

The level nearest to the surface of the ground where water is found.

work

The result of energy expenditure. Common examples of work are movement, chemical reactions, and changes from one physical state to another.

Y

yeast

A unicellular nonmycelial fungus. Some yeasts are of commercial importance in the brewing and baking industries.

Z

zoology

The study of animals; a branch of BIOLOGY.

Answer Sheet

Chemistry and Physics Test 1

1. Ⓐ Ⓑ Ⓒ Ⓓ
2. Ⓐ Ⓑ Ⓒ Ⓓ
3. Ⓐ Ⓑ Ⓒ Ⓓ
4. Ⓐ Ⓑ Ⓒ Ⓓ
5. Ⓐ Ⓑ Ⓒ Ⓓ
6. Ⓐ Ⓑ Ⓒ Ⓓ
7. Ⓐ Ⓑ Ⓒ Ⓓ
8. Ⓐ Ⓑ Ⓒ Ⓓ
9. Ⓐ Ⓑ Ⓒ Ⓓ
10. Ⓐ Ⓑ Ⓒ Ⓓ
11. Ⓐ Ⓑ Ⓒ Ⓓ
12. Ⓐ Ⓑ Ⓒ Ⓓ
13. Ⓐ Ⓑ Ⓒ Ⓓ

14. Ⓐ Ⓑ Ⓒ Ⓓ
15. Ⓐ Ⓑ Ⓒ Ⓓ
16. Ⓐ Ⓑ Ⓒ Ⓓ
17. Ⓐ Ⓑ Ⓒ Ⓓ
18. Ⓐ Ⓑ Ⓒ Ⓓ
19. Ⓐ Ⓑ Ⓒ Ⓓ
20. Ⓐ Ⓑ Ⓒ Ⓓ
21. Ⓐ Ⓑ Ⓒ Ⓓ
22. Ⓐ Ⓑ Ⓒ Ⓓ
23. Ⓐ Ⓑ Ⓒ Ⓓ
24. Ⓐ Ⓑ Ⓒ Ⓓ
25. Ⓐ Ⓑ Ⓒ Ⓓ
26. Ⓐ Ⓑ Ⓒ Ⓓ

27. Ⓐ Ⓑ Ⓒ Ⓓ
28. Ⓐ Ⓑ Ⓒ Ⓓ
29. Ⓐ Ⓑ Ⓒ Ⓓ
30. Ⓐ Ⓑ Ⓒ Ⓓ
31. Ⓐ Ⓑ Ⓒ Ⓓ
32. Ⓐ Ⓑ Ⓒ Ⓓ
33. Ⓐ Ⓑ Ⓒ Ⓓ
34. Ⓐ Ⓑ Ⓒ Ⓓ
35. Ⓐ Ⓑ Ⓒ Ⓓ
36. Ⓐ Ⓑ Ⓒ Ⓓ
37. Ⓐ Ⓑ Ⓒ Ⓓ
38. Ⓐ Ⓑ Ⓒ Ⓓ
39. Ⓐ Ⓑ Ⓒ Ⓓ

40. Ⓐ Ⓑ Ⓒ Ⓓ
41. Ⓐ Ⓑ Ⓒ Ⓓ
42. Ⓐ Ⓑ Ⓒ Ⓓ
43. Ⓐ Ⓑ Ⓒ Ⓓ
44. Ⓐ Ⓑ Ⓒ Ⓓ
45. Ⓐ Ⓑ Ⓒ Ⓓ
46. Ⓐ Ⓑ Ⓒ Ⓓ
47. Ⓐ Ⓑ Ⓒ Ⓓ
48. Ⓐ Ⓑ Ⓒ Ⓓ
49. Ⓐ Ⓑ Ⓒ Ⓓ
50. Ⓐ Ⓑ Ⓒ Ⓓ
51. Ⓐ Ⓑ Ⓒ Ⓓ
52. Ⓐ Ⓑ Ⓒ Ⓓ

53. Ⓐ Ⓑ Ⓒ Ⓓ
54. Ⓐ Ⓑ Ⓒ Ⓓ
55. Ⓐ Ⓑ Ⓒ Ⓓ
56. Ⓐ Ⓑ Ⓒ Ⓓ
57. Ⓐ Ⓑ Ⓒ Ⓓ
58. Ⓐ Ⓑ Ⓒ Ⓓ
59. Ⓐ Ⓑ Ⓒ Ⓓ
60. Ⓐ Ⓑ Ⓒ Ⓓ
61. Ⓐ Ⓑ Ⓒ Ⓓ
62. Ⓐ Ⓑ Ⓒ Ⓓ
63. Ⓐ Ⓑ Ⓒ Ⓓ
64. Ⓐ Ⓑ Ⓒ Ⓓ
65. Ⓐ Ⓑ Ⓒ Ⓓ

Chemistry and Physics Test 2

1. Ⓐ Ⓑ Ⓒ Ⓓ
2. Ⓐ Ⓑ Ⓒ Ⓓ
3. Ⓐ Ⓑ Ⓒ Ⓓ
4. Ⓐ Ⓑ Ⓒ Ⓓ
5. Ⓐ Ⓑ Ⓒ Ⓓ
6. Ⓐ Ⓑ Ⓒ Ⓓ
7. Ⓐ Ⓑ Ⓒ Ⓓ
8. Ⓐ Ⓑ Ⓒ Ⓓ

9. Ⓐ Ⓑ Ⓒ Ⓓ
10. Ⓐ Ⓑ Ⓒ Ⓓ
11. Ⓐ Ⓑ Ⓒ Ⓓ
12. Ⓐ Ⓑ Ⓒ Ⓓ
13. Ⓐ Ⓑ Ⓒ Ⓓ
14. Ⓐ Ⓑ Ⓒ Ⓓ
15. Ⓐ Ⓑ Ⓒ Ⓓ
16. Ⓐ Ⓑ Ⓒ Ⓓ

17. Ⓐ Ⓑ Ⓒ Ⓓ
18. Ⓐ Ⓑ Ⓒ Ⓓ
19. Ⓐ Ⓑ Ⓒ Ⓓ
20. Ⓐ Ⓑ Ⓒ Ⓓ
21. Ⓐ Ⓑ Ⓒ Ⓓ
22. Ⓐ Ⓑ Ⓒ Ⓓ
23. Ⓐ Ⓑ Ⓒ Ⓓ
24. Ⓐ Ⓑ Ⓒ Ⓓ

25. Ⓐ Ⓑ Ⓒ Ⓓ
26. Ⓐ Ⓑ Ⓒ Ⓓ
27. Ⓐ Ⓑ Ⓒ Ⓓ
28. Ⓐ Ⓑ Ⓒ Ⓓ
29. Ⓐ Ⓑ Ⓒ Ⓓ
30. Ⓐ Ⓑ Ⓒ Ⓓ
31. Ⓐ Ⓑ Ⓒ Ⓓ
32. Ⓐ Ⓑ Ⓒ Ⓓ

33. Ⓐ Ⓑ Ⓒ Ⓓ
34. Ⓐ Ⓑ Ⓒ Ⓓ
35. Ⓐ Ⓑ Ⓒ Ⓓ
36. Ⓐ Ⓑ Ⓒ Ⓓ
37. Ⓐ Ⓑ Ⓒ Ⓓ
38. Ⓐ Ⓑ Ⓒ Ⓓ
39. Ⓐ Ⓑ Ⓒ Ⓓ
40. Ⓐ Ⓑ Ⓒ Ⓓ

answer sheet

Human Anatomy and Physiology Test 3

1. Ⓐ Ⓑ Ⓒ Ⓓ   12. Ⓐ Ⓑ Ⓒ Ⓓ   23. Ⓐ Ⓑ Ⓒ Ⓓ   34. Ⓐ Ⓑ Ⓒ Ⓓ   45. Ⓐ Ⓑ Ⓒ Ⓓ
2. Ⓐ Ⓑ Ⓒ Ⓓ   13. Ⓐ Ⓑ Ⓒ Ⓓ   24. Ⓐ Ⓑ Ⓒ Ⓓ   35. Ⓐ Ⓑ Ⓒ Ⓓ   46. Ⓐ Ⓑ Ⓒ Ⓓ
3. Ⓐ Ⓑ Ⓒ Ⓓ   14. Ⓐ Ⓑ Ⓒ Ⓓ   25. Ⓐ Ⓑ Ⓒ Ⓓ   36. Ⓐ Ⓑ Ⓒ Ⓓ   47. Ⓐ Ⓑ Ⓒ Ⓓ
4. Ⓐ Ⓑ Ⓒ Ⓓ   15. Ⓐ Ⓑ Ⓒ Ⓓ   26. Ⓐ Ⓑ Ⓒ Ⓓ   37. Ⓐ Ⓑ Ⓒ Ⓓ   48. Ⓐ Ⓑ Ⓒ Ⓓ
5. Ⓐ Ⓑ Ⓒ Ⓓ   16. Ⓐ Ⓑ Ⓒ Ⓓ   27. Ⓐ Ⓑ Ⓒ Ⓓ   38. Ⓐ Ⓑ Ⓒ Ⓓ   49. Ⓐ Ⓑ Ⓒ Ⓓ
6. Ⓐ Ⓑ Ⓒ Ⓓ   17. Ⓐ Ⓑ Ⓒ Ⓓ   28. Ⓐ Ⓑ Ⓒ Ⓓ   39. Ⓐ Ⓑ Ⓒ Ⓓ   50. Ⓐ Ⓑ Ⓒ Ⓓ
7. Ⓐ Ⓑ Ⓒ Ⓓ   18. Ⓐ Ⓑ Ⓒ Ⓓ   29. Ⓐ Ⓑ Ⓒ Ⓓ   40. Ⓐ Ⓑ Ⓒ Ⓓ   51. Ⓐ Ⓑ Ⓒ Ⓓ
8. Ⓐ Ⓑ Ⓒ Ⓓ   19. Ⓐ Ⓑ Ⓒ Ⓓ   30. Ⓐ Ⓑ Ⓒ Ⓓ   41. Ⓐ Ⓑ Ⓒ Ⓓ   52. Ⓐ Ⓑ Ⓒ Ⓓ
9. Ⓐ Ⓑ Ⓒ Ⓓ   20. Ⓐ Ⓑ Ⓒ Ⓓ   31. Ⓐ Ⓑ Ⓒ Ⓓ   42. Ⓐ Ⓑ Ⓒ Ⓓ   53. Ⓐ Ⓑ Ⓒ Ⓓ
10. Ⓐ Ⓑ Ⓒ Ⓓ   21. Ⓐ Ⓑ Ⓒ Ⓓ   32. Ⓐ Ⓑ Ⓒ Ⓓ   43. Ⓐ Ⓑ Ⓒ Ⓓ   54. Ⓐ Ⓑ Ⓒ Ⓓ
11. Ⓐ Ⓑ Ⓒ Ⓓ   22. Ⓐ Ⓑ Ⓒ Ⓓ   33. Ⓐ Ⓑ Ⓒ Ⓓ   44. Ⓐ Ⓑ Ⓒ Ⓓ   55. Ⓐ Ⓑ Ⓒ Ⓓ

Human Anatomy and Physiology Test 4

1. Ⓐ Ⓑ Ⓒ Ⓓ   11. Ⓐ Ⓑ Ⓒ Ⓓ   21. Ⓐ Ⓑ Ⓒ Ⓓ   31. Ⓐ Ⓑ Ⓒ Ⓓ   41. Ⓐ Ⓑ Ⓒ Ⓓ
2. Ⓐ Ⓑ Ⓒ Ⓓ   12. Ⓐ Ⓑ Ⓒ Ⓓ   22. Ⓐ Ⓑ Ⓒ Ⓓ   32. Ⓐ Ⓑ Ⓒ Ⓓ   42. Ⓐ Ⓑ Ⓒ Ⓓ
3. Ⓐ Ⓑ Ⓒ Ⓓ   13. Ⓐ Ⓑ Ⓒ Ⓓ   23. Ⓐ Ⓑ Ⓒ Ⓓ   33. Ⓐ Ⓑ Ⓒ Ⓓ   43. Ⓐ Ⓑ Ⓒ Ⓓ
4. Ⓐ Ⓑ Ⓒ Ⓓ   14. Ⓐ Ⓑ Ⓒ Ⓓ   24. Ⓐ Ⓑ Ⓒ Ⓓ   34. Ⓐ Ⓑ Ⓒ Ⓓ   44. Ⓐ Ⓑ Ⓒ Ⓓ
5. Ⓐ Ⓑ Ⓒ Ⓓ   15. Ⓐ Ⓑ Ⓒ Ⓓ   25. Ⓐ Ⓑ Ⓒ Ⓓ   35. Ⓐ Ⓑ Ⓒ Ⓓ   45. Ⓐ Ⓑ Ⓒ Ⓓ
6. Ⓐ Ⓑ Ⓒ Ⓓ   16. Ⓐ Ⓑ Ⓒ Ⓓ   26. Ⓐ Ⓑ Ⓒ Ⓓ   36. Ⓐ Ⓑ Ⓒ Ⓓ   46. Ⓐ Ⓑ Ⓒ Ⓓ
7. Ⓐ Ⓑ Ⓒ Ⓓ   17. Ⓐ Ⓑ Ⓒ Ⓓ   27. Ⓐ Ⓑ Ⓒ Ⓓ   37. Ⓐ Ⓑ Ⓒ Ⓓ   47. Ⓐ Ⓑ Ⓒ Ⓓ
8. Ⓐ Ⓑ Ⓒ Ⓓ   18. Ⓐ Ⓑ Ⓒ Ⓓ   28. Ⓐ Ⓑ Ⓒ Ⓓ   38. Ⓐ Ⓑ Ⓒ Ⓓ   48. Ⓐ Ⓑ Ⓒ Ⓓ
9. Ⓐ Ⓑ Ⓒ Ⓓ   19. Ⓐ Ⓑ Ⓒ Ⓓ   29. Ⓐ Ⓑ Ⓒ Ⓓ   39. Ⓐ Ⓑ Ⓒ Ⓓ   49. Ⓐ Ⓑ Ⓒ Ⓓ
10. Ⓐ Ⓑ Ⓒ Ⓓ   20. Ⓐ Ⓑ Ⓒ Ⓓ   30. Ⓐ Ⓑ Ⓒ Ⓓ   40. Ⓐ Ⓑ Ⓒ Ⓓ   50. Ⓐ Ⓑ Ⓒ Ⓓ

Biology Test 5

1. Ⓐ Ⓑ Ⓒ Ⓓ	13. Ⓐ Ⓑ Ⓒ Ⓓ	25. Ⓐ Ⓑ Ⓒ Ⓓ	37. Ⓐ Ⓑ Ⓒ Ⓓ	49. Ⓐ Ⓑ Ⓒ Ⓓ
2. Ⓐ Ⓑ Ⓒ Ⓓ	14. Ⓐ Ⓑ Ⓒ Ⓓ	26. Ⓐ Ⓑ Ⓒ Ⓓ	38. Ⓐ Ⓑ Ⓒ Ⓓ	50. Ⓐ Ⓑ Ⓒ Ⓓ
3. Ⓐ Ⓑ Ⓒ Ⓓ	15. Ⓐ Ⓑ Ⓒ Ⓓ	27. Ⓐ Ⓑ Ⓒ Ⓓ	39. Ⓐ Ⓑ Ⓒ Ⓓ	51. Ⓐ Ⓑ Ⓒ Ⓓ
4. Ⓐ Ⓑ Ⓒ Ⓓ	16. Ⓐ Ⓑ Ⓒ Ⓓ	28. Ⓐ Ⓑ Ⓒ Ⓓ	40. Ⓐ Ⓑ Ⓒ Ⓓ	52. Ⓐ Ⓑ Ⓒ Ⓓ
5. Ⓐ Ⓑ Ⓒ Ⓓ	17. Ⓐ Ⓑ Ⓒ Ⓓ	29. Ⓐ Ⓑ Ⓒ Ⓓ	41. Ⓐ Ⓑ Ⓒ Ⓓ	53. Ⓐ Ⓑ Ⓒ Ⓓ
6. Ⓐ Ⓑ Ⓒ Ⓓ	18. Ⓐ Ⓑ Ⓒ Ⓓ	30. Ⓐ Ⓑ Ⓒ Ⓓ	42. Ⓐ Ⓑ Ⓒ Ⓓ	54. Ⓐ Ⓑ Ⓒ Ⓓ
7. Ⓐ Ⓑ Ⓒ Ⓓ	19. Ⓐ Ⓑ Ⓒ Ⓓ	31. Ⓐ Ⓑ Ⓒ Ⓓ	43. Ⓐ Ⓑ Ⓒ Ⓓ	55. Ⓐ Ⓑ Ⓒ Ⓓ
8. Ⓐ Ⓑ Ⓒ Ⓓ	20. Ⓐ Ⓑ Ⓒ Ⓓ	32. Ⓐ Ⓑ Ⓒ Ⓓ	44. Ⓐ Ⓑ Ⓒ Ⓓ	56. Ⓐ Ⓑ Ⓒ Ⓓ
9. Ⓐ Ⓑ Ⓒ Ⓓ	21. Ⓐ Ⓑ Ⓒ Ⓓ	33. Ⓐ Ⓑ Ⓒ Ⓓ	45. Ⓐ Ⓑ Ⓒ Ⓓ	57. Ⓐ Ⓑ Ⓒ Ⓓ
10. Ⓐ Ⓑ Ⓒ Ⓓ	22. Ⓐ Ⓑ Ⓒ Ⓓ	34. Ⓐ Ⓑ Ⓒ Ⓓ	46. Ⓐ Ⓑ Ⓒ Ⓓ	58. Ⓐ Ⓑ Ⓒ Ⓓ
11. Ⓐ Ⓑ Ⓒ Ⓓ	23. Ⓐ Ⓑ Ⓒ Ⓓ	35. Ⓐ Ⓑ Ⓒ Ⓓ	47. Ⓐ Ⓑ Ⓒ Ⓓ	59. Ⓐ Ⓑ Ⓒ Ⓓ
12. Ⓐ Ⓑ Ⓒ Ⓓ	24. Ⓐ Ⓑ Ⓒ Ⓓ	36. Ⓐ Ⓑ Ⓒ Ⓓ	48. Ⓐ Ⓑ Ⓒ Ⓓ	60. Ⓐ Ⓑ Ⓒ Ⓓ

General Science Test 6

1. Ⓐ Ⓑ Ⓒ Ⓓ	15. Ⓐ Ⓑ Ⓒ Ⓓ	29. Ⓐ Ⓑ Ⓒ Ⓓ	43. Ⓐ Ⓑ Ⓒ Ⓓ	56. Ⓐ Ⓑ Ⓒ Ⓓ
2. Ⓐ Ⓑ Ⓒ Ⓓ	16. Ⓐ Ⓑ Ⓒ Ⓓ	30. Ⓐ Ⓑ Ⓒ Ⓓ	44. Ⓐ Ⓑ Ⓒ Ⓓ	57. Ⓐ Ⓑ Ⓒ Ⓓ
3. Ⓐ Ⓑ Ⓒ Ⓓ	17. Ⓐ Ⓑ Ⓒ Ⓓ	31. Ⓐ Ⓑ Ⓒ Ⓓ	45. Ⓐ Ⓑ Ⓒ Ⓓ	58. Ⓐ Ⓑ Ⓒ Ⓓ
4. Ⓐ Ⓑ Ⓒ Ⓓ	18. Ⓐ Ⓑ Ⓒ Ⓓ	32. Ⓐ Ⓑ Ⓒ Ⓓ	46. Ⓐ Ⓑ Ⓒ Ⓓ	59. Ⓐ Ⓑ Ⓒ Ⓓ
5. Ⓐ Ⓑ Ⓒ Ⓓ	19. Ⓐ Ⓑ Ⓒ Ⓓ	33. Ⓐ Ⓑ Ⓒ Ⓓ	47. Ⓐ Ⓑ Ⓒ Ⓓ	60. Ⓐ Ⓑ Ⓒ Ⓓ
6. Ⓐ Ⓑ Ⓒ Ⓓ	20. Ⓐ Ⓑ Ⓒ Ⓓ	34. Ⓐ Ⓑ Ⓒ Ⓓ	48. Ⓐ Ⓑ Ⓒ Ⓓ	61. Ⓐ Ⓑ Ⓒ Ⓓ
7. Ⓐ Ⓑ Ⓒ Ⓓ	21. Ⓐ Ⓑ Ⓒ Ⓓ	35. Ⓐ Ⓑ Ⓒ Ⓓ	49. Ⓐ Ⓑ Ⓒ Ⓓ	62. Ⓐ Ⓑ Ⓒ Ⓓ
8. Ⓐ Ⓑ Ⓒ Ⓓ	22. Ⓐ Ⓑ Ⓒ Ⓓ	36. Ⓐ Ⓑ Ⓒ Ⓓ	50. Ⓐ Ⓑ Ⓒ Ⓓ	63. Ⓐ Ⓑ Ⓒ Ⓓ
9. Ⓐ Ⓑ Ⓒ Ⓓ	23. Ⓐ Ⓑ Ⓒ Ⓓ	37. Ⓐ Ⓑ Ⓒ Ⓓ	51. Ⓐ Ⓑ Ⓒ Ⓓ	64. Ⓐ Ⓑ Ⓒ Ⓓ
10. Ⓐ Ⓑ Ⓒ Ⓓ	24. Ⓐ Ⓑ Ⓒ Ⓓ	38. Ⓐ Ⓑ Ⓒ Ⓓ	52. Ⓐ Ⓑ Ⓒ Ⓓ	65. Ⓐ Ⓑ Ⓒ Ⓓ
11. Ⓐ Ⓑ Ⓒ Ⓓ	25. Ⓐ Ⓑ Ⓒ Ⓓ	39. Ⓐ Ⓑ Ⓒ Ⓓ	53. Ⓐ Ⓑ Ⓒ Ⓓ	66. Ⓐ Ⓑ Ⓒ Ⓓ
12. Ⓐ Ⓑ Ⓒ Ⓓ	26. Ⓐ Ⓑ Ⓒ Ⓓ	40. Ⓐ Ⓑ Ⓒ Ⓓ	54. Ⓐ Ⓑ Ⓒ Ⓓ	67. Ⓐ Ⓑ Ⓒ Ⓓ
13. Ⓐ Ⓑ Ⓒ Ⓓ	27. Ⓐ Ⓑ Ⓒ Ⓓ	41. Ⓐ Ⓑ Ⓒ Ⓓ	55. Ⓐ Ⓑ Ⓒ Ⓓ	68. Ⓐ Ⓑ Ⓒ Ⓓ
14. Ⓐ Ⓑ Ⓒ Ⓓ	28. Ⓐ Ⓑ Ⓒ Ⓓ	42. Ⓐ Ⓑ Ⓒ Ⓓ		

answer sheet

CHEMISTRY AND PHYSICS TEST 1

65 Questions • 65 Minutes

Directions: Read each question carefully and consider all possible answers. When you have decided which choice is best, blacken the corresponding space on your answer sheet. There is only one best answer for each question.

1. Oxygen gas can be obtained in appreciable quantities by heating all of the following EXCEPT
   - (A) H_2O
   - (B) H_2O_2
   - (C) HgO
   - (D) PbO_2

2. All of the reactions between the following pairs will produce hydrogen EXCEPT
   - (A) copper and hydrochloric acid.
   - (B) iron and sulfuric acid.
   - (C) magnesium and steam.
   - (D) sodium and alcohol.

3. When hydrochloric acid is added to sodium sulfite, and the gas that is formed is bubbled through barium hydroxide, the salt formed is
   - (A) $BaCl_2$
   - (B) $BaSO_3$
   - (C) NaCl
   - (D) NaOH

4. If 3,480 calories of heat are required to raise the temperature of 300 grams of a substance from 50°C to 70°C, the substance would be:

   Use the formula: $c = Q/M\Delta T$

   c = specific heat
   Q = number of calories
   M = mass
   T = temperature

	Substances	Specific Heat
(A)	ethyl alcohol	0.581
(B)	aluminum	0.214
(C)	liquid ammonia	1.125
(D)	water	1.0

5. Ozone is a molecular variety of
   - (A) oxygen.
   - (B) chlorine.
   - (C) hydrogen.
   - (D) sulfur.

6. If an eudiometer tube is filled with 26 milliliters of hydrogen and 24 milliliters of oxygen and the mixture exploded, which of the following would remain uncombined?
   - (A) 2 milliliters hydrogen
   - (B) 14 milliliters hydrogen
   - (C) 23 milliliters hydrogen
   - (D) 11 milliliters oxygen

7. The gas resulting when hydrochloric acid is added to a mixture of iron filings and sulfur is
   - (A) H_2S
   - (B) SO_2
   - (C) SO_3
   - (D) H_2

8. Calculate the time required for 100 milligrams of I^{131} (dissociation constant, K = 0.086625) to decay to 50 milligrams. Use the formula

$$K = \frac{0.693}{t^{\frac{1}{2}}}$$

(A) 0.5 days
(B) 0.4 days
(C) 64 days
(D) 8 days

9. What is the percentage composition of oxygen in a mole of glucose ($C_6H_{12}O_6$)?

(C = 12, H = 1, O = 16)
(A) 53
(B) 35
(C) 6
(D) 20

10. In sulfuric acid, the valence number of sulfur is
(A) + 2
(B) – 2
(C) – 4
(D) + 6

11. The boiling points of the following gases are as follows: argon, –185.7°C; helium, –268.9°C; nitrogen, –195.8°C; oxygen, –183°C. In the fractional distillation of liquid air, the gas that boils off last is
(A) argon.
(B) helium.
(C) nitrogen.
(D) oxygen.

12. The chemical reaction $2Zn + 2HCl = 2ZnCl + H_2$ is an example of
(A) double displacement.
(B) synthesis.
(C) analysis.
(D) single displacement.

13. When carbon dioxide gas is bubbled through water in a test tube, the product is
(A) ozone.
(B) methane.
(C) hydrogen peroxide.
(D) carbonic acid.

14. Bronze is an alloy of copper and
(A) iron.
(B) lead.
(C) zinc.
(D) tin.

15. Which of the following substances will raise the pH of a solution of hydrochloric acid?
(A) NaCl
(B) H_2CO_3
(C) $NaHCO_3$
(D) HNO_3

16. An oxide whose water solution will turn litmus red is
(A) BaO
(B) Na_2O
(C) P_2O_3
(D) CaO

17. 100 ml of a H_2SO_4 solution is completely neutralized with 50 ml of 1.0 M NaOH. What is the molarity of the H_2SO_4 solution? (S = 32, O = 16, Na = 23, H = 1).
(A) 1.0 M
(B) 0.25 M
(C) 0.5 M
(D) None of the above.

18. A solution of zinc chloride should NOT be stored in a tank made of aluminum because
(A) aluminum will displace the zinc in the zinc chloride solution.
(B) the zinc will become contaminated.
(C) the chloride ion will react with impurities in the solution.
(D) the two metals will react to produce an undesirable compound.

19. The valence number of sulfur in the ion SO_4^{-2} is
    (A) –2
    (B) +2
    (C) +6
    (D) +10

20. The chemical name for sulfuric acid is
    (A) hydrogen sulfate.
    (B) hydrogen sulfite.
    (C) sulfur trioxide.
    (D) hydrogen sulfide.

21. The number of grams of hydrogen formed by the action of 6 grams of magnesium (atomic weight = 24) on an appropriate quantity of acid is
    (A) 0.5
    (B) 8
    (C) 22.4
    (D) 72

22. The symbol for 2 molecules of hydrogen is
    (A) H_2
    (B) 2H
    (C) 2H+
    (D) $2H_2$

23. The formula for sodium bisulfate is
    (A) $NaBiSO_4$
    (B) $NaHSO_4$
    (C) NaH_2SO_4
    (D) Na_2SO_4

24. The law of multiple proportions was first proposed by
    (A) Dalton.
    (B) Davy.
    (C) Priestley.
    (D) Williams.

25. One liter of a certain gas, under standard conditions, weighs 1.16 grams. A possible formula for the gas is
    (A) C_2H_2
    (B) CO
    (C) NH_3
    (D) O_2

26. Which of the following compounds would be classified as a salt?
    (A) Na_2CO_3
    (B) $Ca(OH)_2$
    (C) H_2CO_3
    (D) CH_3OH

27. Of the following, which is an aromatic compound?
    (A) Benzene
    (B) Ethyl alcohol
    (C) Iodoform
    (D) Methane

28. Of the following, which is a monosaccharide?
    (A) Dextrose
    (B) Glycogen
    (C) Lactose
    (D) Sucrose

29. Fats belong to the class of organic compounds represented by the general formula, RCOOR', where R and R' represent hydrocarbon groups; therefore, fats are
    (A) ethers.
    (B) soaps.
    (C) esters.
    (D) lipases.

30. Oil and water are immiscible (do not mix) because
    (A) oil is polar and water is polar.
    (B) oil is nonpolar and water is polar.
    (C) water is nonpolar and oil is polar.
    (D) water is nonpolar and oil is nonpolar.

31. The chemical bond that forms between the carboxyl (RCOOH) group of one amino acid and the amino (RC-NH$_2$) of another is a(n)

    (A) peptide bond.

    (B) coordinate covalent.

    (C) ionic bond.

    (D) high energy bond.

32. Two atoms have the same atomic number but different atomic weights (masses); therefore, these atoms are

    (A) compounds.

    (B) isotopes.

    (C) neutrons.

    (D) different elements.

33. Commercial bleach has the formula

    (A) CaCl$_2$

    (B) CaOCL

    (C) Ca(OCl)$_2$

    (D) Ca(ClO$_3$)$_2$

34. In forming an ionic bond with an atom of chlorine, a sodium atom will

    (A) receive 1 electron from the chlorine atom.

    (B) receive 2 electrons from the chlorine atom.

    (C) give up 1 electron to the chlorine atom.

    (D) give up 2 electrons to the chlorine atom.

35. Which of the following is an example of a transition element? (Refer to the periodic table on page 312.)

    (A) Aluminum

    (B) Astatine

    (C) Nickel

    (D) Rubidium

36. A gas lighter than air is

    (A) CH$_4$

    (B) C$_6$H$_6$

    (C) HCl

    (D) N$_2$O

37. Of the following gases, which is odorless and heavier than air?

    (A) CO

    (B) CO$_2$

    (C) H$_2$S

    (D) N$_2$

38. In a volume of air at a pressure of one atmosphere at sea level, the partial pressure of oxygen is equal to

    (A) 593 mm of mercury.

    (B) 494 mm of mercury.

    (C) 380 mm of mercury.

    (D) 160 mm of mercury.

39. The complete combustion of carbon disulfide would yield carbon dioxide and

    (A) sulfur.

    (B) sulfur dioxide.

    (C) sulfuric acid.

    (D) water.

40. Alcoholic beverages contain

    (A) wood alcohol.

    (B) isopropyl alcohol.

    (C) glyceryl alcohol.

    (D) ethyl alcohol.

41. Of the following compounds, which is more difficult to decompose than lithium fluoride?

    (A) Lithium bromide

    (B) Lithium chloride

    (C) Lithium iodide

    (D) None of the above

42. Which of the following molecules would be classified as a ketone?

(A)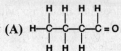

(B) H—C—C—C—C—C—H with H H H OH H substituents

(C) H—C—C—C—C—H with double-bonded O

(D) H—C—C—C—C—C=O

43. The periodic table (page 312) shows that the atomic number of fluorine is 9; this indicates that the fluoride atom contains

   (A) 9 neutrons in its nucleus.
   (B) 9 protons in its nucleus and 9 electrons in orbit around the nucleus.
   (C) a total of 9 protons and neutrons.
   (D) a total of 9 protons and electrons.

44. The element neon is considered an inert gas because it has __ electrons in its outermost energy shell.

   (A) 8
   (B) 7
   (C) 4
   (D) 2

45. Of four copper wires with the following dimensions, which one would have the greatest resistance to electrical current?

   (A) Length of 1 meter and diameter of 4 millimeters
   (B) Length of 2 meters and diameter of 8 millimeters
   (C) Length of 1 meter and diameter of 8 millimeters
   (D) Length of 2 meters and diameter of 2 millimeters

46. The general formula for an organic acid is

   (A) RCOOR
   (B) ROH
   (C) ROR
   (D) RCOOH

47. An example of a strong electrolyte is

   (A) sugar.
   (B) calcium chloride.
   (C) glycerin.
   (D) boric acid.

48. A lead ball, a wooden ball, and a styrofoam ball, all with a mass of 1 kilogram, are thrown at a wall 16 meters away, and all of them hit the wall in 2 seconds. Which ball will strike the wall with the greatest force?

   (A) Lead ball
   (B) Wooden ball
   (C) Styrofoam ball
   (D) All strike with the same force.

49. Identify the 2 atoms with the same number of electrons in their outermost energy level. (Use the periodic table on page 312.)

   (A) Na/K
   (B) K/Ca
   (C) Na/Mg
   (D) Ca/Na

50. When copper oxide is heated with charcoal, the reaction that occurs is an example of

   (A) reduction only.
   (B) oxidation only.
   (C) both oxidation and reduction.
   (D) neither oxidation nor reduction.

51. Nonmetal oxides, when dissolved in water, tend to form

   (A) acids.
   (B) bases.
   (C) salts.
   (D) hydrides.

52. The most important of the greenhouse gases contributing to global warning and altering the marine carbon cycle is
    (A) SO_2
    (B) CO
    (C) NH_3
    (D) CO_2

53. The best reducing agent is
    (A) mercury.
    (B) hydrogen.
    (C) copper.
    (D) carbon dioxide.

54. For a solution of H_2SO_4, the equivalency between molarity and normality would be (H = I, S = 32, O = 16)
    (A) IM = IN
    (B) IM = 2N
    (C) IN = 2M
    (D) IM = 0.5N

55. The test for a nitrate results in
    (A) a precipitate.
    (B) a red flame.
    (C) a brown ring.
    (D) litmus turning blue.

56. A solution that contains all the solute it can normally dissolve at a given temperature must be
    (A) concentrated.
    (B) supersaturated.
    (C) saturated.
    (D) unsaturated.

57. The oxides of barium and sulfur combine to form a(n)
    (A) salt.
    (B) base.
    (C) acid.
    (D) anhydride.

58. A pencil is dropped into a glass half filled with water. It looks as if the end that is underwater does not match up with the end that is in the air. This optical illusion is the result of
    (A) diffraction of light.
    (B) convection of light.
    (C) diffusion of light.
    (D) refraction of light.

59. The reason why concentrated H_2SO_4 is used extensively to prepare other acids is that concentrated sulfuric acid
    (A) is highly ionized.
    (B) is an excellent dehydrating agent.
    (C) has a high specific gravity.
    (D) has a high boiling point.

60. In a 0.001 M solution of HCl, the pH is:
    (A) 2
    (B) −3
    (C) 1
    (D) 3

61. By use of the periodic table on page 312, it can be determined that the atoms with the greatest affinity would be
    (A) Na and Cl
    (B) K and F
    (C) Na and F
    (D) K and Cl

62. Using the periodic table on page 312, determine if the valence of a sodium ion is:
    (A) +1
    (B) 0
    (C) −1
    (D) +12

63. The portion of an atom directly involved in the ionic bonding is the

(A) protons in the nucleus.

(B) neutrons in the nucleus.

(C) electrons in the outer energy level.

(D) electrons in the innermost energy level.

64. If the toxicity of a pesticide or a herbicide is in the range that a few drops could be fatal, the label should read

(A) Warning.

(B) Caution.

(C) Avoid.

(D) Danger.

65. A tornado passed over a house and destroyed it, primarily because

(A) the air pressure over the roof was lower than the pressure in the attic.

(B) the air pressure over the roof was equal to the pressure in the attic.

(C) the air pressure over the roof was higher than the pressure in the attic.

(D) None of the above

STOP

IF YOU FINISH BEFORE TIME IS CALLED, YOU MAY CHECK YOUR WORK ON THIS SECTION ONLY. DO NOT TURN TO ANY OTHER SECTION IN THE TEST.

CHEMISTRY AND PHYSICS TEST 2

40 Questions • 40 Minutes

Directions: Read each question carefully and consider all possible answers. When you have decided which choice is best, fill in the corresponding space on your answer sheet. There is only one best answer for each question.

1. Which of the following properties is considered a physical property?
   (A) Flammability
   (B) Boiling point
   (C) Reactivity
   (D) Osmolarity

2. Which one of the following substances is a chemical compound?
   (A) Blood
   (B) Water
   (C) Oxygen
   (D) Air

3. What are the differentiating factors between potential and kinetic energy?
   (A) Properties—physical or chemical
   (B) State—solid or liquid
   (C) Temperature—high or low
   (D) Activity—in motion or in storage

4. How many calories are required to change the temperature of 2 grams of H_2O from 20°C to 38°C?
   (A) 36 calories
   (B) 24 calories
   (C) 18 calories
   (D) 12 calories

5. The oxidation of 1 gram of CHO produces 4 calories. How much CHO must be oxidized in the body to produce 36 calories? (CHO is a carbohydrate.)
   (A) 4 grams
   (B) 7 grams
   (C) 9 grams
   (D) 12 grams

6. What is the atomic weight of the element in the figure below?

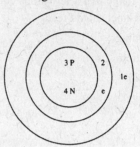

   (A) 2
   (B) 3
   (C) 4
   (D) 7

7. Which of the following kinds of radiation is most penetrating?
   (A) Alpha
   (B) Beta
   (C) Gamma
   (D) X-rays

8. I^{131} has a half-life of eight days. A 100-milligram sample of this radioactive element would decay to what amount after eight days?
   (A) 50 milligrams
   (B) 40 milligrams
   (C) 30 milligrams
   (D) 20 milligrams

9. A direct physiological effect of radiation on human tissues is
   (A) impairment of cellular metabolism.
   (B) proliferation of white blood cells.
   (C) formation of scar tissue.
   (D) reduction of body fluids.

10. What is the gram molecular weight of $C_6H_{12}O_6$? ($C = 12$, $H = 1$, $O = 16$)

    (A) 29 grams

    (B) 174 grams

    (C) 180 grams

    (D) 696 grams

11. Which one of the following equations is balanced?

    (A) $H_2O \rightarrow H_2 \uparrow + O_2 \uparrow$

    (B) $Al + H_2SO_4 \rightarrow Al_2(SO_4)_3 + H_2 \uparrow$

    (C) $S + O_2 \rightarrow SO_3$

    (D) $2HgO \rightarrow 2Hg + O_2 \uparrow$

12. A person with a fever would be expected to have

    (A) an increase in pulse rate.

    (B) a decrease in pulse rate.

    (C) no change in pulse rate.

    (D) All of the above

13. Which of the following bodily substances is a catalyst?

    (A) Bile

    (B) Hemoglobin

    (C) Enzyme

    (D) Mucus

14. In order to increase the temperature of a gas in a closed unit, it would be necessary to

    (A) increase the pressure.

    (B) decrease the density.

    (C) decrease the volume.

    (D) increase the space.

15. Which of the following equations represents an oxidation-reduction reaction?

    (A) $2Na + Cl_2 \rightarrow NaCl$

    (B) $CO_2 + H_2O \rightarrow H_2CO_3$

    (C) $HNO_3 + KOH \rightarrow KNO_3 + H_2O$

    (D) $CaO + H_2O \rightarrow Ca(OH)_2$

16. Which one of the following equations represents neutralization?

    (A) $2Na + Cl_2 \rightarrow 2NaCl$

    (B) $CO_2 + H_2O \rightarrow H_2CO_3$

    (C) $HNO_3 + KOH \rightarrow KNO_3 + H_2O$

    (D) $CaO + H_2O \rightarrow Ca(OH)_2$

17. What happens when a small amount of soap is added to hard water?

    (A) Copious suds are formed.

    (B) A scum is formed.

    (C) All sediments filter out.

    (D) Sediments diffuse equally throughout the solution.

18. A 10-percent solution of glucose will contain

    (A) 1 gram of glucose per 1,000 milliliters of solution.

    (B) 1 gram of glucose per 100 milliliters of solution.

    (C) 1 gram of glucose per 10 microliters of solution.

    (D) 10 grams of glucose per 100 milliliters of solution.

QUESTIONS 19–22 REFER TO THE DIAGRAMS BELOW.

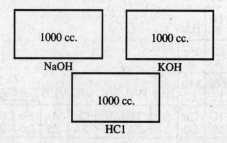

Each diagram represents one solution: One gram molecular weight of NaOH, one of KOH, and one of HCl, each dissolved in enough H_2O to make 1 liter.

19. What is the weight of NaOH in the solution diagram?

    (A) 40

    (B) 20

    (C) 23

    (D) 16

facebook.com/petersonspublishing

20. These are molar quantities because

(A) their molecular weights are equal to each other.

(B) the volume for each solution is the same.

(C) each solution contains 1 gram molecular weight.

(D) the percentage of solute to solvent is equal in each solution.

21. Identify the products of the chemical reaction between 1 cubic centimeter of KOH and 1 cubic centimeter of HCl.

(A) $K^+ + Cl_2 + 2H + OH$

(B) $KCl + H_2 + O_2$

(C) $K + Cl + HOH$

(D) $KCl + H_2O$

22. CA^{++} (atomic weight 40) is bivalent; hence, 1 gram equivalent weighs

(A) 40 grams.

(B) 30 grams.

(C) 20 grams.

(D) 10 grams.

23. A covalent bond between 2 amino acid molecules can be created by

(A) inserting a water molecule between them.

(B) removing a water molecule from them.

(C) inserting a carbon atom between them.

(D) removing a carbon atom from one of them.

24. Identify those elements in the periodic table that are inert gases (refer to columns).

(A) IA

(B) Zero

(C) IIIB–VIIB

(D) VIII

25. The basic inorganic raw materials for photosynthesis are

(A) water and oxygen.

(B) water and carbon dioxide.

(C) oxygen and carbon dioxide.

(D) sugar and carbon dioxide.

PERIODIC TABLE

IA																	VIIA	Zero
H 1	IIA											IIIA	IVA	VA	VIA		H 1	He 2
Li 3	Be 4											B 5	C 6	N 7	O 8		F 9	Ne 10
Na 11	Mg 12	IIIB	IVB	VB	VIB	VIIB		VIII		IB	IIB	Al 13	Si 14	P 15	S 16		Cl 17	Ar 18
K 19	Ca 20	Sc 21	Ti 22	V 23	Cr 24	Mn 25	Fe 26	Co 27	Ni 28	Cu 29	Zn 30	Ga 31	Ge 32	As 33	Se 34		Br 35	Kr 36
Rb 37	Sr 38	Y 39	Zr 40	Nb 41	Mo 42	Tc 43	Ru 44	Rh 45	Pd 46	Ag 47	Cd 48	In 49	Sn 50	Sb 51	Te 52		I 53	Xe 54
Cs 55	Ba 56	*La 57	Hf 72	Ta 73	W 74	Re 75	Os 76	Ir 77	Pt 78	Au 79	Hg 80	Tl 81	Pb 82	Bi 83	Po 84		At 85	Rn 86
Fr 87	Ra 88	**Ac 89																

*LANTHANIDE SERIES	Ce 58	Pr 59	Nd 60	Pm 61	Sm 62	Eu 63	Gd 64	Tb 65	Dy 66	Ho 67	Fr 68	Tm 69	Yb 70	Lu 71
**ACTINIDE SERIES	Th 90	Pa 91	U 92	Np 93	Pu 94	Am 95	Cm 96	Bk 97	Cf 98	Es 99	Fm 100	Md 101	No 102	Lr 103

26. Production of Salk vaccine against polio depended upon discovery of a method for
    (A) growing the polio virus outside the human body.
    (B) killing the polio virus.
    (C) observing the polio virus in the human body.
    (D) producing a polio antitoxin.

27. Ringworm is caused by a(n)
    (A) alga.
    (B) bacterium.
    (C) fungus.
    (D) protozoan.

28. The process responsible for the continuous removal of carbon dioxide from the atmosphere is
    (A) respiration.
    (B) metabolism.
    (C) oxidation.
    (D) photosynthesis.

29. All of the following concepts in genetics were first clearly stated by Gregor Mendel EXCEPT
    (A) dominance.
    (B) independent assortment.
    (C) segregation.
    (D) hybrid vigor.

30. The relation between termites and their intestinal protozoa is an example of
    (A) trophism.
    (B) parasitism.
    (C) mutualism.
    (D) commensalism.

31. When completed, the number of DNA base pairs comprising the human genome is expected to be approximately
    (A) 10 thousand.
    (B) 10 million.
    (C) 3 billion.
    (D) 3 trillion.

32. A completed human genomic map identifies the nucleotide sequences on the following chromosomal pairs:
    (A) 22 autosomes + 1 sex chromosome
    (B) 48 autosomes + 1 sex chromosome
    (C) 23 autosomes + 1 sex chromosome
    (D) 92 autosomes + 2 sex chromosomes

33. A technique (in which a catheter is inserted into the uterus to retrieve tissue samples) for the prenatal diagnosis of genetic diseases is called
    (A) amniocentesis.
    (B) positional cloning.
    (C) chorionic villus sampling (CVS).
    (D) None of the above

34. Identify the correct statement about DNA fingerprinting analysis of human tissues.
    (A) It is effective with small samples (e.g., less than 100 microliters of blood).
    (B) It produces identical bond patterns from all tissues in an individual.
    (C) It is effective on tissues more than 1,000 years old.
    (D) All of the above

35. In a DNA fingerprinting analysis of blood samples from a mother (M), a child (C), and an alleged father (F), the banding pattern in the child's blood was 50 percent (F), 27.3 percent (M), and 22.3 percent (FM). The statistical probability that the man is the child's father is
    (A) 50 percent.
    (B) greater than 50 percent.
    (C) less than 50 percent.
    (D) zero.

36. Glycogenesis occurs primarily in the
    (A) blood cells and spleen.
    (B) pancreas and gallbladder.
    (C) small intestines and stomach.
    (D) liver and muscles.

37. The end products of the Krebs cycle are
    (A) carbon dioxide and water.
    (B) urea and bile pigments.
    (C) lactic acid and pyruvic acid.
    (D) ketones and acetones.

38. The functional unit (or nephron) of the human kidney consists of
    (A) Bowman's capsule and veins.
    (B) Bowman's capsule, the glomerulus, and renal tubule.
    (C) the ureter and renal tubule.
    (D) the ureter, urethra, and renal tubule.

39. An organ that functions both as an endocrine and an exocrine gland is the
    (A) salivary gland.
    (B) gall bladder.
    (C) thyroid gland.
    (D) pancreas.

40. Aerobic oxidation of glucose occurs in two major stages; these are
    (A) glycolysis and reduction.
    (B) synthesis and the Krebs cycle.
    (C) glycolysis and the Krebs cycle.
    (D) degradation and hydrolysis.

STOP

IF YOU FINISH BEFORE TIME IS CALLED, YOU MAY CHECK YOUR WORK ON THIS SECTION ONLY. DO NOT TURN TO ANY OTHER SECTION IN THE TEST.

HUMAN ANATOMY AND PHYSIOLOGY TEST 3

55 Questions • 55 Minutes

Directions: Read each question carefully and consider all possible answers. When you have decided which choice is best, fill in the corresponding space on your answer sheet. There is only one best answer for each question.

Cells and Tissues

1. Cholesterol, in spite of its bad reputation, is an essential component of
   (A) microtubules.
   (B) the cell membrane.
   (C) ribosomes.
   (D) cytosol.

2. Synthesis of phospholipids, steroid hormones, and glycogen occurs within
   (A) rough endoplasmic reticulum.
   (B) mitochondria.
   (C) smooth endoplasmic reticulum.
   (D) golgi apparatus.

3. Following synthesis at the rough endoplasmic reticulum, new proteins are stored and "packaged" by
   (A) smooth endoplasmic reticulum.
   (B) the cell membrane.
   (C) golgi apparatus.
   (D) lysosomes.

4. Cell membranes control the movement of substances into and out of the cell and are best described as
   (A) selectively permeable.
   (B) freely permeable.
   (C) impermeable.
   (D) totally permeable.

5. Mammalian cells suspended within a hypertonic solution will
   (A) swell and possibly rupture.
   (B) lose water by osmosis.
   (C) take on water by osmosis.
   (D) remain unchanged since intracellular fluid is also hypertonic.

6. Glucose, a primary energy source for skeletal muscle, is insoluble in lipids and is too large to pass through membrane channels. Movement of glucose into skeletal muscle cells occurs via
   (A) active transport.
   (B) exocytosis.
   (C) diffusion.
   (D) facilitated diffusion.

7. The _____ are the control centers of cellular operations and usually contain nucleoli.
   (A) nuclei
   (B) mitochondria
   (C) ribosomes
   (D) lysosomes

8. _____, a multifunctional tissue, is comprised of layers of cells that cover both internal and external structures, including all exposed body surfaces. Although avascular, it is characterized by a high level of regeneration.
   (A) Muscle tissue
   (B) Neural tissue
   (C) Epithelia
   (D) Connective tissue

9. Connection of skeletal muscle to bones is made by tendons, which consist primarily of _____ fibers.
   (A) collagen
   (B) elastic
   (C) reticular
   (D) nerve

10. Joint cavities are found at articulations, are fluid-filled, and are lined by _____ membranes.
    (A) mucous
    (B) serous
    (C) cutaneous
    (D) synovial

Integumentary System

11. Protection of the skin from the harmful effects of ultraviolet light is provided by the pigment _____, which is produced by specialized cells within the stratum germanitivum.
    (A) carotene
    (B) melanin
    (C) keratin
    (D) hemoglobin

12. Lines of cleavage result from the parallel arrangements of _____ within the skin. They are significant in that incisions made parallel to a cleavage line tend to remain closed whereas incisions crossing lines of cleavage tend to pull open.
    (A) sebaceous glands
    (B) smooth muscle
    (C) blood vessels
    (D) collagen

13. The ear canal is protected against the invasion of foreign particles by a material produced by _____ glands.
    (A) ceruminous
    (B) sebaceous
    (C) apocrine
    (D) merocrine

14. _____ sweat glands become functional at puberty. Its product supports bacterial growth, which intensifies its odor.
    (A) Merocrine
    (B) Apocrine
    (C) Sebaceous
    (D) Ceruminous

15. Merkel discs and Meisnner corpuscles in the skin are functionally involved in
    (A) sweat production.
    (B) transport of blood.
    (C) sensation.
    (D) oil production.

Skeletal System

16. New bone matrix accompanied by increased strength and mass is the result of activity of
    (A) osteoblasts.
    (B) osteoclasts.
    (C) osteocytes.
    (D) lacuna.

17. Blood cell formation in adults is a function of red bone marrow primarily located within
    (A) periosteum.
    (B) endosteum.
    (C) compact bone.
    (D) spongy bone.

18. When blood calcium levels fall to below normal levels, osteoclast activity is stimulated and calcium excretion is decreased under the influence of elevated levels of
    (A) calcitonin.
    (B) parathyroid hormone.
    (C) calcitriol.
    (D) thyroxine.

19. The fetal skeleton begins as a model formed by cartilage. Replacement of cartilage by bone is the process of
    (A) intramembranous ossification.
    (B) endochondral ossification.
    (C) osteoclast activation.
    (D) osteoblast inhibition.

20. Freely moveable joints, such as those found at the elbow and ankle, are functionally categorized as
    (A) synarthrosis.
    (B) amphiarthrosis.
    (C) diarthrosis.
    (D) arthritis.

21. Movement at a joint that takes a body part away from the long axis of the body is
    (A) flexion.
    (B) extension.
    (C) abduction.
    (D) adduction.

Muscle

22. Following release of transmitter substance at the neuromuscular junction, the action of that transmitter is terminated by
    (A) acetylcholine.
    (B) acetylcholinesterase.
    (C) epinephrine.
    (D) monoamine oxidase.

23. Following production of an action potential at the end plate, that electrical activity is conducted to the interior of the cell via the
    (A) motor neuron.
    (B) muscle capillaries.
    (C) epimysium.
    (D) transverse tubules.

24. Skeletal muscle contraction, resulting from the interaction of myosin and actin, is a consequence of the release of calcium ions from the
    (A) motor neuron.
    (B) end plate.
    (C) mitochondria.
    (D) sarcoplasmic reticulum.

25. In a(n) _____ voluntary contraction, muscle length changes, movement occurs, and work is done.
    (A) isometric
    (B) isotonic
    (C) paralytic
    (D) flaccid

26. Relaxed muscles produce more energy than is required for resting metabolism. That energy is stored in the form of
    (A) ATP.
    (B) ADP.
    (C) creatine.
    (D) creatine phosphate.

27. Lifting progressively heavier weight requires the activation of an increased number of motor units, which is
    (A) complete tetanus.
    (B) recruitment.
    (C) muscle tone.
    (D) a twitch.

28. Slow muscle fibers are particularly resistant to fatigue, a property due, in part to the presence of _____, a protein that reversibly binds oxygen.
    (A) hemoglobin
    (B) myoglobin
    (C) ATP
    (D) ADP

29. Intercalated discs form connections between adjacent _____ muscle cells and play a major role in the function of that type of muscle.
    (A) striated
    (B) voluntary
    (C) cardiac
    (D) smooth

30. Individual muscle fibers and motor units either produce maximal tension in response to a stimulus or develop no tension at all. This is referred to as the _____ principle.
    (A) muscle tone
    (B) tetanus
    (C) twitch
    (D) all-or-none

Nervous System

31. _____ are glial cells within the central nervous system that play a role in maintaining the blood-brain barrier.
    (A) Ependymal cells
    (B) Microglia
    (C) Astrocytes
    (D) Oligodendrocytes

32. Following an action potential, sodium is returned to the extracellular space through the process of
    (A) diffusion.
    (B) filtration.
    (C) osmosis.
    (D) active transport.

33. An increase in potassium permeability at the postsynaptic membrane will result in a(n)
    (A) depolarization.
    (B) action potential.
    (C) excitatory postsynaptic potential.
    (D) inhibitory postsynaptic potential.

34. Spinal cord transection will result in a loss of respiration if the trauma is at upper _____ levels interrupting outflow of the phrenic nerve.
    (A) cervical
    (B) thoracic
    (C) lumbar
    (D) sacral

35. Sensitivity of muscle spindles is controlled by the central nervous system through its ability to activate
    (A) alpha motor neurons.
    (B) gamma motor neurons.
    (C) large diameter afferent axons.
    (D) the neuromuscular junction.

36. Damage to the _____ lobe of the cerebral cortex may result in deficits in conscious perception of auditory stimuli.
    (A) frontal
    (B) parietal
    (C) occipital
    (D) temporal

37. Sensory and motor innervation of the face is the domain of the ophthalmic, maxillary, and mandibular branches of the _____ nerve.
    (A) trochlear
    (B) trigeminal
    (C) facial
    (D) vestibulocochlear

38. Information regarding fine touch to the body surface ascends the spinal cord within the
    (A) spinothalamic tracts.
    (B) lateral corticospinal tracts.
    (C) posterior (dorsal) columns.
    (D) spinocerebellar tracts.

39. Active dreaming and autonomic alterations of blood pressure along with EEG tracings resembling the awake state are characteristic of
    (A) slow wave sleep.
    (B) rapid eye movement (REM) sleep.
    (C) coma.
    (D) arousal.

40. Parasympathetic autonomic outflow to the heart, lungs, and digestive system is a primary function of cranial nerve number
    (A) I.
    (B) II.
    (C) X.
    (D) XII.

Endocrinology and Reproduction

41. Release of thyroid hormones is triggered by _____ from the anterior pituitary gland.
    (A) thyrotropin releasing hormone
    (B) thyrotropin
    (C) thyroxine
    (D) iodide

42. In response to the release of _____ by the adenohypophysis, levels of glucocorticoids are elevated.
    (A) corticotropin releasing hormone
    (B) cortisol
    (C) aldosterone
    (D) adrenocorticotropic hormone

43. _____ stimulates the smooth muscle of the uterine wall during the labor and delivery process. After delivery, it promotes the ejection of milk.
    (A) Oxytocin
    (B) Vasopressin
    (C) Somatotropin
    (D) Prolactin

44. In females, _____ promotes estrogen secretion from cells within the ovaries, while in males, it stimulates sperm production within the testes.
    (A) testosterone
    (B) melanotropin
    (C) follicle stimulating hormone
    (D) luteinizing hormone

45. Pancreatic beta cells produce the hormone _____, which lowers blood glucose levels by promoting glucose uptake and utilization.
    (A) glucagon
    (B) insulin
    (C) epinephrine
    (D) renin

46. An individual with an abnormally high basal metabolic rate accompanied by weight loss and unusual temperature sensitivity is probably suffering from
    (A) high levels of growth hormone.
    (B) low levels of growth hormone.
    (C) high levels of thyroid hormones.
    (D) low levels of thyroid hormones.

47. Insulin is released by the beta cells of the pancreas in response to
    (A) low blood glucose levels.
    (B) high blood glucose levels.
    (C) high prolactin levels.
    (D) high growth hormone levels.

48. The mineralocorticoid _____ is a product of the adrenal cortex.
    (A) epinephrine
    (B) norepinephrine
    (C) ACTH
    (D) aldosterone

49. Abnormally low levels of parathyroid hormone could result in
    (A) convulsions.
    (B) hyperglycemia.
    (C) hypoglycemia.
    (D) excess water loss via the kidneys.

50. Type I diabetes mellitus is characterized by
    (A) high insulin levels.
    (B) ineffective insulin receptors.
    (C) low blood glucose levels.
    (D) decreased insulin production.

51. Glycogenesis occurs primarily in the
    (A) blood cells and spleen.
    (B) pancreas and gallbladder.
    (C) small intestines and stomach.
    (D) liver and muscles.

52. The end products of the Krebs cycle are
    (A) carbon dioxide and water.
    (B) urea and bile pigments.
    (C) lactic acid and pyruvic acid.
    (D) ketones and acetones.

53. The functional unit (or nephron) of the human kidney consists of
    (A) Bowman's capsule and veins.
    (B) Bowman's capsule, the glomerulus, and renal tubule.
    (C) the ureter and renal tubule.
    (D) the ureter, urethra, and renal tubule.

54. An organ that functions both as an endocrine and an exocrine gland is the
    (A) salivary gland.
    (B) gallbladder.
    (C) thyroid gland.
    (D) pancreas.

55. Aerobic oxidation of glucose occurs in two major stages; these are
    (A) glycolysis and reduction.
    (B) synthesis and the Krebs cycle.
    (C) glycolysis and the Krebs cycle.
    (D) degradation and hydrolysis.

STOP

IF YOU FINISH BEFORE TIME IS CALLED, YOU MAY CHECK YOUR WORK ON THIS SECTION ONLY. DO NOT TURN TO ANY OTHER SECTION IN THE TEST.

HUMAN ANATOMY AND PHYSIOLOGY TEST 4

50 Questions • 50 Minutes

Directions: Read each question carefully and consider all possible answers. When you have decided which choice is best, fill in the corresponding space on your answer sheet. There is only one best answer for each question.

Blood

1. Maintenance of the osmotic pressure of plasma is a major role of
   (A) albumin.
   (B) globulins.
   (C) fibrinogen.
   (D) platelets.

2. Anemia is a condition resulting from abnormally low levels of
   (A) platelets.
   (B) plasma proteins.
   (C) leukocytes.
   (D) erythrocytes or hemoglobin.

3. Production of red blood cells is stimulated by the release of _____ from specialized cells of the kidneys in response to hypoxia (low oxygen levels).
   (A) platelets
   (B) erythrocytes
   (C) erythropoietin
   (D) leukocytes

4. Blood typing is a classification determined by the identification of
   (A) erythrocyte surface antigens.
   (B) erythrocyte surface antibodies.
   (C) plasma antigens.
   (D) plasma antibodies.

5. Rh-positive blood indicates the presence of the
   (A) Rh antigen in plasma.
   (B) Rh antigen on the surfaces of erythrocytes.
   (C) Rh antibody on erythrocyte surfaces.
   (D) Rh antibody in plasma.

6. Transfusion of blood from a Type A donor to a Type B recipient will result in
   (A) agglutination.
   (B) blood vessel spasm.
   (C) platelet plug formation.
   (D) slowly progressive anemia.

7. The most numerous leukocytes are _____. They are granulocytes and represent one of the earliest defenses against infection.
   (A) lymphocytes
   (B) monocytes
   (C) basophils
   (D) neutrophils

8. T cells, B cells, and NK cells are classes of _____, agranulocytes involved in immunity processes.
   (A) monocytes
   (B) lymphocytes
   (C) neutrophils
   (D) eosinophils

9. Release of ADP, thromboxane A_2, and serotonin are events associated with the _____ phase of hemostasis.
   (A) vascular
   (B) platelet
   (C) coagulation
   (D) inflammation

10. The last step in the final common pathway of coagulation involves the production of insoluble strands of the protein
    (A) prothrombin.
    (B) thrombin.
    (C) fibrinogen.
    (D) fibrin.

Cardiovascular

11. Action potentials in cardiac cells are longer in duration than those in skeletal muscle. The long plateau seen in cardiac action potentials is primarily due to
    (A) calcium entry into the cell.
    (B) calcium exit from the cell.
    (C) sodium entry into the cell.
    (D) sodium exit from the cell.

12. Conducting cells of the heart do not maintain a stable resting membrane potential. The rate of spontaneous depolarizations is greatest within
    (A) the A-V node.
    (B) the S-A node.
    (C) bundle branch fibers.
    (D) purkinje fibers.

13. Depolarization of the ventricles is reflected in the _____ of the electrocardiogram.
    (A) P wave
    (B) QRS complex
    (C) T wave
    (D) P-R segment

14. The maximum ventricular volume within a cardiac cycle is expressed as the
    (A) stroke volume.
    (B) ejection fraction.
    (C) end-systolic volume.
    (D) end-diastolic volume.

15. The amount of tension the ventricles must produce in order to open semilunar valves and eject blood is the
    (A) preload.
    (B) afterload.
    (C) cardiac output.
    (D) stroke volume.

16. Norepinephrine acts at _____ receptors of the heart, resulting in an increase in heart rate.
    (A) alpha 1
    (B) alpha 2
    (C) beta 1
    (D) beta 2

17. Exchange of materials from the vascular system to surrounding interstitial fluids is a property of
    (A) arteries.
    (B) arterioles.
    (C) capillaries.
    (D) veins.

18. Pressure in veins is low and significantly influenced by the force of gravity. In the extremities, unidirectional blood flow is maintained by
    (A) venous valves.
    (B) venous smooth muscle.
    (C) precapillary sphincters.
    (D) semilunar valves.

19. Pulse pressure, the difference between systolic and diastolic pressure, is greatest within
    (A) arteries.
    (B) arterioles.
    (C) capillaries.
    (D) veins.

20. The primary responsibility for rapid correction of blood pressure alterations involves
    (A) angiotensin.
    (B) antidiuretic hormone.
    (C) chemoreceptors.
    (D) baroreceptor reflexes.

Respiration

21. During the act of swallowing, entry of liquids and solid materials into the respiratory tract is prevented by the
    (A) glottis.
    (B) epiglottis.
    (C) pharynx.
    (D) hard palate.

22. Septal (Type II) cells in the lung produce _____, which reduces the surface tension within alveoli. Infant respiratory distress syndrome results in individuals producing an inadequate amount of the substance.
    (A) serous fluid
    (B) pleural fluid
    (C) surfactant
    (D) mucous

23. _____ is the volume of air moved into or out of the respiratory system during a single respiratory cycle.
    (A) Tidal volume
    (B) Minute volume
    (C) Residual volume
    (D) Inspiratory reserve volume

24. The volume of air in the respiratory conduction passages that does NOT participate in gas exchange is the
    (A) vital capacity.
    (B) expiratory reserve volume.
    (C) anatomical dead space.
    (D) total lung capacity.

25. Movement of respiratory gases is primarily dependent upon the presence of a(n) _____ gradient.
    (A) concentration
    (B) osmotic
    (C) partial pressure
    (D) temperature

26. Contraction of the diaphragm results in inspiration as a result of
    (A) increased thoracic cavity volume.
    (B) decreased thoracic cavity volume.
    (C) increased abdominal cavity volume.
    (D) decreased abdominal cavity volume.

27. Oxygen unloading at the tissue level is accelerated by
    (A) elevated blood pressure.
    (B) lowered blood pressure.
    (C) elevated pH.
    (D) decreased pH.

28. Although most carbon dioxide is transported as bicarbonate, and some is dissolved in plasma, about 20% is carried
    (A) by leukocytes.
    (B) by plasma proteins.
    (C) as carbaminohemoglobin.
    (D) on the surface of erythrocytes.

29. The reaction of carbon dioxide and water leading to the formation of carbonic acid is catalyzed by
    (A) antigens on the surface of erythrocytes.
    (B) antibodies within plasma.
    (C) enzymes in plasma.
    (D) carbonic anhydrase within erythrocytes.

30. Length of inspiration is shortened by inhibitory impulses originating within the
    (A) apneustic center.
    (B) pneumotaxic center.
    (C) inspiratory center.
    (D) precentral gyrus.

Renal

31. Decline in systemic blood pressure leads to the release of renin, which results in the production of
    (A) angiotensinogen.
    (B) angiotensin I.
    (C) angiotensin II.
    (D) carbonic anhydrase.

32. Angiotensin II has multiple direct and indirect effects, including
    (A) vasoconstriction.
    (B) vasodilation.
    (C) inhibition of aldosterone release.
    (D) increased urine output.

33. _____ are examples of substances that are NOT significantly reabsorbed by the kidneys and are therefore excreted.
    (A) Amino acids
    (B) Vitamins
    (C) Nitrogenous by-products of protein catabolism
    (D) Water and electrolytes

34. Glucose and most other nutrients, such as amino acids and vitamins, are reabsorbed within the _____ of the nephron.
    (A) collecting duct
    (B) proximal convoluted tubule
    (C) loop of Henle
    (D) distal convoluted tubule

35. The movement of urine from the kidneys to the bladder is driven by
    (A) gravity alone.
    (B) peristalsis.
    (C) bladder pressure.
    (D) blood pressure.

36. Urinary continence is maintained by contraction of the external urethral sphincter, which is innervated by the
    (A) sympathetic division of the ANS.
    (B) parasympathetic division of the ANS.
    (C) phrenic nerve.
    (D) pudendal nerve.

37. The cation in the highest concentration within extracellular fluid that plays a major role in water distribution is
    (A) sodium.
    (B) potassium.
    (C) calcium.
    (D) magnesium.

38. The hormone most responsible for the renal regulation of sodium is
    (A) thyroxine.
    (B) insulin.
    (C) glucagon.
    (D) aldosterone.

39. Acid-base regulation is most powerful and most complete by
    (A) buffers.
    (B) respiratory mechanisms.
    (C) renal mechanisms.
    (D) urinary bladder activity.

40. Uncontrolled diabetes mellitus results in
    (A) respiratory acidosis.
    (B) respiratory alkalosis.
    (C) metabolic acidosis.
    (D) metabolic alkalosis.

Digestion

41. Absorption of vitamin B_{12} (required for erythrocyte production) is promoted by intrinsic factor—a product of cells found within the
    (A) small intestine.
    (B) stomach.
    (C) pancreas.
    (D) large intestine.

42. Bile that is NOT immediately needed for digestion is stored and concentrated within the
    - **(A)** liver.
    - **(B)** gallbladder.
    - **(C)** pancreas.
    - **(D)** ileum.

43. Secretion of pancreatic juice is stimulated by _____, released in response to proteins and fats within the small intestine.
    - **(A)** secretin
    - **(B)** cholecystokinin
    - **(C)** insulin
    - **(D)** aldosterone

44. Diarrhea and constipation result primarily from altered motility of the
    - **(A)** stomach.
    - **(B)** small intestine.
    - **(C)** liver.
    - **(D)** large intestine.

45. In order to be absorbed, carbohydrates must be reduced to the form of
    - **(A)** monosaccharides.
    - **(B)** disaccharides.
    - **(C)** polysaccharides.
    - **(D)** oligosaccharides.

46. Protein digestion begins in the stomach by a group of proteolytic enzymes referred to as
    - **(A)** lipase.
    - **(B)** sucrase.
    - **(C)** pepsin.
    - **(D)** amylase.

47. Vitamin _____ is water-soluble and readily absorbed from the intestine by diffusion.
    - **(A)** A
    - **(B)** D
    - **(C)** E
    - **(D)** C

48. Gastric ulcers occur when the protective inner layer of the stomach is damaged and the _____ layer, with its blood vessels and nerve cells, is exposed to acid.
    - **(A)** serosal
    - **(B)** mucosal
    - **(C)** submucosal
    - **(D)** muscular

49. Saliva contains mucus, water, and _____, which partially digests polysaccharides.
    - **(A)** lipase
    - **(B)** amylase
    - **(C)** pepsin
    - **(D)** insulin

50. Smooth muscle activity of the digestive system is stimulated by increased levels of _____ activity.
    - **(A)** parasympathetic autonomic
    - **(B)** sympathetic autonomic
    - **(C)** thyroid gland
    - **(D)** aldosterone

STOP

IF YOU FINISH BEFORE TIME IS CALLED, YOU MAY CHECK YOUR WORK ON THIS SECTION ONLY. DO NOT TURN TO ANY OTHER SECTION IN THE TEST.

BIOLOGY TEST 5

60 Questions • 60 Minutes

Directions: Read each question carefully and consider all possible answers. When you have decided which choice is best, fill in the corresponding space on your answer sheet. There is only one best answer for each question.

1. Passage of water through the membrane of a cell is called
   - (A) assimilation.
   - (B) osmosis.
   - (C) circulation.
   - (D) transpiration.

2. The largest portion of the iron supplied to the body by foods is used by the body for the
   - (A) growth of hard bones and teeth.
   - (B) manufacture of insulin.
   - (C) development of respiratory enzymes.
   - (D) formation of hemoglobin.

3. Phenylketonuria is a genetic disorder that involves an inability of
   - (A) blood to clot properly.
   - (B) one amino acid to be convened to another.
   - (C) blood cells to carry a sufficient load of oxygen.
   - (D) lung alveoli to stay open.

4. A new drug for treatment of tuberculosis was being tested in a hospital. Patients in group A received doses of the new drug; those in group B were given only sugar pills. Group B represents a(n)
   - (A) scientific experiment.
   - (B) scientific method.
   - (C) experimental error.
   - (D) experimental control.

5. Which is most closely associated with the process of transpiration?
   - (A) Spiracles of a grasshopper
   - (B) Root of a geranium
   - (C) Leaf of a maple
   - (D) Gills of a fish

6. Which term includes all the others?
   - (A) Organ
   - (B) Tissue
   - (C) System
   - (D) Organism

7. When several drops of pasteurized milk were placed in a petri dish containing sterilized nutrient agar, many colonies developed. This experiment shows the milk
   - (A) contained some bacteria.
   - (B) contained harmful bacteria.
   - (C) should have been sterilized.
   - (D) was incorrectly stamped "pasteurized."

8. The growth of green plants toward light is related most specifically to the distribution of _____ in the plant.
   - (A) minerals
   - (B) enzymes
   - (C) auxins
   - (D) amino acids

9. In humans, the digestion of carbohydrates begins in the
   - (A) stomach.
   - (B) small intestine.
   - (C) mouth.
   - (D) liver.

10. To determine whether an unknown black guinea pig is pure or hybrid black, it should be crossed with

    (A) a white guinea pig.

    (B) a hybrid black guinea pig.

    (C) a pure black guinea pig.

    (D) another unknown.

11. In a series of rock layers arranged one on top of another, fossils found in the lowest layers are

    (A) completely different from fossils found in the upper layers.

    (B) older than the fossils found in the upper layers.

    (C) of organisms simpler than the organisms fossilized in the upper layers.

    (D) of organisms more complex than the organisms fossilized in the upper layers.

12. The principal way in which forests help to prevent soil erosion is that the

    (A) trees provide homes for wildlife.

    (B) leaves of the trees manufacture food.

    (C) forest floors absorb water.

    (D) forest shields the soil from the sun's heat.

13. Which factor in the environment of an organism causes it to react?

    (A) A stimulus

    (B) A response

    (C) A reflex

    (D) An impulse

14. A breeder wanted to develop a strain of beef cattle with high-quality meat and the ability to thrive in a hot, dry climate. How can she best accomplish this?

    (A) Continued selection among the members of a prize herd

    (B) Crossbreeding followed by selection

    (C) Inbreeding to bring out desirable hidden traits

    (D) Inbreeding followed by selection

15. The inhaling and exhaling of air by the human lungs is mainly an application of

    (A) Boyle's Law—the inverse relationship between the pressure and the volume of a gas.

    (B) the volume of a gas at standard temperature and pressure (STP).

    (C) Charles' Law—the direct relationship between the temperature and the volume of a gas.

    (D) the number of O_2 and CO_2 particles per mole.

16. Which plant tissues are mostly concerned with storage?

    (A) Phloem and xylem

    (B) Phloem and cambium

    (C) Palisade cells and epidermis

    (D) Pith and spongy cells

17. The Hubble Telescope is able to produce images of very distant celestial objects more clearly than other telescopes because

    (A) its reflector is able to concentrate more light on the lens.

    (B) its images are enhanced by computer.

    (C) its view is not obstructed by atmosphere.

    (D) it has a larger lens.

18. Which reagent should be used in the urine test for diabetes?

    (A) Iodine

    (B) Nitric acid

    (C) Ammonia

    (D) Benedict's solution

19. The major benefit of buffer systems is that they

    (A) increase pH significantly.

    (B) resist significant changes in pH.

    (C) decrease pH significantly.

    (D) None of the above

20. The Krebs cycle produces
    (A) H_2O and NADH.
    (B) CO_2 and H_2.
    (C) pyruvic acid and lactic acid.
    (D) amino acids.

21. The removal for microscopic examination of a small bit of living tissue from a patient is called
    (A) biopsy.
    (B) surgery.
    (C) dissection.
    (D) therapy.

22. The presence of which substance is most important for all cell activity?
    (A) Light
    (B) Carbon dioxide
    (C) Water
    (D) Chlorophyll

23. The end products of digestion that enter the lacteals are
    (A) glucose.
    (B) amino acids.
    (C) minerals.
    (D) fatty acids.

24. A student in the laboratory tossed two pennies from a container 100 times and recorded these results: both heads, 25; one head and one tail, 47; both tails, 28. Which cross between plants would result in approximately the same ratio?
    (A) Aa × AA
    (B) Aa × Aa
    (C) AA × aa
    (D) Aa × aa

25. In the following equation for photosynthesis, the oxygen comes
    $$CO_2 + H_2O \rightarrow C_6H_{12}O_6 + O_2$$
    (A) entirely from CO_2.
    (B) from a simple sugar molecule.
    (C) partially from CO_2 and H_2O.
    (D) entirely from H_2O.

26. Tissue culture has been extensively used as a research method in all of the following fields of biological investigation EXCEPT
    (A) photosynthesis.
    (B) virology.
    (C) development of nerve cells.
    (D) experimental embryology.

27. After each transfer of a culture of bacteria, the wire loop should be
    (A) dipped into alcohol.
    (B) held in a flame.
    (C) dipped into liquid soap.
    (D) washed repeatedly in water.

28. Identify the statement that is NOT true of cellular respiration.
    (A) It is a downhill process.
    (B) It occurs in both plant and animal cells.
    (C) It uses CO_2 and H_2O for reactants.
    (D) It is an exergonic process.

29. In which one of the following ways does combustion differ from cellular respiration?
    (A) More heat is produced.
    (B) More energy is wasted.
    (C) It is less rapid.
    (D) It occurs at a higher temperature.

30. Of the following, an enzyme responsible for the digestion of proteins is
    (A) maltase.
    (B) trypsin.
    (C) ptyalin.
    (D) steapsin.

31. Failure of blood to clot readily when exposed to air may be due to a(n)
    (A) oversupply of erythrocytes.
    (B) deficiency of leucocytes.
    (C) overabundance of fibrin.
    (D) inadequacy of thrombokinase.

32. Cone cells are most closely associated with the function of
    (A) digestion.
    (B) absorption.
    (C) vision.
    (D) secretion.

33. The part of the vertebrate eye that controls the amount of light entering the eye is the
    (A) cornea.
    (B) ciliary body.
    (C) iris.
    (D) conjunctiva.

34. Most of the carbon dioxide in the blood is carried in the
    (A) liquid portion.
    (B) leucocytes.
    (C) erythrocytes.
    (D) platelets.

35. Increased blood pressure may be brought about by excess secretion of
    (A) thyroxin.
    (B) insulin.
    (C) ACTH.
    (D) adrenaline.

36. Of the following, the plant hormone concerned with growth is
    (A) auxin.
    (B) estrogen.
    (C) testosterone.
    (D) ATP.

37. Bread mold resembles ferns in that both develop
    (A) mycelia.
    (B) hyphae.
    (C) pinnules.
    (D) spores.

38. Sap rises in woody stems because of root pressure and
    (A) transpiration pull.
    (B) enzyme action.
    (C) molecular adhesion.
    (D) photosynthesis.

39. Vascular tissues present in the body of a flowering plant are xylem and
    (A) cambium.
    (B) phloem.
    (C) meristem.
    (D) lenticels.

40. Stored food for the embryo of a bean seed is found in the
    (A) plumule.
    (B) hypocotyl.
    (C) cotyledons.
    (D) testa.

41. Which of the following is NOT a characteristic of cancer cells?
    (A) High power for self-affinity
    (B) Altered genetic material
    (C) Uncontrolled division
    (D) Loss of normal functions

42. In the structure of a flower, the stigma is most closely positioned to the
    (A) style.
    (B) ovary.
    (C) sepal.
    (D) ovule.

43. The basic structure of cell membranes is a
    (A) protein bilayer.
    (B) protein-impregnated phospholipid bilayer.
    (C) carbohydrate bilayer.
    (D) phospholipid bilayer.

44. When catalyzed by sucrase, sucrose decomposes to yield glucose + fructose. The reaction is
    (A) fermentation.
    (B) hydrolysis.
    (C) denaturation.
    (D) condensation.

45. Continental drift is caused by
    (A) fluctuations in the Earth's magnetic field.
    (B) extrusion of molten rock through cracks in sea floors.
    (C) fragmentation of larger land masses into smaller ones.
    (D) Coriolis force generated by the rotation of the Earth.

46. Carbohydrates are a combination of carbon, hydrogen, and oxygen in an approximate ratio of
    (A) 2:1:2
    (B) 3:2:1
    (C) 1:2:1
    (D) 1:1:1

47. Rod-shaped bacteria are classified as
    (A) bacilli.
    (B) cocci.
    (C) vibrios.
    (D) spirilla.

48. A stain used in classifying bacteria is
    (A) Gram's.
    (B) Wright's.
    (C) Loeffler's.
    (D) Giemsa.

49. A bacteriophage is a kind of
    (A) enzyme.
    (B) toxin.
    (C) bacterium.
    (D) virus.

50. Of the following, the marsupial native to the United States is the
    (A) raccoon.
    (B) wombat.
    (C) opossum.
    (D) armadillo.

51. The first fully terrestrial vertebrates were the
    (A) amphibians.
    (B) reptiles.
    (C) birds.
    (D) mammals.

52. Enzyme molecules are all of the following EXCEPT
    (A) lipids.
    (B) proteins.
    (C) macromolecules.
    (D) biological catalysts.

53. The size of most eukaryotic cells is
    (A) 0.1–1.0 microns.
    (B) 10–100 microns.
    (C) 1.0–10 microns.
    (D) greater than 100 microns.

54. Sickle cell anemia is a genetic disorder that involves an inability of
    (A) erythrocytes to contain a sufficient amount of hemoglobin.
    (B) bone marrow to produce a sufficient number of erythrocytes.
    (C) bone marrow to produce erythrocytes of normal size.
    (D) erythrocytes to carry a sufficient load of oxygen.

55. Of the following, a crustacean that lives on land is the
    (A) centipede.
    (B) millipede.
    (C) sow bug.
    (D) tick.

56. Where would you find a leucoplast?

    (A) In a liver cell

    (B) In white blood cell

    (C) In a white potato

    (D) In a bacterium

57. Of the following, the hydra is most closely related to

    (A) coral.

    (B) flatworm.

    (C) sponge.

    (D) roundworm.

58. An unforeseen result of the widespread use of DDT is the

    (A) control of mosquitoes.

    (B) development of insects immune to DDT.

    (C) development of fishes immune to DDT.

    (D) destruction of harmful birds.

59. Cytoplasmic structures that contain powerful hydrolysis enzymes, which could lead to cell destruction in the absence of surrounding membranes, are

    (A) lysosomes.

    (B) golgi.

    (C) ribosomes.

    (D) None of the above

60. If the carrying capacity (k-value) represents the maximum number of individuals of a species that a habitat can support, it suggests that the population

    (A) is regulated by density-dependent factors.

    (B) will ultimately become extinct.

    (C) is regulated by density-independent factors.

    (D) can increase at an exponential rate, indefinitely.

STOP

IF YOU FINISH BEFORE TIME IS CALLED, YOU MAY CHECK YOUR WORK ON THIS SECTION ONLY. DO NOT TURN TO ANY OTHER SECTION IN THE TEST.

GENERAL SCIENCE TEST 6

68 Questions • 68 Minutes

Directions: For each of the following items, select the choice that best answers the question or completes the statement. Fill in the corresponding space on your answer sheet.

1. A tree native to China and NOT to the United States is the
   - (A) silvery maple.
   - (B) chestnut.
   - (C) gingko.
   - (D) tulip tree.

2. Mammals are believed to have evolved directly from
   - (A) fish.
   - (B) amphibians.
   - (C) reptiles.
   - (D) birds.

3. The biochemical technique that would be used to separate differently-sized pieces of DNA created by digesting a sample of DNA with a restriction enzyme is
   - (A) diapedesis.
   - (B) liquid scintillation.
   - (C) electrophoresis.
   - (D) kinesthesia.

4. Which of the following groups, in primate phylogeny, includes the primate most closely related to humans?
   - (A) Old World monkeys
   - (B) Great apes
   - (C) New World monkeys
   - (D) Lemurs

5. Stanley Miller obtained evidence supporting the possibility of spontaneous generation by achieving laboratory synthesis of
   - (A) amino acids.
   - (B) DNA.
   - (C) RNA.
   - (D) glucose.

6. The part of a compound light microscope that focuses light before it passes through the specimen is the
   - (A) objective.
   - (B) micrometer.
   - (C) ocular.
   - (D) condenser.

7. Choose the correct structural formula for acetylene, C_2H_2.
   - (A) $HC = CH$
   - (B) $HC - CH$
   - (C) $HC \equiv CH$
   - (D) $HC \equiv CH$

8. We can see only one side of the moon because the
   - (A) Earth rotates on its own axis.
   - (B) moon makes one rotation as it makes one revolution around the Earth.
   - (C) moon has no refractive atmosphere.
   - (D) sun does not shine on the moon's unseen side.

9. Which of the following is NOT an essential biotic element of all ecosystems?
   - (A) Producers
   - (B) Water
   - (C) Consumers
   - (D) Decomposers

10. The deadly property of carbon monoxide, if inhaled, is due to its
    - (A) high affinity for O_2.
    - (B) low affinity for hemoglobin.
    - (C) high affinity for hemoglobin.
    - (D) conversion to cyanide gas.

11. Of the following, vitamin B_{12} is most useful in combating
    (A) pernicious anemia.
    (B) night blindness.
    (C) rickets.
    (D) goiter.

12. Choose the correct description, relative to scolar and vector quantities.
    (A) Vectors = magnitude and direction
    (B) Scolar = direction
    (C) Vector = magnitude
    (D) Scolar = magnitude and direction

13. An emission device in modern cars that uses platinum beads to oxidize carbon monoxide and hydrocarbons to carbon dioxide and water is the
    (A) carburetor.
    (B) catalytic converter.
    (C) PCV valve.
    (D) air filter.

14. Of the following electrical devices, the one that develops the highest voltage is the
    (A) electric broiler.
    (B) radio tube.
    (C) television picture tube.
    (D) electric steam-iron.

15. Most soluble food substances enter the bloodstream through the
    (A) small intestine.
    (B) duodenum.
    (C) capillaries in the stomach.
    (D) hepatic vein.

16. Air-polluting sulfa dioxide (SO_2) results primarily from
    (A) natural gas furnaces.
    (B) leaded gasoline.
    (C) paper waste.
    (D) coal-burning power plants.

17. The "dark" side of the moon refers to the
    (A) craters, into which no sunlight has ever reached.
    (B) south pole of the moon's axis.
    (C) hemisphere that has never reflected the sun's rays on the Earth.
    (D) moon itself in the early phases of the month.

18. Of the following, the one NOT characteristic of poison ivy is
    (A) milky juice.
    (B) shiny leaves.
    (C) three-leaflet clusters.
    (D) white berries.

19. Glucose is a reducing sugar, which if boiled in Benedict's reagent, produces an orange to brick-red color. Choose the chemical species it reduces.
    (A) OH^-
    (B) $C\Phi^{++}$
    (C) $C\Phi$
    (D) $C\Phi^{--}$

20. A patient whose total body complement of physiological reactions has reached equilibrium is best described as
    (A) dead.
    (B) stable.
    (C) moribund.
    (D) healthy.

21. Of the following, the one present in greatest amounts in dry air is
    (A) carbon dioxide.
    (B) oxygen.
    (C) water vapor.
    (D) nitrogen.

22. Which is NOT a characteristic of enzymes?
    (A) They are proteins.
    (B) They catalize metabolics reactions.
    (C) They act on substances.
    (D) They are phospholipids.

23. Nerve cells transmit impulses by varying the permeability of their membranes primarily to
    (A) Na^+ and K^+
    (B) Cl^- and K^+
    (C) Na^+ and Cl^-
    (D) K^+ and Mg^{++}

24. Identify the statement which is NOT characteristic of exergonic reactions.
    (A) They are downhill reactions.
    (B) They have a negative energy change (–H).
    (C) They are uphill reactions.
    (D) The products have less energy than the reactants.

25. As electrons from aerobic respiration are moved through the electron transport system (ETS), the final electron acceptor is
    (A) hydrogen.
    (B) carbon dioxide.
    (C) oxygen.
    (D) water.

26. The normal height of a mercury barometer at sea level is
    (A) 15 inches.
    (B) 30 inches.
    (C) 32 feet.
    (D) 34 feet.

27. One of the necessary parameters for supporting the theory of evolution by natural selection is the age of the Earth, which is, by geographical indices, approximately (in years)
    (A) 1 billion.
    (B) 400 million.
    (C) 4 billion.
    (D) 100 million.

28. Of the following, the statement that best describes a "high" on a weather map is that the air
    (A) extends farther up than normal.
    (B) pressure is greater than normal.
    (C) temperature is higher than normal.
    (D) moves faster than normal.

29. The nerve endings for the sense of sight are located in the part of the eye called the
    (A) cornea.
    (B) sclera.
    (C) iris.
    (D) retina.

30. Malaria is caused by
    (A) bacteria.
    (B) mosquitoes.
    (C) protistans.
    (D) bad air.

31. A 1,000-ton ship must displace a weight of water equal to
    (A) 500 tons.
    (B) 1,000 tons.
    (C) 1,500 tons.
    (D) 2,000 tons.

32. Of the following instruments, the one that can convert light into an electric current is the
    (A) radiometer.
    (B) dry cell.
    (C) electrolysis apparatus.
    (D) photoelectric cell.

33. On the film in a camera, the lens forms an image that by comparison with the original subject, is
    (A) right side up and reversed from left to right.
    (B) upside down and reversed from left to right.
    (C) right side up and not reversed from left to right.
    (D) upside down and not reversed from left to right.

34. The development of insecticide resistant insects is based on

(A) inheritance of acquired characteristics.

(B) gradualism.

(C) natural selection.

(D) sexual selection.

35. Which of the following insects belongs to the order of insects containing the largest number of species?

(A) Housefly

(B) Flour beetle

(C) Grasshopper

(D) Cockroach

36. Which of the following could react chemically with ammonia?

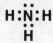

(A) H

(B) Cl⁻

(C) Na

(D) H⁺

37. Photosynthesis is a cellular process that

(A) is an exergonic reaction.

(B) produces simple sugar and O_2.

(C) is initiated by chemical energy.

(D) produces CO_2 and H_2O.

38. One-celled eukaryotes belong to the group of living things known as

(A) protistans.

(B) poriferans.

(C) annelids.

(D) arthropods.

39. Spiders can be distinguished from insects because spiders have

(A) hard outer coverings.

(B) large abdomens.

(C) four pairs of legs.

(D) biting mouth parts.

40. The greenhouse effect is believed to be primarily due to

(A) pesticide accumulation in soil.

(B) carbon dioxide increase in the atmosphere.

(C) oxygen increase in the atmosphere.

(D) pesticide increase in the water.

41. The lightest element known on Earth is

(A) hydrogen.

(B) helium.

(C) oxygen.

(D) air.

42. Of the following gases in the air, the most plentiful is

(A) argon.

(B) nitrogen.

(C) oxygen.

(D) carbon dioxide.

43. The time it takes for light from the sun to reach the Earth is approximately

(A) four years.

(B) four months.

(C) eight minutes.

(D) sixteen years.

44. The composition of edible sodium chloride (NaCl) from an explosive metal (Na) and a poisonous gas (Cl) illustrates which characteristic of matter?

(A) Impenetrability

(B) Malleability

(C) Density

(D) Emergent properties

45. The time it takes for the Earth to rotate 45 degrees is

(A) one hour.

(B) three hours.

(C) four hours.

(D) ten hours.

46. Of the following glands, the one that regulates the metabolic rate is the
    (A) adrenal.
    (B) salivary.
    (C) thyroid.
    (D) thymus.

47. In the small intestine, a digestive enzyme can break the peptide bond between 2 amino acids in a protein molecule by
    (A) removing a water molecule from them.
    (B) inserting a water molecule between them.
    (C) removing a carbon atom from one of them.
    (D) inserting a carbon atom between them.

48. The major cause for seasonal changes in temperature and light on Earth is
    (A) distance of the Earth from the sun.
    (B) a 23.5 inclination of the Earth on its axis.
    (C) alignment between the Earth, sun, and moon.
    (D) rotation of the Earth on its axis.

49. Passive immunity to diphtheria may be achieved by taking an injection of a(n)
    (A) vaccine.
    (B) toxin.
    (C) toxoid.
    (D) antitoxin.

50. Of the following, the only safe blood transfusion would be
    (A) group A blood into a group O person.
    (B) group B blood into a group A person.
    (C) group O blood into a group AB person.
    (D) group AB blood into a group B person.

51. If the effect of two or more factors is greater than the sum of the individual effects (e.g., $2 + 2 > 4$), the phenomenon is called
    (A) synergism.
    (B) coopeativity.
    (C) antagonism.
    (D) None of the above

52. The water-conducting tissue in an angiosperm is
    (A) phloem.
    (B) xylem.
    (C) pith.
    (D) cambium.

QUESTIONS 53 AND 54 REFER TO THE DIAGRAM BELOW.

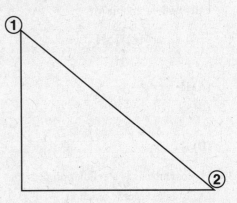

The boulder at the top of an inclined plane has potential energy, $E_p = mgh$, and if it rolls down the plane the energy becomes kinetic, $E_k = \frac{1}{2}mV^2$. Therefore, $mgh = \frac{1}{2}mV^2$.

53. Choose the correct formula for calculating the boulder's velocity when it reaches position 2.
    (A) $V = \sqrt{2gh}$
    (B) $V = 2gh$
    (C) $V = mgh^2$
    (D) $V = \sqrt{mg^2h}$

54. The expression $mgh = \frac{1}{2}mV^2$ on the previous page represents
   (A) conservation of momentum.
   (B) constancy of velocity.
   (C) variability of acceleration.
   (D) conservation of energy.

55. Completion of the human genome project gave further proof that genes are
   (A) nucleic acid.
   (B) phospholipids.
   (C) protein.
   (D) protein and nucleic acid.

56. Of the following, the process that will result in water most nearly chemically pure is
   (A) aeration.
   (B) chlorination.
   (C) distillation.
   (D) filtration.

57. The number of degrees on the Fahrenheit thermometer between the freezing point and the boiling point of water is
   (A) 100 degrees.
   (B) 180 degrees.
   (C) 212 degrees.
   (D) 273 degrees.

58. One is most likely to feel the effects of static electricity on a
   (A) cold, damp day.
   (B) cold, dry day.
   (C) warm, humid day.
   (D) warm, dry day.

59. Of the following planets, the one that has the largest number of satellites is
   (A) Jupiter.
   (B) Mercury.
   (C) Neptune.
   (D) Earth.

60. The deserts of the Earth generally occur on the _____ side of the continents.
   (A) west
   (B) north
   (C) east
   (D) south

61. Atmospheric moisture (H_2O) combines with oxides of carbon, nitrogen, and sulfur (CO_2, NO_3^-, and SO_2) to produce
   (A) alkaline precipitation.
   (B) acid rain.
   (C) alcohol.
   (D) None of the above

62. As water is warmed, its solubility of oxygen (O_2)
   (A) increases.
   (B) decreases.
   (C) remains constant.
   (D) fluctuates randomly.

63. The chlorinated hydrocarbon pesticide DDT was banned from use in the United States during the 1970s because it
   (A) has high affinity for milk and adipose tissues.
   (B) is deleterious to eggs of several species of birds.
   (C) is a biological concentration in ecosystem food chains.
   (D) All of the above

64. Of the 92 naturally occurring elements, the number found in the human body is closer to
   (A) 50
   (B) 10
   (C) 25
   (D) 75

65. Inasmuch as the molecular formula for glucose is $C_6H_{12}O_6$ and the molecular formula for fructose is $C_6H_{12}O_6$, the two substances are

   (A) hextomers.

   (B) isomers.

   (C) heteromers.

   (D) anomers.

66. Which of the following elements is the most abundant in the human body?

   (A) Carbon

   (B) Potassium

   (C) Nitrogen

   (D) Oxygen

67. The density of gold (Au) is 19.3g/cm^3 and that of iron (Fe) is 7.9g/com^3. A comparison of the volumes (V) of 50-gram samples of each metal would show that

   (A) $V_{Au} = V_{Fe}$

   (B) $V_{Au} < V_{Fe}$

   (C) $V_{Au} > V_{Fe}$

   (D) There is no predictable relationship between volumes.

68. The genomic diversity between *E. coli,* fruit flies, and humans results from

   (A) different types of chemical bases.

   (B) different types of amino acids.

   (C) same number of bases with different sequences.

   (D) different numbers and different sequences of bases.

STOP

IF YOU FINISH BEFORE TIME IS CALLED, YOU MAY CHECK YOUR WORK ON THIS SECTION ONLY. DO NOT TURN TO ANY OTHER SECTION IN THE TEST.

ANSWER KEY AND EXPLANATIONS

Chemistry and Physics Test 1

1. A	14. D	27. A	40. D	53. B
2. A	15. C	28. A	41. D	54. B
3. B	16. C	29. C	42. C	55. C
4. A	17. B	30. B	43. B	56. C
5. A	18. A	31. A	44. A	57. A
6. D	19. C	32. B	45. D	58. D
7. D	20. A	33. C	46. D	59. D
8. D	21. A	34. C	47. B	60. D
9. A	22. D	35. C	48. D	61. B
10. D	23. B	36. A	49. A	62. A
11. D	24. A	37. B	50. C	63. C
12. D	25. A	38. D	51. A	64. D
13. D	26. A	39. B	52. D	65. A

1. **The correct answer is (A).** Heating water to a very high temperature (about 2,000°C) will cause only about 2 percent of the water to dissociate into hydrogen and oxygen—not a very economical or efficient way of obtaining oxygen. Electrolysis will decompose water at a much lower temperature. Hydrogen peroxide and many oxides or metals can be decomposed more easily by heating alone.

2. **The correct answer is (A).** All acids contain hydrogen, which may be displaced by certain metals. However, copper ranks below hydrogen in the *electromotive* or *activity series*. *Activity* refers to the activity of a metal in displacing hydrogen in acids and in water. Metals ranked below hydrogen in the series do not displace hydrogen from acids.

3. **The correct answer is (B).** Hydrochloric acid can react with sodium hydrogen sulfite to produce sodium chloride, water, and sulfur dioxide. Sulfur dioxide can react with barium hydroxide to form barium sulfite and water.

4. **The correct answer is (A).** The problem can be solved by using the formula: $c = Q/M\Delta T$. Inasmuch as Q, M, D, and T are given, no algebraic rearrangement is necessary to solve for c (specific heat).

5. **The correct answer is (A).** Ozone is a molecule variety of oxygen in which 3 oxygen atoms bond to make 1 molecule of O_3. Ozone is easily formed by the action of electricity or ultraviolet radiation on the normal diatomic form (O_2) of oxygen.

6. **The correct answer is (D).** Since there is twice as much hydrogen as there is oxygen in a molecule of water (H_2O), the 26 milliliters of hydrogen could combine with only 13 milliliters of oxygen. This would leave 11 of the 24 milliliters of oxygen uncombined.

7. **The correct answer is (D).** Hydrochloric acid reacts with active metals, forming the chloride of that metal and releasing hydrogen.

8. **The correct answer is (D).** Inasmuch as 100 milligrams will decay to 50.0 milligrams, the formula: $K = \dfrac{0.693}{t_{\frac{1}{2}}}$ should be algebraically rearranged to solve for $t_{\frac{1}{2}}$ (half-life). To do this, multiply both sides by $t_{\frac{1}{2}}$ and divide both sides by K.

9. **The correct answer is (A).** The percentage composition of oxygen in 1 mole of glucose (180 grams) is calculated as follows

Atomic Mass				No. of Atoms
Carbon 12	×	6	=	72
Hydrogen 1	×	12	=	12
Oxygen 16	×	6	=	96
				180

$$\% \text{ Comp. } O_2 = \frac{96}{180} \times 100 \approx 53$$

10. **The correct answer is (D).** Sulfuric acid (H_2SO_4) contains 4 oxygens, each with a valence of -2; the total negative valence is 8. Each of the 2 hydrogens has a valence of $+1$; the total hydrogen valence equals $+2$. Therefore, sulfur would need a valence of $+6$ to equalize the positive and negative valences in the molecule.

11. **The correct answer is (D).** Fractional distillation can be used to separate the components of a mixture; the mixture is heated to boiling and the temperature is constantly raised. The component with the lowest boiling point vaporizes first; the component with the highest boiling point will vaporize last. Liquid oxygen has a boiling point of $-183°C$, which is higher than the boiling point of the other components; therefore, oxygen will boil off last.

12. **The correct answer is (D).** Only one substance (HCl) is dissociated; therefore, the reaction is a single displacement.

13. **The correct answer is (D).** Free carbon dioxide and water will combine to produce carbonic acid (H_2CO_3). Different reactants would be needed to produce ozone (O_3), methane (CH_4), or hydrogen peroxide (H_2O_2).

14. **The correct answer is (D).** Bronze is an alloy of copper and tin. An alloy is made by mixing two or more metals while in molten condition and then allowing the mixture to cool and solidify. The metals remain completely dissolved in one another after solidification, forming a homogenous substance with properties different from any of the constituent metals in their pure forms. For example, bronze is both harder and more resistant to corrosion than pure copper.

15. **The correct answer is (C).** $NaHCO_3$ will combine with HCl (hydrochloric acid) to form NaCl and H_2CO_3. H_2CO_3 is a weaker acid than HCl; therefore, the net effect of replacing HCl molecules with H_2CO_3 molecules is to raise the pH of the solution. In causing this reaction, $NaHCO_3$ is acting as a *buffer*. NaCl is a salt that will have no effect on the pH of an HCl solution. The other two compounds are acids that would lower the pH of the solution further if added.

16. **The correct answer is (C).** Litmus turns red in acid solution. When phosphorus trioxide dissolves in water, phosphorus acid is formed. The other compounds named form alkaline solutions.

17. **The correct answer is (B).** The 50 ml of a 1.0 M NaOH soulution required to neutralize an unknown amount of H_2SO_4 contains 0.05 Moles of NaOH. Since each mole of H_2SO_4 has 2 protons that are neutralized in the reaction, the number of Moles of H_2SO_4 in the 100 ml solution is 0.05 divided by 2 = 0.025 Moles of H_2SO_4. Since Molarity is the # Moles per 1000 ml and we have 0.025 moles H_2SO_4 per 100 ml, multiplying 0.025 moles × 10 = 0.25 Moles per liter or 0.25 M, which is the answer.

18. **The correct answer is (A).** Zinc is ranked above the others but below aluminum in the activity series of metals. The higher

the metal is ranked, the more energetic it is in its displacement ability. Therefore, aluminum could displace zinc in the zinc chloride solution, forming aluminum chloride. For this reason, zinc chloride should not be stored in a tank made of aluminum because aluminum will displace the zinc in the zinc chloride.

19. **The correct answer is (C).** The 4 oxygen ions would have a total *valence* of –8 (each oxygen, –2); if the valence of the SO_4 ion is –2, the remaining valence of 6 would be matched to a positive valence. Therefore, sulfur must have a valence of +6.

20. **The correct answer is (A).** Sulfuric acid is composed of 2 hydrogen ions and 1 sulfate ion. The chemical formula is H_2SO_4; thus, its chemical name is hydrogen sulfate.

21. **The correct answer is (A).** Magnesium has an atomic weight of 24; hydrogen's atomic weight is approximately 1. As is true with many metals, magnesium can react with an acid, such as hydrochloric acid, to produce hydrogen ($Mg + 2HCl \rightarrow MgCl_2 + H_2$). The amount of hydrogen produced can be calculated by using the following equation:

$$\frac{\text{amount Mg}}{\text{atomic weight}} = \frac{\text{amount } H_2}{\text{atomic weight}}$$

Substituting in the equation, we get the following:

$$\frac{6 \text{ grams}}{24} = \frac{x \text{ grams}}{2} = 0.5 \text{ grams}$$

In working out problems in which one must determine the amount of a substance derived from a given reaction, the chemical equation must be balanced and molecular weight must be used. Thus, for diatomic gases, use twice the atomic weight.

22. **The correct answer is (D).** Hydrogen in molecular form is composed of 2 atoms; the formula for 1 molecule of hydrogen is H_2. Therefore, 2 molecules of hydrogen is $2H_2$.

23. **The correct answer is (B).** Sodium bisulfate differs from sodium sulfate in having hydrogen as a part of the molecule. Since the sulfate ion has a valence of –2, and hydrogen and sodium each have a valence of +1, then one sodium and one hydrogen must be in combination with the sulfate ion ($NaHSO_4$).

24. **The correct answer is (A).** John Dalton discovered the facts concerning chemical combinations and suggested that materials are composed of atoms. He first proposed the law of multiple proportions in 1804. The law states that in a series of compounds formed by the same two or more elements, given a definite weight for one element, the different weights of the second element are in the ratio of small whole numbers to the weight of the first. For example, in sulfur dioxide (SO_2), the weight of oxygen is 32 (atomic weight = 16); in sulfur trioxide (SO_3), the weight of oxygen is 48. Therefore, the ratio is 2:3.

25. **The correct answer is (A).** One mole (*gram molecular weight*) of a gas occupies 22.4 liters under standard conditions. Since 1 liter of the gas in question is $\frac{1}{22.4}$ of 1 mole, it is $\frac{1}{22.4}$ of its gram molecular weight. Knowing this, the molecular weight of the gas can be determined. We can set up the equation as follows:

$$\frac{x \text{ unknown gram mol. wt.}}{22.4 \text{ liters}} = \frac{1.16 \text{ grams}}{1 \text{ liters}}$$

Solving the equation, we get 26 as 1 gram molecular weight. C_2H_2 (ethane) fits this weight ($C = 12 \times 2$, $H = 1 \times 2$).

26. **The correct answer is (A).** A salt is an ionic compound that yields ions other than hydrogen ions (H^+) or hydroxide ions ($OH–$) when it dissociates. Na_2CO_3 will yield neither when it dissociates into 2 $Na^+ + CO_3^{2-}$. $Ca(OH)_2$ will yield hydroxide ions when it dissociates, and H_2CO_3 will yield hydrogen ions. CH_3OH is a covalent compound and will not dissociate.

27. The correct answer is (A). *Aromatic* compounds are so named because of their odors; they occur in ring structure (molecular structure) and include such compounds as benzene, tolulene, and xylene.

28. The correct answer is (A). Dextrose is a *monosaccharide,* in that its molecule is composed of one "sugar unit" and cannot be hydrolyzed into simpler sugars. Lactose and sucrose are *disaccharides,* each yielding two monosaccharides by hydrolysis. Glycogen is a *polysaccharide* composed of a large number of monosaccharide units.

29. The correct answer is (C). Fats are glyceryl esters that, when hydrolized, yield glycerol and fatty acids. The cleavage of the ester linkage upon hydrolysis can be achieved by saponification, acids, superheated steam, or lipase, which is an enzyme that hydrolyzes fats. This may be represented as follows:

$$RCOOR' + H_2O \rightarrow RCOOH + R'OH$$

30. The correct answer is (B). As a rule, polar liquids dissolve in polar liquids and nonpolar liquids dissolve in nonpolar liquids. Water is polar and oil is nonpolar. Therefore, oil and water are immiscible.

31. The correct answer is (A). The bond formed between the carboxy (RCOOH) and the amino $(R - (NH_2))$ of two amino acids is a peptide bond, and the resulting compound is a depeptide.

32. The correct answer is (B). The *atomic number* represents the number of protons within the nucleus of an atom; since an atom is electrically neutral, the atomic number also equals the number of electrons of the atom. The atomic weight (*mass number*) represents the total number of nuclear particles (protons plus neutrons). All atoms of the same element have the same number of protons and, thus, the same atomic number. If the number of neutrons differ, the mass number is different; these atoms, then, are *isotopes.*

33. The correct answer is (C). Calcium hypochlorite $(Ca(OCl)_2)$ is effective as a bleach due to the oxidizing activity of hypochlorous acid (HClO), which is produced from calcium hypochloride, and from which chlorine gas can also be liberated.

34. The correct answer is (C). An ionic bond will form between 2 atoms if the loss of electrons from one to the other will result in both atoms having a completely filled outer electron orbit. A sodium atom has 11 electrons, 2 in its first electron orbit, 8 in its second electron orbit, and 1 in its outer electron orbit. The loss of 1 electron from the sodium atom will eliminate its outer electron orbit, making the next orbit in toward the nucleus the new outer orbit with a full complement of 8 electrons. A chlorine atom has 17 electrons, 2 in its first electron orbit, 8 in its second, and 7 in its outer electron orbit. The acceptance of 1 electron by the chlorine atom will fill its outer electron orbit with the full complement of 8 electrons.

35. The correct answer is (C). Transition elements are characterized by their 4s electron shell being completely filled, but the 3d shell is not completely filled.

36. The correct answer is (A). Air is a mixture of gases; the gases present in greatest quantity are nitrogen and oxygen. The quantity of nitrogen in the air is almost four times that of oxygen. Of the compounds listed, methane (CH_4), with a molecular weight of 16, is lighter than air.

37. The correct answer is (B). Carbon dioxide is an odorless gas in relatively low concentrations. High concentrations of carbon dioxide have an acidic odor.

38. The correct answer is (D). The pressure of a gas is measured by the distance in millimeters that it will lift a column of mercury in a barometer. The pressure of air is 760 mm of mercury at sea level. Air is a mixture of gases, and the pressure of each gas in such a mixture, referred to as its *partial pressure,* is equal to its concentration in the mixture. Oxygen constitutes 21% of air; therefore, its partial pressure at sea level would be 21% of 760 mm of mercury of pressure, or 160 mm of mercury.

39. **The correct answer is (B).** Carbon disulfide is highly flammable; its complete combustion yields carbon dioxide and sulfur dioxide.

$$CS_2 + 3O_2 \rightarrow CO_2 + 2SO_2$$

40. **The correct answer is (D).** The ethyl alcohol of alcoholic beverages is produced by fermentation of monosaccharides; usually yeast is used to supply the enzymes needed, and the fermentation process supplies the energy needed by the yeast.

$$C_6H_{12}O_6 \rightarrow 2C_2H_5OH + 2CO_2$$

41. **The correct answer is (D).** Because fluorine is extremely active, it does not occur freely in nature but combines naturally with all elements except the inert gases, forming very stable compounds. Because it is a vigorous oxidizing agent, it cannot be oxidized by other oxidizing agents. For these reasons, fluorides are more difficult to decompose than are compounds of the other halogens.

42. **The correct answer is (C).** A *ketone* is an organic molecule that contains a carbon atom double-bonded to an oxygen atom located between 2 other carbon atoms $-\overset{|}{\underset{\overset{\|}{O}}{C}}-C-C-$. The compound shown in choice

    (A) is an aldehyde because it contains a terminal CHO $\overset{H}{\underset{-C=O}{|}}$ group. The compound shown in choice **(B)** is an alcohol because it contains an OH group bonded to a carbon. The compound shown in choice **(D)** is both an alcohol and an aldehyde.

43. **The correct answer is (B).** The atomic number indicates the number of *protons* (positively charged particles) within the nucleus of an atom. Since an atom is electrically neutral, the number of protons is equal to the number of *electrons* (negatively charged particles) of the atom. Thus, the atomic number can indicate the number of electrons as well as the number of protons.

44. **The correct answer is (A).** Inert gases, such as neon, have a complete octet (8 electrons) in the outer shell of electrons.

45. **The correct answer is (D).** The resistance of a metal wire is directly proportional to its length and inversely proportional to its cross-sectional area. The longest wire with the smallest diameter will therefore have the greatest resistance.

46. **The correct answer is (D).** An *organic* acid is characterized by the presence of a carboxyl group (—COOH), or $-\overset{O}{\underset{OH}{C}}$. R represents a hydrocarbon group or a radical derived from a hydrocarbon.

47. **The correct answer is (B).** An *electrolyte* is a substance that forms an electrically conducting solution when dissolved in water. This is caused by the dissociation of the compound into ions, or *ionization*. The greater the ionization, the stronger the electrolyte. Calcium chloride ionizes to a much greater degree than the others and is a strong electrolyte.

48. **The correct answer is (D).** Force is a function of mass, distance, and acceleration. Since all of these factors are equal in this example, all of the balls strike the wall with the same force. The force is calculated as $1 \text{ kg} \times 16 \text{ m}/(2 \text{ sec})^2 = 4$ newtons.

49. **The correct answer is (A).** Sodium (Na) and potassium (K) are both in group IA, with 1 electron in the outer energy level. Sodium and potassium have three and four energy levels, respectively.

50. **The correct answer is (C).** Charcoal is an amorphous form of carbon, and carbon can react with oxides of many metals and other substances to form CO, CO_2, and the carbides of the metals. Thus, the oxides would be reduced by the removal of oxygen, and carbon would be oxidized to carbon monoxide or carbon dioxide; therefore, oxidation and reduction would occur.

51. **The correct answer is (A).** Nonmetal oxides, such as oxides of sulfur, carbon, and nitrogen, can react with water to form acids. The equations below are examples:

$$CO_2 + H_2O \rightarrow H_2CO_3$$

$$SO_2 + H_2O \rightarrow H_2SO_3$$

52. **The correct answer is (D).** Carbon dioxide (CO_2) comprises only approximately 0.04 percent of the earth's atmospheric gases. When this percentage increases, it prevents sun rays that strike the Earth from radiating back into space. This produces warming of the atmosphere and the Earth's surface, causing the greenhouse effect.

53. **The correct answer is (B).** Although hydrogen is relatively inert at ordinary temperatures, it can combine with free oxygen, with oxygen that is in chemical combination, with some metallic elements, and with many nonmetallic elements. The addition of hydrogen reduces a substance.

54. **The correct answer is (B).** A 1-molar solution of H_2SO_4 is prepared by dissolving 98g into water and adjusting the volume to 1-liter. However, H_2SO_4 has two (2) titratable or reactive protons per mole and the normality is equal to two (2).

55. **The correct answer is (C).** The nitrate test involves the use of a sulfate, such as iron sulfate, and sulfuric acid. The nitrate and sulfate ions react, forming nitric oxide. Nitric oxide then combines with the ferrous ion to form a ferrous-nitrogen-oxygen complex, which produces a brown color.

56. **The correct answer is (C).** A *saturated* solution is one that is in equilibrium; a condition of equilibrium exists between the solvent and the solute, and no more of the solute can dissolve.

57. **The correct answer is (A).** Oxides of barium and sulfur can combine to produce barium sulfate, a salt.

$$BaO + SO_3 \rightarrow BaSO_4$$

58. **The correct answer is (D).** The optical illusion described is the result of refraction, the abrupt bending of a ray of light when it passes at an angle from a medium of one density to a medium of a different density. Air and water have very different densities, resulting in the refraction of light. Diffraction is the separation of light into bands of different wavelengths, as in a rainbow. Diffusion is the scattering of light, such as the effect produced when light passes through frosted glass. Convection does not apply to light; it is the transfer of heat by circulation of air or water.

59. **The correct answer is (D).** Sulfuric acid has a high boiling point: 317°C. Because of this, it is not very volatile and can be used to prepare more volatile acids, such as hydrochloric and nitric acids.

$$NaCl + H_2SO_4 \rightarrow NaHSO_4 + HCl$$

60. **The correct answer is (D).** The pH of a solution is a measure of the negative logarithm of the hydrogen ion concentration (e.g., $pH = -\log[H^+]$). The H+ in question is 1×10^{-3}. Therefore, the pH = $^+3$.

61. **The correct answer is (B).** Reactivity of elements in group IA increases from top to bottom because valence electrons are progressively further from the positive charges in the nucleus of atoms. Reactivity of elements in group VIIA increases from bottom to top because valence electrons are progressively closer to the positive charges of the nucleus.

62. **The correct answer is (A).** Sodium (Na) is a metal in group IA, with 1.0 electron in its outermost shell. Its most stable configuration is achieved by donating 1.0 electron, resulting in a +1 valence.

63. **The correct answer is (C).** The electrons in the outer energy level comprise the portion of an atom directly involved in ionic bonding. The outer energy level will either gain or lose electrons in order to achieve a complete octet (8 electrons).

64. The correct answer is (D). The Federal Government requires that all pesticides have a label with a signal word. The pesticide will read DANGER (highly toxic) if only a few drops could be fatal.

65. The correct answer is (A). The circular winds that form a tornado create an area of extremely low pressure in the center. When rotating areas of low pressure move over most structures that have areas of higher air pressure, the structure explodes outward, as air is forced down a pressure gradient.

Chemistry and Physics Test 2

1. B	9. A	17. B	25. B	33. C
2. B	10. C	18. D	26. A	34. D
3. D	11. D	19. A	27. C	35. B
4. A	12. A	20. C	28. D	36. D
5. C	13. C	21. D	29. D	37. A
6. D	14. A	22. C	30. C	38. B
7. C	15. A	23. B	31. C	39. D
8. A	16. C	24. B	32. A	40. C

1. The correct answer is (B). Physical properties are those that do not involve any change in the nature or chemical composition of the substance. Heating a substance to the temperature at which it boils (its *boiling point*) will change its physical state but will not alter its chemical state.

2. The correct answer is (B). Water is a compound formed by oxygen and hydrogen in chemical combination. Blood and air are mixtures, and oxygen is an element.

3. The correct answer is (D). *Potential energy* is, in effect, energy in storage that can be released when conditions are conducive. *Kinetic energy* is energy of activity; it is released as the activity occurs.

4. The correct answer is (A). One calorie (kilocalorie) will raise 1 kilogram (1 grams) of water 1 degree Celsius. It would take 18 calories to raise 1,000 grams of water 18 degrees ($38° - 20°$), or 36 calories to raise 2 grams of water 18 degrees Celsius.

5. The correct answer is (C). If 1 gram of carbohydrate produces 4 calories, 9 grams are required to produce 36 calories. 36 calories $\div$ 4 calories/gram = 9 grams.

6. The correct answer is (D). The atomic weight (or mass number of an atom) equals the total of the number of protons and neutrons in the nucleus of the atom, or the total number of particles in the nucleus.

7. The correct answer is (C). Nearly every unstable nucleus of an atom gives off one or more of the three kinds of radiation: alpha, beta, and gamma. *Alpha* and *beta* radiation are particle emission; *gamma rays* are shortwave energy rays similar to X-rays, but stronger and more penetrating. Both gamma rays and X-rays are more penetrating than alpha and beta radiation.

8. The correct answer is (A). The *half-life period* can be defined as the time needed for half of a given amount of a substance to undergo spontaneous decomposition. This varies with different radioactive elements. There would be 50 milligrams left of a 100 milligram sample of material with a half-life of eight days after the eight days pass.

9. **The correct answer is (A).** Radiation can cause *mutations,* or genetic change. Any change in the genetic code would alter or destroy the trait associated with that particular gene. This could involve changes in enzymes produced and other factors associated with cellular metabolism.

10. **The correct answer is (C).** Gram molecular weight may be defined as the weight of the molecule expressed in grams. The molecular weight of glucose ($C_6H_{12}O_6$) is 180, as the following indicates: The weight of the six atoms of carbon equals 72 (6×12); twelve hydrogens weigh 12 (12×1); the weight of the six oxygens equals 96 (6×16). The total is 180; thus, the gram molecular weight of glucose is 180 grams.

11. **The correct answer is (D).** Equation (D) is balanced, because the amount of each substance is equal on both sides of the equation. There are two mercury atoms and two oxygen atoms on each side.

12. **The correct answer is (A).** A person with a fever has a higher temperature than normal. This reflects an increase in metabolic activities, since heat is given off as a waste product when energy in the form of ATP is used for metabolic purposes. Consequently, the pulse rate of a person with a fever is higher than normal because the heart is pumping blood at a greater rate so that the transport of materials like oxygen and glucose in the blood can accommodate this increased metabolic activity. Also, the circulatory system has to work harder to carry the greater amount of heat generated away from the tissues to be radiated from the surface of the body.

13. **The correct answer is (C).** Enzymes are called *organic catalysts,* in that they are produced by the organisms and catalyze reactions that occur within that organism. The other substances named do not function as catalysts.

14. **The correct answer is (A).** Gases are affected by temperature and pressure. If the gas is in a closed system, it cannot change its volume if temperature or pressure changes. Therefore, in a closed system, increasing the pressure would increase the temperature.

15. **The correct answer is (A).** For every oxidation, there must be a reduction. Oxidation can involve the removal of electrons, the removal of hydrogen, or the addition of oxygen; reduction, the opposite. In equation (A) metallic sodium loses an electron to become a positively charged ion; chlorine gains an electron to become a negatively charged chloride ion. Thus, sodium is oxidized and chlorine is reduced.

16. **The correct answer is (C).** Nitric acid reacts with the base potassium hydroxide to form potassium nitrate and water. For each hydrogen ion of the acid, there is a hydroxyl ion of the base to combine with it to form water. Therefore, neutralization occurs.

17. **The correct answer is (B).** Hard water contains calcium sulfate, calcium bicarbonate, or magnesium compounds. Soap is a mixture of sodium salts of organic acids that will react with these dissolved minerals. The insoluble calcium salt of the organic acid is precipitated out. This is the *scum,* or insoluble curdy material, that forms first. If enough soap is added, the soap acts as a cleansing agent after the first portion has precipitated the calcium ion.

18. **The correct answer is (D).** The concentration of a solution, on a percentage basis, contains a specific amount of solute in grams per 100 milliliters of solution. Thus, a 10-percent solution would have 10 grams of solute per 100 milliliters of solution.

19. **The correct answer is (A).** A 1-molar solution is the amount of (NaOH) per liter as defined by its gram molecular weight, which can be calculated by adding the weights of the individual chemical elements.

20. **The correct answer is (C).** A molar solution contains 1 gram *molecular weight* (the molecular weight of the molecule expressed in grams), or 1 mole per liter of solution. Therefore, each is a 1-molar solution.

21. **The correct answer is (D).** Potassium hydroxide (KOH) and hydrochloric acid (HCl) react to form potassium chloride (KCl) and water. This is a double displacement.

$$KOH + HCl \rightarrow K^+ Cl- + H_2O$$

22. **The correct answer is (C).** An *equivalent weight* of an element is that weight of the element that combines with or displaces 1 atomic weight of hydrogen. Since calcium has a valence of +2 while hydrogen has a valence of +1, one half of the atomic weight of calcium will displace 1 atomic weight of hydrogen. Calcium has an atomic weight of 40; therefore, its equivalent weight is 20, or, expressed as grams, 20 grams. The following equation can apply:

equivalent weight = [atomic weight/valence]

23. **The correct answer is (B).** Two amino acid molecules can be bonded together by removing a hydrogen atom from the amino group (NH$_2$) of 1 amino acid molecule and removing a hydroxyl ion (OH–) from the carboxyl group (COOH) of the other. The result is a molecule of water removed from the 2 amino acids and a covalent bond between the nitrogen atom in the amino group of one amino acid and the carbon atom in the carboxyl group of the other. This type of reaction is called *dehydration synthesis* and results in the production of water within cells that is called *metabolic water*. Creation of a bond between 2 amino acids can be illustrated as follows (R represents any of the 20 different side chains that can be included in amino acids):

Removing this water molecule will create a bond between the nitrogen and carbon.

24. **The correct answer is (B).** The periodic table places elements according to similarities in properties due to the number and arrangement of electrons in the atom. Group Zero is the inert gases. Metals and nonmetals are included in the remaining groups.

25. **The correct answer is (B).** Carbon dioxide and water, in the presence of light and the chlorophylls, yield glucose and oxygen. The water is absorbed by the root system of green plants and translocated through xylem to the leaves and other parts, which are the photosynthetic organs. Carbon dioxide enters the plants through epidermal stomates.

26. **The correct answer is (A).** Salk vaccine is prepared from inactivated polio virus. Viruses are obligate intracellular parasites; therefore, a method for growing viruses outside the human body had to be discovered and refined. Viruses typically are cultured in chick embryos.

27. **The correct answer is (C).** Ringworm is caused by fungi known as dermatophytes. These are sometimes known as the *Tineas*.

28. **The correct answer is (D).** *Photosynthesis* is the process characteristic of green plants by which carbon dioxide and water react to produce glucose and oxygen. The carbon dioxide used in the process enters the tissue from the air, passing in through stomata of the epidermis; oxygen produced by the reaction passes through the stomata into the air. This process occurs only in the presence of light, and therefore, continuous carbon dioxide removal occurs only in the presence of light.

29. **The correct answer is (D).** Mendel's Laws clearly stated the concepts of dominance and segregation (first law—Law of Segregation) and of independent assortment (second law—Law of Independent Assortment), but did not deal with the concept of hybrid vigor.

30. **The correct answer is (C).** Any relationship between two individual species is *symbiosis*. The word *symbiosis* means "life together." There are several kinds of symbiotic relationships, including commensalism, parasitism, and mutualism. A *mutualistic* relationship is one in which strong bonds exist between the two species, and each member benefits from the relationship. This kind of symbiotic relationship exists between termites and the protozoans (flagellates) of their intestinal tract. There is evidence that some bacteria in the termite's intestinal tract also play a role in the relationship. The flagellates and bacteria digest the cellulose that the termites consume.

31. **The correct answer is (C).** The Human Genome Project, which is funded by the National Institutes of Health and the Department of Energy, was initiated in 1990 and was completed in April 2003.

32. **The correct answer is (A).** The human genomic contains 22 pairs of autosomes and 1 pair of sex chromosomes in each somatic cell.

33. **The correct answer is (C).** Chorionic villus sampling (CVS) involves inserting a catheter into the uterus to take samples of the fetal chorion.

34. **The correct answer is (D).** DNA fingerprinting analyses produce identical band patterns from all tissues of an individual and can be done with less than 100 microliters of tissue. These techniques have been done on samples from Egyptian mummies more than 2,000 years old.

35. **The correct answer is (B).** All bands in the child's blood were inherited from either the father or the mother. Inasmuch as the father, in this case, produced half of the bands and contributed to an additional one quarter of them, paternity can be assigned with high statistical confidence.

36. **The correct answer is (D).** *Glycogenesis* is the formation of glycogen from glucose; glycogen is the form in which carbohydrates are stored in animals. Glycogen is stored in larger quantities and more permanently in the liver; some is produced and stored temporarily in muscle.

37. **The correct answer is (A).** Carbon dioxide and water are the end products of the Krebs cycle, which is the second phase of aerobic cellular oxidation of glucose for the release of energy.

38. **The correct answer is (B).** The kidney has the function of filtering wastes from the blood. Each nephron performs this function; thus, it is the functional unit. Wastes and water are filtered out from the blood in the glomerulus, a mass of capillaries lying in Bowman's capsule; the water and wastes pass through the capsule wall into the renal tubule. Much of the water is reabsorbed into the bloodstream through the walls of the capillaries surrounding the loop of Henle of the renal tubule. The remaining liquid, or urine, passes into the renal pelvis, to the ureter and bladder, and is eventually eliminated through the urethra.

39. **The correct answer is (D).** An endocrine (or ductless) gland secretes hormone(s) directly into the bloodstream. The hormone is transported by the blood and will affect only the target tissue. An exocrine gland passes its secretion through a duct to a specific site. The pancreatic islet cells secrete the hormone insulin; other cells of the pancreas secrete pancreatic juice, containing enzymes, through the pancreatic duct into the duodenum.

40. **The correct answer is (C).** In the first stage of aerobic oxidation, glucose is oxidized to pyruvic acid; this is known as *glycolysis*. The two pyruvates resulting from glycolysis of a molecule of glucose enter into the Krebs cycle (Citric Acid cycle) and are oxidized to carbon dioxide and water.

Human Anatomy and Physiology Test 3

1. B	12. D	23. D	34. A	45. B
2. C	13. A	24. D	35. B	46. C
3. C	14. B	25. B	36. D	47. B
4. A	15. C	26. D	37. B	48. D
5. B	16. A	27. B	38. C	49. A
6. D	17. D	28. B	39. B	50. D
7. A	18. B	29. C	40. C	51. D
8. C	19. B	30. D	41. B	52. A
9. A	20. C	31. C	42. D	53. B
10. D	21. C	32. D	43. A	54. D
11. B	22. B	33. D	44. C	55. C

1. **The correct answer is (B).** Cholesterol is an essential component of cell membranes. Microtubules are composed of proteins arranged in very small diameter tubes. Ribosomes contain proteins and RNA. Cytosol is the fluid component of cytoplasm.

2. **The correct answer is (C).** The function of smooth endoplasmic reticulum is lipid and carbohydrate synthesis. Rough endoplasmic reticulum is involved in the production of proteins. Mitochondria are devoted to energy (ATP) production and golgi apparatus function in the storage and packaging of cellular secretory products.

3. **The correct answer is (C).** Golgi apparatus function on the storage and packaging of secretory products and lysosomal enzymes. The function of smooth endoplasmic reticulum is lipid and carbohydrate synthesis. Control of the entry and exit of materials is the primary function of the cell's membrane and lysosomes are responsible for the removal of unwanted intracellular items.

4. **The correct answer is (A).** Cell membranes are selective permeable, which determines which substances may cross and which may not. Freely permeable

and totally permeable membranes would allow any substances to pass through, and an impermeable membrane is one through which nothing can pass.

5. **The correct answer is (B).** The cell will lose water by osmosis down water's concentration gradient, which is lower in a hypertonic solution. Cells will swell when placed in a hypotonic solution. Osmosis cannot move water from an area of low concentration (the hypertonic solution) into the cell interior with its higher water concentration. Intracellular fluid is not hypertonic.

6. **The correct answer is (D).** Glucose enters skeletal muscle cells by facilitated diffusion via a carrier protein, which must be activated by insulin. Active transport is not involved in glucose movement into muscle cells. Exocytosis is a process of removing substances from the cell's interior. Glucose cannot enter these cells by simple diffusion because of its lipophobic properties and its size.

7. **The correct answer is (A).** The nucleus stores information to control protein synthesis and determines the structure and function of the cell. Mitochondria are

sites of energy production. Ribosomes manufacture proteins intracellularly and lysosomes are intracellular vesicles containing enzymes.

8. **The correct answer is (C).** Epithelia line all body surfaces and provide a multiplicity of functions, including protection and control of permeability. Muscle is primarily characterized by the ability to contract, and neural tissue provides for the rapid conduction of action potentials. Connective tissues are found throughout the body, but they are never exposed to the external environment.

9. **The correct answer is (A).** Tendons consist primarily of collagen fibers, which are characterized by extreme flexibility and strength. Elastic fibers return to their original length after stretching. Reticular fibers provide the structural framework of organs, such as the spleen and liver. Nerve tissue is not connective in function.

10. **The correct answer is (D).** Synovial membranes surround the joint cavities, which are filled with synovial fluid. Mucous membranes line cavities that communicate with the external environment, while serous membranes line the components of the ventral body cavity and do not communicate with the external environment. The cutaneous membrane is skin.

11. **The correct answer is (B).** Melanin is the brown/black protective pigment produced by melanocytes within the deepest layer of the epidermis. Carotene is an orange-yellow pigment most commonly found in the stratum corneum of light-skinned individuals. Keratin is a protective protein that begins to appear in the middle layers of the epidermis. Hemoglobin is the oxygen-carrying substance found within red blood cells.

12. **The correct answer is (D).** Collagen and elastic fibers in the skin are arranged in parallel bundles orientated to resist applied forces. Smooth muscle within the skin does not have a directional orientation.

Sebaceous glands, or oil glands, produce sebum. Blood vessels within the skin do not alter the opening properties of an incision and do not have a parallel pattern of organization.

13. **The correct answer is (A).** Ceruminous glands produce cerumen (ear wax). Sebaceous glands produce sebum, which protects and conditions hair shafts and skin. Apocrine and merocrine glands are forms of sweat glands.

14. **The correct answer is (B).** Apocrine glands do not become functional until puberty when sex hormone levels rise; merocrine gland activity is lifelong. Sebaceous glands produce sebum, and ceruminous glands produce cerumen (ear wax).

15. **The correct answer is (C).** Merkel discs and Meisnner corpuscles are sensory receptors found within cutaneous tissue. Sweat production is provided by sudoriferous glands and oil production is provided by sebaceous glands. Blood transport is provided by components of the vascular system.

16. **The correct answer is (A).** Osteoblasts produce and release the components of bone matrix, leading to increased bone mass and strength. Osteoclasts remove bone matrix, causing bone to weaken. Osteocytes are mature bone cells, which maintain and monitor protein and mineral content of bone. Lacunae are fluid-filled pockets within which osteocytes are found.

17. **The correct answer is (D).** Red bone marrow, found within the trabecular network of spongy bone, is a major site of blood cell formation in adults. Periosteum is the membrane covering the outer surface of bone and endosteum is the membranous lining of the medullary cavity. Compact bone comprises the shafts of long bones and does not contain blood-forming functions.

18. **The correct answer is (B).** Parathyroid hormone levels increase in response to hypocalcemia to promote bone resorption and reduce renal elimination of calcium.

Calcitonin lowers blood calcium by inhibiting osteoclast activity. Calcitriol acts within the digestive tract to promote calcium absorption. Thyroxine stimulates osteoblast activity and lowers blood calcium levels.

19. **The correct answer is (B).** Endochondral ossification is the process of replacing hyaline cartilage with bone. Intramembranous ossification is the formation of bone on or within loose fibrous connective tissue. Osteoclast activation and osteoblast inhibition would both slow the rate of bone formation.

20. **The correct answer is (C).** Diarthrosis refers to freely movable (synovial) joints. Synarthroses refers to immovable joints such as the sutures of the skull. Amphiarthroses are slightly movable joints exemplified by the symphysis at the junction of the left and right pubic bones of the pelvis. Arthritis refers to a group of pathologies of the joints.

21. **The correct answer is (C).** Abduction is movement away from the axis and away from the anatomical position. Flexion is movement of the anterior-posterior plane resulting in a decreased angle of the joint. Extension increases the angle at a joint and returns the body to the anatomical position. Adduction is movement toward the longitudinal axis and restoration of the anatomical position.

22. **The correct answer is (B).** Acetylcholinesterase breaks down the transmitter substance, acetylcholine, into acetate and choline, which are inactive at the neuromuscular junction. Epinephrine is not involved with the neuromuscular junction, and monoamine oxidase is an enzyme that regulates levels of available catechol amines.

23. **The correct answer is (D).** Electrical activity initiated on the muscle surface sweeps across the membrane and descends each transverse tubule into the muscle interior. Motor neurons deliver action potential activity to the neuromuscular junction.

Blood vessels are not involved in electrical activity propagation. Epimysium is the connective tissue covering of an entire muscle.

24. **The correct answer is (D).** Sarcoplasmic reticulum stores calcium ions released upon the arrival of action potential activity via the transverse tubules. The motor neuron delivers action potentials to the end plate on the surface of the muscle. Mitochondria are involved in energy production and are not calcium storage sites.

25. **The correct answer is (B).** Isotonic contractions are characterized by muscle shortening accompanied by constant muscle tone throughout the contraction. During isometric contractions, muscle tone increases but muscle length remains unchanged and no movement results. Paralytic implies the absence of voluntary motor activity, and flaccid refers to a loss of muscle tone.

26. **The correct answer is (D).** Muscles at rest transfer high-energy phosphate groups from ATP to creatine, forming creatine phosphate and ADP. When needed, that energy is transferred back to ADP, resulting in production of ATP.

27. **The correct answer is (B).** Recruitment is the process of activating additional motor units to meet the demand for increased contraction force. Complete tetanus refers to muscle contraction in which there is no relaxation phase. Muscle tone is the partial contracture of resting muscle. A twitch is a single stimulus-contraction-relaxation sequence.

28. **The correct answer is (B).** Myoglobin is a red pigment that reversibly binds oxygen in muscle. It is structurally related to hemoglobin, the oxygen-carrying pigment found in blood. ATP and ADP are involved in phosphate energy group utilization.

29. **The correct answer is (C).** Cardiac muscle cells influence the electrical activity of adjacent cells through intercalated discs. "Striated" and "voluntary" are synony-

mous with skeletal muscle, which does not have intercalated discs. Smooth muscle cells communicate through dense bodies.

30. **The correct answer is (D).** The all-or-none principle states that a muscle fiber (or motor unit) is either maximally contracted or not contracted at all. Muscle tone is the partial contracture present in a resting muscle. Tetanus occurs when stimuli are produced so rapidly that there is no muscle relaxation. A twitch is a single stimulus-contraction-relaxation sequence.

31. **The correct answer is (C).** Astrocytes interface with neurons and blood vessels, regulating movement of substances between those compartments. Ependymal cells are involved in the production and circulation of cerebrospinal fluid. Microglia function to remove unwanted materials from the brain and oligodendrocytes myelinate CNS axons.

32. **The correct answer is (D).** Following action potential activity, sodium and potassium are returned to their respective starting compartments by the active transport of the sodium-potassium pump. Since these movements are against concentration gradients, diffusion would be ineffective. Filtration is a process of capillaries, and osmosis refers to the movement of water.

33. **The correct answer is (D).** Increasing postsynaptic permeability to potassium will permit potassium to exit the cell, resulting in a more negative intracellular space. Depolarization, action potentials, and excitatory postsynaptic potentials require an increase in sodium permeability; all would be opposed by increased potassium permeability.

34. **The correct answer is (A).** The phrenic nerve, which supplies the diaphragm, exits the spinal cord at upper cervical levels. While the outflow of lower spinal levels may influence respiration, they are unable to sustain adequate ventilation.

35. **The correct answer is (B).** Gamma motor neurons (efferents), when activated, render the muscle spindles more sensitive to stretch. Alpha motor neurons and large diameter afferents are axons going away from muscle to the CNS. The neuromuscular junction does not normally influence reflex activity.

36. **The correct answer is (D).** The temporal lobe functions in the conscious perception of auditory and olfactory stimuli. The frontal lobe contains centers for voluntary control of skeletal muscle and plays a role in emotion. Parietal lobe function includes conscious perception of skin sensations such as touch, pain, and temperature. The occipital lobe is involved in the conscious perception of visual stimuli.

37. **The correct answer is (B).** The trigeminal nerve is the major component of sensory and motor innervation to the face. Trochlear function involves control of eye movements. The facial nerve subserves taste receptors from the anterior $\frac{2}{3}$ of the tongue, and the vestibulocochlear nerve functions in auditory and vestibular activities.

38. **The correct answer is (C).** The posterior columns contain the ascending pathways for fine touch and pressure to the body surface. Spinothalamic tract axons carry information about pain, temperature, and crude touch. The lateral corticospinal tract is part of the motor system (descending), and the spinocerebellar tracts subserve proprioception.

39. **The correct answer is (B).** REM sleep is characterized by active, often visual dreaming, accompanied by changes in autonomic activity; the EEG shows a high frequency and resembles the awake EEG. The EEG in slow wave (non-REM) sleep shows a characteristic low-frequency wave. Arousal is the awakening from sleep, and dreaming is not a component of coma.

40. **The correct answer is (C).** The tenth (vagus) nerve contains the primary autonomic outflow to the organs of the thoracic and abdominopelvic cavities. The first (olfac-

tory) cranial nerve functions in the sense of smell (olfaction). The second (optic) cranial nerve subserves the sense of vision, while the twelfth (hypoglossal) nerve controls the musculature of the tongue.

41. **The correct answer is (B).** Thyrotropin from the anterior pituitary regulates the growth and development of the thyroid gland and controls its release of thyroid hormones. Thyrotropin releasing hormone, from the hypothalamus, promotes the release of thyrotropin. Thyroxine is one of the hormones released by the thyroid gland. Iodide is a constituent of thyroid hormones.

42. **The correct answer is (D).** Adrenocorticotropic hormone (ACTH) from the adenohypophysis (anterior pituitary) stimulates the release of glucocorticoids, including cortisol, from the adrenal cortex. Corticotropin releasing hormone (CRH) is produced by the hypothalamus and promotes the release of ACTH. Aldosterone is a mineralocorticoid produced by the adrenal cortex.

43. **The correct answer is (A).** Oxytocin promotes labor and delivery by inducing uterine smooth muscle contraction. Vasopressin (antidiuretic hormone—ADH) promotes water reabsorption by the kidneys. Somatotropin (growth hormone) stimulates cell growth by accelerating protein synthesis. Prolactin participates in the stimulation of mammary gland development and promotes milk production.

44. **The correct answer is (C).** Follicle stimulating hormone (FSH), a gonadotropin from the anterior pituitary, promotes follicle development and estrogen secretion in females, whereas in males it promotes sperm cell production. Testosterone is an androgen with most of its effects seen in males. Melanotropin activates melanocytes within the skin. Luteinizing hormone is responsible for initiating ovulation.

45. **The correct answer is (B).** Insulin is the hormone that lowers blood glucose levels through a number of mechanisms including activating receptors involved in the facilitated diffusion of glucose into muscle. Glucagon is the pancreatic hormone responsible for elevating blood glucose levels; epinephrine also elevates blood glucose. Renin, a hormone from the kidneys, initiates the renin-angiotensin system, which is involved in blood pressure control.

46. **The correct answer is (C).** These symptoms suggest high levels of thyroid hormones (hyperthyroidism); opposite symptoms (i.e., low basal metabolic rate, weight gain, and sensitivity to cold) would be symptomatic of hypothyroidism. Neither high nor low levels of growth hormone would produce these symptoms.

47. **The correct answer is (B).** Insulin is released by beta cells when blood glucose exceeds normal levels (70–110 mg/dL). Low blood glucose triggers the release of glucagon from the pancreas. Prolactin is not involved in the control of blood glucose. Elevated growth hormone levels cause elevations of blood glucose.

48. **The correct answer is (D).** Aldosterone is the hormone from the adrenal cortex that participates in the regulation of sodium and potassium levels. Epinephrine and norepinephrine are products of the adrenal medulla. ACTH is produced by the anterior pituitary.

49. **The correct answer is (A).** Low parathyroid hormone levels would lead to hypocalcemia, which in turn could cause convulsions. Parathyroid hormone is not involved in the regulation of blood glucose levels, nor does it influence water retention/loss mechanisms in the kidneys.

50. **The correct answer is (D).** Type I diabetes mellitus results from inadequate insulin production by the beta cells of the pancreas; high insulin levels would reflect just the opposite. Ineffective insulin receptors are associated with Type II diabetes. Both Type I and Type II diabetic patients display high blood glucose levels.

51. **The correct answer is (D).** *Glycogenesis* is the formation of glycogen from glucose; glycogen is the form in which carbohydrates are stored in animals. Glycogen is stored in larger quantities and more permanently in the liver; some is produced and stored temporarily in muscle.

52. **The correct answer is (A).** Carbon dioxide and water are the end products of the Krebs cycle, which is the second phase of aerobic cellular oxidation of glucose for the release of energy.

53. **The correct answer is (B).** The kidney has the function of filtering wastes from the blood. Each nephron performs this function; thus, it is the functional unit. Wastes and water are filtered out from the blood in the glomerulus, a mass of capillaries lying in Bowman's capsule; the water and wastes pass through the capsule wall into the renal tubule. Much of the water is reabsorbed into the bloodstream through the walls of the capillaries surrounding the loop of Henle of the renal tubule. The remaining liquid, or urine, passes into the renal pelvis, to the ureter and bladder, and is eventually eliminated through the urethra.

54. **The correct answer is (D).** An endocrine (or ductless) gland secretes hormone(s) directly into the bloodstream. The hormone is transported by the blood and will affect only the target tissue. An exocrine gland passes its secretion through a duct to a specific site. The pancreatic islet cells secrete the hormone insulin; other cells of the pancreas secrete pancreatic juice, containing enzymes, through the pancreatic duct into the duodenum.

55. **The correct answer is (C).** In the first stage of aerobic oxidation, glucose is oxidized to pyruvic acid; this is known as glycolysis. The two pyruvates resulting from glycolysis of a molecule of glucose enter into the Krebs cycle (Citric Acid cycle) and are oxidized to carbon dioxide and water.

Human Anatomy and Physiology Test 4

1. A	11. A	21. B	31. B	41. B
2. D	12. B	22. C	32. A	42. B
3. C	13. B	23. A	33. C	43. B
4. A	14. D	24. C	34. B	44. D
5. B	15. B	25. C	35. B	45. A
6. A	16. C	26. A	36. D	46. C
7. D	17. C	27. D	37. A	47. D
8. B	18. A	28. C	38. D	48. C
9. B	19. A	29. D	39. C	49. B
10. D	20. D	30. B	40. C	50. A

1. **The correct answer is (A).** Albumin is the major plasma protein and is responsible for maintaining osmotic pressure and plasma volume. Globulins function in the transport of materials and have immune functions. Fibrinogen is a clotting factor. Platelets do not significantly alter plasma osmotic pressure.

2. **The correct answer is (D).** Anemia, a decrease in oxygen delivery, results from deficiencies in erythrocytes or hemoglobin within erythrocytes. Platelets, plasma proteins, and leukocytes do not participate in oxygen transport.

3. **The correct answer is (C).** Erythropoietin is released by cells in the kidneys when they are faced with low oxygen levels; erythropoietin promotes erythropoiesis, red blood cell formation. Neither platelets nor leukocytes are involved in oxygen delivery. Erythrocytes are red blood cells.

4. **The correct answer is (A).** Blood typing is based on the identification of antigens (agglutinogens) located on the surfaces of erythrocytes. Antibodies relevant to blood typing (agglutinins) are found in plasma, but blood type is based on red blood cell surface antigens.

5. **The correct answer is (B).** Rh+ indicates the presence of the Rh (D) antigen on the surfaces of erythrocytes; Rh– indicates the absence of that antigen. Rh antigens are not found in plasma, nor are Rh antibodies. Rh antibodies are found in plasma.

6. **The correct answer is (A).** The anti-A antibodies from the plasma of the Type B blood will attack the A-antigens of the Type A blood, leading to agglutination, the clumping and breakdown of erythrocytes. Blood vessel spasm and platelet plug formation are processes involved in hemostasis. The onset of decreased oxygen delivery would be very rapid.

7. **The correct answer is (D).** Neutrophils are granulocytes and are usually the first white blood cells to arrive at an injury site or infection. Lymphocytes and monocytes are agranulocytes. Basophils, accounting for less than 1% of the circulating leukocyte population, produce histamine and heparin.

8. **The correct answer is (B).** T cells, B cells, and NK cells are classes of lymphocytes (indistinguishable under the light microscope), which are involved in immune processes. Neutrophils and eosinophils are granulocytes and are not involved in immunity.

9. **The correct answer is (B).** During the platelet phase of hemostasis, platelets stick to damaged endothelium and become activated, releasing ADP, thromboxane A_2, and serotonin, substances that participate in the hemostasis process. The vascular phase is characterized by contraction of the smooth muscle of the blood vessel wall. Coagulation refers to blood clotting. There is no inflammation phase of hemostasis.

10. **The correct answer is (D).** The last step in the final common pathway produces insoluble strands of fibrin that form the matrix of the blood clot. The conversion of prothrombin to thrombin is the initial step in the final common pathway. Fibrinogen, a plasma protein, is the precursor to fibrin.

11. **The correct answer is (A).** Calcium entry into cardiac cells results in a plateau of about 175 m/sec. Calcium exit from the cell would shorten the action potential. Sodium entry into the cell leads to the rapid initial depolarization, and sodium exit occurs after the action potential is completed.

12. **The correct answer is (B).** Spontaneous depolarizations occur most rapidly within the S-A node, and it is therefore the normal pacemaker of the heart. The A-V node, bundle branch fibers, and purkinje fibers also depolarize spontaneously but at a slower rate than the S-A cells.

13. **The correct answer is (B).** The QRS complex results from ventricular depolarization. The P wave reflects atrial depolarization and the T wave relates to ventricular repolarization. The P-R segment reflects the time between atrial and ventricular depolarization.

14. **The correct answer is (D).** End-diastolic volume is the quantity of blood in the ventricles just before the initiation of ventricular contraction (systole). Stroke volume is the quantity of blood ejected during ventricular contraction. Ejection fraction evaluates the efficiency of ventricular emptying during systole. End-diastolic volume is the quantity of blood remaining within the ventricles after ventricular contraction.

15. **The correct answer is (B).** Afterload reflects the forces that the ventricles must overcome in order to eject blood. Preload is the degree of stretching during ventricular diastole and is directly proportional to the end-diastolic volume. Cardiac output measures the volume of blood pumped by the ventricles in one minute. Stroke volume is the quantity of blood ejected during ventricular contraction.

16. **The correct answer is (C).** Beta 1 receptor activation by norepinephrine results in increased heart rate and increased force of contraction. Alpha 1 receptor activation leads to vasoconstriction. Alpha 2 receptors in the CNS cause vasodilation. Beta 2 receptors primarily influence bronchioles, producing bronchodilation.

17. **The correct answer is (C).** Capillaries are the only blood vessels involved in exchange of materials. Arteries carry blood from the heart under high pressure. Arterioles control the flow of blood into capillary beds. Veins return blood to the heart.

18. **The correct answer is (A).** Venous valves prohibit backflow of blood toward the capillaries. Smooth muscle in veins alters vessel diameter but does not impede backflow. Precapillary sphincters control blood flow into capillary beds. Semilunar valves are found within the heart.

19. **The correct answer is (A).** Pulse pressure is much greater in arteries. Arterioles have a small pulse pressure, while blood flow through capillaries and veins is not pulsatile.

20. **The correct answer is (D).** Baroreceptor reflexes are responsible for rapid adjustments of blood pressure. Chemoreceptors are primarily concerned with control of respiration. Angiotensin II and antidiuretic hormone are involved in long-term regulation of blood pressure.

21. **The correct answer is (B).** During swallowing, material is kept out of the respiratory tract by the folding of the epiglottis over the glottis. The pharynx is the chamber shared by the digestive and respiratory systems. The hard palate forms the anterior roof of the mouth.

22. **The correct answer is (C).** Surfactant reduces surface tension within alveoli and prevents alveolar collapse. Serous fluid is produced by serous membranes that line surfaces not accessing the external environment. Pleural fluid increases the surface tension within the pleural space (between the visceral and parietal pleura). Mucus increases surface tension.

23. **The correct answer is (A).** Tidal volume is the volume of a single breath. Minute volume is the volume of air moved within 1 minute. Residual volume is the amount of air remaining in the lungs after a maximal expiration. Inspiratory reserve volume is the amount of air that can be inhaled in excess of a tidal inspiration.

24. **The correct answer is (C).** Anatomical dead space never goes further than the conducting passages and is not involved in gas exchange. Vital capacity is the maximal amount of air that an individual can move into or out of the lungs in a single respiratory cycle. Total lung capacity is the total volume of the lungs.

25. **The correct answer is (C).** Gases diffuse down a partial pressure gradient, not a concentration gradient. Osmotic pressures and gradients refer to properties of fluids. Within normal limits, temperature plays a minimal role in gas movement.

26. **The correct answer is (A).** Increasing thoracic volume leads to decreased intra-

thoracic pressure and inspiration. Decreasing thoracic volume increases intrathoracic pressure, leading to expiration. Changes in abdominal volumes do not directly affect respiration except through their influences on thoracic volumes.

27. **The correct answer is (D).** Declining blood pH weakens the hemoglobin-oxygen bond (the Bohr Effect) and promotes oxygen release to tissues. Conversely, elevated pH will strengthen the bond. Changes in blood pressure do not appreciably affect oxygen unloading.

28. **The correct answer is (C).** A significant portion of carbon dioxide is transported within erythrocytes as carbaminohemoglobin. Blood gases are not transported by plasma proteins or leukocytes, nor are they transported on the surface of red blood cells.

29. **The correct answer is (D).** Carbonic anhydrase within erythrocytes reversibly catalyzes the reaction of carbon dioxide and water, a reaction that is very slow in the absence of the enzyme. Antigens, antibodies, and plasma enzymes do not influence the reaction.

30. **The correct answer is (B).** The pneumotaxic center of the pons sends inhibitory signals to the inspiratory center, resulting in shortened duration of inspiration.

31. **The correct answer is (B).** Angiotensin I is the result of the action of renin on angiotensinogen. Angiotensin II is subsequently formed from angiotensin I. Carbonic anhydrase is the enzyme that catalyzes the reaction of carbon dioxide and water.

32. **The correct answer is (A).** Angiotensin II is a potent vasoconstrictor and an important component in reversing a hypotensive condition; it is not a vasodilator. Angiotensin II promotes aldosterone release and acts to conserve water rather than eliminate water.

33. **The correct answer is (C).** Nitrogenous by-products of protein catabolism (including uric acid, creatinine, and urea) are not significantly reabsorbed and therefore appear in urine. Amino acids, vitamins, water, and electrolytes are all reabsorbed within the nephron.

34. **The correct answer is (B).** Nutrients are reabsorbed from the proximal convoluted tubule. The other segments of the nephron are primarily involved in the regulation of the blood levels of electrolytes and of water.

35. **The correct answer is (B).** Peristaltic waves of the smooth muscle of the ureters propel urine from the kidneys to the bladder; gravity does not play a significant role. Bladder pressure would not promote flow toward the bladder, and blood pressure is not a factor in ureters action.

36. **The correct answer is (D).** The somatic motor fibers of the pudendal nerve regulate the contracture of the external sphincter. As a skeletal muscle structure, the external sphincter is not innervated by the autonomic nervous system. The phrenic nerve innervates the diaphragm.

37. **The correct answer is (A).** Sodium is the major positive-charged ion within extracellular fluid and is a primary controller of water distribution. Potassium and magnesium are more concentrated within intracellular fluid. Calcium does not play a major role in water distribution.

38. **The correct answer is (D).** Aldosterone promotes the reabsorption of sodium within the kidneys. Thyroxine is a thyroid hormone and is not involved with sodium levels. Insulin and glucagon are involved in the control of blood glucose levels.

39. **The correct answer is (C).** Although generally slower, the kidneys are the most powerful and complete correctors of pH imbalance. Buffers are the most rapid but the weakest mechanisms. Although more powerful than buffers, respiratory mechanisms rarely complete a correction of pH imbalance. The bladder is not involved in acid-base balance.

40. **The correct answer is (C).** Lack of insulin leads to the utilization of fats for energy. Byproducts include ketone bodies, which

are acidic and responsible for the acidosis seen in these patients. Diabetic patients are not alkalotic, and diabetes does not result in acid production through actions on the respiratory system.

41. **The correct answer is (B).** Intrinsic factor is produced by cells of the stomach and promotes the absorption of vitamin B_{12}. The small intestine is the site of action of intrinsic factor but not the source. The pancreas and large intestine do not participate in vitamin B_{12} absorption.

42. **The correct answer is (B).** The gallbladder stores bile and concentrates it up to tenfold. Bile is manufactured in the liver but not stored there. Neither the pancreas nor the ileum are involved in bile storage.

43. **The correct answer is (B).** Cholecystokinin (CCK) is released from the intestine in response to the presence of proteins or fats. Secretin is released in response to the presence of acid from the stomach. Neither insulin nor aldosterone are released from intestinal tissues.

44. **The correct answer is (D).** Because of its role in water reabsorption, excess motility of the large intestine may lead to diarrhea, while decreased motility may lead to constipation. The stomach, liver, and small intestine are not controllers of water reabsorption.

45. **The correct answer is (A).** Carbohydrates must be reduced to monosaccharides in order for intestinal absorption to occur. Disaccharides are enzymatically broken down in the small intestine, as are polysaccharides (glycogen and starch), which are broken down into oligosaccharides.

46. **The correct answer is (C).** Pepsin results in the breakdown of proteins into polypeptides. Lipase participates in fat digestion. Sucrase breaks sucrose down into monosaccharides. Amylase initiates the digestion of starch.

47. **The correct answer is (D).** Vitamin C is a water-soluble vitamin. Vitamins A, D, E, and K are fat-soluble.

48. **The correct answer is (C).** Pain and bleeding associated with gastric ulcers result from erosion of the mucosal layer, which exposes the vascular and highly innervated submucosal layer. The muscular layer and the outer (serosal) layer generally are not involved in ulcer production.

49. **The correct answer is (B).** Amylase is an enzyme found in saliva, which begins the breakdown of starch. Lipase is involved in fat digestion; pepsin begins the digestion of proteins; and insulin is involved in glucose processes.

50. **The correct answer is (A).** Digestive smooth muscle is activated by the parasympathetic division of the autonomic nervous system. The sympathetic division inhibits digestive activity. Neither the thyroid gland nor aldosterone are involved in control of gastrointestinal smooth muscle.

Biology Test 5

1. B	13. A	25. D	37. D	49. D
2. D	14. B	26. A	38. A	50. C
3. B	15. A	27. B	39. B	51. B
4. D	16. D	28. C	40. C	52. A
5. C	17. C	29. D	41. A	53. B
6. D	18. D	30. B	42. A	54. D
7. A	19. B	31. D	43. B	55. C
8. C	20. B	32. C	44. B	56. C
9. C	21. A	33. C	45. B	57. A
10. A	22. C	34. A	46. C	58. B
11. B	23. D	35. D	47. A	59. A
12. C	24. B	36. A	48. A	60. A

1. **The correct answer is (B).** Although other mechanisms may be involved in passage of materials through a cell membrane, the passage of some materials, especially water, occurs by *diffusion*; diffusion occurs from regions of higher concentration of the substance to regions of lower concentration. Diffusion through a membrane, such as the cell membrane, is known as *osmosis*.

2. **The correct answer is (D).** Iron is a part of the hemoglobin molecule, and, as such, is essential for its formation. Hemoglobin is the oxygen-carrying pigment found in red corpuscles.

3. **The correct answer is (B).** *Phenylketonuria (PKU)* is a genetic disorder characterized by the inability of the affected person to convert excess molecules of the amino acid phenylalanine to molecules of the amino acid tyrosine. It is caused by inheriting a defect in the gene for the enzyme that catalyzes the conversion.

4. **The correct answer is (D).** A *control* is used with experiments for comparison. The control is treated in the same manner as is the experimental group except for one variable. In this case, the variable would be the administering of the drug or sugar pills. Thus, any differences between the groups in experimental results could be attributed to this one variable.

5. **The correct answer is (C).** *Transpiration* is the loss of water in a gaseous state, through epidermal stomata, from the aerial parts of a plant. Most transpiration occurs through the leaf epidermis. Stomata are not found in root epidermis.

6. **The correct answer is (D).** An organism is a living thing or individual. An organism consists of "systems," which are made up of organs. Organs consist of tissues, especially in the case of higher organisms. This statement would not apply to lower organisms that have not reached the system level of phylogenetic development.

7. **The correct answer is (A).** Milk is not sterile; it contains numerous bacteria. Pasteurization does not sterilize milk, but does destroy certain harmful bacteria that can be carried in milk.

8. **The correct answer is (C).** *Auxins* are growth hormones found in plants; in stems, auxins stimulate growth. If a plant is unevenly illuminated, auxins are more concentrated on the side of the stem that is more poorly illuminated, stimulating growth on that side. This will cause the stem to bend toward the light.

9. **The correct answer is (C).** In humans, carbohydrate digestion begins in the mouth with the enzyme ptyalin, produced by the salivary glands.

10. **The correct answer is (A).** Black is dominant over white in this case; therefore, the white guinea pig carries only white genes and is *homozygous,* or pure recessive. When such a test cross is made, the offspring will indicate the genotype of the black guinea pig. If the black guinea pig is hybrid, or *heterozygous* black (carrying one white gene), black and white offspring will result in a theoretical ratio of 1:1; if the black guinea pig is pure, or homozygous black, all offspring will be black because of dominance, although all of the offspring will be hybrid because they carry a white gene.

11. **The correct answer is (B).** Fossils found in the lowest rock layers are the oldest because these layers were deposited before the ones above. Fossils in upper layers are not always different from the lower layers. Some species have very long histories and leave fossils in more than one layer. Conversely, fossils in upper layers are never completely the same as fossils in lower layers. At least some species of organisms whose fossils lie in lower layers would have become extinct and been replaced by fossils of different organisms by the time upper layers were deposited. Older organisms were not always simpler than modern organisms and were certainly not more complex.

12. **The correct answer is (C).** The roots of plants help to hold the soil in place and prevent soil erosion; the ground can absorb water. Eroded lands do not absorb water readily. Water may run off, carrying with it some of the topsoil. This reduces the quality of the land. Where plants are present, the run-off is reduced or diminished, and the ground absorbs water.

13. **The correct answer is (A).** A *stimulus* is anything that can cause a *reaction* or response by the organism. The reaction may be involuntary, such as batting the eye when an object approaches, or voluntary, such as moving from an area of discomfort.

14. **The correct answer is (B).** Crossbreeding between strains with the desired traits, followed by selection of the offspring for future breeding and establishing the herd, is the best way to accomplish the breeder's goal. Inbreeding is just as likely to bring out undesirable hidden traits.

15. **The correct answer is (A).** The inhaling and exhaling of air by the human lungs demonstrates Boyle's Law. Inhaling results from the expansion of the chest cavity (increase in volume and decrease in air pressure) and exhaling results from compression of the chest cavity (decrease in volume and increase in air pressure). These changes are accomplished by movement of the ribs and diaphragm.

16. **The correct answer is (D).** Pith typically consists of *parenchyma* cells, which store starch in typical green plants. Spongy cells, characteristic of dicot leaves, also store starch, but temporarily.

17. **The correct answer is (C).** The Hubble Telescope is able to produce sharper images of objects than other telescopes because it is in orbit around Earth and does not have its view obstructed by atmosphere. Images seen through telescopes on Earth's surface are always obscured to some degree by the scattering of light as it passes through the atmosphere and by the passage of air currents created by heating of the atmosphere.

18. **The correct answer is (D).** A symptom of diabetes is sugar (glucose) in the urine. *Benedict's solution* is a reagent used to test for the presence of reducing sugars such as glucose.

19. **The correct answer is (B).** Buffer systems resist significant changes in pH. When a strong acid or a strong base is added to a buffer system, it produces a weak acid and a salt or a weak base and water, respectively. In each case, the pH would change only slightly.

20. **The correct answer is (B).** Each turn of the Krebs cycle generates 2 moles of CO_2 and four pairs of H_2.

21. **The correct answer is (A).** The removal of a small bit of living tissue from a patient for microscopic examination is called a *biopsy,* a useful diagnostic tool—especially for diseases of a cancerous nature.

22. **The correct answer is (C).** Water constitutes about 75–85 percent of the typical living cell. No activities associated with life can occur without water.

23. **The correct answer is (D).** Fats are *emulsified,* or broken down into small droplets, by bile secreted from the liver into the small intestine. The enzyme lipase then digests the fat droplets into fatty acids and glycerin. These products are not absorbed through capillary walls directly into the bloodstream, but enter the small lymph vessels, or *lacteals,* located in the villi of the intestine.

24. **The correct answer is (B).** The results of the penny toss approximate a 1:2:1 ratio, which is the same ratio that is obtained from a monohybrid cross:

    $Aa \times Aa \rightarrow 1AA:2Aa:1aa$

25. **The correct answer is (D).** In the light phase of photosynthesis, H_2O is dissociated into $H_2 + O_2$. The O_2 comes entirely from the water molecules. The resulting H_2 is then used to reduce CO_2 to simple sugar.

26. **The correct answer is (A).** Tissue culture is the technique of growing tissues or cells in solutions of water and nutrients. This technique is especially useful in studying growth, differentiation, and morphology.

27. **The correct answer is (B).** Incineration is an effective method of sterilization; holding a loop in a flame sterilizes the loop, preventing contamination of surfaces on work areas, etc., and the possible spread of infectious bacteria.

28. **The correct answer is (C).** Cellular respiration oxidizes digested food molecules and produces CO_2 and H_2O as end products. It is a downhill reaction and occurs in both plant and animal cells.

29. **The correct answer is (D).** *Combustion,* or burning, is a rapid reaction giving off much heat and light in a short period of time. The energy is expended more rapidly; thus, the reaction occurs at a higher temperature since the temperature of the combustible material must be raised to a combustion point. Cellular respiration occurs more slowly, at lower temperatures, and is controlled by enzymes. If cellular respiration occurred at combustion temperatures, cells would be destroyed.

30. **The correct answer is (B).** *Trypsin,* an enzyme found in pancreatic juice, digests proteins, peptones, and proteoses to peptides. The digestion of peptides to amino acids also occurs in the small intestine under the control of the enzyme erepsin. Some protein digestion (to peptones and proteoses) occurs in the stomach, under the control of the enzyme pepsin. Ptyalin and maltase act on carbohydrates; steapsin, on fats.

31. **The correct answer is (D).** Thrombocytes disintegrate when ruptured, as when blood flows from an injured blood vessel, releasing thrombokinase (thromboplastin), which acts to convert prothrombin to thrombin. Thrombin acts on fibrinogen in the plasma, converting it to insoluble fibrin, the material that forms the clot. Inadequacy of thrombokinase would prevent the first step of clotting, the formation of thrombin from prothrombin.

32. **The correct answer is (C).** *Cone cells* are photoreceptor cells found in the retina of the eye. They are responsible for color vision. Cone cells are functional only in bright light; therefore, color is not perceived in dim light.

33. **The correct answer is (C).** The *iris* is a circular muscle that regulates the diameter of the *pupil,* the aperture that allows light

to enter the posterior chamber of the eye where the light-sensitive retina is located. The *cornea* allows light to enter the eye but does not regulate the amount of light entering. The *ciliary body* is a muscle that changes either the position or shape of the lens to focus the light coming through the pupil. The *conjunctiva* is a thin, protective layer of epithelium that covers the exposed surface of the eyeball.

34. **The correct answer is (A).** Most of the carbon dioxide is transported in the blood plasma in the form of sodium bicarbonate ($NaHCO_3$). *Erythrocytes, leucocytes,* and *platelets* (thrombocytes) are blood cells suspended in the plasma.

35. **The correct answer is (D).** *Adrenalin,* a hormone secreted by the adrenal glands, causes increases in blood pressure, heart rate, breathing, blood glucose levels, etc., preparing the body for heightened situations.

36. **The correct answer is (A).** *Auxins* are plant growth hormones; *testosterone* and *estrogen* are animal sex hormones. ATP (adenosine triphosphate) is an energy-transport compound found in cells.

37. **The correct answer is (D).** Bread mold is a fungus, while ferns are vascular plants. Both bread mold and ferns, however, produce spores as asexual reproductive cells. A *mycelium* is a mass of fungal hyphae and is not a part of the fern-plant body. *Pinnules* are the "leaflets" of a fern frond and are not part of a fungus.

38. **The correct answer is (A).** *Transpiration* is the loss of gaseous water from a plant through epidermal stomata of the aerial parts of the plant, especially the leaves. Water forms a continuous column in the xylem tissue. The pull of water effected by transpiration is a factor in the rise of *sap* (water plus dissolved materials). The process is much the same as drinking liquid through a straw.

39. **The correct answer is (B).** Xylem and phloem serve the purpose of transporting materials in vascular tissues. Upward translocation of plant sap is accomplished mainly through vessels (in angiosperms) and tracheids of xylem. Downward translocation is accomplished through the sieve tubes of phloem.

40. **The correct answer is (C).** The cotyledons of dicotyledonous plants (such as beans) store food for use by the plant embryo as it develops into a seedling that can carry on photosynthesis. The *plumule* is composed of the embryonic or first leaves of the embryo; the *hypocotyl* is the lower embryonic stem; and the *testa* is the seed coat.

41. **The correct answer is (A).** Normal cells have a high power of self-affinity (tendency to adhere to their own kind). Cancer cells lose this ability, as demonstrated by the spreading of cancer from one organ to another (malignancy).

42. **The correct answer is (A).** The *stigma* is the top portion of the pistil on which pollen lands in pollination. The *style* is the neck-like portion of the pistil, located between the stigma and the ovary, the basal part. *Ovules* are potential seeds.

43. **The correct answer is (B).** Intensive research has demonstrated that the basic structure of cell membranes is a mosaic of proteins in an outer and inner layer of phospholipids.

44. **The correct answer is (B).** The enzyme sucrase adds a molecule of water (hydrolysis to the band that binds the monosaccharides forming sucrose) to decompose the dissaccharide to simple sugars.

45. **The correct answer is (B).** The movement of continents relative to one another is mostly the result of the spreading apart of sea floor between continental masses caused by the extrusion of molten rock through cracks in the sea floor. Fluctuations in Earth's magnetic field and Coriolis force are real events, but neither has any effect on continental drift. Fragmentation of large land masses to make

smaller ones has sometimes been a part of continental drift, but it qualifies as a result rather than a cause.

46. **The correct answer is (C).** The generic formula for carbohydrates is $(CH_2O)^n = 1C:2H:1O$ (1:2:1).

47. **The correct answer is (A).** There are three morphological types, or shapes, of bacteria: spherical-shaped bacteria are called *cocci*; rod-shaped bacteria are called *bacilli*; curved or spiral-shaped bacteria are usually known as *spirilla*.

48. **The correct answer is (A).** Bacteria are classified as gram positive or gram negative; this depends on their ability to retain crystal violet, the primary stain of the gram stain. Those bacteria that cannot be decolorized with ethanol, but retain crystal violet, are classified as gram positive. Those that can be decolorized are gram negative. The difference is due to the chemical composition of the cell wall.

49. **The correct answer is (D).** A *bacteriophage* is a kind of virus that attacks and destroys the bacterial cell. The viruses can pass their DNA into the bacterial cells and cause the cells to manufacture vital DNA and viral protein.

50. **The correct answer is (C).** A *marsupial* is a viviparous mammal that gives birth to immature embryos; the development of the young is completed in the female's pouch, located on her ventral side. Nourishment for the embryo is from the mammary glands, the nipples of which are located in the pouch.

51. **The correct answer is (B).** Reptiles are the first vertebrates in evolutionary development that spend the early or developmental part of their lives, as well as adult stages, on land. They do not possess gills for breathing in water as do the larval stages of amphibians.

52. **The correct answer is (A).** Enzymes are macromolecular proteins that serve as biological catalysts that lower activation energy requirements in cellular reactions.

53. **The correct answer is (B).** Most eukaryotic cells are in the range of 10 microns to 100 microns.

54. **The correct answer is (D).** *Sickle cell anemia* is caused by inheriting the defective form of a gene that codes for part of the protein portion of the hemoglobin molecule. The number of erythrocytes produced and the amount of hemoglobin in each erythrocyte are normal, but the altered structure of the hemoglobin molecules causes them to stick together in a manner that distorts erythrocytes into an abnormal crescent shape, making them less able to carry oxygen. Other types of anemia are due to insufficient hemoglobin within erythrocytes, too few erythrocytes, or erythrocytes that are abnormally small.

55. **The correct answer is (C).** All named are members of the phylum Arthropoda, but only the sow bug is a crustacean. The characteristics of the class Crustacea are two pairs of antennae, three pairs of mouth parts, and a three-part body. Most crustaceans are aquatic, gilled animals, but a few live on land. The sow bug is one of these.

56. **The correct answer is (C).** Leucoplasts are cellular plastids that store starches and are found only in plant cells.

57. **The correct answer is (A).** The hydra and corals are coelenterates, diploblastic animals characterized by a gastrovascular cavity.

58. **The correct answer is (B).** Many insects have developed an immunity to or tolerance of DDT, so it does not kill them. However, DDT can accumulate in the bodies of insects and then be transferred to the tissues of birds, fishes, and other insect predators. These predators can accumulate DDT and, when consumed by their predators, pass on the DDT. Thus, this harmful insecticide can be passed up the food chain with the concentration in animal tissues increasing at each level, and it can have harmful effects on higher animals that consume the lower DDT-containing animals.

59. The correct answer is (A). Lysosomes store powerful hydrolysis enzymes.

60. The correct answer is (A). All environments have limited amounts of food and space, allowing animal populations to increase up to these limits, and regulating the populations by the number of individuals per unit of space (density-dependent).

General Science Test 6

1. C	15. A	29. D	43. C	56. C
2. C	16. D	30. C	44. D	57. B
3. C	17. C	31. B	45. B	58. B
4. B	18. A	32. D	46. C	59. A
5. A	19. B	33. B	47. B	60. A
6. D	20. A	34. C	48. B	61. B
7. C	21. D	35. B	49. D	62. B
8. B	22. D	36. D	50. C	63. D
9. B	23. A	37. B	51. A	64. C
10. C	24. C	38. A	52. B	65. B
11. A	25. C	39. C	53. A	66. D
12. A	26. B	40. B	54. D	67. B
13. B	27. C	41. A	55. A	68. D
14. C	28. B	42. B		

1. **The correct answer is (C).** The gingko is native to the Orient but has been imported into the United States and now is in widespread use as an ornamental tree.

2. **The correct answer is (C).** Evidence indicates that a primitive reptile known as a therapsid is the ancestor of mammals. These early reptiles of the Triassic period had acquired some mammalian characteristics, such as warm-bloodedness, hair, and mammary glands. They are sometimes referred to as "premammals."

3. **The correct answer is (C).** *Electrophoresis* is a technique that takes advantage of the fact that molecules in solution will migrate through a porous gel when an electrical current is passed through it. A mixture of differently sized molecules is placed into a depression at one end of the gel, and the current is turned on. Smaller molecules will travel farther through the gel than larger molecules, with the result that bands of molecules will accumulate at various distances from the starting point according to their size. These bands can be made visible by staining, allowing the results of one electrophoretic separation to be compared to another.

4. **The correct answer is (B).** Fossil evidence indicates that there was an isolation of ape-like forms, including hominids (human-like creatures), during the Pliocene period. These seemingly originated from the same "branch" of the evolutionary "tree." Lemurs, New World monkeys, and

Old World monkeys apparently evolved earlier.

5. **The correct answer is (A).** It was found that if a mixture of methane, ammonia, and hydrogen is continuously bombarded with spark discharges as an energy source, amino acids are formed. If inorganic phosphate is added to the mixture, ATP, the energy compound of cells, is formed also. The earth, at its very early age, had the inorganic substances, and the sun could have provided the energy source.

6. **The correct answer is (D).** The *condenser* is an adjustable lens that focuses light before it reaches the specimen. This enhances the sharpness of the image produced by the magnifying lenses of the microscope. The *objective* and the *ocular* are the lenses used to create a magnified image of the light after it has passed through the specimen. A *micrometer* is a device used to measure objects viewed through the microscope.

7. **The correct answer is (C).** Triple bonds, sharing six electrons between two carbon atoms, provide each with a complete octet.

8. **The correct answer is (B).** As the moon revolves around the Earth, it rotates on its axis so that only one side of the moon faces Earth. Because the moon makes one rotation with one revolution around the Earth, one side of the moon never faces the Earth.

9. **The correct answer is (B).** In all ecosystems, producers (green plants or algae) convert CO_2 and H_2O into sugars, which serve as food for consumers (animals) whose bodies are ultimately degraded by decomposers (bacteria and fungi). Water, although vital, is an inorganic substance.

10. **The correct answer is (C).** Carbon monoxide has a greater affinity than oxygen for hemoglobin. This binding blocks hemoglobin from binding oxygen for transport to body cells for metabolic needs.

11. **The correct answer is (A).** A deficiency of vitamin B_{12} leads to *pernicious anemia,* a condition in which red blood cells fail to mature. Vitamin B_{12} is essential for the formation of red blood cells.

12. **The correct answer is (A).** Scalar quantities have only magnitude; vectors have magnitude and direction.

13. **The correct answer is (B).** The catalytic converter uses platinum to convert carbon monoxide and hydrocarbons to carbon dioxide and water, resulting in reduced air pollution.

14. **The correct answer is (C).** In a cathode-ray tube, such as found in television sets (picture tube), a *cathode* (negative terminal) and an *anode* (positive terminal) are present. There is no material between the two through which electricity (electrons) can flow from one terminal to another: a vacuum exists in the tube. A heated cathode generates electrons, which become excited by heat and can acquire enough energy to leave the cathode. Once they do, they are attracted to the anode because of the difference in charges (electrons have a negative charge) and flow across the gap toward the anode. In other appliances, the material through which the electricity flows may produce some resistance; in a picture tube, the electrons are flowing across a space in a vacuum and encounter no resistance.

15. **The correct answer is (A).** The small-intestine lining is characterized by millions of *villi,* small, thin-walled projections into the lumen. Each villus is supplied with capillaries and a lacteal. The large number of villi greatly increase the absorptive area of the small intestine, and the blood vessels and lacteal are close to the food supply. Thus, digested foods are absorbed with ease through the thin-walled villus and thin capillary walls into the bloodstream or, in the case of fats, into the opened ends of the lacteals.

16. **The correct answer is (D).** Coal is the major source of SO_2 because gasoline, natural gas, and paper waste contain only small amounts of sulfur.

17. The correct answer is (C). The moon shines by the reflected light of the sun. Because the moon rotates on its axis as it revolves around the Earth, one side of the moon never faces the Earth. This side, the dark side of the moon, can never reflect the sun's light onto the Earth.

18. The correct answer is (A). Poison ivy has a clear juice rather than a milky sap. Three-leaflet clusters, white berries, and shiny leaves are all characteristic of poison ivy.

19. The correct answer is (B). The divalent (Cu^{+2}) cupric ion is the species capable of receiving electrons.

20. The correct answer is (A). When an organism dies, eventually all functions cease and the body reaches equilibrium.

21. The correct answer is (D). Air is a mixture of gases; dry air consists of about 78 percent nitrogen and 21 percent oxygen. The remaining 1 percent consists of other gases, including carbon dioxide.

22. The correct answer is (D). Enzymes are proteins that catalyze reactions of substances known as substrates.

23. The correct answer is (A). The reverse outside-inside concentration and membrane crossing of Na^+ and K^+ are the major ions responsible for resting potentials and action potentials.

24. The correct answer is (C). Exergonic reactions are downhill reactions.

25. The correct answer is (C). As oxygen accepts electrons from the ETS, it acquires a -2 valence, which attracts $2H^+$ to form HOH.

26. The correct answer is (B). Air pressure at sea level is 14.7 pounds/square inch. This pressure, at 0 degrees C, supports a barometer mercury column of 76 centimeters, or 30 inches. This is equivalent to 1 atmosphere of pressure.

27. The correct answer is (C). Radioactive elements suggest that the Earth is 4.5 billion years old.

28. The correct answer is (B). A *high* indicates an area of high air pressure, while a *low* indicates an area of low air pressure. Weather can be predicted by measuring differences between pressures. A high usually indicates fair weather, whereas low pressure areas indicate storms and bad weather.

29. The correct answer is (D). The retina of the eye contains rods and cones; these are the photoreceptors of the eye, so named because of their shape. Rods are concerned with perception of gray to black in dim light, while cones respond to light of high intensity and are concerned with color perception. Nerve fibers from these receptors eventually converge to form the optic nerves leading to the brain.

30. The correct answer is (C). Malaria is a parasitic disease caused by protists in the genus *Plasmodium*. Some of the life cycle stages of *Plasmodium* are passed in mosquitoes of the genus *Anopheles,* which transmit the disease.

31. The correct answer is (B). Archimedes' Principle indicates that an object will displace its weight in water. Thus, a 1,000-ton ship would displace 1,000 tons of water.

32. The correct answer is (D). A photoelectric cell works on the principle that light can be used to produce electric currents in some metals. When light energy strikes the metal (usually cesium) in the photoelectric cell, it is converted into electric energy. The cesium emits electrons. The greater the amount of light striking the metal, the more electric energy produced.

33. The correct answer is (B). A camera lens is convex; light passing through such a lens is bent toward the center of the lens. Light reflected near the object and passing through the thinner outer edges of a convex lens bends more than light passing through the thicker areas, and light passing through the exact center of the lens does not bend at all. Because light reflected from an object is focused through such a lens and bent, rather than passing in a straight line, as it would if passing through plain glass, the image formed is reversed and is smaller than the original object.

34. **The correct answer is (C).** Insecticide resistance is acquired and developed through natural selection. Some insects are not affected by the chemical; they are "resistant."

35. **The correct answer is (B).** The flour beetle belongs to the Order Coleoptera which, with approximately 350,000 described species, is the largest order of insects. The housefly belongs to the Order Diptera, containing approximately 120,000 described species. The grasshopper belongs to the Order Orthoptera, containing approximately 20,000 species. The cockroach belongs to the Order Blattaria, containing only 4,000 species.

36. **The correct answer is (D).** The H^+ has no electrons, which enables it to use 2 unshared electrons from N to form a coordinate covalent bond.

37. **The correct answer is (B).** Photosynthesis is an endergonic reaction that uses CO_2 + H_2O to produce simple sugar and O_2. It is driven by radiant energy from sunlight.

38. **The correct answer is (A).** Unicellular eukaryotes, including colonial forms, belong to the Kingdom *Protista*. The other organisms belong to phyla in the Kingdom *Animalia,* of which all members are multicellular. Phylum *Annelida* includes segmented worms, such as the earthworm. Phylum *Porifera* includes sponges. Phylum *Arthropoda* includes animals such as insects, spiders, crabs, crayfish, and millipedes that have a chitinous exoskeleton and jointed appendages.

39. **The correct answer is (C).** Spiders are characterized by a two-part body and four pairs of legs, while insects have a three-part body and three pairs of legs.

40. **The correct answer is (B).** The CO_2 from the burning of fossil fuels prevents heat from escaping the Earth's surface, thus raising temperatures.

41. **The correct answer is (A).** Hydrogen is the lightest element known, having an atomic weight of 1.008. The atom contains 1 proton, no neutrons, and 1 electron.

42. **The correct answer is (B).** Nitrogen composes nearly four fifths of the air; oxygen nearly one fifth. The remainder of air consists of other gases.

43. **The correct answer is (C).** Light travels at a speed of about 186,000 miles per second; the sun is approximately 93,000,000 miles from the Earth. Thus, calculations (93,000,000 miles divided by 186,000 miles per second) show that it takes about 500 seconds, or a bit more than eight minutes, for light from the sun to reach the Earth.

44. **The correct answer is (D).** Emergent properties of matter cause atoms that react to form compounds to lose their original properties and gain properties of the new substance.

45. **The correct answer is (B).** The Earth makes one complete rotation on its axis (360 degrees) in 24 hours; 45 degrees is one eighth of 360 degrees. Therefore, it would take one eighth of 24 hours, or three hours, for the Earth to rotate 45 degrees.

46. **The correct answer is (C).** The thyroid regulates metabolic rate under normal conditions. A deficiency of thyroid hormone will cause a low basal metabolism, while an excess of the hormone will increase the metabolic rate.

47. **The correct answer is (B).** A *peptide bond* is the covalent bond that links the nitrogen atom on the end of 1 amino acid molecule with the carbon atom on the opposite end of another amino acid molecule. A peptide bond is formed by removing a molecule of water from the 2 amino acid molecules. Therefore, inserting a water molecule between 2 amino acids linked by a peptide bond will break the bond by putting a hydrogen atom back onto the nitrogen atom of 1 amino acid and a hydroxyl ion (OH–) back onto the terminal carbon atom of the other amino acid. Breaking a bond between 2 molecules by inserting a water molecule between them is called *hydrolysis* and is a common way

of digesting large organic molecules such as starches and proteins.

48. **The correct answer is (B).** The 23.5 inclination of the Earth on its axis causes it to tilt toward and away from the sun as it revolves around the sun.

49. **The correct answer is (D).** Passive immunity involves administering an antibody (an antitoxin, in the case of diphtheria) to the patient. This immunity is temporary, since the patient's body is not stimulated to form antibodies, as it would be if an antigen were administered. The temporary immunity is considered *passive* because the body is not active in forming antibodies. If an antigen stimulates the body to form its own antibodies against it, the immunity produced is *active*. Passive immunity provides temporary protection to one who has been exposed to a disease, or a method of treatment until the patient's body has started producing its own antibodies if the disease has been contracted. Active immunity imparts more lasting protection.

50. **The correct answer is (C).** Group O blood lacks antigen A and antigen B. Although it can form antibodies against both A and B, it cannot stimulate the formation of antibodies against A and B. Persons of group O are known as *universal donors*. Group AB blood has both antigens A and B but cannot form antibodies against either. Persons of group AB are known as *universal recipients*. Since group O has neither antigen, and AB cannot form either antibody, the only safe transfusion of those listed is choice (C). Persons of group A contain antigen A and can form antibodies against antigen B; blood group B contains antigen B and can form antibodies against A.

51. **The correct answer is (A).** Synergism is a phenomenon in which the whole is greater than the sum of the individual parameters.

52. **The correct answer is (B).** Xylem, characterized in angiosperms by vessels, conducts material upward in the plant. Most of the material conducted upward is water that has been absorbed from the soil by the root system. The water contains dissolved minerals and may contain, especially in deciduous perennials in the spring, sugar that has been formed by the digestion of starch stored in the lower plant parts.

53. **The correct answer is (A).** After the common multiplier **(M)** was removed from $mgh = \frac{1}{2}mV^2$, the equation was multiplied by 2 to eliminate the $\frac{1}{2}$, and the square root of both sides was extracted.

54. **The correct answer is (D).** Total potential energy was connected to kinetic energy.

55. **The correct answer is (A).** Genes are composed of segments of nucleotide bases of DNA molecules.

56. **The correct answer is (C).** Distillation involves *evaporation,* or changing the water from a liquid to a gaseous state (usually by heating), and collecting and *condensing* the gaseous water back to a liquid. The water, because it is in a gaseous state, is separated from any impurities since they cannot evaporate with the water.

57. **The correct answer is (B).** On the Fahrenheit scale, the boiling point of water is 212 degrees; the freezing point is 32 degrees. Subtracting 32 degrees from 212 degrees results in a difference of 180 degrees, the number of degrees between the boiling and the freezing points of water.

58. **The correct answer is (B).** *Static electricity* is a non-moving electrical charge that accumulates on the surface of an object. A substance that contains an equal number of *protons* (positively charged particles) and *electrons* (negatively charged particles) is electrically neutral. If electrons are gained or lost, the substance becomes charged. When one object loses electrons and becomes positively charged, another must gain electrons and become negatively charged. If electrons are not in motion, the electricity is static. However, warm, moist air is a good conductor of electricity; moisture collects on the surfaces of objects and conducts electrons away from the surface, preventing the object from becoming charged. Cold air acts as a

good insulator, preventing the movement of electrons away from the object. Therefore, static electricity can best be felt on a cold, dry day, when the electrons can accumulate on an object or surface.

59. **The correct answer is (A).** As of 2009, Jupiter has 49 official and 14 unofficial moons, which is the most in the solar system.

60. **The correct answer is (A).** Deserts of the Earth generally occur on the west side of continents, as influenced by prevailing westerly winds and nearby mountains. As the Earth rotates from west to east, winds that approach continents from the west side lose moisture in ascending mountains and evaporate moisture from the opposite side—resulting in dry regions known as deserts.

61. **The correct answer is (B).** Atmospheric moisture combines with oxides of carbon, nitrogen, and sulfur to produce acid rain, as illustrated by the following reactions:

$$H_2O + CO_2 \rightarrow H_2CO_3$$

$$H_2O + 2NO_2 \rightarrow 2HNO_3$$

$$H_2O + SO_2 \rightarrow H_2SO_3$$

62. **The correct answer is (B).** As water is warmed, its solubility of oxygen decreases, resulting in a lower O_2 content and producing unfavorable conditions for animals.

63. **The correct answer is (D).** The pesticide DDT was banned from the United States during the 1970s because research studies had shown it to be present in milk, fatty tissues, and the eggs of eagles and other birds. It was also proven to be a biological concentration—building up to higher concentration in succeeding levels of food chains.

64. **The correct answer is (C).** The human body is composed primarily of oxygen, carbon, hydrogen, and nitrogen, which comprise approximately 96 percent of the body's mass, with about 15 other elements comprising the rest.

65. **The correct answer is (B).** Glucose and fructose are isomers because they are composed of identical numbers of carbon, hydrogen, and oxygen atoms, with different structural arrangements and different functional groups. The carbon-oxygen bonding in glucose and fructose form aldehydes and ketones, respectively.

66. **The correct answer is (D).** The approximate percentages of oxygen, carbon, nitrogen, and potassium in the human body are: 65, 18.5, 3.5, and 0.5, respectively.

67. **The correct answer is (B).** Density is defined as mass per unit volume ($D = \frac{m}{v}$).

The mathematical relationship shows that when equal masses of two substances of different densities are compared, the one with greater density occupies less space (volume).

68. **The correct answer is (D).** The same four bases A, T, C, and G are in all living organisms. Organisms differ according the numbers and arrangements.

FINAL SCIENCE EXAMINATION ANSWER SHEET

1. Ⓐ Ⓑ Ⓒ Ⓓ	16. Ⓐ Ⓑ Ⓒ Ⓓ	31. Ⓐ Ⓑ Ⓒ Ⓓ	46. Ⓐ Ⓑ Ⓒ Ⓓ	61. Ⓐ Ⓑ Ⓒ Ⓓ
2. Ⓐ Ⓑ Ⓒ Ⓓ	17. Ⓐ Ⓑ Ⓒ Ⓓ	32. Ⓐ Ⓑ Ⓒ Ⓓ	47. Ⓐ Ⓑ Ⓒ Ⓓ	62. Ⓐ Ⓑ Ⓒ Ⓓ
3. Ⓐ Ⓑ Ⓒ Ⓓ	18. Ⓐ Ⓑ Ⓒ Ⓓ	33. Ⓐ Ⓑ Ⓒ Ⓓ	48. Ⓐ Ⓑ Ⓒ Ⓓ	63. Ⓐ Ⓑ Ⓒ Ⓓ
4. Ⓐ Ⓑ Ⓒ Ⓓ	19. Ⓐ Ⓑ Ⓒ Ⓓ	34. Ⓐ Ⓑ Ⓒ Ⓓ	49. Ⓐ Ⓑ Ⓒ Ⓓ	64. Ⓐ Ⓑ Ⓒ Ⓓ
5. Ⓐ Ⓑ Ⓒ Ⓓ	20. Ⓐ Ⓑ Ⓒ Ⓓ	35. Ⓐ Ⓑ Ⓒ Ⓓ	50. Ⓐ Ⓑ Ⓒ Ⓓ	65. Ⓐ Ⓑ Ⓒ Ⓓ
6. Ⓐ Ⓑ Ⓒ Ⓓ	21. Ⓐ Ⓑ Ⓒ Ⓓ	36. Ⓐ Ⓑ Ⓒ Ⓓ	51. Ⓐ Ⓑ Ⓒ Ⓓ	66. Ⓐ Ⓑ Ⓒ Ⓓ
7. Ⓐ Ⓑ Ⓒ Ⓓ	22. Ⓐ Ⓑ Ⓒ Ⓓ	37. Ⓐ Ⓑ Ⓒ Ⓓ	52. Ⓐ Ⓑ Ⓒ Ⓓ	67. Ⓐ Ⓑ Ⓒ Ⓓ
8. Ⓐ Ⓑ Ⓒ Ⓓ	23. Ⓐ Ⓑ Ⓒ Ⓓ	38. Ⓐ Ⓑ Ⓒ Ⓓ	53. Ⓐ Ⓑ Ⓒ Ⓓ	68. Ⓐ Ⓑ Ⓒ Ⓓ
9. Ⓐ Ⓑ Ⓒ Ⓓ	24. Ⓐ Ⓑ Ⓒ Ⓓ	39. Ⓐ Ⓑ Ⓒ Ⓓ	54. Ⓐ Ⓑ Ⓒ Ⓓ	69. Ⓐ Ⓑ Ⓒ Ⓓ
10. Ⓐ Ⓑ Ⓒ Ⓓ	25. Ⓐ Ⓑ Ⓒ Ⓓ	40. Ⓐ Ⓑ Ⓒ Ⓓ	55. Ⓐ Ⓑ Ⓒ Ⓓ	70. Ⓐ Ⓑ Ⓒ Ⓓ
11. Ⓐ Ⓑ Ⓒ Ⓓ	26. Ⓐ Ⓑ Ⓒ Ⓓ	41. Ⓐ Ⓑ Ⓒ Ⓓ	56. Ⓐ Ⓑ Ⓒ Ⓓ	71. Ⓐ Ⓑ Ⓒ Ⓓ
12. Ⓐ Ⓑ Ⓒ Ⓓ	27. Ⓐ Ⓑ Ⓒ Ⓓ	42. Ⓐ Ⓑ Ⓒ Ⓓ	57. Ⓐ Ⓑ Ⓒ Ⓓ	72. Ⓐ Ⓑ Ⓒ Ⓓ
13. Ⓐ Ⓑ Ⓒ Ⓓ	28. Ⓐ Ⓑ Ⓒ Ⓓ	43. Ⓐ Ⓑ Ⓒ Ⓓ	58. Ⓐ Ⓑ Ⓒ Ⓓ	73. Ⓐ Ⓑ Ⓒ Ⓓ
14. Ⓐ Ⓑ Ⓒ Ⓓ	29. Ⓐ Ⓑ Ⓒ Ⓓ	44. Ⓐ Ⓑ Ⓒ Ⓓ	59. Ⓐ Ⓑ Ⓒ Ⓓ	74. Ⓐ Ⓑ Ⓒ Ⓓ
15. Ⓐ Ⓑ Ⓒ Ⓓ	30. Ⓐ Ⓑ Ⓒ Ⓓ	45. Ⓐ Ⓑ Ⓒ Ⓓ	60. Ⓐ Ⓑ Ⓒ Ⓓ	75. Ⓐ Ⓑ Ⓒ Ⓓ

answer sheet

FINAL SCIENCE EXAMINATION

75 Questions • 75 Minutes

Directions: After carefully reading each test item, select the best answer. Fill in the corresponding space on your answer sheet.

1. Of the following human traits, the one under both genetic and hormonal control is
   (A) hemophilia.
   (B) color blindness.
   (C) baldness.
   (D) blood type.

2. If a sexually reproducing animal has a diploid number of 12, how many chromosomes would a mature sperm have?
   (A) 3
   (B) 24
   (C) 4
   (D) 6

3. The tissue to which gland cells belong is
   (A) connective.
   (B) epithelial.
   (C) secretory.
   (D) nerve.

4. Of the following, which is closest to the speed of sound in air at sea level?
   (A) $\frac{1}{5}$ mile per second
   (B) $\frac{1}{2}$ mile per second
   (C) 1 mile per second
   (D) 5 miles per second

5. The general formula for the acetylene series of hydrocarbons is
   (A) $C_nH_2n + 2$.
   (B) C_nH_2n.
   (C) $C_nH_2n - 2$.
   (D) None of the above

6. How many molecules of ATP are required to activate a molecule of glucose in glycolysis?
   (A) 2
   (B) 6
   (C) 3
   (D) None

7. The vitamin that helps clotting of the blood is
   (A) C.
   (B) D.
   (C) E.
   (D) K.

8. Each nucleotide in a DNA molecule contains
   (A) a sugar.
   (B) a nitrogen base.
   (C) a phosphate group.
   (D) All of the above

9. The wavelength (nm) of the visible portion of the electromagnetic spectrum is in the range of
   (A) 350–700.
   (B) 800–1,000.
   (C) 200–350.
   (D) 550–900.

10. A person is more buoyant when swimming in salt water than in fresh water because
    (A) the person keeps his or her head out of salt water.
    (B) salt water has greater tensile strength.
    (C) salt coats the person's body with a floating membrane.
    (D) salt water is denser than an equal volume of fresh water.

11. Two parameters (e.g., the volume and the temperature of a gas) are directly proportional if a constant value can be calculated from their
    (A) product.
    (B) ratio.
    (C) sum.
    (D) difference.

12. Cellular proteins are synthesized by
    (A) ribosomes.
    (B) mitochondria.
    (C) lysosomes.
    (D) golgi.

13. All of the following mechanisms affect the amount of glucose in the blood EXCEPT
    (A) adrenaline secretion.
    (B) insulin secretion.
    (C) level of oxygen intake.
    (D) level of physical activity.

14. The most active mixing of many digestive juices occurs in the
    (A) stomach.
    (B) duodenum.
    (C) ileum.
    (D) jejunum.

15. A *cold-blooded* animal is one that
    (A) has a body temperature colder than that of other types of animals.
    (B) uses heat from its blood to warm other tissues of the body, lowering the blood temperature.
    (C) depends on external heat sources to regulate its body temperature.
    (D) is incapable of regulating its body temperature.

16. The basic mechanism of hereditary transmission is
    (A) sexual reproduction.
    (B) polyploidy.
    (C) separation, rearrangement, and distribution of chromosomes.
    (D) the mitotic mechanism.

17. If sound waves have the following pattern, what is the frequency?

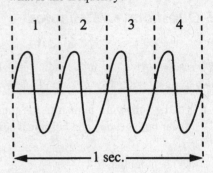

    (A) 4 hertz
    (B) 8 hertz
    (C) 12 hertz
    (D) 16 hertz

18. Of the following, the highest bactericidal activity of light occurs at a wavelength in angstrom units of
    (A) 2,536.
    (B) 3,256.
    (C) 5,236.
    (D) 6,532.

19. In the diagram below, the refraction of the light rays indicates that the lens is

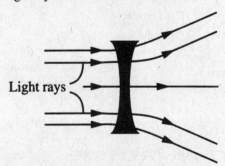

    (A) thicker in the center than the edges.
    (B) thinner at the center than the edges.
    (C) uniform in thickness.
    (D) consistent in dimensions.

20. Which of the following compounds is an ether?

    (A) CH_2CHO

    (B) $CH_3–O–CH_3$

    (C) $CH_3–COOH$

    (D) $CH_3–CH_2OH$

21. Which of the following statements about wavelengths is true?

    (A) Visible wavelengths vary in lengths.

    (B) The wavelength of green is the longest.

    (C) Radio waves are electromagnetic waves shorter than infrared.

    (D) Infrared rays are shorter than red light rays.

22. An object appears white, or colorless, when it

    (A) absorbs the light reaching it.

    (B) transmits only blue light.

    (C) rejects all colors.

    (D) reflects all colors at the same time.

23. Another name for animal starch is

    (A) cellulose.

    (B) lecithin.

    (C) glycogen.

    (D) chitin. .

24. Of the following, a human blood disease that has been definitely shown to be due to a hereditary factor or factors is

    (A) pernicious anemia.

    (B) sickle cell anemia.

    (C) polycythemia.

    (D) leukemia.

25. All of the following elements are major constituents of a cell EXCEPT

    (A) carbon.

    (B) potassium.

    (C) hydrogen.

    (D) phosphorus.

26. If a machine listed for 1,800 watts is plugged into a 110-volt system, approximately how many amps will it use?

    (A) 6.6

    (B) 13.0

    (C) 16.0

    (D) 19.8

27. The selection of algae as a possible nutritional supplement for humans is based primarily on their ability to carry on

    (A) fermentation.

    (B) digestion.

    (C) photosynthesis.

    (D) oxidation.

28. A nurse administered a medication at 10^{-4} molar concentrated to a patient. The doctor instructed that the dosage be reduced by one-half strength, which was

    (A) $10^{-2}M$

    (B) $5 \times 10^{-5}M$

    (C) $10^{-8}M$

    (D) $10^{-3}M$

29. In eukaryotic cells, the phase of division that produces two daughter cells is

    (A) $G_.$

    (B) mitosis.

    (C) G_2

    (D) cytokinesis.

30. Efficiency (mechanical and biological) is a relationship between input, output, and total available energy for work. Which of the following is the correct formula for efficiency?

    (A) $E = \dfrac{Input}{Output} \times 100$

    (B) $E = \dfrac{Input \times Output}{100}$

    (C) $E = \dfrac{Output - Input}{100}$

    (D) $E = \dfrac{Output}{Input} \times 100$

31. When a molecule of glucose in humans is degraded, the percent of its energy capable of generating ATP is nearest to

    (A) 100.

    (B) 50.

    (C) 25.

    (D) 80.

32. Velocity, defined as the rate of displacement of an object, is

    (A) scalar.

    (B) inertia.

    (C) vector.

    (D) centripetal.

33. The fundamental principle expressed by the Einstein Equation ($E = mc^2$) on mass-energy equivalency is that

    (A) small mass = much energy.

    (B) small mass = little energy.

    (C) little energy = great mass.

    (D) All of the above

34. Exophthalmic goiter is caused by

    (A) hypoactivity of the thyroid.

    (B) hyperactivity of the thyroid.

    (C) deficiency of vitamin A.

    (D) radioactive iodine.

35. If other factors are compatible, a person who can most safely receive blood from any donor belongs to this basic blood group.

    (A) O

    (B) A

    (C) B

    (D) AB

36. The Schick test indicates whether or not a person is probably immune to

    (A) tuberculosis.

    (B) diptheria.

    (C) poliomyelitis.

    (D) scarlet fever.

37. Evaporation of water is likely to be greatest on days of

    (A) high humidity.

    (B) low humidity.

    (C) little or no wind.

    (D) low pressure.

38. The generic formula for alkane, aliphatic hydrocarbons is $C_NH_{2N}+2$, from which the formula for propane is derived, is what?

    (A) C_2H_4

    (B) C_3H_8

    (C) NaNO

    (D) C_3H_4

39. The percentage of oxygen by weight in $Al_2(SO_4)_3$ (atomic weights: Al = 27, S = 32, O = 16) is approximately

    (A) 19.

    (B) 21.

    (C) 56.

    (D) 92.

40. In backcrossing, a hybrid is always mated with

    (A) its own parent.

    (B) another hybrid.

    (C) a pure dominant.

    (D) a pure recessive.

41. The diameter of a light microscope on low power is 2 mm. The number of 50Φ wide paramecia (side-by-side) that stretches across the entire field is

    (A) 400.

    (B) 500.

    (C) 40.

    (D) 4.

42. Of the following, a structure found in mammals but NOT in reptiles is the

    (A) lung.

    (B) brain.

    (C) diaphragm.

    (D) ventricle.

43. If the osmotic pressure of human blood is determined by the number of dissolved particles, and a 0.315 molar glucose solution is isotonic to blood, the concentration of isotonic sodium chloride (NaCl) would be
    (A) 0.630M.
    (B) 0.3M.
    (C) 0.157M.
    (D) 0.2M.

44. The resistance of matter to changes in motion is
    (A) elasticity.
    (B) inertia.
    (C) momentum.
    (D) inflexible.

45. Some substances are transported across cell membranes by proteins known as
    (A) ligases.
    (B) permeases.
    (C) hydrolases.
    (D) monomers.

46. Which sequence correctly illustrates a food chain?
    (A) algae – insect larvae – fish – human
    (B) algae – fish – insect larvae – human
    (C) insect larvae – algae – fish – human
    (D) fish – insect larvae – algae – human

47. Grasses are usually pollinated by
    (A) wind.
    (B) water.
    (C) birds.
    (D) insects.

48. Among vertebrates, the embryonic ectoderm gives rise to which of the following?
    (A) Nervous system
    (B) Digestive system
    (C) Skeletal system
    (D) Respiratory system

49. Generally, life depends directly or indirectly for food, energy, and oxygen upon
    (A) parasitic organisms.
    (B) green plants.
    (C) fungi.
    (D) animals.

50. Pathogenic bacteria responsible for food poisoning are becoming resistant to the antibiotic Cipro. This phenomenon illustrates that the populations are
    (A) photosynthesizing nutrients.
    (B) encapsulating practices.
    (C) evolving.
    (D) dominating amino acids.

51. The weight in grams of 22.4 liters of nitrogen (atomic weight = 14) is
    (A) 3
    (B) 7
    (C) 14
    (D) 28

52. In the production of sounds, the greater the number of vibrations per second, the
    (A) greater the volume.
    (B) higher the tone.
    (C) lower the volume.
    (D) lower the tone.

53. A segment of a DNA molecule transcribes a base sequence, AGAUAU, on an mRNA codon. Which of the following is the compatible sequence on the tRNA anticodon?
    (A) UUAGCG
    (B) UCUAUA
    (C) AAUAUA
    (D) CGCAAA

54. Which of the following species will combine with a chloride ion to produce ammonium chloride?
    (A) NH_3
    (B) K^+
    (C) NH_4^+
    (D) Al^{+++}

55. The newest vaccine for a human cancer controls the HPV-16 virus of the
    (A) cervix.
    (B) lungs.
    (C) colon.
    (D) breasts.

56. Which one of the following graphs represents Boyle's Law?

    (A)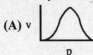

    (B)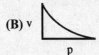

    (C)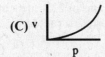

    (D)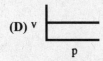

57. Which of the following minerals is restored to the soil by plants of the pea and bean family?
    (A) Sulfates
    (B) Nitrates
    (C) Carbonates
    (D) Phosphates

58. In humans, any hereditary defect caused by a gene on the Y chromosome would occur
    (A) only in males.
    (B) only in females.
    (C) only if the gene were recessive.
    (D) about equally in males and females.

59. There is no oxidation-reduction in a reaction that involves
    (A) single replacement.
    (B) double replacement.
    (C) simple decomposition.
    (D) direct combination of elements.

60. A cross between two black guinea pigs yields 3 black and 1 white offspring. The white allele in the parents was
    (A) dominant.
    (B) recessive.
    (C) sex-linked.
    (D) absent.

61. The cellular organelle where respiratory reactions for the release of energy occurs is a
    (A) centrosome.
    (B) chromosome.
    (C) chromoplast.
    (D) mitochondrion.

62. Members of a population that are reproductively isolated from other populations form a
    (A) race.
    (B) species.
    (C) community.
    (D) genus.

63. The most efficient cellular respiratory process, in terms of energy-yield per molecule of glucose, is
    (A) aerobic respiration.
    (B) anaerobic respiration.
    (C) fermentation.
    (D) phosphorylation.

64. Which of the following is/are not a requirement(s) for photosynthesis?
    (A) Oxygen
    (B) Carbon dioxide and water
    (C) Sunlight
    (D) Chlorophyll

65. A cellular organelle found in typical plant cells but not in typical animal cells is the
    (A) chloroplast.
    (B) ribosome.
    (C) mitochondrion.
    (D) centrosome.

66. In the absence of oxygen, plants and microbes convert pyruvic acid into
    (A) alcohol and CO_2.
    (B) lactic acid.
    (C) CO_2 and H_2O.
    (D) amino acids.

67. Every cell contains
    (A) a cell membrane and cytoplasm.
    (B) a cell wall and cytoplasm.
    (C) a nucleus and cell wall.
    (D) plastids and pigments.

68. Digestion in humans is
    (A) extracellular.
    (B) intracellular.
    (C) vacuolar.
    (D) intercellular.

69. An example of an obligate intracellular parasitic microorganism is a
    (A) tapeworm.
    (B) virus.
    (C) bacterium.
    (D) spirochaete.

QUESTIONS 70–72 REFER TO THE FOLLOWING GRAPH AND EQUATION.

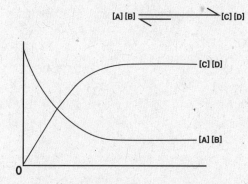

70. At time zero, the percentage of substance that is [A] [B] is approximately
    (A) 100.
    (B) 0.
    (C) 50.
    (D) 25.

71. The comparative affinity of the reactants and products is
    (A) [C] [D] > [A] [B].
    (B) [A] [B] = [C] [D].
    (C) [A] [B] > [C] [D].
    (D) None of the above

72. Choose the incorrect statement, relative to the reaction at equilibrium.
    (A) Concentration of reactants and products remains constant.
    (B) Reaction is shifted to the right.
    (C) Forward and reverse reactions occur at equal rates.
    (D) Reaction is shifted to the left.

73. The second law of thermodynamics (entropy) states that systems (ranging from a single organism to the entire universe) become increasingly disordered or random with time. Early scientists erroneously believed that the human body, by maintaining its structural and functional integrity, violated this law.

    It is currently understood that the human body conforms to the second law of thermodynamics because it is a(an)
    (A) closed system.
    (B) assembly of organic molecules.
    (C) open system.
    (D) composite of inorganic and organic molecules.

74. Data from the human genome project have shown that the total number of genes in humans is close to
    (A) 30
    (B) 1,000,000
    (C) 3,000
    (D) 30,000

75. The smallest chromosome in the human
genome is
   (A) 1
   (B) 51
   (C) 21
   (D) Y

STOP

IF YOU FINISH BEFORE TIME IS CALLED, YOU MAY CHECK YOUR WORK ON THIS SECTION ONLY. DO NOT TURN TO ANY OTHER SECTION IN THE TEST.

ANSWER KEY AND EXPLANATIONS

Final Science Examination

1. C	16. C	31. B	46. A	61. D
2. D	17. A	32. C	47. A	62. B
3. B	18. A	33. A	48. A	63. A
4. A	19. B	34. B	49. B	64. A
5. C	20. B	35. D	50. C	65. A
6. A	21. A	36. B	51. D	66. A
7. D	22. D	37. B	52. B	67. A
8. D	23. C	38. B	53. B	68. A
9. A	24. B	39. C	54. C	69. B
10. D	25. B	40. A	55. A	70. A
11. B	26. C	41. C	56. B	71. A
12. A	27. C	42. C	57. B	72. D
13. C	28. B	43. C	58. A	73. C
14. B	29. D	44. B	59. B	74. D
15. C	30. D	45. B	60. B	75. C

1. **The correct answer is (C).** All conditions are under genetic control; however, hereditary baldness is also under hormonal control. Baldness is expressed as a dominant characteristic in males but recessive in females because of the hormones present. Thus, a male and female may inherit the same genes for baldness, but the expression of the genes will depend on the sex hormones.

2. **The correct answer is (D).** Diploid cells in the testes undergo meiosis to reduce the chromosome number by one half to the haploid condition.

3. **The correct answer is (B).** There are only four basic kinds of tissues: epithelial, connective, muscle, and nerve. Gland cells are among the epithelial tissues that cover the internal and external surfaces of various parts of the body.

4. **The correct answer is (A).** The speed of sound in air varies slightly with temperature, increasing slightly as temperature increases. For convenience, the speed of sound in air is referred to as 1,100 feet per second. This is an approximate value that can be used despite various conditions. 1,100 feet is approximately one fifth of a mile (1 mile = 5,280 feet).

5. **The correct answer is (C).** A member of the acetylene series is unsaturated, with a triple bond between two carbons. The formula for acetylene, for example, is H–C $\equiv$ C–H; because of the triple bond between 2 carbons, the number of hydrogens is reduced by 2. Thus, the general formula is $C_n H_2 n - 2$.

6. **The correct answer is (A).** A molecule of glucose uses 2 molecules of ATP to supply activation energy to initiate the glycolytic pathway.

7. **The correct answer is (D).** Prothrombin is produced in insufficient quantities if there is a deficiency of vitamin K; prothrombin produces thrombin, which acts as an enzyme to convert fibrinogen to fibrin, the mesh that traps blood cells, forming the clot. Thus, if vitamin K is deficient, prothrombin is deficient, and clotting is delayed or does not occur.

8. **The correct answer is (D).** Each nucleotide of a DNA molecule contains a molecule of deoxyribose sugar, a nitrogen base, and a phosphate group, which is attached to the 3' carbon of 1 sugar molecule and the 5' carbon of a second sugar.

9. **The correct answer is (A).** The wavelength of energy in the electromagnetic spectrum ranges from 10^{-3} nM to 10^{14} nM, with visible light between 350 nM and 700 nm.

10. **The correct answer is (D).** The buoyancy of an object in water or air is determined by its *density* relative to the surrounding medium: thus, objects less dense than the surrounding medium will float, and those more dense will sink. Salt water is denser than fresh water because of the much greater amount of dissolved substances. Therefore, a person will float more easily in salt water because there is a greater difference between the density of the person's body and that of the water.

11. **The correct answer is (B).** Two parameters are directly proportional if their ratio is a mathematical constant $(K = \frac{x}{y})$.

12. **The correct answer is (A).** Cellular proteins are synthesized by the ribosomes where codon triplets of m-RNA are paired with anticodon triplets of t-RNA to direct amino acid sequences.

13. **The correct answer is (C).** Insulin increases the permeability of the cell membrane to glucose, thus increasing the rate of glucose uptake by the cells from the bloodstream. Adrenalin promotes an increase in cardiac activity, respiratory rate, and the breakdown of glycogen (stored in the liver) to glucose, thus raising the glucose level of the blood. With physical activity, glucose is more rapidly utilized by cells, which must remove glucose from the blood, thus reducing the blood level of glucose.

14. **The correct answer is (B).** The digestion and absorption of most nutrients occurs in the *duodenum,* the first portion of the small intestine. Therefore, digestive juices are most active at this site.

15. **The correct answer is (C).** The term *cold-blooded* is commonly used in reference to animals such as reptiles that depend on external sources of heat to help regulate their body temperature. Cold-blooded animals, more properly called *ectotherms,* must bask in sunlight or lie on warm ground to raise their body temperature. Conversely, they must lie in the shade or shelter beneath an object such as a rock to cool off their bodies. By contrast, warm-blooded animals, more properly called *endotherms,* are more or less independent of external sources of heat, relying on a combination of heat generated by their metabolism and insulation on the surface of the body to keep their internal temperature constant.

16. **The correct answer is (C).** Chromosomes contain genetic material, or carry genes; the separation of the chromosomes of each pair is involved in *meiosis,* or reduction division, in the production of sexual reproductive cells. The *gametes* (egg and sperm) will each receive one half the chromosomes carried by the parent, or one chromosome of each pair carried by the parent. Thus, the gametes will be *haploid.* When fertilization occurs, the zygote becomes *diploid,* having received one chromosome of each pair from each parent. Therefore, each individual inherits one half of its chromosomes and genes from its father and one half from its mother.

17. **The correct answer is (A).** A *hertz* can be defined as the number of wavelengths per second. A wave or wavelength is the distance between successive values, for example, from crest to crest. The diagram shows 4 waves in the one-second period, or 4 hertz.

18. **The correct answer is (A).** Light consists of colors of varying wavelengths. Visible light ranges from red, with a wavelength of about 7,000 angstrom units, down to violet, with a wavelength of about 4,000 angstroms. Ultraviolet has shorter wavelengths (150–3,900 Å) and is bactericidal; the highest bactericidal activity occurs between 2,000 Å and 3,000 Å.

19. **The correct answer is (B).** The lens is concave; therefore, it is thicker at the edges. Light rays passing through a concave lens are refracted or bent outward, so they spread apart. A light ray passing through the center of the lens is not bent.

20. **The correct answer is (B).** The functional group for ethers is R–O–R.

21. **The correct answer is (A).** Visible light consists of different colors of light, producing a spectrum of red (with the longest wavelength), orange, yellow, green, blue, indigo, and violet (with the shortest wavelength).

22. **The correct answer is (D).** White light consists of the colors or wavelengths of the visible spectrum—red, orange, yellow, green, blue, indigo, and violet. An object appears to be a certain color when it is reflecting light of this wavelength, and absorbing all others. A white object is reflecting all of the colors or wavelengths at the same time.

23. **The correct answer is (C).** Liver glycogen, which is a polymer of glucose molecules, is called animal starch.

24. **The correct answer is (B).** Persons with sickle cell anemia carry a variant hemoglobin molecule in the red blood cells, instead of the normal hemoglobin A. The production of hemoglobin is under genetic control.

25. **The correct answer is (B).** All elements listed are found in cells. Carbon, hydrogen, and phosphorus are three of the six major elements from which most organic molecules are built. Potassium is one of the five essential minor elements.

26. **The correct answer is (C).** An *ampere* (amp) is a unit for measuring the rate of flow of electricity. A *watt* is the metric unit of power; it is the power produced by 1 amp in a 1 volt circuit. Thus, the formula $watt = amp \times volt,$ can be used, or $amp = \dfrac{watt}{volt}$. If the problem is worked using this formula, the answer is choice (C), 16 amps.

27. **The correct answer is (C).** Photosynthesis is the process by which an organic, energy-containing compound (sugar or glucose) is produced from inorganic materials. This is a process basic to the production of organic compounds that can be used for food. Algae and other green plants exhibit photosynthesis.

28. **The correct answer is (B).** A half of the dosage is 5×10^{-5}M.

29. **The correct answer is (D).** Cytokinesis is the stage in eukaryotic cell division in which the cytoplasm divides to produce daughter cells.

30. **The correct answer is (D).** Efficiency is the ratio of work-out per work-in.

31. **The correct answer is (B).** Eukaryotic cells have high efficiency, relative to mechanical device. They are capable of extracting approximately 50 percent of the energy in glucose molecules for biological work.

32. **The correct answer is (C).** Vector quantities must have both magnitude and direction for complete description. An object cannot have a velocity without direction.

33. **The correct answer is (A).** The equation $E = mc^2$ demonstrates mass and energy are interchangeable and that small amounts of mass can yield large amounts of energy under specific conditions.

34. **The correct answer is (B).** The overproduction of the thyroid hormones causes a condition known as exophthalmic goiter, or Graves' disease. The thyroid may or may not be enlarged, but increased metabolic rate, protrusion of eyes (exophthalmus), increased blood pressure, increased heart rate, loss of weight, etc., are symptoms of Graves' disease. This disease may be treated by surgical removal or destruction of part of the thyroid gland.

35. **The correct answer is (D).** A person of blood group AB has antigen A and antigen B, but cannot produce antibodies against A or B. Therefore, such a person can receive blood from any of the four blood groups and is often called a "universal recipient."

36. **The correct answer is (B).** The Schick test, developed by Bela Schick, is administered by injecting a weak solution of the diphtheria toxin cutaneously. A reddening of the site of injection indicates susceptibility to diphtheria; lack of reddening indicates immunity and the presence of sufficient antitoxin to protect the person against diphtheria.

37. **The correct answer is (B).** *Evaporation* is the physical change of a substance from a liquid to a gas. The rate of movement of gas molecules into the air is more rapid in dry air, or when the humidity is low, and decreases with increased humidity. The movement of air currents (wind) carries away the vapor above the surface of the liquid, thus increasing evaporation rate.

38. **The correct answer is (B).** Propane (C_3H_8) satisfies the generic aliphatic hydrocarbon formula (C_nH_{2n+2}).

39. **The correct answer is (C).** Of the 17 atoms making up a molecule of $Al_2(SO_4)_3$, there are 2 atoms of aluminum, 3 atoms of sulfur, and 12 atoms of oxygen (4 oxygens in each of the 3 sulfate ions). The weight of the oxygen is 192; the total weight of the molecule is 342. Thus, the percentage of oxygen by weight is $\frac{192}{342}$, or 56 percent.

40. **The correct answer is (A).** Backcrossing of a hybrid with one of the parents or a genetically similar individual yields offspring similar to the parent.

41. **The correct answer is (C).** A microscope field 2 mm in diameter is 2,000Φ. Paramecia (50Φ) could be placed 40Φ side-by-side across the field.

42. **The correct answer is (C).** Reptiles do not possess a diaphragm but have the other structures listed.

43. **The correct answer is (C).** Sodium chloride is an ionic substance that dissociates in aqueous solutions, to give 2 times the number of particles per mole in molecular substances such as glucose.

44. **The correct answer is (B).** Inertia is the tendency of a body at rest or in motion to remain constant unless acted upon by an outside force.

45. **The correct answer is (B).** Permease are cellular proteins that transport substances across plasma membranes.

46. **The correct answer is (A).** In a food chain, algae are the primary "producers," occupying the bottom level of the food chain since they produce organic materials through photosynthetic processes. Insect larvae are some of the animals that can feed on algae; fish, which prey on animals such as insect larvae, are in turn consumed by humans.

47. **The correct answer is (A).** Grasses are usually pollinated by wind; the grass flower typically does not attract insects or birds. Since grasses are mostly land plants, water would not play a significant role in their pollination.

48. **The correct answer is (A).** The *ectoderm* is the outer germ layer, which gives rise to the nervous and integumentary systems of the embryo.

49. **The correct answer is (B).** Only green plants can produce organic materials (food) from inorganic materials (carbon dioxide and water) through the process of

photosynthesis. Oxygen and a by-product are returned to the air by means of this process. Animals may consume green plants (direct dependence) or may consume animals that consume green plants (indirect dependence) for food and energy.

50. **The correct answer is (C).** This illustrates the concept of survival-of-the-fittest from a bacterial population.

51. **The correct answer is (D).** One mole (gram molecular weight) of nitrogen is 28 grams, since 2 nitrogen atoms form a nitrogen molecule (N_2). One mole of gas occupies a volume of 22.4 liters at standard conditions.

52. **The correct answer is (B).** The frequency, or number of vibrations per second, determines pitch, or tone. The greater the frequency, the higher the pitch; the lower the frequency, the lower the pitch.

53. **The correct answer is (B).** In DNA and RNA molecules, adenine (A) must pair with thymine (T) or uracil (U). Guanine (G) always pairs with cytosine (C). This specificity is based on complementarity of molecular geometry, relative to the formation of double or triple bonds.

54. **The correct answer is (C).** The NH^+ species has a positive valence, which has affinity for a negative chloride (Cl^-) ion.

55. **The correct answer is (A).** Cervical cancer has been determined to be caused by the HPV-16 virus. A vaccine against this virus has been shown to be effective in preventing this disease.

56. **The correct answer is (B).** Boyle's Law illustrates the relationship between the pressure and volume of a mass of gas at a fixed temperature. The law can be simply stated: at a given fixed temperature and mass of gas, pressure, and volume are inversely proportional. For example, volume will increase as pressure decreases, or volume will decrease as pressure increases. Therefore, pressure × volume = a constant.

57. **The correct answer is (B).** Peas and beans are members of the legume family and have nitrogen-fixing bacteria in nodules on their roots. Nitrogen-fixing bacteria convert atmospheric gaseous nitrogen into nitrates, thus restoring nitrates to the soil. It is only in the form of nitrates that plants generally can obtain nitrogen from the soil.

58. **The correct answer is (A).** The male sex chromosome is referred to as the Y chromosome. It is inherited only by male offspring; thus, a male is XY and a female is XX, as far as inheritance of sex is concerned. Therefore, any gene located on the Y chromosome is inherited only by males since females will inherit an X from the male parent.

59. **The correct answer is (B).** Oxidation-reduction reactions are those in which one substance is oxidized by the loss of electrons, and another substance is reduced by the gain of electrons. In double replacement reactions, this does not occur. Ions are exchanged between reactants and do not lose or gain electrons.

60. **The correct answer is (B).** The cross indicates that the parents were heterozygous blacks (1 black and 1 white allele). The cross would yield 1 homozygous black, 2 heterozygous blacks, and 1 homozygous white offspring.

61. **The correct answer is (D).** The mitochondrion is called the powerhouse of the cell; most of the respiratory process involving the release of energy occurs in this organelle.

62. **The correct answer is (B).** Reproductive isolation is the major criterion for determination of speciation.

63. **The correct answer is (A).** Aerobic metabolism is 19 times more efficient than anaerobic metabolism (which yields 2 mol ATP per 1 mol glucose).

64. **The correct answer is (A).** Oxygen is a waste product of photosynthesis. Green plants use carbon dioxide and water as raw materials to produce sugar in the presence of chlorophyll and sunlight as follows:

$$CO_2 + H_2O \xrightarrow[\text{chlorophyll}]{\text{sunlight}} C_6H_{12}O_6 + O_2$$

65. **The correct answer is (A).** Chloroplasts contain the chlorophylls, the green pigments, and are characteristic of green plants but not of animals.

66. **The correct answer is (A).** In the absence of oxygen, plants and microbes convert pyruvic acid into alcohol and carbon dioxide by a process called fermentation.

67. **The correct answer is (A).** The cell wall and plastids are characteristic of plant cells but not of animal cells. A nucleus may not be present in some cells, such as mature human red blood cells. But all cells have cytoplasm surrounded by a plasma or cell membrane.

68. **The correct answer is (A).** Digestion in humans occurs primarily in the lumen of the stomach and small intestine where macromolecules are degraded to small molecules capable of being absorbed.

69. **The correct answer is (B).** A virus does not exhibit reproduction, synthesis, and other characteristics of life outside a living host cell; thus, it is an obligate intracellular parasite.

70. **The correct answer is (A).** At the initiation of the reaction, all substances are reactants (A and B).

71. **The correct answer is (A).** The affinity of [C] and [D] is greater than that of [A] and [B], resulting in a greater concentration of products versus reactants at equilibrium.

72. **The correct answer is (D).** The reaction is shifted to the right.

73. **The correct answer is (C).** The human body is an open system—exchanging nutrients, CO_2 and O_2, nitrogenous waste, water, and heat with the external environment.

74. **The correct answer is (D).** The current estimate of genes is about 24,000–40,000 genes.

75. **The correct answer is (C).**

Reading Comprehension

OVERVIEW

TECHNIQUES

Reading comprehension presents problems to many test-takers. To avoid this, make every effort to improve your ability to interpret reading passages.

First, understand that there are two aspects of success in reading interpretation:

1. Reading speed

2. Reading understanding

Too many individuals read with excellent comprehension but read too slowly. Remember, there is a time limit on your test. On the other hand, some people read rapidly, but, for reasons that we shall cite later, do not thoroughly understand what they are reading. Both speed of reading and comprehension of the material read are important during an exam.

Practice Reading Intensively

You were probably taught to read letter-by-letter. Gradually, as you matured, you learned to read word-by-word. As an adult, however, you should be able to read a complete phrase as quickly as you once read just one letter. If you cannot do this, or if you have trouble understanding what you read, you should practice reading intensively.

There is no need to be discouraged if this is the case. Most students can increase the speed of their reading significantly with little effort. The old idea that slow readers make up for their slowness by better comprehension of what they read has been proved untrue. Your ability to comprehend what you read should keep pace with your increase in speed. You can absorb as many ideas per page, and get many more ideas per unit of reading time, by applying specific techniques of reading.

unit 4

It has been demonstrated that those who read best also read quickly. This is probably due to the fact that heavier concentration is required for rapid reading, and concentration is what enables a reader to grasp important ideas contained in the reading material.

A good paragraph generally has one central thought—that is, a *topic sentence*. Your main task is to locate and absorb that thought while reading the paragraph. The correct interpretation of the paragraph is based upon that thought, and not upon your personal opinions, prejudices, or preferences. If a selection consists of two or more paragraphs, its correct interpretation is based on the central idea of the entire passage. The ability to grasp the central idea of a passage can be acquired by practice—practice that will also increase the speed with which you read.

An important rule to follow in order to improve reading ability is to force yourself to increase your speed. Just as you once stopped reading letter-by-letter, now learn to stop reading word-by-word. Force yourself to read rapidly across the line of type, skimming it. Don't permit your eyes to stop for individual words; try instead to reconstruct the whole idea even if a word has been missed. Proceed quickly through the paragraph in this skimming fashion, without rereading or backtracking to a missed word.

If you find yourself failing to comprehend what you read, read the material over several times rapidly until you do understand. Do *not* slow down on rereading. At first, you may find yourself missing some of the ideas. With persistent practice, however, you will step up both your reading speed and your ability to comprehend.

You may need to overcome certain handicaps or unhelpful reading habits at once. Do not move your lips, pronounce words individually silently or aloud, or think of each word separately as you read. These habits can be overcome almost automatically if you learn to leap from phrase to phrase. You can synchronize your eye movements with your mind, both of which are nimbler than your lips.

Certain physical factors affect reading. You should always read sitting in a comfortable position, erect, with head slightly inclined. The light should be excellent, with both an indirect and a direct source available; direct light should come from behind you and slightly above your shoulder, in such a way that the type is evenly lit. Hold the reading matter at your own best reading distance and at a convenient height, so you don't stoop or squint. If you need reading glasses, you should certainly use them.

How to Increase Reading Speed

Problem: Word-by-word reading

Our earliest reading, since it is done aloud, is, of necessity, word-by-word reading. Unfortunately, this method of reading sometimes becomes so firmly implanted that it persists as a bad reading habit.

Cure: Use the eye-span method.

Look at the first part of a sentence that consists of a thought-unit. Then, look for the next thought-unit, if there is another one in the same sentence—then, look for still another thought-unit. For example, consider this sentence:

Reading maketh a full man, conference a ready man, and writing an exact man. How many ideas are there in the sentence? Three. Now, employ the eye-span method in reading this sentence.

Reading maketh a full man,
EYE-SPAN 1

conference a ready man,
EYE-SPAN 2

and writing an exact man.
EYE-SPAN 3

Problem: Vocalizing

Some readers move their lips or whisper while they read "silently." This practice slows down silent reading time considerably.

Cure

You must consciously refrain from moving your lips or whispering during silent reading. Have someone watch you while you read. Are you vocalizing?

Problem: One-speed reading

You should vary your reading speed according to what you are reading.

Cure

The pace of your reading should change not only from book to book, but even within a reading selection. Be flexible so that you can change speed from paragraph to paragraph, even from sentence to sentence. Adjust your reading rate according to the purpose for which you are reading. Scanning a passage for main ideas may be accomplished with rapid reading. Reading a novel for enjoyment would allow you to read at a medium rate. Reading to obtain detailed information would require you to read at a slower pace.

Increasing Reading Comprehension

The following are ten good techniques to use on *any* reading interpretation question.

1. Read through the selection quickly to get the general sense.

2. Reread the selection, concentrating on the central idea.

3. Attempt to pick out the *topic sentence* in each paragraph.

4. If the selection consists of more than one paragraph, determine the *central idea* of the entire selection.

5. Examine the four choices for each test item carefully yet rapidly. Eliminate immediately those choices that are far-fetched, ridiculous, irrelevant, false, or impossible.

6. Eliminate those choices that may be true but have nothing to do with the sense of the selection.

7. Check those few choices that now remain as possibilities.

8. Refer back to the original selection and determine which one of these remaining possibilities is best in view of
   a. information *stated* in the selection
   b. information *implied* in the selection

9. Be sure to consider only the facts *given* or *definitely implied* in the selection.

10. Be especially careful of trick expressions or catch-words, which sometimes destroy the validity of a seemingly acceptable answer. These include the expressions "under all circumstances," "at all times," "always," "under no conditions," "absolutely," "completely," and "entirely."

Avoid Traps

Trap 1

Sometimes, the questions cannot be answered on the basis of the stated facts. You may be required to make a deduction from the facts given. Making a deduction requires you to draw conclusions from something already known.

Trap 2

Some reading passages are designed to arouse the reader's emotion, or describe situations with which the reader can identify. Be certain to base an answer selection on the information presented in the passage. Eliminate your personal opinions.

Trap 3

Many questions, and the appropriate responses to these questions, are based on important details that are nestled in the paragraph. Reread the paragraph as many times as necessary (keeping an eye on your watch) to find significant facts that will provide answers to the questions.

Get Plenty of Practice

Read:

- Editorial pages of various newspapers

- Book, drama, and movie reviews

- Magazine articles

For each selection that you read, do the following:

- Jot down the main idea of the article.

- Look up the meanings of words of which you are unfamiliar or unsure.

A Sample Question

Here is a sample question followed by analysis. Try to understand the process of arriving at the correct answer.

> Too often, indeed, have scurrilous and offensive allegations by underworld figures been sufficient to blast the careers of irreproachable and incorruptible executives who, because of their efforts to serve the people honestly and faithfully, incurred the enmity of powerful political forces and lost their positions.

Judging from the contents of the preceding sentence, which conclusion might be most valid?

(A) The large majority of executives are irreproachable and incorruptible.

(B) Criminals often swear in court that honest officials are corrupt in order to save themselves.

(C) Political forces are always clashing with government executives.

(D) False statements by criminals sometimes cause honest officials to lose their positions or ruin their careers.

ANALYSIS

Choice (A) can generally be said to be a true statement, but it cannot be derived from the paragraph. Nothing is said in the paragraph about "the large majority" of executives.

Choice (B) may also be a true statement and can, to a certain extent, be derived from the paragraph. However, the phrase "in order to save themselves" is not relevant to the sense of the paragraph, and even if it were, this choice does not sum up its central thought.

Choice (C) cannot be derived from the paragraph. The catch-word "always" makes this choice entirely invalid.

Choice (D) is the best conclusion that can be drawn from the contents of the paragraph, in light of the four choices given. It is open to no exceptions and adequately sums up the central thought of the paragraph.

Analysis of the Reading Comprehension Test Item

There are standardized tests designed to assess reading comprehension skills and provide an evaluation of the test-taker's independent reading level, instructional reading level, frustration reading level, and reading rate. Reading comprehension test items usually elicit a response that would indicate the test-taker's ability to identify directly stated details, indirectly stated details, main ideas, inferences, and generalizations. Other target skills may include making judgments, drawing conclusions, and determining the author's purpose.

There are two types of reading comprehension test items. The first type is a long reading passage, usually a few paragraphs in length, followed by a series of questions. The second type is a short passage, usually a single paragraph in length, alongside one question. Several paragraphs in succession may treat the same topic, but the questions will always deal with the adjacent paragraph.

In order to determine your reading rate, the proctor will tell test-takers to stop after exactly 1 minute of exam time. Test-takers will then be asked to mark the point at which they were reading when they were told to stop, and this marking will be used for the determination.

Long Reading Passage Sample

This sample long reading passage, followed by a set of 6 questions, will help you to analyze comprehension test items and to understand why a particular response is the correct or appropriate one.

Studying the questions before reading a passage will cause you to be more alert when reading the passage; that is, you will be aware of what information in the passage will best help you answer the questions. Now read the 6 questions at the end of the passage, and then read the passage and answer the questions. Note that the questions are followed by explanations that indicate the skill addressed and strategies to use in your approach to a particular type of question.

"The Land of Frost and Fire" is no misnomer for the elliptic island republic in the North Atlantic known as Iceland. The island is so called because erupting volcanoes and steaming hot springs lie adjacent to its glaciers and ice fields. The official name of the country in Icelandic is Lydveldid Island, or the Republic of Iceland.

The "frost" is frigidly evident in the island's numerous ice fields that traverse the hoary landscape. Approximately one eighth of the island is covered by glaciers. In the southeast, a glacier known as Vatnajokull makes an area of about 8,550 square kilometers (about 3,300 square miles). Iceland, just south of the Arctic Circle, has more than 120 glaciers.

Lydveldid Island's "fire" leaps from the many hot springs and spouting geysers that cloud the panorama of the seventeen-province republic. To add heat to the "fire" are some 100 volcanoes, including at least twenty-five that have erupted and been recorded in the annals of the island's autocratic history. Lava and rocks erupting from volcanoes have contoured much of the land. The central highlands reflect the barren wilderness of lava fields. Hekla, in the southwest, is the best-known Icelandic volcano because of its many eruptions. The years 1766, 1940, 1947, and 1980 mark its explosive appearances.

Thermal springs are also common in Iceland. The springs occur as geysers, sizzling mud lakes, and various other forms. The most famous geyser here is Great Geysir, which is situated in southwest Iceland. The natives of this island of swift-flowing rivers boast of Geysir's spectacular and frequent eruptions occurring at irregular intervals of 5 to 36 hours. The torrid spring reportedly thrusts a column of boiling water upward to about 60 meters, or 200 feet.

Volcanic in origin, Iceland is indeed a land of contrast. Dazzling ice and jet black lava covering most of Iceland's surface attest to the appropriateness of its nickname—"Land of Frost and Fire."

1. Where are Iceland's hot springs and geysers located?

   (A) In the central highlands

   (B) In the southwest

   (C) Next to the glaciers

   (D) In the southeast

The correct answer is (C). This is a directly stated detail question. When answering this type of question, always consider the *wh* word with which the question begins. *Who* can be answered by the name of a person. *When* is answered by a word or phrase that tells at what time or in what sequence something happens. *Why* is answered by a word or phrase that tells the reason something happens. *What* is usually answered by the name of a thing or event. *Which* is answered by choosing the correct person, place, or thing from two or more persons, places, or things. *Where* is answered by the name of a place or a phrase that describes the location of one person or thing in relation to another (spatial relationships). *How* is answered by the way in which something is done. Question 1 is a *where* question denoting a spatial relationship. The correct answer is (C). Since adjacent means "next to" and encompasses the location of both the glaciers and geysers, this is the appropriate response. Choices (A), (B), and (D) could be ruled out immediately because they do not describe the location of both the glaciers and the geysers.

2. An appropriate title for this passage would be
   (A) Volcanoes and Geysers.
   (B) Iceland: The Island Republic.
   (C) Iceland: A Land of Contrast.
   (D) Thermal Springs.

   The correct answer is (C). This is a main idea question. This type of question requires the test-taker to consider what the passage is mostly about. Read the question first. Then scan the entire passage to find out what it is mostly about. A word of caution: Some answer choices are merely details from the passage. It is not difficult to choose (C) as the best title.

3. It is apparent that this passage is intended to
   (A) inform.
   (B) entertain.
   (C) persuade.
   (D) share an experience.

   The correct answer is (A). The skill addressed in this question is identifying author's purpose. The test-taker must determine what the author is trying to accomplish by writing this selection. What kind of response does he or she want from the reader? If the reader can say that he or she enjoyed this passage or thought it was hilarious, obviously the passage was meant to entertain. If the reader's reaction is, "Well, I think I'll try that," or "I have to agree with that," then the passage was written to persuade. If the passage is a narration or a storytelling written in the first person (I, me, my, myself—all references to the writer), the passage is probably aimed at sharing an experience. If the reader's reaction is, "I didn't know that," or "I never heard of this before," there is a good chance that the author intended to inform.

4. The sentiments of people of Iceland toward the presence of geysers in their native land is one of
   (A) mixed emotions.
   (B) pride.
   (C) dread and fear.
   (D) indifference.

   The correct answer is (B). This question requires the test-taker to infer a meaning or idea. In other words, "read between the lines." In the fourth paragraph of this passage, it is mentioned that the natives "boast of Geysir's spectacular and frequent eruptions." Usually, people boast about something when they are proud of it. The correct response would therefore be choice (B).

5. According to this passage, Iceland's form of government at one time reflected

   (A) total rule by the state.

   (B) rule by and for the people.

   (C) rule by royalty.

   (D) rule by dictator.

   The correct answer is (D). This test question is an example of indirectly stated detail. In paragraph three of this passage the phrase "the annals of the island's autocratic history" appears. The adjective "autocratic," though irrelevant to the main idea of the passage, and even to the sentence in which it appears, does provide an informational detail. The term autocratic suggests government by one person having unlimited power. The correct answer, therefore, would be (D). In completing this type of question, the test-taker should scan the passage to eliminate answer choices that are obviously related to the main idea. In some cases, the reader should also be careful of negative words in the question (no, not, not any).

6. Iceland is a difficult place to

   (A) grow crops.

   (B) raise a family.

   (C) get an education.

   (D) start a business.

   The correct answer is (A). Question 6 requires that you make a judgment or draw a conclusion. Since the passage does not mention family life, education, or industry, it would be safe to eliminate choices (B), (C), and (D). The passage also does not mention agriculture; however, it does describe the land as being "barren wilderness" and "covered by glaciers." These conditions are unsuitable for farming. Therefore, (A) is an appropriate answer.

Short Reading Passage Samples

Here are two sample short reading passages and questions, followed by analyses of the test items. Try to determine the answers on your own before reading the explanations.

A

At birth, you more than likely weighed less than 10 pounds. As an adult, you may weigh anywhere from 90 to 200 pounds or more. Obviously, there is much more of you as an adult. Despite your growth, the cells that make up your adult body are no larger than those that made up your body in infancy. This means that your adult body has billions more cells. You might question the source of these new cells. To satisfy your curiosity, they came from old cells via a process known as cell division.

31. The main idea of Paragraph A:

   (A) Most infants weigh less than 10 pounds.

   (B) Growth in human beings is accomplished by cell division.

   (C) Living cells increase in number by a process called cell division.

   (D) The cells that make up an adult body are larger than those of an infant body.

B

At a certain time during its existence, a cell divides into two cells. At the start of cell division, the nucleus becomes more dense and grainier than it was earlier. The grainy material, known as chromatin, eventually divides into short, cordlike structures called chromosomes. The chromosomes travel through the cell, forming a double line near the center of the cell.

32. As a result of the movement of chromosomes through the cell,

(A) a grainy material is formed.

(B) a cell divides into two cells.

(C) the chromatin divides into short, cordlike structures.

(D) a double line of them is formed near the center of the cell.

C

Boatmen who catch wild fish and shellfish are often more strictly regulated than seafood farmers, whose wholesome image has helped them resist government oversight. But after eight years of discussion, shrimp farmers around the world are considering adoption of a universal certification process that would require them to comply with standards on the siting of ponds, effluent treatment, the reduction of chemicals, and disease management. In exchange, their products would be labeled eco-friendly. By 2004, labels indicating whether seafood is farmed or wild will become mandatory in the U.S. (though they won't be required on restaurant menus). Jason Clay, 51, a senior fellow at World Wildlife Fund who helped develop the standards, is optimistic that they will be accepted. "As the industry gets more competitive, those who survive will be those who do it better and cleaner," he says.

—Copyright © 2002 Time Inc. Reprinted by permission.
From *Time*, Nov. 25, 2002. "A Fishy Business,"
by Terry McCarthy and Campbell River.

33. "Effluent" may be defined as

(A) wealthy.

(B) a fluid or liquid state.

(C) flowing out from a larger body of water.

(D) bubbling.

QUESTION 31

The correct answer is (B). In question 31, you are clearly asked to find the main idea of Paragraph A. This means that you are to consider what the paragraph is mostly about. If you chose (B), "Growth in human beings is accomplished by cell division," you have cited the correct response. A review or second reading of the paragraph will show that choice (A) could be supported by the paragraph; however, you should question the word "most." This statement merely provides a detail that leads to the principal concept. Choice (C) is factual, but it only supplies a major detail to the overall concept. Choice (D), according to the paragraph, is incorrect information since the passage states that "despite your growth, the cells that comprise your adult body are no larger than those that made up your body in infancy." Choice (B) most clearly ties together the two remaining details, choices (A) and (C), and states what the paragraph is mostly about.

QUESTION 32

The correct answer is (D). In question 32, the word "result" indicates a cause/effect response ("result" and "effect" are synonymous in this case). The paragraph clearly states that "the chromosomes travel through the cell, forming a double line near the center of the cell" (paraphrase: *causing* a double line to form). A review of the paragraph would prove that adding any of the activities described in choices (A), (B), or (C) to the question stem would not yield the proper sequence of the cell division process.

QUESTION 33

The correct answer is (C). If you're thinking Paragraph C is definitely a short passage reading comprehension question, you're right. If you're saying to yourself, "but this looks like a verbal ability question," you're right again! Reading comprehension is closely related to and dependent upon the understanding of words that test-makers often include; verbal ability questions are often integrated into reading comprehension test items. This type of question requires you to think in terms of the precise meaning of a word as used in the passage. We call the answer to this question "vocabulary in context."

As for the answer to question 33, you should begin by eliminating choice (A). There is clearly no mention of money or financial assets in this passage. Choice (B) is also doubtful since only larger bodies of water are mentioned rather than the liquid state of matter. Choice (D) hints that the author is trying to trick you with the resemblance of the word effervescent to effluent. Use your "word power" and take the word "effluent" apart. Remember that the stem *flu* means flowing and that the prefix *e-* means out or out from.

ALERT!

Time matters. Don't just keep rereading.

Reading in the Content Area

Efficient reading requires that the reader be flexible. As you already read, it is necessary to adjust your reading rate according to the purpose for which you are reading. It is equally important to adapt your reading style to the material being read. Before investigating effective strategies to use in making such reading adjustments, it is necessary to examine and recognize the structure and patterns of writing unique to each subject area. This study of various reading materials will help you get a feel for their differences and determine which reading style to apply to any given reading task.

Reading comprehension test items are frequently designed to reflect the course content of the field of study targeted by the entrance examination. For instance, entrance exams for educational programs leading to health careers may feature reading passages with scientific topics and information.

Unlike the humanities—which deal with emotions, attitudes, and sympathies of human beings via the study of philosophy, religion, music, art, and literature—science is the accumulation of knowledge by means of the study, observation, and classification of data justifiable by general laws or concrete truths. Scientists look for and acquire information regarding forms and processes of nature. They search for an undistorted view of reality and, therefore, cannot allow their values, feelings, attitudes, beliefs, and prejudices—or those of society—to interfere with their work.

Due to the nature of the subject matter, a scientist's writings follow a certain style. Descriptions are very exacting, factual, and detailed. They are void of background mood or setting, and are unemotional. As you read scientific material, you must concentrate on the following five reading skills:

1. Developing vocabulary.

2. Finding the main concepts.

3. Determining and remembering supporting details.

4. Understanding the organization or major pattern of writing in science (examination, classification, generalization, problem solution, comparison or contrast, sequence).

5. Drawing conclusions.

The Verbal Ability section of this book provides strategies for understanding and developing specialized scientific vocabulary. One method encourages vocabulary expansion through the use of a glossary, dictionary, thesaurus, etc., as well as through context clues. Another encourages the recognition of words that stand for concepts instead of facts. Other approaches include the study of word roots and affixes and the recognition of symbols.

The design or style of the text in science reading materials makes finding the main concepts simple. There are usually titles, opening comments in boldface type, headings, a summary, and questions at the end of the chapter or chapter section. In your initial reading, read only the text features just mentioned. This will allow you to explore and get a sense of the main ideas presented in the chapter, article, or selection. It will also prepare you for a second and closer reading.

Once you have identified the main ideas in a scientific passage, the next step in understanding what you are reading is to determine the supporting details. Supporting details answer the who, what, why, where, and when surrounding the main idea. Ask yourself these questions once you have completed a paragraph. In science, you should also question how much or to what extent.

Understanding the organization or major pattern of writing in science is vital to your reading comprehension. First of all, you should concentrate on examining the material you are about to read *before* you actually read it. Know the topic(s) that will be addressed and sum up the vocabulary in the particular reading selection. Next, identify the writing pattern that stands out in the material. There are four patterns:

1. **Classification** places into groups and subgroups a variety of objects or areas. For instance, in the explanation of plant life, a writer may outline the classification of plants. The breakdown could begin with vascular and nonvascular and seedless nonvascular plants. From here, the author could branch out to descriptions of mosses and liverworts, etc. In this pattern, watching for structural parts in order of importance is a must. Be aware of subheadings and all font treatments.

2. **Process-description** requires you to be aware of what the process is and exactly how it works. Studying illustrations and diagrams is helpful in this pattern.

3. **Factual-statement** involves the presentation of facts to define, compare or contrast, and illustrate. When reading for facts, remember that "fact" in the world of science means a statement that can be supported by scientific observation and experimentation and that has not yet been disproved. A fact defines something or explains its actions.

4. **Problem-solving** usually appears in science passages that give an account of past scientific problems and discoveries achieved through experimentation. There are 3 helpful questions that you should ask yourself when analyzing a problem-solving passage: (1) What is the problem or question? (2) How does the author answer or respond to the question? (3) How do I know the question was answered?

TIP

Don't give up on a passage, no matter how hard. A third of the questions about that passage are likely to be easy for you to answer.

Drawing conclusions is basic to the study of the sciences. A sound conclusion is a judgment based on facts. Consider what you need to know in order to make a sound judgment about something you read. Check the given facts. Think about what these facts are based on (experimentation, observation, etc.) to make certain of their reliability. Then consider the facts that are not given. Reread the passage to gather information that may be implied rather than stated. This method should help you in your test-taking venture. Speaking of tests, by now you have probably drawn some conclusions about the entrance exam you are about to take, and about the specialized vocabulary that may appear on it. However, do not conclude that scientific reading material is extremely difficult; instead, think of it as a kind of reading material that requires a very different approach.

Answer Sheet

Test 1

1. Ⓐ Ⓑ Ⓒ Ⓓ   4. Ⓐ Ⓑ Ⓒ Ⓓ   7. Ⓐ Ⓑ Ⓒ Ⓓ   10. Ⓐ Ⓑ Ⓒ Ⓓ   13. Ⓐ Ⓑ Ⓒ Ⓓ
2. Ⓐ Ⓑ Ⓒ Ⓓ   5. Ⓐ Ⓑ Ⓒ Ⓓ   8. Ⓐ Ⓑ Ⓒ Ⓓ   11. Ⓐ Ⓑ Ⓒ Ⓓ   14. Ⓐ Ⓑ Ⓒ Ⓓ
3. Ⓐ Ⓑ Ⓒ Ⓓ   6. Ⓐ Ⓑ Ⓒ Ⓓ   9. Ⓐ Ⓑ Ⓒ Ⓓ   12. Ⓐ Ⓑ Ⓒ Ⓓ   15. Ⓐ Ⓑ Ⓒ Ⓓ

Test 2

1. Ⓐ Ⓑ Ⓒ Ⓓ   3. Ⓐ Ⓑ Ⓒ Ⓓ   5. Ⓐ Ⓑ Ⓒ Ⓓ   7. Ⓐ Ⓑ Ⓒ Ⓓ   8. Ⓐ Ⓑ Ⓒ Ⓓ
2. Ⓐ Ⓑ Ⓒ Ⓓ   4. Ⓐ Ⓑ Ⓒ Ⓓ   6. Ⓐ Ⓑ Ⓒ Ⓓ

Test 3

1. Ⓐ Ⓑ Ⓒ Ⓓ   3. Ⓐ Ⓑ Ⓒ Ⓓ   5. Ⓐ Ⓑ Ⓒ Ⓓ   7. Ⓐ Ⓑ Ⓒ Ⓓ   9. Ⓐ Ⓑ Ⓒ Ⓓ
2. Ⓐ Ⓑ Ⓒ Ⓓ   4. Ⓐ Ⓑ Ⓒ Ⓓ   6. Ⓐ Ⓑ Ⓒ Ⓓ   8. Ⓐ Ⓑ Ⓒ Ⓓ

Test 4

1. Ⓐ Ⓑ Ⓒ Ⓓ   3. Ⓐ Ⓑ Ⓒ Ⓓ   5. Ⓐ Ⓑ Ⓒ Ⓓ   7. Ⓐ Ⓑ Ⓒ Ⓓ   9. Ⓐ Ⓑ Ⓒ Ⓓ
2. Ⓐ Ⓑ Ⓒ Ⓓ   4. Ⓐ Ⓑ Ⓒ Ⓓ   6. Ⓐ Ⓑ Ⓒ Ⓓ   8. Ⓐ Ⓑ Ⓒ Ⓓ   10. Ⓐ Ⓑ Ⓒ Ⓓ

Test 5

1. Ⓐ Ⓑ Ⓒ Ⓓ   3. Ⓐ Ⓑ Ⓒ Ⓓ   5. Ⓐ Ⓑ Ⓒ Ⓓ   7. Ⓐ Ⓑ Ⓒ Ⓓ   8. Ⓐ Ⓑ Ⓒ Ⓓ
2. Ⓐ Ⓑ Ⓒ Ⓓ   4. Ⓐ Ⓑ Ⓒ Ⓓ   6. Ⓐ Ⓑ Ⓒ Ⓓ

Test 6

1. Ⓐ Ⓑ Ⓒ Ⓓ   3. Ⓐ Ⓑ Ⓒ Ⓓ   4. Ⓐ Ⓑ Ⓒ Ⓓ   5. Ⓐ Ⓑ Ⓒ Ⓓ   6. Ⓐ Ⓑ Ⓒ Ⓓ
2. Ⓐ Ⓑ Ⓒ Ⓓ

answer sheet

READING COMPREHENSION TEST 1

15 Questions • 35 Minutes

Directions: Carefully read the following paragraphs and then answer the accompanying questions, basing your answer on what is stated or implied in the paragraphs. When you have decided which choice is best, fill in the corresponding space on your answer sheet. There is only one best answer for each question.

Taking It to Heart

A

Prior to 1628, when William Harvey published his book on the circulation of the blood and the operation of the heart, no one really knew or understood the function of the heart or how it worked. There was some speculation about it having something to do with the blood; however, people generally thought of it as the place in the body from which love and courage were generated.

B

Until Harvey's discovery, no one was aware that the heart is one of the toughest muscles in the human body and one of the most awesome pumps in the world. It is the heart that pumps the blood throughout the body night and day. This mighty muscle, though only the size of a clenched fist, does enough work in one 24-hour period to lift a man weighing 150 pounds to an altitude of almost 1,000 feet into the air.

C

Actually, the heart is two pumps, side by side—one on the right and one on the left. The right pump sends blood from the veins to the lungs. Then it pumps blood through the lungs to the pump on the left, which sends it through the body.

1. Based upon paragraph A, which of these statements is true?
   (A) One function of the heart is to generate love and courage in a human being.
   (B) The purpose and function of the heart was not understood until 1628.
   (C) Harvey published a book that dealt with performing operations on the heart.
   (D) The fact that the heart is instrumental in the circulation of the blood is merely speculation.

2. According to paragraph B, it is understood that
   (A) the heart is a muscle that pumps blood throughout the body.
   (B) Harvey discovered the heart.
   (C) the heart can lift a man weighing 150 pounds to a height of 1,000 feet.
   (D) all muscles in the human body perform as pumps.

3. The main idea of paragraph C is that
   (A) the right pump of the heart sends blood from the veins to the lungs.
   (B) the pumps that make up the heart are situated side by side.
   (C) the left pump sends the blood through the body.
   (D) the heart is two pumps that work to send blood throughout the body.

D

Although the right- and left-hand sides of the heart are two different pumps with no direct connection between them, they squeeze and relax in just about the same rhythm. Together they pump approximately 13,000 quarts of blood through the body daily.

E

The most amazing thing about the heart is that it continues beating throughout life, resting only a fraction of a second after each beat. Considering that this entails 100,000 beats per day, the durability of this organ is undoubtedly phenomenal.

4. Paragraph D makes the point that
   - (A) the human body contains 13,000 quarts of blood.
   - (B) despite the fact that they squeeze and relax in just about the same rhythm, the two pumps do not have a connection.
   - (C) the rhythm of the two pumps is synchronized.
   - (D) the two pumps operate as one.

5. Which statement is supported by paragraph E?
   - (A) The third part of the heartbeat is a period of rest.
   - (B) A steady heartbeat is characteristic of a strong and healthy heart.
   - (C) The heart beats about 70 times per minute.
   - (D) You can easily detect your own heartbeat.

The Skin You're In

F

The first thing you see when you look at the human body is the skin. The average adult human body is covered with about 18 square feet of skin. Skin varies in thickness. It is very thin over the eyelids and considerably thicker on the palms of the hands and the soles of the feet.

G

The skin is composed of two layers. The outer layer of skin is called the epidermis. This name comes from ancient Greek meaning "outer layer." This layer is made up of dead, flattened cells that are continually sloughing off as we move around. The bottom of the epidermis is made of live cells that die and replace those that wear off on the surface. Throughout the body's lifetime, the under layer of skin continually creates new cells. This is the reason why cuts and scrapes heal in a short period of time.

H

Beneath the outer layer is another layer called the dermis. This is a much deeper layer made entirely of living cells. There are several small blood vessels and nerve endings in the dermis. There are coiled tubes in this layer that open into the epidermis layer through openings called pores. The pores are openings to the coiled tubes or sweat glands. Hairs, which grow out of the skin, are rooted in the dermis. They grow out of openings called hair follicles. Oil glands in the skin connected with the hair roots constantly oil the outer skin, keeping it supple and strong.

6. From paragraph F, the reader can conclude that

    (A) the skin is the one organ readily visible on the human body.

    (B) adults have thicker skin than children.

    (C) skin on the human body is thicker on parts of the body most likely to come in contact with foreign objects and surfaces.

    (D) 18 square feet of skin would be adequate to cover and protect all adult human beings.

7. From paragraph G, it may be inferred that

    (A) the production of new cells constitutes healing in the human being.

    (B) the ancient Greeks were probably the first to study skin.

    (C) the bottom of the epidermis is comprised of flattened cells that gradually wear away.

    (D) skin is the organ responsible for growth in the human body.

8. Which statement is supported by paragraph H?

    (A) The skin needs oil to remain pliant and durable.

    (B) The coiled tubes in the epidermis are actually pores.

    (C) Dry skin may be an indication of a problem in the hair follicle.

    (D) The epidermis provides the body with adequate temperature control.

I

The functions of the skin are numerous. The skin is a protective covering for the body that is airtight and waterproof. When it is unbroken it is a barrier to harmful bacteria. The coloring matter of the skin, known as pigment, serves to screen out certain harmful rays of the sun. The skin helps to regulate the temperature of the body and also functions as a sense organ. There are many nerve endings in the skin that caution us to stay away from things that are too hot or too cold and cause us to have a sense of touch. They enable us to detect sensation in our immediate surroundings and transmit impulses to the brain where the sensations are identified.

9. According to paragraph I, it is understood that

    (A) skin coloring is the result of harmful rays of the sun.

    (B) sensations are directly perceived by the skin.

    (C) the function of the skin is merely that of a protective covering.

    (D) the skin is a deterrent to harmful bacteria only if it is unbroken.

Nursing Interventions

J

The term "nursing interventions" encompasses and describes activities that reflect nursing responsibility in the execution of health treatment. More specifically, it refers to nursing treatments, nursing observations, health teaching, and medical treatment performed by nurses. A nursing intervention is a single course of action intended to fulfill the unmet human needs that are ascertained from the patient's problem. A nursing diagnosis is, therefore, a prerequisite to implementing the appropriate care to meet the needs of the patient. It is apparent that in order to determine and initiate nursing intervention, one must have a scientific background and extensive education in nursing.

10. The main idea of paragraph J is that

    (A) the role of an individual who has a scientific and nursing education background, and who performs a single course of action to satisfy the unmet human needs of a patient, is known as nursing intervention.

    (B) a nursing diagnosis is synonymous with nursing intervention.

    (C) nursing responsibility includes health teaching.

    (D) nursing assessment is necessary for effective nursing intervention.

Blood Donors Available—No Thanks! I'll Do It Myself!

K

With the advent of AIDS and other communicable diseases, people are reluctant to submit to blood transfusions as a measure of medical treatment, even in emergency situations. Many individuals are opting to store their own blood in case it is ever needed.

L

New blood cells are constantly being produced in the body. This is the reason that lost blood in a healthy person is replaced quickly. This rapid production of blood cells also enables a person to donate to others who might need blood. When blood is taken from one person and given to another, the procedure is called a homologous blood transfer. When a person's own blood is used for transfusion, having been stored in anticipation of surgery, the procedure is known as autologous blood transfer. This blood is collected prior to surgery.

M

Though the concept of being transfused with one's own blood is very comforting, there are many factors that discourage the use of this technology. First is the expense of storing the blood. Another drawback is that a patient may be thousands of miles away from his or her blood supply or blood bank when the need for blood arises.

11. The accelerated interest in autologous transfusion is due to

    (A) a lack of blood donors.

    (B) an attempt to stimulate rapid production of new blood cells.

    (C) the time-saving element in the event of emergency surgery.

    (D) a rise in fear of communicable diseases.

N

In an attempt to satisfy patients' requests to be transfused with their own blood, regardless of the medical emergency, doctors have developed two forms of autologous blood transfusion. One form utilizes suction devices to collect blood lost during surgery. After this blood has been cleansed, it may be put back into the body. Blood lost during surgery can also be collected with sponges. The sponges are then squeezed out into a container of saline solution, a kind of salt solution. This blood is processed within 15 minutes and is again introduced into the patient's circulation. Doctors believe that by using both methods they can retrieve up to 90 percent of blood that would otherwise be lost.

O

Despite these efforts to make autologous blood transfer feasible for most patients, there still remain those situations that make it virtually impossible to collect blood. For instance, in the case of an auto accident victim, much blood is often lost before medical treatment is obtainable. To help in an incident such as this, doctors are researching ways to develop artificial hemoglobin that would temporarily transport oxygen and carbon dioxide throughout the body. Another solution being explored is the reproduction of a hormone that causes the body to produce blood cells much more rapidly than it would normally. This would mean that the body could replace most of its own blood and therefore reduce the need for transfusion. Even though researchers are doing extensive work to develop new techniques to protect people from blood tainted by disease, reserving one's own blood for future use seems to be the safest method of transfusion for now.

12. This passage supports the concept that

   (A) autologous transfer is a practical and easily accessible alternative to blood transfusion.

   (B) any type of blood transfusion places a patient in a high-risk health situation.

   (C) hemoglobin carries oxygen and carbon dioxide throughout the body.

   (D) lost blood, even in a healthy person, is replaced only after a long period of time.

13. From this passage it may be inferred that

   (A) saline is a cleansing or sterilizing agent.

   (B) the storing of one's own blood supply is affordable for all.

   (C) homologous transfusion requires blood typing and matching.

   (D) the option of autologous transfusion is not feasible in instances of elective surgery.

14. A fact expressed in this passage is that

   (A) artificial hemoglobin could permanently supply the body with oxygen and carbon dioxide.

   (B) suction devices and sponges are two surgical implements used in the collection of blood lost during surgery.

   (C) laser surgery is being used more frequently in an effort to minimize blood loss during surgery.

   (D) autologous transfusion, in the event of surgery, requires that the blood always be collected prior to surgery.

15. This article suggests that

   (A) homologous transfusions are on the decline.

   (B) the effort by researchers to protect patients from blood contaminated by disease cannot guarantee safe blood transfusion.

   (C) autologous transfusion is impractical.

   (D) surgical patients who are transfused autonomously are assured a more rapid recovery.

STOP

IF YOU FINISH BEFORE TIME IS CALLED, YOU MAY CHECK YOUR WORK ON THIS SECTION ONLY. DO NOT TURN TO ANY OTHER SECTION IN THE TEST.

READING COMPREHENSION TEST 2

8 Questions • 12 Minutes

Directions: Carefully read the following passage and then answer the accompanying questions, basing your answers on what is stated or implied in the passage. When you have decided which choice is best, fill in the corresponding space on your answer sheet. There is only one best answer for each question.

Live and Learn

A

It has been a difficult year. As our country and the world continue to cope with the aftermath of September 11, 2001, some people have boldly chosen to take their lives back. Many others, though, are finding it extremely difficult to move on.

1. Paragraph A implies that the events of September 11, 2001 were
   (A) devastating.
   (B) unavoidable,
   (C) pragmatic.
   (D) intolerable.

2. The event(s) alluded to impacted
   (A) nationally.
   (B) globally.
   (C) positively.
   (D) moderately.

B

It is troubling that thousands of lives were taken in a heartbeat, and now we're witnessing a domino effect across the globe as a result of the attacks on America. It's no secret that the U.S. is an ally of Israel and that this position has been the fuel for terrorist attacks on our soil. But war in the Middle East has been brewing for years, so now we explore other issues that contribute to the conflict.

3. According to the writer, the loss of lives was
   (A) instantaneous.
   (B) by heart malfunction.
   (C) ephemeral.
   (D) predictable.

C

Are immigration and integration in Palestine to blame? What about U.S. dollars going to Israel? Or Muslim extremists? Whatever the reasons, every nation is adjusting its policies to ready themselves for what might be coming. Recently, the United States and a bloc of Southeast Asian nations signed a treaty aimed at making the region—a second front in the war against terrorism—more responsive to future threats. Sadly, it took a tragedy of this magnitude to get America to realize that it's not invincible and that we really are living in an interdependent world.

4. It is suggested that the attacks of 9/11 may be directly related to

    (A) the ongoing Middle East oil dispute.

    (B) the absence of a treaty between the United States and Southeast Asian nations.

    (C) Palestinians' hatred of the United States.

    (D) U.S. aid to and friendship with Israel.

5. America's realization of its vulnerability

    (A) has prompted Middle East peace talks.

    (B) has resulted in more gun control laws.

    (C) is a significant outcome of 9/11.

    (D) has resulted in relaxed national security.

6. The author mentions "domino effect" to describe

    (A) the falling of the towers.

    (B) the mass physical destruction that came out of this event.

    (C) the far-reaching consequences that stem from 9/11.

    (D) the political turmoil that was caused by 9/11.

D

The nation's economy is in a serious slump. The failures of such high-performing companies as Enron, and the government investigations of others, including AOL Time Warner and MCI WorldCom, Inc., which was charged with fraud after the company admitted to hiding almost $4 billion in costs, has contributed to the stock market nosedive.

E

The ripple effects of the U.S. economic woes are widespread. Stress is on the rise for good reasons. The Dow Jones industrial average recently reached its largest weekly decline (nearly 700 points) since last September. Retirees are having to re-enter the work force, and who doesn't know someone who's recently lost his or her job? People continue to file claims for unemployment insurance, and a study released roughly four months after the attacks predicted that the effects of the more than 1.6 million jobs that will probably be lost in 2002 will reverberate through the U.S. economy for years to come.

F

The jobless are penny-pinching and postponing vacations, which is a dire dilemma for many tourism-dependent nations. Caribbean countries like Jamaica and St. Lucia are expected to lose $3 billion tourism revenue—money that is normally used for health care and other services and accounts for roughly 70 percent of the gross domestic product of many Caribbean countries.

G

Everyone has been affected by September 11 in one way or another. Even though we've struggled through the past year, we, as Americans, are truly blessed. What is most important now is to accept what has taken place, and to learn and grow from it. It takes faith, and it is that faith that has guided our people for centuries. So take pride in this country and help make it a better place for you and your children.

—Reprinted with permission of Upscale
from Founder's Desk, Live and Learn,
by Bernard Bronner, Founder.
Upscale, October 2002.

7. The tragedy of 9/11 has
   (A) left all of humankind emotionally scarred.
   (B) drastically changed our lives and the way we view life.
   (C) helped the economy rally.
   (D) strengthened relations between the United States and the Middle East.

8. The attitude of the author is one of
   (A) defeat.
   (B) hopefulness.
   (C) indifference.
   (D) despair.

STOP

IF YOU FINISH BEFORE TIME IS CALLED, YOU MAY CHECK
YOUR WORK ON THIS SECTION ONLY. DO NOT TURN TO ANY
OTHER SECTION IN THE TEST.

READING COMPREHENSION TEST 3

9 Questions • 12 Minutes

Directions: Carefully read the following passage and then answer the accompanying questions, basing your answers on what is stated or implied in the passage. When you have decided which choice is best, fill in the corresponding space on your answer sheet. There is only one best answer for each question.

Is It Your Fault If You're Fat?

A

Why are more Americans overweight and developing diabetes? Is it fast food? No regular meals and precious little exercise? Our love affair with the TV and computer? The wrong advice about what to eat?

B

Very likely it's all these things—combined with something about the genetic make-up in many of us. Genes may program some to feel hungry when they aren't and others to be less able to tell when they are full.

1. The generalization could be made that obesity is caused by

   (A) eating fast foods.

   (B) lack of exercise.

   (C) lack of education as to which foods to eat.

   (D) lifestyle and genetic makeup.

2. People are programmed to feel hungry (when they actually are not) by

   (A) therapists.

   (B) genes.

   (C) nutritional counseling.

   (D) dining trends.

C

Some extreme obesity in children is caused by an identifiable, single gene defect. Obesity is no more their "fault" than developing cystic fibrosis is the "fault" of a child who has the CF gene. Admittedly, perhaps only 5 percent of obesity is purely genetic. But research suggests that multiple genes control appetite and metabolism, and defects in one or more may make someone more prone to being overweight. Fat cells, particularly in the abdomen, in turn release substances that can make people more prone to insulin resistance, which leads to Type 2 diabetes.

D

Some people are genetically blessed and never gain much weight. Those with gene defects must expend huge effort to overcome messages their bodies are sending their brains to eat more.

3. People who are more prone to insulin resistance are

   (A) candidates for stomach problems.

   (B) those with no weight problem.

   (C) those who are likely to develop Type 2 diabetes.

   (D) in danger of becoming obese.

4. When great effort is put forth, people with gene defects can

   (A) overcome urges to eat more.

   (B) overcome diabetes.

   (C) live a normal life.

   (D) be overweight.

5. The author's purpose in this passage is to

   (A) inform.

   (B) persuade.

   (C) entertain.

   (D) analyze.

E

For example, research at Rockefeller University and elsewhere suggests that people who lack leptin or lack receptors to make their cells sensitive to leptin have uncontrolled hunger, overeat, and become extremely obese. The melanocortin pathway in the brain has recently been identified by scientists at Beth Israel Deaconess Medical Center and elsewhere as another target influencing both obesity and anorexia.

F

In addition, some researchers have shown that the absence of a peptide called MSH, which suppresses eating, leads to obesity. Research at Joslin Diabetes Center in Boston and elsewhere suggests that another peptide, MCH, which stimulates eating, may also play a role.

6. Researchers have found that

   (A) an overabundance of leptin causes obesity.

   (B) the absence of a certain substance in the body results in uncontrolled eating.

   (C) MHS is a peptide.

   (D) overeating is a habit.

7. Obesity may be defined as

   (A) fat.

   (B) a state of being significantly overweight.

   (C) a genetic condition.

   (D) a disease related to overeating.

G

Ghrelin, a stomach hormone that signals hunger, is another potential target. Interestingly, extremely obese individuals who undergo stomach bypass surgery (stomach stapling) may be less inclined to eat afterwards because food no longer passes through the section of the stomach that produces ghrelin.

H

Some overeating may be trigged by stress, boredom, or depression. For example, food smells may stimulate production of certain peptides that make one want to eat—even if not hungry. Behavior modification may be needed to combat these stimulants of weight gain.

I

As our genes haven't changed in the last 20–30 years, societal influences are still the major culprit for growing obesity. We are more sedentary. Super-sizing meals makes it harder not to eat for those trying mightily to ignore the errant signals their bodies are sending. Until we can identify who has what gene defects, and the medications are developed to treat them, we must remember that it is much easier to prevent weight gain than to lose weight once gained. Your body adjusts quickly to these extra calories.

J

Life as overweight adults often has its roots in life as a child. For the moment, the best approach to obesity, and the Type 2 diabetes it causes, is prevention—in ourselves and our children. As nationwide studies show, even modest weight loss—15 pounds—and 30 minutes of daily exercise, are the best ways to prevent diabetes in those most likely to develop it.

—Copyright © Joslin Diabetes Center.
Reprinted with permission from *Time*,
"Is It Your Fault If You're Fat?"
by Eleftheria Marasthos-Flier, M.D., and Jeffrey S. Flier, M.D.
Time Magazine Special Advertising
Section, November 4, 2002.

8. The main idea of this passage is that

   (A) overeating can be controlled with diet and exercise.

   (B) diabetes is related to obesity.

   (C) current research reveals a number of contributing factors to obesity.

   (D) there are cures for obesity.

9. From this passage one can draw the conclusion that

   (A) being overweight is unhealthy.

   (B) children, too, can have weight problems.

   (C) being fat may not necessarily be the fault of the obese individual.

   (D) obesity can be attributed solely to genetics.

STOP

IF YOU FINISH BEFORE TIME IS CALLED, YOU MAY CHECK YOUR WORK ON THIS SECTION ONLY. DO NOT TURN TO ANY OTHER SECTION IN THE TEST.

READING COMPREHENSION TEST 4

10 Questions • 13 Minutes

Directions: Carefully read the following passage and then answer the accompanying questions, basing your answers on what is stated or implied in the passage. When you have decided which choice is best, fill in the corresponding space on your answer sheet. There is only one best answer for each question.

With the recent use of DNA (deoxyribonucleic acid) as a means of providing evidence in a number of world-renowned criminal cases, the general public views this carrier of genetic information as a modern-day scientific discovery. However, a glimpse at the history of DNA will prove the notion of a "modern-day miracle" quite to the contrary.

To investigate the discovery of DNA, one would have to research the laboratory and work of the Swiss biochemist, Johan Friedrich Miescher, back in 1868. Miescher had been involved in the study of the cell nucleus, the round control center that contains the chromosomes as well as other elements. He believed that cells were made of protein and attempted to break down this protein with a digestive enzyme. As Miescher continued this investigation, he was perplexed by the fact that the enzyme would break down the cell but not the nucleus. He then launched an investigation of the substance that comprised the cell. As he analyzed it, he saw that it contained large amounts of a strange material that was very unlike protein. Miescher chose to call this substance nuclein. He had no idea of its significance, nor did he recognize that he had discovered what came to be known in later years as nucleic acid. Nucleic acid is the chemical family to which DNA belongs.

In 1944, a team of scientists from the Rockefeller Institute proved for the first time that DNA was the carrier of hereditary information. Oswald T. Avery, Colin M. MacLeod, and Maclyn McCarty accomplished this by extracting some of the DNA in pure form from a bacterium and substituting it for a defective gene in another related bacterium.

Some ten years later, the intricate molecular structure of DNA was described by Harvard biochemist James D. Watson and physicist Francis Crick of Great Britain. However, prior to this, scientist Rosalind Franklin discovered that the DNA molecule was a strand of molecules in a spiral form. Dr. Franklin demonstrated that the spiral was so large that it was most likely formed by two spirals. Ultimately, Franklin determined that the structure of DNA is similar to the handrails and steps of a spiral staircase.

Equipped with the work and findings of Rosalind Franklin and others, Watson and Crick were able to construct a model of a DNA molecule. This model depicted the sides or "handrails" of the DNA molecules as being made up of two twisted strands of sugar and phosphate molecules. The "stairs" that hold the two sugar phosphate strands apart are made up of molecules called nitrogen bases.

All of this data supports the fact that DNA is by no means a "new discovery"; however, what is the significance of it at all? Why is DNA important to you? The answer is that all of the characteristics you possess are affected by the DNA in your cells. It controls the color of your eyes, the color of your hair, and whether or not you have a tolerance for dairy products. These characteristics are known as traits. The way your traits appear depends on the kinds of proteins your cells make. DNA stores the blueprints for making the proteins. Your DNA is uniquely different from that of anyone else on earth, and you are identifiable by these proteins.

1. It could be concluded that
   (A) Watson and Crick discovered DNA.
   (B) the strands of DNA take the form of a double hexagon.
   (C) DNA is as unique to individuals as a fingerprint.
   (D) Miescher's analysis of nuclein resulted directly in the discovery of DNA.

2. From this passage, it may be deduced that enzymes are
   - **(A)** unstable.
   - **(B)** ineffective.
   - **(C)** catalysts.
   - **(D)** solutions.

3. It may be inferred that an individual's DNA determines
   - **(A)** whether or not he or she can digest milk.
   - **(B)** whether or not he or she is immune to the common cold.
   - **(C)** an individual's choice of residential location.
   - **(D)** a person's inclination toward dishonesty.

4. The types of protein produced by a cell are controlled by the DNA contained in its
   - **(A)** nitrogen bases.
   - **(B)** nucleus.
   - **(C)** cell wall.
   - **(D)** sugar phosphate bands.

5. It is implied that proteins are the
   - **(A)** control center of the cell.
   - **(B)** blueprint of the cell.
   - **(C)** storage center of the cell.
   - **(D)** building blocks of a cell.

6. A reference to the "spiral staircase" constitutes a description of the molecular structure of
   - **(A)** proteins.
   - **(B)** digestive enzymes.
   - **(C)** RNA.
   - **(D)** DNA.

7. Digestive enzymes are effective in breaking up
   - **(A)** nuclein.
   - **(B)** DNA.
   - **(C)** all chemical compounds.
   - **(D)** protein.

8. The word "nucleus" refers to
   - **(A)** the round control center of the cell.
   - **(B)** the walls of the cell.
   - **(C)** a strand of molecules.
   - **(D)** a helix.

9. The scientific disciplines used in determining the structure of the DNA molecule include biology, chemistry, and
    (A) genealogy.
    (B) serology.
    (C) physics.
    (D) embryology.

10. As described in this passage, "model" means
    (A) an exhibitor of fashion.
    (B) a physical form representing a concept.
    (C) a miniature version of an existing object.
    (D) a person on whom an artist bases his or her rendition.

STOP

IF YOU FINISH BEFORE TIME IS CALLED, YOU MAY CHECK
YOUR WORK ON THIS SECTION ONLY. DO NOT TURN TO ANY
OTHER SECTION IN THE TEST.

READING COMPREHENSION TEST 5

8 Questions • 8 Minutes

Directions: Carefully read the following passage and then answer the accompanying questions, basing your answers on what is stated or implied in the passage. When you have decided which choice is best, fill in the corresponding space on your answer sheet. There is only one best answer for each question.

Computer Watch Your Step

A

Can a computer spot a criminal or a terrorist infiltrating an airport tarmac? Face-recognition programs are useless if a person's face is obscured, unlit, or just too far away. So a number of researchers are trying to identify a person simply by the way he or she walks.

B

One approach is to collect video images of the surveillance area and analyze everybody passing through. "We've been trying to measure things like stride length and body shapes," says Aaron Bobick, a computer vision researcher at Georgia Tech in Atlanta. Video cameras still require good light and a clear view, however, so Gene Greneker at the Georgia Tech Research Institute is experimenting with radar. "It can see through clothes, at night, at long ranges," he says.

1. The title of this article
   (A) cautions computers to watch their step.
   (B) cautions readers to watch their step.
   (C) implies that computers will be able to observe the way people walk.
   (D) implies that computers are a threat.

2. "Surveillance" means
   (A) hidden.
   (B) obscure.
   (C) large surface.
   (D) observed.

3. It is implied that
   (A) radar may be an alternative to problems encountered with video cameras.
   (B) good light and clear vision are attainable with video cameras.
   (C) computer vision researchers at Virginia Tech are advancing surveillance technology.
   (D) it will be a long time before this technology is available.

4. The video cameras
   (A) sweep a designated area.
   (B) view the perimeter of the area to be inspected.
   (C) collect images that pass through the surveillance area.
   (D) have zoom lenses that capture close-ups of people in the surveillance area.

C

Greneker and his team use a device that sends out a signal and measures the echo. If the return waves shift to higher frequencies, that means they reflected off something approaching. "There are different shifts for different body parts, because they are moving at different velocities," Greneker says. A computer program analyzes these shifts and creates a radar fingerprint for each person's walk. So far, researchers have collected gait profiles of about 100 test subjects, which the program can identify up to 80 percent of the time. That is not nearly good enough for airport security, but Bobick is convinced gait recognition can be made to work. "If I show you moving light displays of people walking, you can distinguish one person from the next. We know the information is there."

—Reprinted with permission from *Discover*,
"Computer Watch Your Step" by Fenella Saunders,
Discover Special Issue: The Year in Science, January 2003.

5. The device used by Greneker and his team

(A) lowers the frequencies.

(B) sends out a signal and measures the echo.

(C) shifts different body parts.

(D) changes the velocities.

6. The identification accuracy is

(A) very high.

(B) moderately low.

(C) average.

(D) moderately high.

7. The researchers have

(A) approved the device for airport security.

(B) not been able to distinguish one person from the next.

(C) completed their study.

(D) gathered gait profiles of subjects.

8. "Gait" most nearly means

(A) style of walking.

(B) fence.

(C) door.

(D) speed of walking.

STOP

IF YOU FINISH BEFORE TIME IS CALLED, YOU MAY CHECK YOUR WORK ON THIS SECTION ONLY. DO NOT TURN TO ANY OTHER SECTION IN THE TEST.

READING COMPREHENSION TEST 6

6 Questions • 8 Minutes

Directions: Carefully read the following passage and then answer the accompanying questions, basing your answers on what is stated or implied in the passage. When you have decided which choice is best, fill in the corresponding space on your answer sheet. There is only one best answer for each question.

A

During my stay at an expensive hotel in New York City, I woke up in the middle of the night with an upset stomach. I called room service and ordered some soda crackers. When I looked at the charge slip, I was furious. I called room service and fumed, "I know I'm in a luxury hotel, but $11.50 for six crackers is outrageous!"

B

"The crackers are complimentary," the voice at the other end coolly explained. "I believe you are complaining about your room number."

—Reprinted with permission from the
January 2003 *Reader's Digest*, "Life in these United States"
by Robert Menchim.

1. The purpose of this reading selection is to
   (A) persuade.
   (B) explain.
   (C) entertain.
   (D) inform.

2. It may be assumed that
   (A) the writer does not have sufficient reading comprehension skills.
   (B) the format of the bill included several numbers and was difficult to interpret.
   (C) room service had made an error.
   (D) the hotel guest is frugal.

3. The word "complimentary" means that the crackers were
   (A) well suited to the hotel guest.
   (B) served with other crackers.
   (C) free.
   (D) not to be ordered.

4. The author's tone in the call to room service is
   (A) humorous.
   (B) one of outrage.
   (C) sarcastic.
   (D) bland.

5. The author implies that
   (A) the anticipated services were costly at this particular hotel.
   (B) all New York hotels are expensive.
   (C) the hotel was substandard.
   (D) the hotel was not one of his choice.

6. An appropriate title for this story would be
   (A) Things Are Not Always What They Seem.
   (B) Quality and Price Are Synonymous.
   (C) A Room at the Top.
   (D) Look Before You Leap.

STOP

IF YOU FINISH BEFORE TIME IS CALLED, YOU MAY CHECK
YOUR WORK ON THIS SECTION ONLY. DO NOT TURN TO ANY
OTHER SECTION IN THE TEST.

ANSWER KEY AND EXPLANATIONS

Test 1

1. B	4. B	7. A	10. A	13. A
2. A	5. C	8. A	11. D	14. B
3. D	6. C	9. D	12. C	15. B

1. **The correct answer is (B).** Sentence 1 states that "Prior to 1628, . . . no one really knew or understood the function of the heart."

2. **The correct answer is (A).** Sentence 2 states that "the heart is a muscle that pumps the blood throughout the body."

3. **The correct answer is (D).** You are looking for the answer that restates what the paragraph is generally about. Choice (D) is the best, most all-encompassing statement. The other choices restate just one or two details mentioned in the paragraph.

4. **The correct answer is (B).** Choice (B) restates sentence 1, so it is the correct answer. The information neither in choice (C) nor in choice (D) is mentioned in the paragraph, so they are easy to rule out immediately.

5. **The correct answer is (C).** A simple mental math calculation verifies that choice (C) is correct. This question asks you to infer an answer from the information given. You can eliminate Choice (A) because the paragraph doesn't divide heartbeats into thirds. The paragraph doesn't provide or imply information about steady heartbeats, choice (B), or being able to detect your own heartbeat, choice (D).

6. **The correct answer is (C).** The question has the word *conclude* in it, which is a signal that you will need to figure out the answer from the information given; the answer is not directly stated. The only answer that fulfills this requirement is choice (C). Choice (A) is directly stated, so rule it out. There is nothing stated or

implied to indicate that either choice (B) or choice (D) is correct.

7. **The correct answer is (A).** The answer can be inferred from the information presented in sentences 6 and 7. Mentioning that the Greeks named the epidermis doesn't necessarily mean they were the first to study skin. Choices (C) and (D) are neither implied nor directly stated.

8. **The correct answer is (A).** Choice (A) paraphrases the last sentence in paragraph H. Choice (B) misstates information in the paragraph, and choices (C) and (D) provide information neither stated nor implied.

9. **The correct answer is (D).** Choice (D) paraphrases sentence 3. Choices (A), (B), and (C) misstate information in the paragraph.

10. **The correct answer is (A).** Only choice (A) provides an overview of the details in paragraph J. The other answer choices state just a single detail each.

11. **The correct answer is (D).** Choice (D) restates sentence 1 in paragraph K. None of the other choices correctly restate information in the paragraphs.

12. **The correct answer is (C).** The answer is found in paragraph O, sentence 3. Choices (A) and (D) are the opposite of what the passage says. Choice (B) is not mentioned in either paragraph.

13. **The correct answer is (A).** Sentence 4 in paragraph N is the basis for selecting choice (A). There is no information in the passage to support choices (B), (C), or (D) as valid inferences.

14. **The correct answer is (B).** Sentences 1, 2, and 4 in paragraph N provide the basis for selecting choice (B). Choice (A) is the opposite of what the paragraph states, and choice (D) is the opposite of what the paragraph implies. Choice (C) has no basis in any paragraph.

15. **The correct answer is (B).** If you weren't sure of the answer, you could use the process of elimination. Nothing in the article supports choices (A), (C), or (D).

Test 2

1. A	3. A	5. C	7. B
2. B	4. D	6. C	8. B

1. **The correct answer is (A).** *Devastating,* meaning "causing destruction including physical and mental destruction," best fits the sense of paragraph A. Choice (D), *intolerable,* may seem like a good choice, but it means "more than can be put up with, irritating" and doesn't fit the sense as well *devastating."* Choice (B), *unavoidable,* makes no sense and neither does Choice (C), *pragmatic,* meaning "practical."

2. **The correct answer is (B).** Sentence 2 states that the world had to cope, so *globally,* choice (B), is the correct answer.

3. **The correct answer is (A).** "In a heartbeat," sentence 1, implies *instantaneously,* choice (A). Be careful of trick answers like choice (B), *by heart malfunction.* On a quick reading of the passage, you might choose this answer.

4. **The correct answer is (D).** You can infer choice (D) based on sentence 2 in the paragraph. Neither choice (A) nor choice (C) is either stated directly or implied. Choice (B) misstates information in the passage.

5. **The correct answer is (C).** Only choice (C) accurately restates information in the paragraph; the answer is in the final sentence.

6. **The correct answer is (C).** The answer can be found in paragraph B and in sentences 1 to 5 in paragraph C. No mention is made in the passage of information in choices (A) or (B). Choice (C) is a better answer than choice (D) because it contains a wider range of consequences than simply political turmoil.

7. **The correct answer is (B).** Choice (B) can be inferred from the information in paragraphs C, D, E, and F. Nothing in the article supports choices (A) or (D), and choice (C) is the opposite of what the article says.

8. **The correct answer is (B).** Paragraph G supports choice (B) as the correct answer.

Test 3

1. D	4. A	6. B	8. C
2. B	5. A	7. B	9. C
3. C			

1. **The correct answer is (D).** A generalization is defined as "a principle or theory with general application." The only answer that fits this definition is choice (D) because it includes two large, or general, ideas: lifestyle and genetic makeup. The other answers are too narrow in their descriptions of the problem.

2. **The correct answer is (B).** Sentence 2 in paragraph B directly states the answer.

3. **The correct answer is (C).** The final sentence in paragraph C states this answer directly.

4. **The correct answer is (A).** The final sentence in paragraph D states this answer directly.

5. **The correct answer is (A).** The author is stating facts, so choice (A), *inform,* is the best answer. There is nothing *persuasive* or *entertaining,* choices (B) and (C), about the passage. While *analyze,* choice (D), may tempt you, the passage is not examining the data methodically, but explaining it.

6. **The correct answer is (B).** The answer is directly stated in paragraph E, sentence 1.

7. **The correct answer is (B).** If you didn't know this, you could infer it from paragraph C, especially sentence 4, which discusses obesity and being overweight.

8. **The correct answer is (C).** To find a main idea statement, you need to look for the statement that encompasses the most information in the passage. Only choice (C) satisfies this criterion.

9. **The correct answer is (C).** To draw a conclusion about the passage in its entirety, you need to consider what the passage is mainly about. Choices (A) and (B) are only two points made in the passage. Choice (D) can be eliminated because it contradicts what the passage says. That leaves only choice (C), which is the correct answer.

Test 4

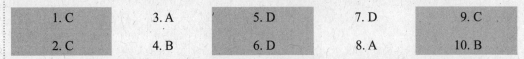

1. C	3. A	5. D	7. D	9. C
2. C	4. B	6. D	8. A	10. B

1. **The correct answer is (C).** The analogy is not stated in the passage, but the last sentence in the article describes DNA as unique and you can infer the analogy from that. The other statements are incorrect and inaccurate.

2. **The correct answer is (C).** This answer can be inferred from information in sentences 3 and 4 in paragraph 2.

3. **The correct answer is (A).** The answer is stated in the last paragraph, sentence 4.

4. **The correct answer is (B).** The answer is found in paragraph 2 in sentences 2 through 4.

5. **The correct answer is (D).** This answer can be inferred from the information in the final paragraph.

6. **The correct answer is (D).** The answer is the last sentence of paragraph 4.

7. **The correct answer is (D).** The answer is in sentence 3 of paragraph 2.

8. **The correct answer is (A).** The answer is in sentence 2 of paragraph 2.

9. **The correct answer is (C).** The answer is in sentence 1 of paragraph 4. Francis Crick is referred to as a physicist.

10. **The correct answer is (B).** The answer can be inferred from the use of the word *construct* in sentence 1 of paragraph 5.

Test 5

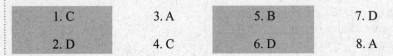

1. C	3. A	5. B	7. D
2. D	4. C	6. D	8. A

1. **The correct answer is (C).** The answer can be inferred from paragraphs 1 and 2. Paragraph 1 sets up the problem and paragraph 2 explores a solution.

2. **The correct answer is (D).** *Surveillance* means "observed, watched over," so choice (D) is the correct answer. Choice (C) makes no sense in the sentence, and while choices (A) and (B), *hidden* and *obscure,* may be tempting, choice (D) is the more precise word.

3. **The correct answer is (A).** The answer is stated in paragraph B, sentences 3 and 4.

4. **The correct answer is (C).** The answer is stated in sentence 1 of paragraph B

5. **The correct answer is (B).** The answer is stated in sentence 1 of paragraph C.

6. **The correct answer is (D).** An 80 percent accuracy rate, stated in sentence 4 of paragraph C, can be categorized as moderately high, choice (D).

7. **The correct answer is (D).** The answer is stated in sentence 4 of paragraph C.

8. **The correct answer is (A).** If you didn't know the answer, you could infer that *gait* means "style of walking" from sentences 2 through 4 in paragraph C. Choice (D) is close, but not as accurate as choice (A).

Test 6

1. C	3. C	4. B	5. A	6. A
2. B				

1. **The correct answer is (C).** The emphasis is on humor in this passage, so choice (C) is the best answer. There is nothing persuasive, explanatory, or informative about the piece.

2. **The correct answer is (B).** You could try the process of eliminate if you weren't sure of the answer. You can eliminate choice (A) immediately because there is nothing to indicate a lack of reading skill by the author, especially since the piece is well written and builds to a climax. Choice (C) is incorrect because the piece indicates that there was no error. While choice (D) may be tempting to choose, Choice (B) makes more sense in the context of the passage.

3. **The correct answer is (C).** Only choice (C) makes sense based on the context of the passage.

4. **The correct answer is (B).** *Outrage* is a near synonym for *furious,* which is how the writer describes himself in paragraph A, sentence 3.

5. **The correct answer is (A).** The answer can be inferred from sentence 4 in paragraph A.

6. **The correct answer is (A).** A title should reflect the main idea of a passage, and choice (A) best describes the scenario recounted in the passage. Choice (D) may be tempting, but the writer did look before he called, but as the answer to question 2 indicates, the bill was confusingly written.

PART IV

PRACTICE FOR ALLIED HEALTH SCHOOL ENTRANCE EXAMINATIONS

Unit 5: Verbal Ability

Unit 6: Quantitative Ability

Unit 7: Science

Unit 8: Reading Comprehension

VERBAL ABILITY ANSWER SHEETS

Synonyms Test 1

1. Ⓐ Ⓑ Ⓒ Ⓓ   8. Ⓐ Ⓑ Ⓒ Ⓓ   15. Ⓐ Ⓑ Ⓒ Ⓓ   22. Ⓐ Ⓑ Ⓒ Ⓓ   29. Ⓐ Ⓑ Ⓒ Ⓓ

2. Ⓐ Ⓑ Ⓒ Ⓓ   9. Ⓐ Ⓑ Ⓒ Ⓓ   16. Ⓐ Ⓑ Ⓒ Ⓓ   23. Ⓐ Ⓑ Ⓒ Ⓓ   30. Ⓐ Ⓑ Ⓒ Ⓓ

3. Ⓐ Ⓑ Ⓒ Ⓓ   10. Ⓐ Ⓑ Ⓒ Ⓓ   17. Ⓐ Ⓑ Ⓒ Ⓓ   24. Ⓐ Ⓑ Ⓒ Ⓓ   31. Ⓐ Ⓑ Ⓒ Ⓓ

4. Ⓐ Ⓑ Ⓒ Ⓓ   11. Ⓐ Ⓑ Ⓒ Ⓓ   18. Ⓐ Ⓑ Ⓒ Ⓓ   25. Ⓐ Ⓑ Ⓒ Ⓓ   32. Ⓐ Ⓑ Ⓒ Ⓓ

5. Ⓐ Ⓑ Ⓒ Ⓓ   12. Ⓐ Ⓑ Ⓒ Ⓓ   19. Ⓐ Ⓑ Ⓒ Ⓓ   26. Ⓐ Ⓑ Ⓒ Ⓓ   33. Ⓐ Ⓑ Ⓒ Ⓓ

6. Ⓐ Ⓑ Ⓒ Ⓓ   13. Ⓐ Ⓑ Ⓒ Ⓓ   20. Ⓐ Ⓑ Ⓒ Ⓓ   27. Ⓐ Ⓑ Ⓒ Ⓓ   34. Ⓐ Ⓑ Ⓒ Ⓓ

7. Ⓐ Ⓑ Ⓒ Ⓓ   14. Ⓐ Ⓑ Ⓒ Ⓓ   21. Ⓐ Ⓑ Ⓒ Ⓓ   28. Ⓐ Ⓑ Ⓒ Ⓓ   35. Ⓐ Ⓑ Ⓒ Ⓓ

Antonyms Test 2

1. Ⓐ Ⓑ Ⓒ Ⓓ Ⓔ   7. Ⓐ Ⓑ Ⓒ Ⓓ Ⓔ   13. Ⓐ Ⓑ Ⓒ Ⓓ Ⓔ   19. Ⓐ Ⓑ Ⓒ Ⓓ Ⓔ   25. Ⓐ Ⓑ Ⓒ Ⓓ Ⓔ

2. Ⓐ Ⓑ Ⓒ Ⓓ Ⓔ   8. Ⓐ Ⓑ Ⓒ Ⓓ Ⓔ   14. Ⓐ Ⓑ Ⓒ Ⓓ Ⓔ   20. Ⓐ Ⓑ Ⓒ Ⓓ Ⓔ   26. Ⓐ Ⓑ Ⓒ Ⓓ Ⓔ

3. Ⓐ Ⓑ Ⓒ Ⓓ Ⓔ   9. Ⓐ Ⓑ Ⓒ Ⓓ Ⓔ   15. Ⓐ Ⓑ Ⓒ Ⓓ Ⓔ   21. Ⓐ Ⓑ Ⓒ Ⓓ Ⓔ   27. Ⓐ Ⓑ Ⓒ Ⓓ Ⓔ

4. Ⓐ Ⓑ Ⓒ Ⓓ Ⓔ   10. Ⓐ Ⓑ Ⓒ Ⓓ Ⓔ   16. Ⓐ Ⓑ Ⓒ Ⓓ Ⓔ   22. Ⓐ Ⓑ Ⓒ Ⓓ Ⓔ   28. Ⓐ Ⓑ Ⓒ Ⓓ Ⓔ

5. Ⓐ Ⓑ Ⓒ Ⓓ Ⓔ   11. Ⓐ Ⓑ Ⓒ Ⓓ Ⓔ   17. Ⓐ Ⓑ Ⓒ Ⓓ Ⓔ   23. Ⓐ Ⓑ Ⓒ Ⓓ Ⓔ   29. Ⓐ Ⓑ Ⓒ Ⓓ Ⓔ

6. Ⓐ Ⓑ Ⓒ Ⓓ Ⓔ   12. Ⓐ Ⓑ Ⓒ Ⓓ Ⓔ   18. Ⓐ Ⓑ Ⓒ Ⓓ Ⓔ   24. Ⓐ Ⓑ Ⓒ Ⓓ Ⓔ   30. Ⓐ Ⓑ Ⓒ Ⓓ Ⓔ

Verbal Ability

OVERVIEW

- Synonyms test 1
- Antonyms test 2
- Answer key and explanations

SYNONYMS TEST 1

35 Questions Time—20 Minutes

Review Unit 1, Synonyms, before attempting this test.

Directions: In each of the following sentences, one word is italicized. For each sentence, select the option that best (or most nearly) corresponds in meaning with the italicized word.

1. It has been recommended that this system to be used in place of *traditional* systems that have been in place for decades.
   - **(A)** unfamiliar
   - **(B)** usual
   - **(C)** flexible
   - **(D)** general

2. In our society, irresponsible behavior often leads to a monetary *penalty*.
   - **(A)** arrangement
   - **(B)** gratification
   - **(C)** punishment
   - **(D)** precaution

3. He spent the *allotted* study time completing his assignments.
   - **(A)** authorized
   - **(B)** designated
   - **(C)** agreed
   - **(D)** alerted

4. The Senate passed the farmland *preservation* bill.
   (A) maintenance
   (B) stratagem
   (C) storage
   (D) incumbency

5. It was apparent that he had attempted to *concoct* an alibi.
   (A) inculcate
   (B) conceal
   (C) reveal
   (D) fabricate

6. The City Council could have avoided this *scenario* by passing the ordinance.
   (A) situation
   (B) setting
   (C) summation
   (D) deficiency

7. The Superior Court judge *imposed* the sentence.
   (A) indicated
   (B) granted
   (C) perpetuated
   (D) prescribed

8. The study was considered *flawed* because the data was self-reported.
   (A) subjective
   (B) inaccurate
   (C) objective
   (D) unscientific

9. Geologists *assure* us that our Earth is a few billion years old.
   (A) guarantee
   (B) instruct
   (C) inform
   (D) advise

10. He was determined to *foil* the scheme of his opponent.
    (A) heighten
    (B) secure
    (C) disencumber
    (D) thwart

11. The examiner *purported* to be an official representative.
    (A) addressed
    (B) claimed
    (C) propitiated
    (D) conciliated

12. The ship carried a *diverse* crowd of vacationers who had come from many countries.
    (A) multitude
    (B) varied
    (C) discrepant
    (D) multiplicity

13. The child could not *recollect* the incident.
    (A) remember
    (B) doubt
    (C) interrogate
    (D) illumine

14. The governor *rescinded* the state of emergency as soon as the roads were cleared of snow.
    (A) negated
    (B) maneuvered
    (C) revoked
    (D) accepted

15. The implementation of the plan was given *scant* consideration.
    (A) audacious
    (B) fervid
    (C) little
    (D) clothed

16. The key speaker, in his lengthy presentation, *scoffed at* the notion of marketing as a public service.
    (A) exonerated
    (B) amplified
    (C) confuted
    (D) mocked

17. She completed the *sprint* with a sudden surge of energy.
    (A) relaxation
    (B) adventure
    (C) run
    (D) convergence

18. The content of the message was *urgent*.
    (A) privileged
    (B) amendable
    (C) pressing
    (D) absolved

19. A *simulated* rescue mission was conducted by the forest rangers.
    (A) pretended
    (B) superficial
    (C) stimulated
    (D) simultaneous

20. Through the course of the day, she became more *agitated* by the noise of the demolition and less focused on her work.
    (A) worried
    (B) upset
    (C) convulsed
    (D) composed

21. Her quickening gait seemed regulated by the *pulse* of the big city.
    (A) utility
    (B) pace
    (C) reverence
    (D) solace

22. The language of the publication is *unsophisticated* but informative.
    (A) ponderous
    (B) elaborate
    (C) simple
    (D) artificial

23. All the evidence presented pointed to *willful* execution of a crime.
    (A) deliberate
    (B) eminent
    (C) amicable
    (D) remorseful

24. There is no *provision* for deadlines in the contract.
    (A) improvement
    (B) convenience
    (C) aggregation
    (D) stipulation

25. The furnishings *impart* an air of elegance to the room.
    (A) communicate
    (B) indemnify
    (C) reinforce
    (D) disguise

26. She exhibited great *valor* in handling the emergency.
    (A) ingeniousness
    (B) courage
    (C) discretion
    (D) optimism

27. Various courses were *fused* in the revision of the curriculum.
    (A) required
    (B) implicated
    (C) combined
    (D) involved

28. He was able to *duplicate* his work even though his hard drive with all his data had died.
    (A) replicate
    (B) synthesize
    (C) fixate
    (D) replenish

29. The task of choosing one from so many qualified applicants *bewildered* the employer.
    (A) perplexed
    (B) aggravated
    (C) subdued
    (D) infuriated

30. The revision of the city plan incorporated adjustments in the projected *modes* of transportation.
    (A) increments
    (B) expenditures
    (C) means
    (D) modifications

31. The politician sought to *aggrandize* himself at the expense of the people.
    (A) exhaust
    (B) subjugate
    (C) sacrifice
    (D) enrich

32. The newcomer made an effort to *mingle* with the crowd.
    (A) argue
    (B) mix
    (C) disrupt
    (D) flout

33. If an organization's programs were described as *philanthropic*, the programs would be
    (A) primitive.
    (B) deleterious.
    (C) extraneous.
    (D) benevolent.

34. If the traits of a nation's leader were *covetous*, they would be
    (A) greedy.
    (B) exemplary.
    (C) disparate.
    (D) adventitious.

35. Rabbits *breed* offspring rapidly.
    (A) raise
    (B) gather
    (C) propagate
    (D) destroy

STOP

IF YOU FINISH BEFORE TIME IS CALLED, YOU MAY CHECK YOUR WORK ON THIS SECTION ONLY. DO NOT TURN TO ANY OTHER SECTION IN THE TEST.

ANTONYMS TEST 2

30 Questions • 15 Minutes

Review Unit 1, Antonyms, before attempting this test.

Directions: Read each question carefully and consider all possible answers. When you have decided which choice is best, fill in the corresponding space on your answer sheet. There is only one best answer for each question.

1. IMMUTABLE
   (A) erudite
   (B) abject
   (C) changeable
   (D) fantastic
   (E) aura

2. DUCTILE
   (A) feted
   (B) aloof
   (C) stubborn
   (D) abnormal
   (E) belabored

3. FASTIDIOUS
   (A) factitious
   (B) absurd
   (C) indifferent
   (D) sloppy
   (E) chary

4. TEMERITY
   (A) affinity
   (B) cherubim
   (C) cautiousness
   (D) degenerate
   (E) scanty

5. ITINERANT
   (A) animosity
   (B) metaphor
   (C) perpetrator
   (D) resident
   (E) cerebrum

6. TACITURN
   (A) malevolent
   (B) loquacious
   (C) paltry
   (D) opaque
   (E) morbid

7. NEFARIOUS
   (A) grotesque
   (B) virtuous
   (C) jovial
   (D) pious
   (E) ceremonious

8. OBSEQUIOUS
   (A) harbinger
   (B) bold
   (C) heredity
   (D) quaff
   (E) fashionable

9. OSTENTATION
   (A) emulsion
   (B) languid
   (C) modesty
   (D) kilogram
   (E) showy

10. CONTENTION
    (A) equation
    (B) guild
    (C) oblivion
    (D) friendliness
    (E) assertion

11. IMPUTATION
    (A) assiduous
    (B) radiant
    (C) accusation
    (D) raiment
    (E) vindication

12. BENIGN
    (A) defensive
    (B) relevant
    (C) robot
    (D) pernicious
    (E) precarious

13. COHERENT
    (A) perspicacious
    (B) organized
    (C) weal
    (D) rational
    (E) changeling

14. DEPREDATION
    (A) plethoric
    (B) gloss
    (C) restoration
    (D) usher
    (E) devastation

15. PROVOCATIVE
    (A) sedentary
    (B) capricious
    (C) vindictive
    (D) tawny
    (E) unexciting

16. SUBMISSION
    (A) authorized
    (B) defiance
    (C) assignment
    (D) defeat
    (E) criticism

17. AFFLUENT
    (A) immigrant
    (B) junction
    (C) insufficient
    (D) kindred
    (E) clandestine

18. CHURLISH
    (A) exiguous
    (B) laudable
    (C) cheerful
    (D) maternal
    (E) sympathetic

19. SYMMETRY
    (A) invocation
    (B) synopsis
    (C) distortion
    (D) satyr
    (E) portrayal

20. DULCET
    (A) extrinsic
    (B) optimistic
    (C) unanimous
    (D) disagreeable
    (E) sweet

21. PIQUANT
    (A) pungent
    (B) vain
    (C) insipid
    (D) vulture
    (E) chromatic

22. OPPORTUNE
    (A) dialectical
    (B) mutable
    (C) clinch
    (D) weird
    (E) inexpedient

23. PETULANT
    (A) irascible
    (B) good-humored
    (C) uncouth
    (D) abnormal
    (E) closure

24. SAVORY
    (A) apathy
    (B) mysterious
    (C) pliant
    (D) unpalatable
    (E) capacious

25. SATIATED
    (A) satirical
    (B) quench
    (C) gorgeous
    (D) delectable
    (E) hungry

26. RECLUSIVE
    (A) reserved
    (B) obscure
    (C) gregarious
    (D) rustic
    (E) sophisticated

27. COURTEOUS
    (A) flaccid
    (B) emollient
    (C) insolent
    (D) scrupulous
    (E) disingenuous

28. USURP
    (A) succinct
    (B) predict
    (C) pacify
    (D) overthrow
    (E) relinquish

29. ACRIMONIOUS
    (A) burning
    (B) bothersome
    (C) debatable
    (D) harmonious
    (E) conclusive

30. OBVIOUS
    (A) discernible
    (B) cryptic
    (C) discursive
    (D) prestigious
    (E) caricature

STOP

IF YOU FINISH BEFORE TIME IS CALLED, YOU MAY CHECK
YOUR WORK ON THIS SECTION ONLY. DO NOT TURN TO ANY
OTHER SECTION IN THE TEST.

ANSWER KEY AND EXPLANATIONS

Synonyms Test 1

1. B	8. B	15. C	22..C	29. A
2. C	9. A	16. D	23. A	30. C
3. B	10. D	17. C	24. D	31. D
4. A	11. B	18. C	25. A	32. B
5. D	12. B	19. A	26. B	33. D
6. A	13. A	20. B	27. C	34. A
7. D	14. C	21. B	28. A	35. C

1. **The correct answer is (B).** *Usual* is a near synonym for *traditional*. A near synonym means almost the same, but not quite. Choice (A), *unfamiliar,* doesn't work because the systems to be replaced have been around for years. *Traditional* typically means something is not adaptable, which is one meaning of *flexible*, so the words are antonyms, not synonyms. *General* doesn't relate to *traditional* in any way.

2. **The correct answer is (C).** *Penalty* and *punishment* are synonyms. Choice (A) is not strong enough for something that is "irresponsible behavior." Choice (B) is the opposite of a penalty. Choice (D), *precaution,* doesn't make sense in the sentence and is not a synonym of *penalty*.

3. **The correct answer is (B).** *Designated* means "allocated, assigned" and so is the correct answer. Nothing indicates that someone gave the person permission to use his study time to do the assignment, so eliminate choice (A). Choice (C) can be eliminated because there is no indication that the person had *agreed* with someone to use the study time for the assignment. Choice (D) makes no sense.

4. **The correct answer is (A).** *Maintenance* is a synonym for *preservation*. Choice (B) might be tempting, but a *stratagem* is "a trick, an underhanded scheme" and that doesn't fit the context nor it is a synonym for *preservation*. Choice (C) doesn't make

sense because how do you store land? Choice (D) doesn't make sense either because an *incumbency* means "a term of office," which is not the same as maintaining something.

5. **The correct answer is (D).** *Concoct* means "to make up" and so does *fabricate*. Choice (A), *inculcate,* means "to instill or drill something into someone's mind by forceful repetition" and doesn't make sense. The same goes for choice (B), *conceal*, meaning "to hide." Choice (C), *reveal*, might be tempting, but the word is not a synonym for *concoct*.

6. **The correct answer is (A).** *Situation* is the best choice among the answers. Choice (A), *setting*, would fit if the test item were about a play or book, but it isn't, so *setting* doesn't make sense in the sentence. Choice (C), *summation*, another word for *summary*, doesn't make sense either. *Deficiency*, choice (D), isn't the right usage of the word, which typically is used to mean "a shortage, a lack of something essential."

7. **The correct answer is (D).** *Prescribe* means "to order, assign" and fits the sense of the sentence. Choice (A) is not strong enough; the judge didn't show or suggest the sentence, but imposed it. A judge doesn't grant a sentence because *grant* has a positive connotation, giving something pleasant to someone, so eliminate choice

(B). Choice (C) doesn't make sense because *perpetuate* is "to make last for a long time."

8. **The correct answer is (B).** *Inaccurate* is a synonym for *flawed*. Choices (A) and (C), *subjective* and *objective*, are opposites of each other, but neither is a synonym for *flawed*. Something may be *unscientific*, but still accurate, so choice (D) is also a wrong answer.

9. **The correct answer is (A).** Choices (B), *instruct*; (C), *inform*; and (D), *advise*, all make sense in the sentence, but only choice (A), *guarantee*, is a synonym for *assure*.

10. **The correct answer is (D).** *Thwart* is a synonym for *foil*, meaning "to prevent from occurring." Choice (A), *heighten*, means "to increase in quality or intensity." Choice (B), *secure*, makes no sense because how would someone take possession of a scheme or connect a scheme securely, both meanings of the word? Choice (C) is incorrect because *disencumber* means "to take away someone's burden, to untangle someone from obligations."

11. **The correct answer is (B).** *Claimed* is a synonym for *purported*. Choice (A), *addressed*, means "to speak to." Choice (C), *propitiated*, means "to appease, to reconcile" and doesn't make sense. For the same reason, *conciliated*, choice (D), doesn't make sense; it means "to reconcile" or "to overcome distrust."

12. **The correct answer is (B).** *Varied* and *diverse* are synonyms. Choices (A) and (D) are incorrect for similar reasons. Both mean "a large number," but neither includes the idea of diversity. Choice (C) is incorrect because *discrepant* means "not in agreement."

13. **The correct answer is (A).** *Remember* is a synonym for *recollect*. None of the other words makes sense in the context. *Illumine*, choice (D), means "to shed light on," and might tempt you, but it doesn't have the same or a similar meaning to *recollect*.

Sometimes, the simplest answer is the right answer.

14. **The correct answer is (C).** To *rescind* is "to *revoke*." Choice (A) is incorrect because typically an official order such as a declaration of a state of emergency is revoked, not *negated*. Choice (B), *maneuver*, means "to carry out a military action," "to change tactics," or "to alter the placement of troops," none of which are synonymous with *rescind*. Choice (D) is incorrect because the governor is ending the state of emergency, not *accepting* it.

15. **The correct answer is (C).** *Scant* means "*little*." Choice (A) is incorrect because *audacious* means "bold, fearless, spirited." Choice (B) is incorrect because *fervid* means "impassioned, intense emotion." Choice (D) is incorrect because *clothed* makes no sense, even in a metaphorical sense.

16. **The correct answer is (D).** To *scoff at* is "to *mock* or make fun of." Choice (A) makes no sense because *exonerate* is "to free someone from blame or responsibility." Choice (B) is incorrect because *amplify* is "to increase," "to exaggerate," or "to make complete." Choice (C), *confute*, is "to prove something or someone wrong."

17. **The correct answer is (C).** *Run* and *sprint* can be synonyms and are in this case. Choice (A) makes no sense because you don't need a surge of energy to *relax*. Choice (B) is incorrect because while *adventure* makes some sense, it is not a synonym for *run*. Choice (D), *convergence*, meaning "where two things come together," makes no sense.

18. **The correct answer is (C).** *Pressing* means "demanding immediate attention," in other words, *urgent*. Choice (A), *privileged*, even meaning "confidential," isn't correct. Choice (B), *amendable*, meaning "capable of being changed," is also incorrect. Choice (D), *absolved*, meaning "pronounced not guilty," is also incorrect.

19. **The correct answer is (A).** *Simulated* is something made to resemble something else; in other words, it is *pretended*. Choice (B) is incorrect because something superficial is something that may be frivolous, perfunctory, or on the surface, none of which are the same simulated. Choice (C) is incorrect because *stimulated* means "aroused or excited emotionally." Choice (D) is incorrect because *simultaneous* means "at the same time."

20. **The correct answer is (B).** Both *worried* and *upset* can be synonyms of *agitated*, but in this sentence, *upset* fits the context better. Choice (C) is incorrect because *convulsed* means "shaking violently"; it can be a synonym of *agitate*, but not in this context. Choice (D) is incorrect because *composed*, meaning "calm," is the opposite of *agitated*.

21. **The correct answer is (B).** A *pulse* is beat or *pace*. Choice (A) is incorrect because *utility* means either "usefulness" or "a power company." Choice (C) is incorrect because *reverence* is a feeling of profound awe or respect and makes no sense and is no a synonym of *pulse*. Choice (D) is incorrect because *solace* is the same as comfort, not a pulse.

22. **The correct answer is (C).** One synonym for *unsophisticated* is *simple*. Choice (A) is incorrect because *ponderous* means "heavy, dull, tedious," none of which is the same as *unsophisticated*. Choice (B) is incorrect because *elaborate* tends to the opposite of *unsophisticated*. Choice (D) is incorrect because *artificial* means "contrived, inauthentic, forced, affected," in other words, the opposite of *unsophisticated*.

23. **The correct answer is (A).** *Willful* and *deliberate* are synonyms. Choice (B) is incorrect because *eminent* means "prominent, great, well-known"; don't confuse it with *imminent*, meaning "about to happen." Choice (C), *amicable*, means "friendly" and makes no sense. Choice (D) is incorrect because *remorseful* means "sorry," and while someone caught for a crime may feel remorseful, it is not a synonym for *willful* and makes no sense.

24. **The correct answer is (D).** *Stipulation* is a synonym for *provision*, meaning "arrangement or plan." Choice (A) is incorrect because *improvement* is not the same as a stipulation and doesn't fit the sense. Choice (B) is incorrect because *convenience* means "benefit, advantage" or "suitability." Choice (C) is incorrect because *aggregation* means "a collection of several things taken as a whole."

25. **The correct answer is (A).** *Impart* and *communicate* are synonyms. Choice (C), *reinforce*, may seem like a good choice, and in terms of context could work, except that *impart* and *reinforce* aren't synonyms. Choice (B) is incorrect because *indemnify* means "to protect against damage or loss." Choice (D) is incorrect because *disguise* isn't a synonym for transmitting information, in this case, a feeling or sense of style.

26. **The correct answer is (B).** *Valor* and *courage* are the same thing. Choice (A) is incorrect because *ingeniousness* is "cleverness," "inventiveness," and "creative thinking." Choice (C) is incorrect because *discretion* is "tactfulness." Choice (D) is incorrect because *optimism* means "expecting that the best will happen.

27. **The correct answer is (C).** To *fuse* is "to mix together," but also "to unite, to join," and among the answer choices, *combine* is the closest in meaning. Choice (A) is incorrect because *required* is not a synonym for *joining*, though courses can be required. Choice (B) is incorrect because *implicated*, meaning "to involve or incriminate someone," makes no sense. Choice (D) is incorrect because while *involved* may make sense in the context, it is not a synonym for *fuse*.

28. **The correct answer is (A).** To *duplicate* is "to *replicate*," or "to make an exact copy." Choice (B) is incorrect because *synthesize* means "to combine pieces to form something new." Choice (C) is incorrect because *fixate* is "to make something stable" or "to

focus attention on something or someone." Choice (D), *replenish*, means "to make something full or complete again."

29. **The correct answer is (A).** To *bewilder* is "to *perplex*," meaning "to confuse." Choice (B) is incorrect because *aggravated* means "made angry" or "made something worse." Choice (C) is incorrect because *subdued* means "conquered, brought under control." Choice (D) is incorrect because *infuriated* means "angry, enraged."

30. **The correct answer is (C).** *Means* can be a synonym of *modes* when they both mean "method, way, or variety," which fits the context of the sentence. Choice (A) is incorrect because *increments* means "the process of increasing in number, size, or quantity." Choice (B) is incorrect because *expenditures* refers to the disbursement of money. Choice (D) is incorrect because *modifications* refers to changes.

31. **The correct answer is (D).** One meaning of *aggrandize* is "to enrich one's self." Choice (A) is incorrect because *exhaust*, "to tire," is not a synonym and doesn't make sense since the politician is exhausting himself, not the people. Choice (B) is incorrect because *subjugate* means "to conquer, to make subservient." This is not only not a synonym, but the politician isn't about to subjugate himself. Choice (C) is incorrect because *sacrifice* is not a synonym, and a politician aggrandizing himself is the opposite of one sacrificing himself for his constituents.

32. **The correct answer is (B).** To *mingle* is "to mix." Choice (A) is incorrect because *argue* is not the same as mingle. Choice (C) is incorrect because *disrupt* is "to interrupt" or "to break up." Choice (D) is incorrect because *flout* is "to show contempt for" or "to brush off, to ignore."

33. **The correct answer is (D).** *Philanthropic* programs are *benevolent,* meaning "generous in helping others, showing kindness." Choice (A) is incorrect because *primitive* means "basic, simple." Choice (B) is incorrect because *deleterious* means "harmful," the opposite of *philanthropic*. Choice (C) is incorrect because *extraneous* means "not essential, unnecessary."

34. **The correct answer is (A).** A *covetous* person is a *greedy* person. Choice (B) is incorrect because *exemplary* means "worthy of being imitated, a model." Choice (C) is incorrect because *disparate* means "something that is very different, unlike." Choice (D) is incorrect because *adventitious* means "added to something by chance or accidentally."

35. **The correct answer is (C).** To *breed* is "to *propagate*" or "to reproduce." Choice (A) is incorrect because *raise* is not the same as *reproduce*. Choice (B), *gather*, is not only not a synonym, but makes no sense. Choice (D), *destroy,* is not a synonym for reproducing.

Antonyms Test 2

1. C	7. B	13. D	19. C	25. E
2. C	8. B	14. C	20. D	26. C
3. D	9. C	15. E	21. C	27. C
4. C	10. D	16. B	22. E	28. E
5. D	11. E	17. C	23. B	29. D
6. B	12. D	18. C	24. D	30. B

1. **The correct answer is (C).** *Immutable* means "not subject to change," so choice (C), *changeable*, is its antonym. Choice (A), *erudite*, means "learned, highly educated," so eliminate it. Choice (B) is incorrect because *abject* means "wretched, forlorn" as well as "despicable," none of which are antonyms for *immutable*. Choice (D) is incorrect because *fantastic* has nothing to do with being able to change. Choice (E) is incorrect because an *aura* is a quality that someone possesses or a bright light around someone's head.

2. **The correct answer is (C).** *Ductile* means "capable of being persuaded or influenced easily, so choice (C), *stubborn*, is an antonym. Choice (A) is incorrect because *feted* means "honored by a celebration." Choice (B) is incorrect because *aloof* means "reserved, remote, distant either physically or emotionally." Choice (D) is incorrect because *abnormal* doesn't relate to either being ductile or stubborn. Choice (E) is incorrect because *belabored* means "having worked at something for an unusually long period of time" or "having criticized someone harshly."

3. **The correct answer is (D).** Being *fastidious* is paying close attention to detail, being fussy, so the opposite is being *sloppy*, choice (D). Choice (A) is incorrect because *factitious* means "lacking in authenticity or genuineness." Choice (B) is incorrect because *absurd* means "ridiculous" or "unreasonable." Choice (C) is incorrect because being indifferent, or not caring or feeling for or against something, is not the

opposite of being *fastidious*. Choice (E) is incorrect because *chary* means "wary, cautious."

4. **The correct answer is (C).** *Temerity* means "foolhardiness, recklessness, daring," which is the opposite of *cautiousness*. Choice (A) is incorrect because *affinity* means "a natural attraction to" as well as "relationship by marriage" and "an inherent similarity between persons and things"; none of the meanings are opposite in meaning to *temerity*. Choice (B) is incorrect because *cherubim* is a category of angels. Choice (D) is incorrect because a *degenerate* means "depraved, perverted, debauched," which isn't the same as *temerity*, but closer to it than opposite of it. Choice (E) is incorrect because *scanty* means "limited, insufficient, small."

5. **The correct answer is (D).** An *itinerant* is someone who moves around from place to place, whereas a *resident* is someone who has a permanent place to stay. Choice (A) is incorrect because *animosity* is hostility. Choice (B) is incorrect because a *metaphor* is a figure of speech implying a comparison. Choice (C) is incorrect because *perpetrator* is someone who commits some act; the connotation is negative. Choice (E) is incorrect because the *cerebrum* is a part of the brain.

6. **The correct answer is (B).** *Taciturn* means "untalkative by habit," whereas *loquacious* means "very talkative." Choice (A) is incorrect because *malevolent* means "evil." Choice (C) is incorrect because *paltry* means "insignificant" or "worth-

less." Choice (D) is incorrect because something that is *opaque* doesn't transmit light through it, not able to reflect light." Choice (E) is incorrect because *morbid* means "having an unusual interest in death" or "gruesome, ghoulish."

7. **The correct answer is (B).** *Nefarious* means "evil, wicked," so *virtuous,* meaning "morally excellent," is its opposite. Choice (A) is incorrect because *grotesque* means "fantastically distorted" or "bizarre." Choice (C) is incorrect because a *jovial* person is a very happy, jolly person. Choice (D) is incorrect because *pious* means "reverent toward God; religious; devout," none of which are exactly the same as being virtuous or the opposite of nefarious. Choice (E) is incorrect because *ceremonious* means "very polite" or "observing formalities."

8. **The correct answer is (B).** *Obsequious* means "obedient or attentive in an ingratiating or flattering way; attempting to gain favor by flattery." Its opposite is being *bold.* Choice (A) is incorrect because *harbinger* means "someone or something that precedes and indicates the approach of someone or something else." Choice (C) is incorrect because *heredity* is the genetic transmission of characteristics from one generation to the next. Choice (D) is incorrect because *quaff* is "to drink." Choice (E) is incorrect because *fashionable*, or stylish, is not an antonym of *obsequious*. Note that *obsequious* is an adjective and *harbinger,* choice (C), is a noun and *quaff,* choice (D), is a verb. Neither would be an antonym for an adjective.

9. **The correct answer is (C).** *Ostentation* means "pretentious display, flamboyance," so *modesty* is an antonym. Choice (A) is incorrect because an *emulsion* is a light-sensitive coating on paper or film, or a chemical colloid. Choice (B) is incorrect because *languid* means "weak, lacking energy or force." Choice (D) is incorrect because *kilogram* is a unit of measure of mass. Choice (E) is incorrect because *showy* is a synonym for *ostentation.*

10. **The correct answer is (D).** A *contention* may be a competition, a dispute, or a point made in an argument. The only answer choice that is an antonym of any of these meanings is *friendliness.* Choice (A) is incorrect because an *equation* is a mathematical statement or a state of equality. Choice (B) is incorrect because a *guild* is an association of workers or merchants. Choice (C) is incorrect because *oblivion* means "the condition of being forgotten or disregarded." Choice (E) is incorrect because an *assertion* is a positive statement and a synonym for *contention.*

11. **The correct answer is (E).** An *imputation* is a statement attributing blame or dishonesty to someone. The opposite is a *vindication,* exonerating or absolving someone of blame. Choice (A) is incorrect because *assiduous* means "diligent": note that this is an adjective and the word for which you need to find an antonym is a noun. That eliminates both choices (A) and (B). Choice (B) is also incorrect because *radiant* is not an antonym of assigning blame to someone. Choice (C) is incorrect because *accusation* is a synonym for *imputation.* Choice (D) is incorrect because *raiment* means "any piece of clothing."

12. **The correct answer is (D).** *Benign* means "favorable," "showing kindness and mildness," or "harmless, not life-threatening." The only answer choice that is the opposite of any of these definitions is *pernicious*, meaning "deadly" or "destructive." Choice (A) is incorrect because *defensive* is not an antonym of *benign*, and neither is *relevant*, choice (B). Choice (C) is incorrect because a *robot* has no connection with being benign. Choice (E) is incorrect because *precarious* means "insecure, dangerous, uncertain."

13. **The correct answer is (D).** "To be coherent" is "to be organized, clear, rational," so chaotic is an antonym. Choices (B) and (E) are incorrect because both *organized* and *rational* are synonyms for *coherent.* Choice (A) is incorrect because *perspicacious* means "having extreme insight and wisdom." Choice (C) is incorrect because

weal means "general welfare of the community" or "happiness or prosperity."

14. **The correct answer is (C).** *Depredation* means "a raid or attack" or "loss." *Restoration* fits as an antonym for the meaning of loss. Choice (A) is incorrect because *plethoric,* the adjectival form of *plethora,* means "an overabundance. Choice (B) is incorrect because *gloss* means either "a shininess on the surface of something" or "to give a shine to something." Choice (D) is incorrect because an *usher* is someone who shows you to your seat. Choice (E) is incorrect because *devastation* is a near synonym for *depredation.*

15. **The correct answer is (E).** *Provocative* means "serving to stimulate, excite, or anger someone," so its antonym is *unexciting.* Choice (A) is incorrect because *sedentary* means "accustomed to sitting, getting little exercise." Choice (B) is incorrect because *capricious* means "impulsive, unpredictable." Choice (C) is incorrect because *vindictive* means "revengeful, spiteful." Choice (D) is incorrect because *tawny* is a light brownish orange color.

16. **The correct answer is (B).** Submission is the act of submitting to the power of someone else; it's being compliant. *Defiance,* boldly resisting, is an antonym. Choice (A) is incorrect because *authorized* means "having been given power or authority." Choice (C) is incorrect because an *assignment* isn't an antonym for *submission.* Choice (D) is incorrect because *defeat* isn't an antonym for *submission.* Choice (E) is incorrect because *criticism,* meaning "a critical, or unfavorable, judgment" is not the same as bold resistance.

17. **The correct answer is (C).** *Affluent* can be a wealthy person or it can mean "having wealth, both money and possessions." The only word that fits as an antonym is *insufficient,* meaning "not having enough." Choice (A) is incorrect because an *immigrant* is a person who moves permanently to another country. Choice (B) is incorrect because a *junction,* or place where two or more points meet or join, is not antonym

for *affluent.* Choice (D) is incorrect because *kindred* means either "a group of related people" or "having the same family." Choice (E) is incorrect because *clandestine* means "done in secret, meant to conceal."

18. **The correct answer is (C).** A *churlish* person is one who is surly, difficult, and/or rude. *Cheerful* is the only word that fits as an antonym. Choice (A) is incorrect because *exiguous* means "meager, stingy." Choice (B) is incorrect because *laudable* means "commendable, worthy of praise." Choice (D) is incorrect because *maternal* is an adjective derived from the word for *mother.* Choice (E) is incorrect because *sympathetic* means "showing sympathy, compassion, or understanding.

19. **The correct answer is (C).** *Symmetry* is the similar or balanced arrangement of parts on opposite sides of something. *Distortion,* or misrepresentation or malformation, is the closest to being the opposite of *symmetry.* Choice (A) is incorrect because an *invocation* is appealing to someone for help, often in the form of a prayer. Choice (B) is incorrect because a *synopsis* is a summary of a report, story, place, etc. Choice (D) is incorrect because a *satyr* is a mythical creature. Choice (E) is incorrect because a *portrayal* is a representation, description, or performance.

20. **The correct answer is (D).** Dulcet describes something soothing or pleasant, sweet, especially sounds. *Disagreeable* is the only word among the answers that fits as a antonym. Choice (A) is incorrect because *extrinsic* means "not essential" or "coming from outside, external." Choice (B) is incorrect because *optimistic* means "typically expecting the best to occur." Choice (C) is incorrect because *unanimous* means "being in complete agreement." Choice (E) is incorrect because *sweet* is a synonym for *dulcet,* not an antonym.

21. **The correct answer is (C).** *Piquant* may mean "spicy or tart," "interesting," or "provocative." *Insipid,* meaning "lacking in flavor" or "lacking in anything that excites or stimulates" is its opposite. Choice

(A) is incorrect because *pungent*, meaning "a strong smell or sharp bitter taste" is a near synonym for *piquant* rather than an antonym. Choice (B) is incorrect because a *vain* person is one who is overly proud. Choice (D) is incorrect because a *vulture* is bird of prey; also, note that it is a noun and *piquant* is an adjective. The antonym also needs to be an adjective. Choice (E) is incorrect because *chromatic* refers to color, not taste.

22. **The correct answer is (E).** *Opportune* means "happening at a suitable or advantageous time" or "being suitable for a particular purpose." *Inexpedient* means "not suitable, inadvisable," so it is an antonym for *opportune*. Choice (A) is incorrect because *dialectical* means "of or relating to dialectics," which is "the process of arriving at the truth through argumentation." Choice (B) is incorrect because *mutable* means "able to change or alter frequently." Choice (C) is incorrect because *clinch* means "to secure, to hold" or as a noun "a hug or embrace." Choice (D) is incorrect because *weird* is not an antonym for *opportune*.

23. **The correct answer is (B).** *Petulant* means "irritable, impatient, sullen," so *good-humored* is an antonym for it. Choice (A) is incorrect because *irascible* is a synonym for *petulant* rather than an antonym. Choice (C) is incorrect because *uncouth* means "crude," or "ungraceful." Choice (D) is incorrect because *abnormal* is not an antonym for *petulant*, and neither is choice (E), *closure,* meaning "something that closes or shuts" or "the end of something."

24. **The correct answer is (D).** *Savory* means "morally wholesome" or "having a pleasing pungent taste." *Unpalatable*, meaning "not pleasing to the taste," is the opposite of the second definition and so is an antonym to *savory*. Choice (A) is incorrect because *apathy* means "lack of interest or emotion." Choice (B) is incorrect because *mysterious* is not an antonym for *savory*. Choice (C) is incorrect because *pliant* means "easily bent" or "able to be influenced easily."

Choice (E) is incorrect because *capacious* means "spacious, large in capacity."

25. **The correct answer is (E).** *Satiated* means "filled to satisfaction," whereas *hungry* is the opposite. Choice (A) is incorrect because *satirical*, the adjective form of *satire*, means "mocking, exposing one to ridicule." Choice (B) is incorrect because *quench*, meaning "to satisfy," is a synonym for *satiated* rather than an antonym. Choice (C) is incorrect because although *gorgeous* might seem like *engorge*, "to stuff one's self," that would be a synonym rather than an antonym, and as it is, *gorgeous* has no relation to *satiated*. Choice (D) is incorrect because *delectable* means "delightful, very pleasing."

26. **The correct answer is (C).** *Reclusive* means "withdrawing from people, living in isolation." The opposite of this is *gregarious*, "seeking out and enjoying the company of others, sociable." Choice (A) is incorrect because *reserved* means "reticent, marked by self-restraint" and is a near synonym for *reclusive*. Choice (B) is incorrect because *obscure* means "unclear, vague," "hidden, secret" and as a verb, "to make unclear" or "to cover over." Choice (D) is incorrect because *rustic* means "relating to country life." Choice (E) is incorrect because *sophisticated* means "refined, cultured."

27. **The correct answer is (C).** The opposite of *courteous* is *insolent,* meaning "arrogant, rude, disrespectful." Choice (A) is incorrect because *flaccid* means "lacking energy, resilience, or muscle tone." Choice (B) is incorrect because an *emollient* is something that softens or soothes skin. Choice (D) is incorrect because *scrupulous* means "conscientious, principled." Choice (E) is incorrect because *disingenuous* means "not straightforward, insincere."

28. **The correct answer is (E).** *Usurp* is "to seize, take over, take control," and its antonym is *relinquish,* meaning "to give up." Choice (A) is incorrect because *succinct* means "clear, brief, concise." Choice (B) is incorrect because *predict* means

"to foretell, to tell about something in advance of its happening." Choice (C) is incorrect because *pacify* means "to calm" or in military terms "to restore peace to an area." Choice (D) is incorrect because *overthrow* is a synonym for *usurp*.

29. **The correct answer is (D).** *Acrimonious* means "bitterness or sharpness in terms of speech, tone, manner, or temper," whereas *harmonious* means "being in agreement, cordial, friendly." Choice (A) is incorrect because *burning* is not an antonym for *acrimonious*. Choice (B) is incorrect because *bothersome* means "causing trouble." Choice (C) is incorrect because *debatable* means "open to disagreement" or "questionable." Choice (E) is incorrect because *conclusive* means "putting an end to doubt, final."

30. **The correct answer is (B).** The antonym of *obvious* is *cryptic*, meaning "having a secret or hidden meaning, mysterious." Choice (A) is incorrect because *discernible*, meaning "able to be perceived," is a synonym for *obvious*, not an antonym. Choice (C) is incorrect because *discursive* means "going from topic to topic in no particular order, long-winded." Choice (D) is incorrect because *prestigious* means "having status or influence." Choice (E) is incorrect because a *caricature* is a representation of person that exaggerates the person's characteristics. *Caricature* is a noun, and remember that you need to choose an answer that is the same part of speech as the word for which you need to choose an antonym.

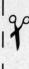

QUANTITATIVE ABILITY ANSWER SHEETS

Nonverbal Arithmetic Test 1

1. Ⓐ Ⓑ Ⓒ Ⓓ   4. Ⓐ Ⓑ Ⓒ Ⓓ   7. Ⓐ Ⓑ Ⓒ Ⓓ   10. Ⓐ Ⓑ Ⓒ Ⓓ   13. Ⓐ Ⓑ Ⓒ Ⓓ
2. Ⓐ Ⓑ Ⓒ Ⓓ   5. Ⓐ Ⓑ Ⓒ Ⓓ   8. Ⓐ Ⓑ Ⓒ Ⓓ   11. Ⓐ Ⓑ Ⓒ Ⓓ   14. Ⓐ Ⓑ Ⓒ Ⓓ
3. Ⓐ Ⓑ Ⓒ Ⓓ   6. Ⓐ Ⓑ Ⓒ Ⓓ   9. Ⓐ Ⓑ Ⓒ Ⓓ   12. Ⓐ Ⓑ Ⓒ Ⓓ

Problem Solving Test 2

1. Ⓐ Ⓑ Ⓒ Ⓓ   4. Ⓐ Ⓑ Ⓒ Ⓓ   7. Ⓐ Ⓑ Ⓒ Ⓓ   10. Ⓐ Ⓑ Ⓒ Ⓓ   13. Ⓐ Ⓑ Ⓒ Ⓓ
2. Ⓐ Ⓑ Ⓒ Ⓓ   5. Ⓐ Ⓑ Ⓒ Ⓓ   8. Ⓐ Ⓑ Ⓒ Ⓓ   11. Ⓐ Ⓑ Ⓒ Ⓓ   14. Ⓐ Ⓑ Ⓒ Ⓓ
3. Ⓐ Ⓑ Ⓒ Ⓓ   6. Ⓐ Ⓑ Ⓒ Ⓓ   9. Ⓐ Ⓑ Ⓒ Ⓓ   12. Ⓐ Ⓑ Ⓒ Ⓓ   15. Ⓐ Ⓑ Ⓒ Ⓓ

Algebra Test 3

1. Ⓐ Ⓑ Ⓒ Ⓓ   3. Ⓐ Ⓑ Ⓒ Ⓓ   5. Ⓐ Ⓑ Ⓒ Ⓓ   7. Ⓐ Ⓑ Ⓒ Ⓓ   8. Ⓐ Ⓑ Ⓒ Ⓓ
2. Ⓐ Ⓑ Ⓒ Ⓓ   4. Ⓐ Ⓑ Ⓒ Ⓓ   6. Ⓐ Ⓑ Ⓒ Ⓓ

Quantitative Comparisons Test 4

1. Ⓐ Ⓑ Ⓒ Ⓓ   5. Ⓐ Ⓑ Ⓒ Ⓓ   9. Ⓐ Ⓑ Ⓒ Ⓓ   13. Ⓐ Ⓑ Ⓒ Ⓓ   17. Ⓐ Ⓑ Ⓒ Ⓓ
2. Ⓐ Ⓑ Ⓒ Ⓓ   6. Ⓐ Ⓑ Ⓒ Ⓓ   10. Ⓐ Ⓑ Ⓒ Ⓓ   14. Ⓐ Ⓑ Ⓒ Ⓓ   18. Ⓐ Ⓑ Ⓒ Ⓓ
3. Ⓐ Ⓑ Ⓒ Ⓓ   7. Ⓐ Ⓑ Ⓒ Ⓓ   11. Ⓐ Ⓑ Ⓒ Ⓓ   15. Ⓐ Ⓑ Ⓒ Ⓓ   19. Ⓐ Ⓑ Ⓒ Ⓓ
4. Ⓐ Ⓑ Ⓒ Ⓓ   8. Ⓐ Ⓑ Ⓒ Ⓓ   12. Ⓐ Ⓑ Ⓒ Ⓓ   16. Ⓐ Ⓑ Ⓒ Ⓓ   20. Ⓐ Ⓑ Ⓒ Ⓓ

answer sheet

Quantitative Ability

OVERVIEW

- Nonverbal arithmetic test 1
- Problem solving test 2
- Algebra test 3
- Quantitative comparisons test 4
- Answer key and explanations

NONVERBAL ARITHMETIC TEST 1

14 Questions • 20 Minutes

Directions: Read each question carefully and consider all possible answers. When you have decided which choice is best, fill in the corresponding space on your answer sheet. There is only one best answer for each question.

1. What fraction of the whole is the shaded area in the figure below?

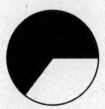

(A) $\frac{1}{2}$

(B) $\frac{3}{4}$

(C) $\frac{2}{3}$

(D) $\frac{2}{5}$

2. Which of the following equations demonstrates that the two figures are equivalent?

(A) $\frac{3}{9} = \frac{1}{3}$

(B) $\frac{9}{3} = \frac{3}{1}$

(C) $\frac{3}{9} = \frac{3}{3}$

(D) $\frac{9}{3} = \frac{1}{3}$

3. Select the answer that represents reduction of the fraction $\frac{630}{140}$ to the lowest term.

(A) $\frac{70}{2}$

(B) $\frac{70}{4}$

(C) $\frac{2}{9}$

(D) $\frac{9}{2}$

4. Which one of the following equations is correct for building up the fraction $\frac{3}{8}$ to have a denominator of 24?

(A) $\frac{3}{8} = \frac{3 \times 3}{3 \times 8} = \frac{9}{24}$

(B) $\frac{3}{8} = 3 \times \frac{24}{8} \times \frac{1}{24} \times \frac{9}{24}$

(C) $8 \times \frac{3}{1} \times \frac{1}{24} = \frac{24}{24}$

(D) $\frac{3}{24} = 3 \times \frac{1}{3} \times \frac{1}{8} = \frac{1}{24}$

5. Which of the following equations expresses the whole number 6 as an equivalent fraction with a denominator of 5?

(A) $\frac{6}{5} = 6 \times \frac{5}{5} \times \frac{1}{5} = \frac{30}{25}$

(B) $\frac{6}{5} = 6 \times \frac{1}{5} \times 1 = \frac{6}{5}$

(C) $\frac{6}{1} = \frac{6 \times 5}{1 \times 5} = \frac{30}{5}$

(D) $\frac{6}{1} = 5 \times \frac{1}{6} \times 1 = \frac{5}{6}$

6. What is the product of $\frac{5}{3} \times \frac{2}{7}$?

(A) $\frac{6}{35}$

(B) $\frac{35}{6}$

(C) $\frac{21}{10}$

(D) $\frac{10}{21}$

7. What is the product of $\frac{25}{36} \times \frac{16}{20}$?

(A) $\frac{10}{8}$

(B) $\frac{8}{10}$

(C) $\frac{9}{5}$

(D) $\frac{5}{9}$

8. What is $\frac{3}{4}$ divided by $\frac{5}{2}$?

(A) $\frac{10}{3}$

(B) $\frac{3}{10}$

(C) $\frac{20}{6}$

(D) $\frac{6}{20}$

9. Select the correct answer for $\frac{72}{50} \div \frac{200}{35}$.

   (A) $\frac{63}{250}$

   (B) $\frac{250}{63}$

   (C) $\frac{288}{35}$

   (D) $\frac{35}{288}$

10. A 12-ounce bottle has 7 ounces of liquid in it. What fraction of the bottle is filled?

    (A) $\frac{3}{4}$

    (B) $\frac{1}{2}$

    (C) $\frac{7}{12}$

    (D) $\frac{12}{7}$

11. What is the solution to the problem $\frac{2}{9} + \frac{5}{6} - \frac{3}{8}$?

    (A) $\frac{72}{60}$

    (B) $\frac{60}{72}$

    (C) $\frac{72}{49}$

    (D) $\frac{49}{72}$

12. When you multiply $2\frac{1}{3} \times 1\frac{1}{2}$, the answer is

    (A) $3\frac{1}{3}$.

    (B) $3\frac{1}{2}$.

    (C) $2\frac{1}{5}$.

    (D) $2\frac{2}{6}$.

13. Change $2\frac{1}{2} \div 3\frac{1}{3}$ to a simple fraction.

    (A) $\frac{3}{4}$.

    (B) $\frac{4}{3}$.

    (C) $\frac{1}{3}$.

    (D) $\frac{1}{4}$.

14. Which one of the following is a solution to the problem $5\frac{3}{4} + 6\frac{5}{9}$?

    (A) $12\frac{5}{12}$

    (B) $11\frac{15}{36}$

    (C) $12\frac{11}{36}$

    (D) $11\frac{8}{13}$

STOP

IF YOU FINISH BEFORE TIME IS CALLED, YOU MAY CHECK YOUR WORK ON THIS SECTION ONLY. DO NOT TURN TO ANY OTHER SECTION IN THE TEST.

PROBLEM SOLVING TEST 2

15 Questions • 20 Minutes

Directions: Read each question carefully and consider all possible answers. When you have decided which choice is best, fill in the corresponding space on your answer sheet. There is only one best answer for each question.

1. If there are 245 sections in a city containing five boroughs, the average number of sections for each of the five boroughs is
   (A) 50 sections.
   (B) 49 sections.
   (C) 47 sections.
   (D) 59 sections.

2. If, in that same city, a section has 45 miles of street to plow after a snowstorm, and nine plows are used, each plow will cover an average of how many miles?
   (A) 7 miles
   (B) 6 miles
   (C) 8 miles
   (D) 5 miles

3. If a crosswalk plow engine is run 5 minutes a day for ten days in a given month, how long will it run in the course of this month?
   (A) 50 minutes
   (B) $1\frac{1}{2}$ hours
   (C) 1 hour
   (D) 30 minutes

4. If the city uses 1,500 laborers in manual street cleaning and half as many more to load and drive trucks, the total number of laborers used is
   (A) 2,200.
   (B) 2,520.
   (C) 2,050.
   (D) 2,250.

5. Of 186 summonses issued, 100 were issued to first offenders. How many summonses were issued to non–first offenders?
   (A) 68
   (B) 90
   (C) 86
   (D) 108

6. A sanitation worker is 40 feet behind a sanitation truck. There is a second sanitation truck 90 feet behind the first truck. How much closer is the worker to the first truck than to the second?
   (A) 30 feet
   (B) 50 feet
   (C) 10 feet
   (D) 70 feet

7. If a flushing machine has a capacity of 1,260 gallons, how many gallons will it contain when it is two-thirds full?
   (A) 809 gallons
   (B) 750 gallons
   (C) 630 gallons
   (D) 840 gallons

8. If an employee earns $160.00 a week and has deductions of $8.00 for the pension fund, $12.00 for medical insurance, and $29.60 withholding tax, his take-home pay is
   (A) $110.40.
   (B) $108.60.
   (C) $102.00.
   (D) $98.40.

9. A city department uses 25 twenty-cent, 35 thirty-cent, and 350 forty-cent metered postage units each day. The total cost of stamps used by the department in a five-day period is
   (A) $29.50.
   (B) $155.00.
   (C) $290.50.
   (D) $777.50.

10. In 2005, a school bought 500 dozen pencils at $0.40 per dozen. In 2008, only 75 percent as many pencils were bought as were bought in 2005, but the price per dozen was 20 percent higher than the 2005 price. The total cost of the pencils bought in 2008 was
    (A) $180.00.
    (B) $187.50.
    (C) $240.00.
    (D) $250.00.

11. If the average cost of sweeping a square foot of a small town's street is $0.75, the cost of sweeping 100 square feet is
    (A) $7.50.
    (B) $750.
    (C) $75.
    (D) $70.

12. If a sanitation department scow is towed at the rate of 3 miles per hour, how many hours will it need to go 28 miles?
    (A) 10 hours 30 minutes
    (B) 12 hours
    (C) 9 hours 20 minutes
    (D) 9 hours 15 minutes

13. If a man is 60 feet away from a sanitation truck, how many feet nearer is he to the truck than a second truck that is 100 feet away?
    (A) 60 feet
    (B) 40 feet
    (C) 50 feet
    (D) 20 feet

14. Six gross of special drawing pencils were purchased for use in a city department. If the pencils were used at the rate of 24 a week, the maximum number of weeks that the six gross of pencils would last is
    (A) 6 weeks.
    (B) 12 weeks.
    (C) 24 weeks.
    (D) 36 weeks.

15. A cogwheel having eight cogs plays into another cogwheel having 24 cogs. When the small wheel has made 42 revolutions, how many has the larger wheel made?
    (A) 14
    (B) 20
    (C) 16
    (D) 10

STOP

IF YOU FINISH BEFORE TIME IS CALLED, YOU MAY CHECK YOUR WORK ON THIS SECTION ONLY. DO NOT TURN TO ANY OTHER SECTION IN THE TEST.

ALGEBRA TEST 3

8 Questions • 20 Minutes

Directions: Read each question carefully and consider all possible answers. When you have decided which choice is best, fill in the corresponding space on your answer sheet. There is only one best answer for each question.

1. In the equation $4a + 5 = 13$, a equals
   (A) 4.
   (B) 2.
   (C) 7.
   (D) 6.

2. In the equation $\frac{10}{m} - 8 = \frac{5}{3}$, m equals
   (A) $\frac{10}{3}$.
   (B) $\frac{3}{10}$.
   (C) $\frac{30}{29}$.
   (D) $\frac{29}{30}$.

3. In the equation $3c^2 = 75d^4$, c equals
   (A) $\pm 5d^2$.
   (B) $\pm 5d^4$.
   (C) $\pm 25d^2$.
   (D) $\pm 25d^4$.

4. If two moles of compound A react with 5 moles of compound B to form compound C, then how many moles of A are required to react completely with 7 moles of B to form compound C?
   (A) 5.7
   (B) 2.8
   (C) 7.5
   (D) 8.2

5. A car traveling at x mph takes 5 hours to go from city A to city B. Traveling at $x - 15$ mph, the car makes the return trip in $6\frac{2}{3}$ hours. What was the speed of the car on the return trip?
   (A) 60 mph
   (B) 55 mph
   (C) 50 mph
   (D) 45 mph

6. In 2003, item A cost $2,500. In 2004, the price of A went up 20 percent because of inflation, while in early 2005 there was a 10 percent increase in the price of A over its 2004 price. In June of 2005, A was put on sale with a 30 percent decrease in price. What was the sale price of A?
   (A) $2,500
   (B) $2,400
   (C) $2,310
   (D) $2,110

7. In the expression $\log_4 \frac{1}{16} = x$, what is the value of x?
   (A) –2
   (B) –4
   (C) +2
   (D) +4

8. What is the volume of a sphere of a radius 3 centimeters?
   (A) 119.05 c³
   (B) 113.04 c³
   (C) 106.00 c³
   (D) 101.08 c³

STOP

IF YOU FINISH BEFORE TIME IS CALLED, YOU MAY CHECK YOUR WORK ON THIS SECTION ONLY. DO NOT TURN TO ANY OTHER SECTION IN THE TEST.

QUANTITATIVE COMPARISONS TEST 4

20 Questions • 30 Minutes

Common Information: In each question, information concerning one or both of the quantities to be compared is given in the ITEM column. A symbol that appears in any column represents the same thing in Column A as it does in Column B.

Figures: Assume that the position of points, angles, regions, and so forth, are in the order shown; that the lines shown as straight are indeed straight; that figures lie in a plane unless otherwise indicated. Figures accompanying questions are intended to provide information you can use in answering the questions. However, unless a note states that a figure is drawn to scale, you should solve the problems by using your knowledge of mathematics, NOT by estimating sizes by sight or by measurement.

Directions: For each of the following questions, two quantities are given: one in Column A and one in Column B. Compare the two quantities and mark your answer sheet with the correct, lettered conclusion. These are your options:

(A) if the quantity in Column A is the greater;
(B) if the quantity in Column B is the greater;
(C) if the two columns are equal;
(D) if the relationship cannot be determined from the information given.

Column A	Column B		Column A	Column

1.

5% of 34	The number that 34 is 5% of

3. $4 > x > -3$

$\dfrac{x}{3}$	$\dfrac{3}{x}$

2.

$\angle 1 < \angle 2$

IR	IT

4.

$\dfrac{2}{3} + \dfrac{3}{7}$	$\dfrac{16}{21} - \dfrac{3}{7}$

SUMMARY DIRECTIONS

Select: **(A)** if Column A is greater;

(B) if Column B is greater;

(C) if the two columns are equal;

(D) if the relationship cannot be determined from the information given.

Column A	Column B	Column A	Column B

5.

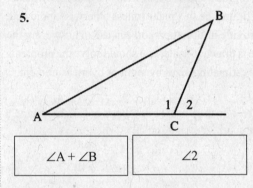

$\angle A + \angle B$	$\angle 2$

9.

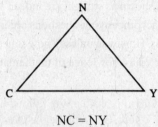

$NC = NY$

$\angle N < \angle C$

NC	CY

6. y = an odd integer

The numerical value of y^2	The numerical value of y^3

10.

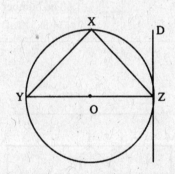

$\angle YXZ$	$\angle DZY$

7.

$8 + (6 \div 3) - 7(2)$	$6 + (8 \div 2) - 7(3)$

8.

$\frac{3}{4}$ of $\frac{9}{9}$	$\frac{9}{9} \times \frac{3}{4}$

11.

A given chord in a given circle	The radius of the same circle

SUMMARY DIRECTIONS		

Select: **(A)**   if Column A is greater;

          (B)   if Column B is greater;

          (C)   if the two columns are equal;

          (D)   if the relationship cannot be determined from the information given.

Column A	**Column B**	**Column A**	**Column B**

12.

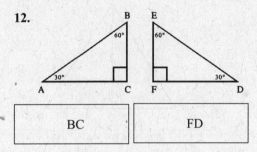

BC	FD

13.

$4 + (3 \times 2) - 7$	$(8 \div 2) + 3 - 1$

14.

50% of $\dfrac{4}{5}$	$\dfrac{4}{5}$ of $\dfrac{1}{2}$

$AC \| BD$

15.

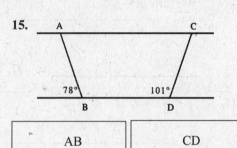

AB	CD

16.

$0.01 \div .1$	$0.01 \times .1$

$OA > OC$

17.

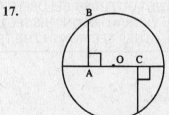

AB	CD

SUMMARY DIRECTIONS

Select: **(A)** if Column A is greater;

(B) if Column B is greater;

(C) if the two columns are equal;

(D) if the relationship cannot be determined from the information given.

Column A	Column B		Column A	Column B

18.

The number that 6 is 20% of	10% of 300

20.

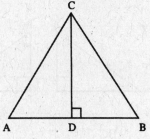

$CD \perp AB; \angle A > \angle B$

AC	CB

19. $3x + 2y = -1; 2x + 3y = 1$

The numerical value of x	The numerical value of y

STOP

IF YOU FINISH BEFORE TIME IS CALLED, YOU MAY CHECK YOUR WORK ON THIS SECTION ONLY. DO NOT TURN TO ANY OTHER SECTION IN THE TEST.

ANSWER KEY AND EXPLANATIONS

Nonverbal Arithmetic Test 1

1. C	4. A	7. D	10. C	13. A
2. A	5. C	8. B	11. D	14. C
3. D	6. D	9. A	12. B	

1. **The correct answer is (C).** Since the whole is divided into 3 units, the denominator is 3. There are 2 units shaded, so the numerator is 2. The shaded part is $\frac{2}{3}$ of the whole.

2. **The correct answer is (A).** The left-hand figure is divided into 9 parts, and is a square. The shaded part can be represented by the fraction $\frac{3}{9}$. The right-hand figure is divided in 3 parts, and is also a square. The fraction $\frac{1}{3}$ represents the shaded part; $\frac{3}{9}$ and $\frac{1}{3}$ represent the same part of the whole and are therefore equivalent, $\frac{3}{9} = \frac{1}{3}$.

3. **The correct answer is (D).**

$$\frac{630}{140} = \frac{63}{14} = \frac{63 \div 7}{14 \div 7} = \frac{9}{2}$$

4. **The correct answer is (A).** Multiply both parts by the same number. 8 multiplied by what number will give 24? Answer: divide 24 by 8 to get 3. The denominator and the numerator are multiplied by 3 to get $\frac{9}{24}$.

$$\frac{3}{8} = \frac{3 \times 3}{3 \times 8} = \frac{9}{24}$$

5. **The correct answer is (C).** Use the same process as in answer number 4.

$$\frac{6}{1} = \frac{6}{1} \times \frac{5}{5} = \frac{30}{5}$$

6. **The correct answer is (D).** Multiply numerators and denominators.

$$\frac{5}{3} \times \frac{2}{7} = \frac{5 \times 2}{3 \times 7} = \frac{10}{21}$$

7. **The correct answer is (D).** Reduce and perform the multiplication.

$$\frac{25}{36} \times \frac{\cancel{16}}{\cancel{20}} = \frac{25}{36} \times \frac{4}{5} \quad \text{(divide by 4)}$$

$$\frac{\cancel{25}}{36} \times \frac{4}{\cancel{5}} = \frac{5}{36} \times \frac{4}{1} \quad \text{(divide by 5)}$$

$$= \frac{5}{36} \times \frac{4}{1} \quad \text{(divide by 4)}$$

$$= \frac{5}{9} \times \frac{1}{1}$$

$$= \frac{5 \times 1}{9 \times 1}$$

$$= \frac{5}{9}$$

8. **The correct answer is (B).** Invert the divisor and change the operation to multiplication, reduce, and perform the multiplication.

$$\frac{3}{4} \div \frac{5}{2} = \frac{3}{4} \times \frac{2}{5}$$

$$\frac{3}{4} \times \frac{2}{5} \quad \text{(divide by 2)}$$

$$\frac{3}{2} \times \frac{1}{5} = \frac{3}{10}$$

9. **The correct answer is (A).** Use the same procedure as in answer number 8.

$$\frac{72}{50} \div \frac{200}{35} = \frac{72}{50} \times \frac{35}{200}$$

$$\frac{72}{50} \times \frac{35}{200} \quad \text{(divide by 8)}$$

$$\frac{9}{50} \times \frac{35}{25} \quad \text{(divide by 5)}$$

$$\frac{9}{50} \times \frac{7}{25} = \frac{63}{250}$$

10. **The correct answer is (C).** The bottle (whole) is divided into 12 ounces (the denominator) of which 7 ounces (the numerator) is filled. Thus, $\frac{7}{12}$ of the bottle is filled.

11. **The correct answer is (D).** Find the lowest common denominator (LCD), which is 72, build up each fraction to have 72 as denominator, and perform addition and subtraction as indicated.

The least common multiple (LCM) of 9 and 6 is 18.

The LCM of 18 and 8 is 72.

Therefore, LCD = 72.

$$\frac{2}{9} = \frac{2}{9} \times \frac{8}{8} = \frac{16}{72}$$

$$\frac{5}{6} = \frac{5 \times 12}{6 \times 12} = \frac{60}{72}$$

$$\frac{3}{8} = \frac{3 \times 9}{8 \times 9} = \frac{27}{72}$$

$$\frac{2}{9} + \frac{5}{6} - \frac{3}{8} = \frac{16}{72} + \frac{60}{72} - \frac{27}{72} = \frac{76}{72} - \frac{27}{72} = \frac{49}{72}$$

12. **The correct answer is (B).** Change both mixed numbers into improper fractions and multiply.

$$2\frac{1}{3} \times 1\frac{1}{2} = \frac{7}{3} \times \frac{3}{2}$$

$$\frac{7}{3} \times \frac{3}{2} = \frac{7}{2} = 3\frac{1}{2}$$

13. **The correct answer is (A).** Use the same procedure as in answer number 12, then change ÷ to × and invert the second fraction.

$$2\frac{1}{2} \div 3\frac{1}{3} = \frac{5}{2} \div \frac{10}{3}$$

$$\frac{\overset{1}{\cancel{5}}}{2} \times \frac{3}{\underset{2}{\cancel{10}}} = \frac{1}{2} \times \frac{3}{2} = \frac{3}{4}$$

14. **The correct answer is (C).** Add the whole numbers and fractional parts separately. Change the improper fraction to a mixed number. Find common denominators for fractional parts, then add.

$$5\frac{3}{4} + 6\frac{5}{9} = 5 + \frac{3}{4} + 6 + \frac{5}{9}$$

$$= 11 + \frac{3}{4} = \frac{5}{9}$$

$$= 11 + \frac{27}{36} + \frac{20}{36}$$

$$= 11 + \frac{47}{36}$$

$$= 11 + 1 + \frac{11}{36}$$

$$= 12 + \frac{11}{36}$$

$$= 12\frac{11}{36}$$

Problem Solving Test 2

1. B	4. D	7. D	10. A	13. B
2. D	5. C	8. A	11. C	14. D
3. A	6. C	9. D	12. C	15. A

1. **The correct answer is (B).** To find the *average* number of sections per borough, take:

   245 sections divided by 5 boroughs = 49

   49 sections/borough

2. **The correct answer is (D).**
   Total miles = 45

   number of plows = 9

   To find the *average* number of miles, divide:

   45 miles by 9 plows = 5 miles/plow

   Average = 5 miles

3. **The correct answer is (A).**

   Total time per day = 5 minutes
   Total days per month = 10 days
   Total time per month =
   $$\frac{5 \text{ minutes}}{\text{day}} \times \frac{10 \text{ days}}{\text{month}} = \frac{50 \text{ minutes}}{\text{month}}$$

4. **The correct answer is (D).**

   Total number for street cleaning = 1,500
   half that number load and drive = +750
                                                         2,250

   2,250 laborers used

5. **The correct answer is (C).**

   Total issued =   186
   subtract:
   first offenders = −100
   non-first offenders   86

6. **The correct answer is (C).** The second truck is 90 feet − 40 feet = 50 feet from the man. The first truck is 40 feet from the man. The first truck is 50 feet − 40 feet = 10 feet closer than the second truck.

7. **The correct answer is (D).** Total capacity = 1,260 gallons

   $$\frac{2}{3} \text{ of } 1,260 = \frac{2}{3} \times 1,260$$
   $$= \frac{2,520}{3}$$
   $$= 840 \text{ gallons}$$

8. **The correct answer is (A).**

   Total earnings = $160.00
   Deductions = $8.00 pension
                        $12.00 medical insurance
                     + $29.60 withholding tax
                        $49.60 total deductions

   The take-home pay can be found by subtracting the total deductions from the salary.

   $160.00 − $49.60 = $110.40

   Take-home pay = $110.40

9. **The correct answer is (D).**

Stamps per day	Cost per day
25 / day × $0.20 =	5.00
35 / day × $0.30 =	10.50
350 × $0.40 =	140.00
Total cost/day	$155.50

   For five days, 5 × $155.50 = $777.50

   Total cost = $777.50

10. **The correct answer is (A).** Total number of pencils bought in 2005 was 500 dozen at $0.40 a dozen; in 2008, 75 percent of the 500 dozen were bought at a 20 percent increase in price.

First, find how many pencils were bought in 2008. Do this by multiplying:

$500 \times 0.75 = 375$ dozen were bought in 2008

Now find the price per dozen. You know that it was 20 percent more than $0.40:

0.40×0.20 increase $= \$0.08$, or 8¢, increase in price

So the price per dozen is:

40¢ + 8¢ = 48¢, or $0.48

To find the cost, multiply the number of dozens of pencils by the cost per dozen.

375 dozen $\times \$0.48$/dozen $= \$180$

Total cost for 2008 = $180

11. **The correct answer is (C).** If it costs $0.75 to sweep 1 square foot, to find the cost for 100 square feet, multiply:

100 square feet $\times 0.75$ per square foot $= \$75$

Total cost = $75

12. **The correct answer is (C).** It takes 1 hour to tow a scow 3 miles. Find the time to tow the scow 28 miles by dividing:

28 miles $\div$ 3 miles/hour $= 9\frac{1}{3}$ hours

$\frac{1}{3}$ hour $\times 60$ minutes/hour $= 20$ minutes

Note: 1 hour = 60 minutes. To change hours to minutes, multiply the fraction of an hour by

$$\frac{60 \text{ minutes}}{\text{hour}}$$

It takes 9 hours, 20 minutes to tow the scow 28 miles.

13. **The correct answer is (B).**

Truck to the other truck	100 feet
Truck to the man	− 60 feet
	40 feet

The difference is 40 feet.

14. **The correct answer is (D).** One gross = 144 pencils

6 gross $= 144$/gross $\times 6$ gross $= 864$ pencils (on hand)

If 24 pencils are used each week, divide to find the number of weeks they will last:

864 divided by 24/week = 36 weeks

Supplies would last 36 weeks.

15. **The correct answer is (A).** If the cogs on two wheels are sized and spaced the same, the smaller of the two wheels will turn faster than the larger one—the fewer cogs a wheel has, the more revolutions it makes. The number of cogs is, therefore, inversely proportional to the number of revolutions.

The smaller wheel will make 3 revolutions for every 1 revolution the larger wheel makes. So when the smaller wheel makes 42 revolutions, the larger wheel will make 42 divided by 3 = 14 revolutions.

Algebra Test 3

1. B	3. A	5. D	7. A	8. B
2. C	4. B	6. C		

1. **The correct answer is (B).**

$$4a + 5 - 5 = 13 - 5$$
$$4a = 8$$
$$\frac{4a}{4} = \frac{8}{4}$$
$$a = 2$$

2. **The correct answer is (C).**

$$\frac{10}{m} - 8 = \frac{5}{3} \quad \text{(multiply by } 3m)$$
$$3m \times \frac{10}{m} - (3m)(8) = \frac{(3m)(5)}{3}$$
$$\frac{30m}{m} - 24m = \frac{15m}{3}$$
$$30 - 24m = 5m$$
$$30 = 29m$$
$$m = \frac{30}{29}$$

3. **The correct answer is (A).**

$$\frac{3c^2}{3} = \frac{75d^4}{3}$$
$$c^2 = 25d^4$$
$$\sqrt{c^2} = \sqrt{25d^4}$$
$$c = \pm 5d^2$$

4. **The correct answer is (B).** In a chemical reaction, the quantities of reactants/products are directly proportional.

Let $x_1 = 2$ moles of A and $y_1 = 5$ moles of B.

Then x_2 = number of moles of A and $y_2 = 7$ moles of B such that:

$$\frac{5}{2} = \frac{7}{x_2}; x_2 = 2.8 \text{ moles of A.}$$

5. **The correct answer is (D).** Since displacement = (speed)(time), $d = vt$, speed and time are inversely proportional for a constant displacement. Let $v_1 = x$ mph and $t_1 = 5$ hours; $v_2 = x - 15$ mph and $t_2 = 6\frac{2}{3}$ hours $= \frac{20}{3}$ hours. Since both displacements are the same:

$$5x = 6\frac{2}{3}(x - 15)$$
$$5x = \frac{20}{3}(x - 15)$$
$$3(5x) = 3\left(\frac{20}{3}\right)(x - 15)$$
$$15x = 20(x - 15)$$
$$15x = 20x - 300$$
$$300 = 5x$$

$x = 60$ mph, speed from A to B

$x - 15 = 45$ mph is the speed on the return trip

6. **The correct answer is (C).**

2003: Cost of A = $2,500

2004: Cost of A $= \$2,500 + \frac{20}{100} \times \$2,500 = \$3,000$

2005: Cost of A $= \$3,000 + \frac{10}{100} \times \$3,000 = \$3,300$

Sale Price (2005) $= \$3,300 - \frac{30}{100} \times \$3,300 = \$2,310$

7. **The correct answer is (A).**

$$\log_4 \frac{1}{16} = x$$
$$4^x = \frac{1}{16}$$
$$x = -2$$

facebook.com/petersonspublishing

8. **The correct answer is (B).** $v = \frac{4}{3}\pi r^3$

Because $r = 3$ and $\pi = 3.14$

$$v = \frac{4}{3}\pi r^3$$

$$= \frac{4}{3}(3.14)(3^3)$$

$$= \frac{4}{3}(3.14)(27)$$

$$= \frac{4(3.14)(27)}{3}$$

$$= 4(3.14)(9)$$

$$= 113.04\ c^3$$

Quantitative Comparisons Test 4

1. B	5. C	9. A	13. B	17. B
2. A	6. D	10. C	14. C	18. C
3. D	7. A	11. D	15. A	19. B
4. A	8. C	12. D	16. A	20. B

1. **The correct answer is (B).** 5% of 34 = $34 \times 0.05 = 1.7$

   The number that 34 is 5% of = 5% of n = 34

   $0.05n = 34$

   $n = \frac{34}{0.05}$
   $n = 680$

   $$\begin{array}{r} 680 \\ .05\overline{)34.00} \\ \underline{30} \\ 40 \\ \underline{40} \\ 0 \\ \underline{0} \end{array}$$

2. **The correct answer is (A).** In a triangle, the greater side lies opposite the greater angle. $\angle 2 > \angle 1$ (given) IR > IT

3. **The correct answer is (D).** Since x could be any number from −3 to 4, the values of the fractions are impossible to determine.

4. **The correct answer is (A).**

   $$\frac{2}{3} + \frac{3}{7} = \frac{14}{21} + \frac{9}{21}$$
   $$= \frac{23}{21}$$
   $$\frac{16}{21} - \frac{3}{7} = \frac{16}{21} - \frac{9}{21}$$
   $$= \frac{7}{21}$$

5. **The correct answer is (C).**

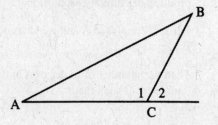

   $\angle 2 = \angle A + \angle B$ (an exterior angle of a triangle is equal to the sum of the two interior remote angles)

6. **The correct answer is (D).** There is not enough information given; y could equal 1, which would make both quantities equal; or y could be greater than 1, which would make y^3 greater than y^2. If y were a negative integer, then y^2 would be greater than y^3.

7. **The correct answer is (A).**

$$8 + (6 \div 3) - 7(2) = 8 + 2 - 14$$
$$= 10 - 14$$
$$= -4$$
$$6 + (8 \div 2) - 7(3) = 6 + 4 - 21$$
$$= 10 - 21$$
$$= -11$$
$$-4 > -11$$

8. **The correct answer is (C).**
$$\frac{3}{4} \text{ of } \frac{9}{9} = \frac{3}{4} \times \frac{9}{9} = \frac{3}{4}$$

9. **The correct answer is (A).**

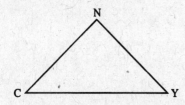

NC = NY given

$\angle C = \angle Y$ angles opposite equal sides are equal

$\angle N < \angle C$ given

$\angle N < \angle Y$ substitution

CY < NC the greater side lies opposite the greater angle

10. **The correct answer is (C).**

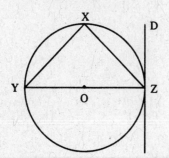

$\angle YXZ = 90°$ an angle inscribed in a semi-circle equals $90°$

$\angle DZY = 90°$ a radius is perpendicular to a tangent at their point of contact

11. **The correct answer is (D).** Impossible to determine from the information given. The radius could be less than, equal to, or greater than the chord.

12. **The correct answer is (D).** Since there are three unknown sides on both triangles, the length of BC or FD is impossible to determine.

13. **The correct answer is (B).**

$$4 + 3 \times 2 - 7 = 4 + 6 - 7$$
$$= 10 - 7$$
$$= 3$$
$$8 \div 2 + 3 - 1 = 4 + 3 - 1$$
$$= 7 - 1$$
$$= 6$$

14. **The correct answer is (C).**

$$50\% \text{ of } \frac{4}{5} = .50 \times \frac{4}{5}$$
$$= \frac{1}{2} \times \frac{4}{5}$$
$$= \frac{2}{5}$$

$$\frac{4}{5} \text{ of } \frac{1}{2} = \frac{4}{5} \times \frac{1}{2}$$
$$= \frac{2}{5}$$

15. **The correct answer is (A).** The shortest line between two parallel lines is a line perpendicular to both lines. Therefore, if there are two transversals between parallel lines, the one whose angle of intersection with the parallel lines is further from $90°$ is the longer transversal.

$$\angle B = 90° - 78° = 12°$$

$$\angle D = 101° - 90° = 11°$$

AB > CD

16. **The correct answer is (A).**

$0.01 \div 0.1 = 0.1$

$0.01 \times 0.1 = 0.001$

$.1 > .001$

17. **The correct answer is (B).** If two perpendiculars are drawn from the circumference of a circle to a diameter of the same circle, the one that is closer to the center of the circle will be longer.

18. **The correct answer is (C).** The number that 6 is 20% of:

$20\% \text{ of } n = 6$

$0.20n = 6$

$n = 6 \div 0.2$

$n = 30$

$10\% \text{ of } 300 = 10\% \times 300$

$= .10 \times 300$

$= 30$

19. **The correct answer is (B).**

$3x + 2y = -1$

$2x + 3y = 1$

$3(3x + 2y = -1)$ (multiply the first equation by 3)

$2(2x + 3y = 1)$ (multiply the second equation by 2)

$9x + 6y = -3$ (subtract the second equation

$\underline{-4x + 6y = \quad 2}$ from the first equation)

$5x \quad = -5$

$x \quad = -1$

$3x + 2y = -1$

$3(-1) + 2y = -1$ (subtract the -1 for x in

$-3 + 2y = -1$ one of the original equations

$2y = 2$ and solve for y)

$y = 1$

20. **The correct answer is (B).** $\angle A > \angle B$ given $CB > AC$. In a triangle, the greater side lies opposite the greater angle.

SCIENCE ANSWER SHEETS

Cells, Structure, and Function Test 1

1. Ⓐ Ⓑ Ⓒ Ⓓ	9. Ⓐ Ⓑ Ⓒ Ⓓ	17. Ⓐ Ⓑ Ⓒ Ⓓ	25. Ⓐ Ⓑ Ⓒ Ⓓ	33. Ⓐ Ⓑ Ⓒ Ⓓ
2. Ⓐ Ⓑ Ⓒ Ⓓ	10. Ⓐ Ⓑ Ⓒ Ⓓ	18. Ⓐ Ⓑ Ⓒ Ⓓ	26. Ⓐ Ⓑ Ⓒ Ⓓ	34. Ⓐ Ⓑ Ⓒ Ⓓ
3. Ⓐ Ⓑ Ⓒ Ⓓ	11. Ⓐ Ⓑ Ⓒ Ⓓ	19. Ⓐ Ⓑ Ⓒ Ⓓ	27. Ⓐ Ⓑ Ⓒ Ⓓ	35. Ⓐ Ⓑ Ⓒ Ⓓ
4. Ⓐ Ⓑ Ⓒ Ⓓ	12. Ⓐ Ⓑ Ⓒ Ⓓ	20. Ⓐ Ⓑ Ⓒ Ⓓ	28. Ⓐ Ⓑ Ⓒ Ⓓ	36. Ⓐ Ⓑ Ⓒ Ⓓ
5. Ⓐ Ⓑ Ⓒ Ⓓ	13. Ⓐ Ⓑ Ⓒ Ⓓ	21. Ⓐ Ⓑ Ⓒ Ⓓ	29. Ⓐ Ⓑ Ⓒ Ⓓ	37. Ⓐ Ⓑ Ⓒ Ⓓ
6. Ⓐ Ⓑ Ⓒ Ⓓ	14. Ⓐ Ⓑ Ⓒ Ⓓ	22. Ⓐ Ⓑ Ⓒ Ⓓ	30. Ⓐ Ⓑ Ⓒ Ⓓ	38. Ⓐ Ⓑ Ⓒ Ⓓ
7. Ⓐ Ⓑ Ⓒ Ⓓ	15. Ⓐ Ⓑ Ⓒ Ⓓ	23. Ⓐ Ⓑ Ⓒ Ⓓ	31. Ⓐ Ⓑ Ⓒ Ⓓ	39. Ⓐ Ⓑ Ⓒ Ⓓ
8. Ⓐ Ⓑ Ⓒ Ⓓ	16. Ⓐ Ⓑ Ⓒ Ⓓ	24. Ⓐ Ⓑ Ⓒ Ⓓ	32. Ⓐ Ⓑ Ⓒ Ⓓ	40. Ⓐ Ⓑ Ⓒ Ⓓ

Biology Test 2

1. Ⓐ Ⓑ Ⓒ Ⓓ	5. Ⓐ Ⓑ Ⓒ Ⓓ	9. Ⓐ Ⓑ Ⓒ Ⓓ	13. Ⓐ Ⓑ Ⓒ Ⓓ	17. Ⓐ Ⓑ Ⓒ Ⓓ
2. Ⓐ Ⓑ Ⓒ Ⓓ	6. Ⓐ Ⓑ Ⓒ Ⓓ	10. Ⓐ Ⓑ Ⓒ Ⓓ	14. Ⓐ Ⓑ Ⓒ Ⓓ	18. Ⓐ Ⓑ Ⓒ Ⓓ
3. Ⓐ Ⓑ Ⓒ Ⓓ	7. Ⓐ Ⓑ Ⓒ Ⓓ	11. Ⓐ Ⓑ Ⓒ Ⓓ	15. Ⓐ Ⓑ Ⓒ Ⓓ	19. Ⓐ Ⓑ Ⓒ Ⓓ
4. Ⓐ Ⓑ Ⓒ Ⓓ	8. Ⓐ Ⓑ Ⓒ Ⓓ	12. Ⓐ Ⓑ Ⓒ Ⓓ	16. Ⓐ Ⓑ Ⓒ Ⓓ	

Biology Test 3

1. Ⓐ Ⓑ Ⓒ Ⓓ	5. Ⓐ Ⓑ Ⓒ Ⓓ	9. Ⓐ Ⓑ Ⓒ Ⓓ	13. Ⓐ Ⓑ Ⓒ Ⓓ	17. Ⓐ Ⓑ Ⓒ Ⓓ
2. Ⓐ Ⓑ Ⓒ Ⓓ	6. Ⓐ Ⓑ Ⓒ Ⓓ	10. Ⓐ Ⓑ Ⓒ Ⓓ	14. Ⓐ Ⓑ Ⓒ Ⓓ	18. Ⓐ Ⓑ Ⓒ Ⓓ
3. Ⓐ Ⓑ Ⓒ Ⓓ	7. Ⓐ Ⓑ Ⓒ Ⓓ	11. Ⓐ Ⓑ Ⓒ Ⓓ	15. Ⓐ Ⓑ Ⓒ Ⓓ	19. Ⓐ Ⓑ Ⓒ Ⓓ
4. Ⓐ Ⓑ Ⓒ Ⓓ	8. Ⓐ Ⓑ Ⓒ Ⓓ	12. Ⓐ Ⓑ Ⓒ Ⓓ	16. Ⓐ Ⓑ Ⓒ Ⓓ	20. Ⓐ Ⓑ Ⓒ Ⓓ

answer sheet

Human Anatomy and Physiology Test 4

1. Ⓐ Ⓑ Ⓒ Ⓓ
2. Ⓐ Ⓑ Ⓒ Ⓓ
3. Ⓐ Ⓑ Ⓒ Ⓓ
4. Ⓐ Ⓑ Ⓒ Ⓓ
5. Ⓐ Ⓑ Ⓒ Ⓓ
6. Ⓐ Ⓑ Ⓒ Ⓓ
7. Ⓐ Ⓑ Ⓒ Ⓓ
8. Ⓐ Ⓑ Ⓒ Ⓓ
9. Ⓐ Ⓑ Ⓒ Ⓓ
10. Ⓐ Ⓑ Ⓒ Ⓓ
11. Ⓐ Ⓑ Ⓒ Ⓓ
12. Ⓐ Ⓑ Ⓒ Ⓓ
13. Ⓐ Ⓑ Ⓒ Ⓓ
14. Ⓐ Ⓑ Ⓒ Ⓓ
15. Ⓐ Ⓑ Ⓒ Ⓓ
16. Ⓐ Ⓑ Ⓒ Ⓓ
17. Ⓐ Ⓑ Ⓒ Ⓓ
18. Ⓐ Ⓑ Ⓒ Ⓓ
19. Ⓐ Ⓑ Ⓒ Ⓓ
20. Ⓐ Ⓑ Ⓒ Ⓓ

21. Ⓐ Ⓑ Ⓒ Ⓓ
22. Ⓐ Ⓑ Ⓒ Ⓓ
23. Ⓐ Ⓑ Ⓒ Ⓓ
24. Ⓐ Ⓑ Ⓒ Ⓓ
25. Ⓐ Ⓑ Ⓒ Ⓓ
26. Ⓐ Ⓑ Ⓒ Ⓓ
27. Ⓐ Ⓑ Ⓒ Ⓓ
28. Ⓐ Ⓑ Ⓒ Ⓓ
29. Ⓐ Ⓑ Ⓒ Ⓓ
30. Ⓐ Ⓑ Ⓒ Ⓓ
31. Ⓐ Ⓑ Ⓒ Ⓓ
32. Ⓐ Ⓑ Ⓒ Ⓓ
33. Ⓐ Ⓑ Ⓒ Ⓓ
34. Ⓐ Ⓑ Ⓒ Ⓓ
35. Ⓐ Ⓑ Ⓒ Ⓓ
36. Ⓐ Ⓑ Ⓒ Ⓓ
37. Ⓐ Ⓑ Ⓒ Ⓓ
38. Ⓐ Ⓑ Ⓒ Ⓓ
39. Ⓐ Ⓑ Ⓒ Ⓓ
40. Ⓐ Ⓑ Ⓒ Ⓓ

41. Ⓐ Ⓑ Ⓒ Ⓓ
42. Ⓐ Ⓑ Ⓒ Ⓓ
43. Ⓐ Ⓑ Ⓒ Ⓓ
44. Ⓐ Ⓑ Ⓒ Ⓓ
45. Ⓐ Ⓑ Ⓒ Ⓓ
46. Ⓐ Ⓑ Ⓒ Ⓓ
47. Ⓐ Ⓑ Ⓒ Ⓓ
48. Ⓐ Ⓑ Ⓒ Ⓓ
49. Ⓐ Ⓑ Ⓒ Ⓓ
50. Ⓐ Ⓑ Ⓒ Ⓓ
51. Ⓐ Ⓑ Ⓒ Ⓓ
52. Ⓐ Ⓑ Ⓒ Ⓓ
53. Ⓐ Ⓑ Ⓒ Ⓓ
54. Ⓐ Ⓑ Ⓒ Ⓓ
55. Ⓐ Ⓑ Ⓒ Ⓓ
56. Ⓐ Ⓑ Ⓒ Ⓓ
57. Ⓐ Ⓑ Ⓒ Ⓓ
58. Ⓐ Ⓑ Ⓒ Ⓓ
59. Ⓐ Ⓑ Ⓒ Ⓓ
60. Ⓐ Ⓑ Ⓒ Ⓓ

61. Ⓐ Ⓑ Ⓒ Ⓓ
62. Ⓐ Ⓑ Ⓒ Ⓓ
63. Ⓐ Ⓑ Ⓒ Ⓓ
64. Ⓐ Ⓑ Ⓒ Ⓓ
65. Ⓐ Ⓑ Ⓒ Ⓓ
66. Ⓐ Ⓑ Ⓒ Ⓓ
67. Ⓐ Ⓑ Ⓒ Ⓓ
68. Ⓐ Ⓑ Ⓒ Ⓓ
69. Ⓐ Ⓑ Ⓒ Ⓓ
70. Ⓐ Ⓑ Ⓒ Ⓓ
71. Ⓐ Ⓑ Ⓒ Ⓓ
72. Ⓐ Ⓑ Ⓒ Ⓓ
73. Ⓐ Ⓑ Ⓒ Ⓓ
74. Ⓐ Ⓑ Ⓒ Ⓓ
75. Ⓐ Ⓑ Ⓒ Ⓓ
76. Ⓐ Ⓑ Ⓒ Ⓓ
77. Ⓐ Ⓑ Ⓒ Ⓓ
78. Ⓐ Ⓑ Ⓒ Ⓓ
79. Ⓐ Ⓑ Ⓒ Ⓓ
80. Ⓐ Ⓑ Ⓒ Ⓓ

81. Ⓐ Ⓑ Ⓒ Ⓓ
82. Ⓐ Ⓑ Ⓒ Ⓓ
83. Ⓐ Ⓑ Ⓒ Ⓓ
84. Ⓐ Ⓑ Ⓒ Ⓓ
85. Ⓐ Ⓑ Ⓒ Ⓓ
86. Ⓐ Ⓑ Ⓒ Ⓓ
87. Ⓐ Ⓑ Ⓒ Ⓓ
88. Ⓐ Ⓑ Ⓒ Ⓓ
89. Ⓐ Ⓑ Ⓒ Ⓓ
90. Ⓐ Ⓑ Ⓒ Ⓓ
91. Ⓐ Ⓑ Ⓒ Ⓓ
92. Ⓐ Ⓑ Ⓒ Ⓓ
93. Ⓐ Ⓑ Ⓒ Ⓓ
94. Ⓐ Ⓑ Ⓒ Ⓓ
95. Ⓐ Ⓑ Ⓒ Ⓓ
96. Ⓐ Ⓑ Ⓒ Ⓓ
97. Ⓐ Ⓑ Ⓒ Ⓓ
98. Ⓐ Ⓑ Ⓒ Ⓓ
99. Ⓐ Ⓑ Ⓒ Ⓓ
100. Ⓐ Ⓑ Ⓒ Ⓓ

Chemistry Test 5

1. Ⓐ Ⓑ Ⓒ Ⓓ
2. Ⓐ Ⓑ Ⓒ Ⓓ
3. Ⓐ Ⓑ Ⓒ Ⓓ
4. Ⓐ Ⓑ Ⓒ Ⓓ
5. Ⓐ Ⓑ Ⓒ Ⓓ

6. Ⓐ Ⓑ Ⓒ Ⓓ
7. Ⓐ Ⓑ Ⓒ Ⓓ
8. Ⓐ Ⓑ Ⓒ Ⓓ
9. Ⓐ Ⓑ Ⓒ Ⓓ

10. Ⓐ Ⓑ Ⓒ Ⓓ
11. Ⓐ Ⓑ Ⓒ Ⓓ
12. Ⓐ Ⓑ Ⓒ Ⓓ
13. Ⓐ Ⓑ Ⓒ Ⓓ

14. Ⓐ Ⓑ Ⓒ Ⓓ
15. Ⓐ Ⓑ Ⓒ Ⓓ
16. Ⓐ Ⓑ Ⓒ Ⓓ
17. Ⓐ Ⓑ Ⓒ Ⓓ

18. Ⓐ Ⓑ Ⓒ Ⓓ
19. Ⓐ Ⓑ Ⓒ Ⓓ
20. Ⓐ Ⓑ Ⓒ Ⓓ
21. Ⓐ Ⓑ Ⓒ Ⓓ

Chemistry and Physical Science Test 6

1. Ⓐ Ⓑ Ⓒ Ⓓ
2. Ⓐ Ⓑ Ⓒ Ⓓ
3. Ⓐ Ⓑ Ⓒ Ⓓ
4. Ⓐ Ⓑ Ⓒ Ⓓ
5. Ⓐ Ⓑ Ⓒ Ⓓ
6. Ⓐ Ⓑ Ⓒ Ⓓ
7. Ⓐ Ⓑ Ⓒ Ⓓ
8. Ⓐ Ⓑ Ⓒ Ⓓ
9. Ⓐ Ⓑ Ⓒ Ⓓ
10. Ⓐ Ⓑ Ⓒ Ⓓ

11. Ⓐ Ⓑ Ⓒ Ⓓ
12. Ⓐ Ⓑ Ⓒ Ⓓ
13. Ⓐ Ⓑ Ⓒ Ⓓ
14. Ⓐ Ⓑ Ⓒ Ⓓ
15. Ⓐ Ⓑ Ⓒ Ⓓ
16. Ⓐ Ⓑ Ⓒ Ⓓ
17. Ⓐ Ⓑ Ⓒ Ⓓ
18. Ⓐ Ⓑ Ⓒ Ⓓ
19. Ⓐ Ⓑ Ⓒ Ⓓ
20. Ⓐ Ⓑ Ⓒ Ⓓ

21. Ⓐ Ⓑ Ⓒ Ⓓ
22. Ⓐ Ⓑ Ⓒ Ⓓ
23. Ⓐ Ⓑ Ⓒ Ⓓ
24. Ⓐ Ⓑ Ⓒ Ⓓ
25. Ⓐ Ⓑ Ⓒ Ⓓ
26. Ⓐ Ⓑ Ⓒ Ⓓ
27. Ⓐ Ⓑ Ⓒ Ⓓ
28. Ⓐ Ⓑ Ⓒ Ⓓ
29. Ⓐ Ⓑ Ⓒ Ⓓ
30. Ⓐ Ⓑ Ⓒ Ⓓ

31. Ⓐ Ⓑ Ⓒ Ⓓ
32. Ⓐ Ⓑ Ⓒ Ⓓ
33. Ⓐ Ⓑ Ⓒ Ⓓ
34. Ⓐ Ⓑ Ⓒ Ⓓ
35. Ⓐ Ⓑ Ⓒ Ⓓ
36. Ⓐ Ⓑ Ⓒ Ⓓ
37. Ⓐ Ⓑ Ⓒ Ⓓ
38. Ⓐ Ⓑ Ⓒ Ⓓ
39. Ⓐ Ⓑ Ⓒ Ⓓ
40. Ⓐ Ⓑ Ⓒ Ⓓ

41. Ⓐ Ⓑ Ⓒ Ⓓ
42. Ⓐ Ⓑ Ⓒ Ⓓ
43. Ⓐ Ⓑ Ⓒ Ⓓ
44. Ⓐ Ⓑ Ⓒ Ⓓ
45. Ⓐ Ⓑ Ⓒ Ⓓ
46. Ⓐ Ⓑ Ⓒ Ⓓ
47. Ⓐ Ⓑ Ⓒ Ⓓ
48. Ⓐ Ⓑ Ⓒ Ⓓ
49. Ⓐ Ⓑ Ⓒ Ⓓ
50. Ⓐ Ⓑ Ⓒ Ⓓ

answer sheet

Science

unit 7

OVERVIEW

- Cells, structure, and function test 1
- Biology test 2
- Biology test 3
- Human anatomy and physiology test 4
- Chemistry test 5
- Chemistry and physical science test 6
- Answer key and explanations

CELLS, STRUCTURE, AND FUNCTION TEST 1

40 Questions • 30 Minutes

Directions: Read each question carefully and consider all possible answers. When you have decided which choice is best, fill in the corresponding space on your answer sheet. There is only one best answer for each question.

1. Which movement requires carrier proteins but no direct cellular energy?
   - (A) Diffusion
   - (B) Osmosis
   - (C) Dialysis
   - (D) Facilitated transport

2. The polymerase chain reaction (PCR) technique is more efficient than cloning for copying large quantities of a gene because it is performed
   - (A) without DNA polymerase.
   - (B) in vitro.
   - (C) without primers.
   - (D) in vivo.

3. Which term denotes the movement of glucose molecules from an area of lower concentration to an area of higher concentration?

(A) Osmosis

(B) Diffusion

(C) Dialysis

(D) Active transport

4. You place a cell in a solution of substance x and water. Substance x is always present in the cell, but you do not know the concentration ratio in either case. The cell increases in size. What is the tonicity of the solution in which you placed the cell?

(A) Hypotonic

(B) Isotonic

(C) Hypertonic

(D) None of the above

5. Substance x passes through a plasma membrane easily. What phrase best describes the probable nature of the substance?

(A) It is hydrophilic and nonpolar.

(B) It is hydrophobic and polar.

(C) It is hydrophilic and polar.

(D) It is hydrophobic and nonpolar.

6. Cells that contain more dissolved salts and sugars than the surrounding solution are called

(A) isotonic.

(B) hypertonic.

(C) hypotonic.

(D) osmosis.

7. Foods containing unsaturated fatty acids are more healthy than those with saturated ones because they contain

(A) more hydrogen.

(B) less oxygen.

(C) more nitrogen.

(D) less hydrogen.

8. You are watching an amoeba engulf another organism. This process is an example of

(A) receptor-mediated endocytosis.

(B) facilitated transport.

(C) pinocytosis.

(D) phagocytosis.

9. The concentration of glucose in blood cells is lower than the concentration of glucose in liver cells. During active transport, glucose moves from blood cells into the liver. Which organelle would you expect to find in large numbers in the liver?

(A) Golgi bodies

(B) Endoplasmic reticulum

(C) Ribosomes

(D) Mitochondria

10. If a red blood cell is placed in sea water, it will be in what kind of solution?

(A) Isotonic

(B) Hypotonic

(C) Hypertonic

(D) Facilitated diffusion

11. Plasmolysis is a term describing

(A) cytoplasmic movement.

(B) cells that become turgid.

(C) cellular shrinkage, which occurs when cells are immersed in hypertonic solution.

(D) amoeboid movement.

12. The movement of substances from lesser concentration to higher concentration is called

(A) osmosis.

(B) diffusion.

(C) active transport.

(D) pinocytosis.

13. Which particular structure is present in both eucaryotic and prokaryotic cells?

(A) Membrane-bound nucleus

(B) Mitochondria

(C) Plastids

(D) Cell membrane

14. In photosynthesis, the reactants CO_2 and H_2O, in the presence of sunlight and chlorophyll, combine chemically to produce glucose and O_2. The O_2 comes from
    (A) H_2O.
    (B) CO_2.
    (C) CO_2 and H_2O.
    (D) N_2.

15. The endoplasmic reticulum and the Golgi body are found in prokaryotes but not eukaryotes.
    (A) True
    (B) False

16. If a radioactive element with a half-life ($t^{1/2}$) of 100 years has 31.5 kg remaining after 400 years of decay, the amount in the original sample was close to
    (A) 2,500 kg.
    (B) 500 kg.
    (C) 50 kg.
    (D) 5,000 kg.

17. As you try to mix water and oil in your salad dressing, they do not mix because
    (A) water is hydrophilic and oil is hydrophobic.
    (B) water is polar and oil is nonpolar.
    (C) both are hydrophilic.
    (D) None of the above

18. Plant cells differ from animal cells in that plant cells
    (A) have a glycoprotein covering their plasma membrane.
    (B) have a cell wall and animal cells do not.
    (C) have mitochondria and animal cells do not.
    (D) do not have a nucleus.

19. Which cell type is characterized by the lack of a true nucleus and the absence of membrane-bound organelles?
    (A) Animal cell type
    (B) Plant cell type
    (C) Fungal cell type
    (D) Prokaryotic cell

20. The cytoskeleton within the cell is thought to function
    (A) in a structural capacity.
    (B) in positioning certain enzymes in close proximity for increased efficiency.
    (C) as a means of enhancing secretion of metabolites within the cell.
    (D) Both (A) and (B)

21. Which organelle is associated with hydrolytic enzymes and is sometimes referred to as a "suicide bag"?
    (A) Golgi apparatus
    (B) Lysosome
    (C) Mitochondrion
    (D) Ribosome

QUESTIONS 22 AND 23 REFER TO THE FOLLOWING STRUCTURAL FORMULA.

$$H\overset{H}{\underset{H}{C}}\!-\!-\!\overset{H}{\underset{NH_2}{C}}\!-\!COOH$$

22. This compound is an
    (A) amino acid.
    (B) aldehyde.
    (C) alpha-keto acid.
    (D) alcohol.

23. In human digestion, this compound is the end product of
    (A) fats.
    (B) vitamins.
    (C) proteins.
    (D) carbohydrates.

24. The virus belongs to which one of the following kingdoms?

(A) Monera

(B) Plantae

(C) Protista

(D) None of the above

25. Organisms that live on dead organic matter are called

(A) parasites.

(B) carnivorous.

(C) autotrophs.

(D) saprophytes.

QUESTIONS 26 AND 27 REFER TO THE FOLLOWING DIAGRAMS.

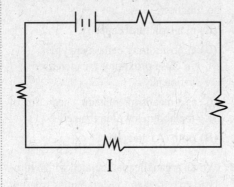

I   II

26. A person who turns off the television does not also cause the refrigerator to stop because they are

(A) in circuit I; TV in series and refrigerator in parallel.

(B) in circuit II; TV in parallel and refrigerator in series.

(C) in circuit II; both the TV and refrigerator are in parallel circuits.

(D) in circuit I; both TV and refrigerator are in series.

27. Along a string of lights on a Christmas tree, if one half goes out, they all go out. Use the above diagram to determine which of the following illustrates this circuitry.

(A) Both I and II

(B) I

(C) II

(D) Neither I nor II

28. Pinocytosis is the process of

(A) enclosing a food source or other substance in a membrane and bringing it into a cell.

(B) enclosing a liquid substance in a membrane and bringing it into the cell.

(C) enclosing a manufactured substance in a membrane and secreting it from the cell.

(D) binding a substance and a receptor and bringing it into the cell.

29. The AIDS virus is transported in bodily fluids. The Surgeon General of the United States sends out information about the disease and its transmission. In one section, there is a recommendation that one should use latex (a form of plastic) condoms rather than those made of natural membranes. This recommendation is probably based upon the principal of

(A) diffusion.

(B) facilitated transport.

(C) active transport.

(D) varied selectivity, permeability of membranes.

30. The plasma membrane of the eukaryotic cell determines selectively which substances can enter and leave the cell. Such a membrane is said to be

    (A) impermeable.

    (B) selectively permeable.

    (C) isotonic.

    (D) hypotonic.

31. What primarily determines the shape of cells that lack cell walls?

    (A) Microtubules and microfilaments

    (B) Nucleus

    (C) Endoplasmic reticulum (ER)

    (D) Ribosomes

32. Which pair of organelles is responsible for energy supply to eukaryotic cells?

    (A) Ribosomes and mitochondria

    (B) Chloroplasts and mitochondria

    (C) Nuclei and ribosomes

    (D) Mitochondria and nuclei

QUESTIONS 33 AND 34 RELATE TO THE FOLLOWING EQUATION AND GRAPH OF AN ENZYME-CATALYZED CELLULAR REACTION.

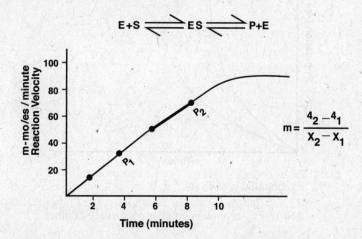

33. The linear distance between P_1 and P_2 on the above graph is the initial velocity of the reaction, as expressed by the slope **(m)** of the line (see above formula), which is

    (A) 60.

    (B) 10.

    (C) 40.

    (D) 6.

34. Choose the correct statement, relative to 10 minutes of reaction time.

    (A) Enzyme has been denatured.

    (B) All ES has been converted to [P].

    (C) All enzyme [E] is occupied with substrate [S].

    (D) All product has been converted to substrate.

35. You collect some pond water and filter out the different organisms into separate jars. You add no food to the water, but one kind of organism is still alive long after the others have died. That species is best described as being

(A) autotrophic.

(B) hydrophilic.

(C) autonomous.

(D) heterotrophic.

36. When you mix salt with water, what is the water called?

(A) Solute

(B) Solvent

(C) Solution

(D) Ionizer

QUESTIONS 37 AND 38 REFER TO THE FOLLOWING DIAGRAM.

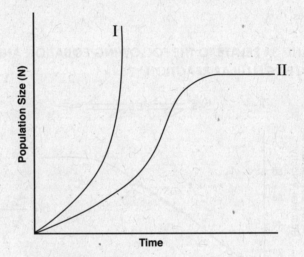

Exponential growth (I):

$\Delta N/\Delta t = r_N$—change in number per change in time

Logistic growth (II):

$\Delta N/\Delta t = r_N(k - N/K)$

r = intrinsic rate of increase

K = carrying capacity of the environment

37. Choose the correct statement expressed by curve II, as N approaches K.

(A) r approaches maximum.

(B) K expands upward.

(C) $\Delta N/\Delta t$ approaches zero.

(D) Resources remain unlimited.

38. Choose the correct statement about curve I.

(A) It assumes unlimited resources.

(B) It expresses limited growth.

(C) It expresses a K value.

(D) It assumes limited resources.

39. With which organelle is the synthesis of ATP associated?

   (A) Ribosome

   (B) Plastid

   (C) Mitochondrion

   (D) Lysosome

40. The plasma membrane is soluble to

   (A) lipids.

   (B) proteins.

   (C) acids.

   (D) nucleic acids.

STOP

IF YOU FINISH BEFORE TIME IS CALLED, YOU MAY CHECK YOUR WORK ON THIS SECTION ONLY. DO NOT TURN TO ANY OTHER SECTION IN THE TEST.

BIOLOGY TEST 2

19 Questions • 15 Minutes

Directions: Read each question carefully and consider all possible answers. When you have decided which choice is best, fill in the corresponding space on your answer sheet. There is only one best answer for each question.

1. The process whereby muscle cells produce lactic acid is called
   (A) aerobic respiration.
   (B) glycolysis.
   (C) fermentation.
   (D) electron transport chain.

2. During aerobic respiration, which one of the following substances is released?
   (A) 22 ATP
   (B) 32 ATP
   (C) 2 ATP
   (D) 36 ATP

QUESTIONS 3 AND 4 REFER TO THE FOLLOWING DIAGRAM.

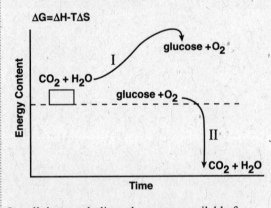

In cellular metabolism, the energy available for doing biological work is called free energy (G). It is equal to the molecular energy, enthalpy (H) minus the disorder, entropy (S) times the absolute temperature (T).

3. Choose the correct statement describing reaction I.
   (A) The reaction is exergonic.
   (B) ΔG is negative.
   (C) Glucose and O_2 have less energy than CO_2 and H_2O.
   (D) The reaction is endergonic.

4. Choose the correct statement describing reaction II.
   (A) ΔG is positive.
   (B) CO_2 and H_2O have more energy than glucose and O_2.
   (C) The reaction is exergonic.
   (D) The reaction is endergonic.

5. In exergonic reactions, the energy is
   (A) used.
   (B) stored.
   (C) released.
   (D) lost.

6. Most human enzymes function best in the temperature range of
   (A) 5–15 degrees C.
   (B) 20–30 degrees C.
   (C) 35–40 degrees C.
   (D) 45–50 degrees C.

7. Vitamins are important to the human diet because they are incorporated into
   (A) enzyme substitutes.
   (B) ATP.
   (C) co-enzymes.
   (D) inhibitors.

8. Stored energy is referred to as
   (A) activation energy.
   (B) kinetic energy.
   (C) potential energy.
   (D) electrical energy.

9. Noncyclic-photophosphorylation takes place inside the
   (A) stroma.
   (B) cytoplasm.
   (C) thylakoids.
   (D) Golgi bodies.

10. The products of the light reaction of photosynthesis are
    (A) carbohydrate + CO_2.
    (B) $NADPH_2$ + ATP + O_2.
    (C) PGAL + CO_2 + H_2O.
    (D) starch + CO_2.

11. The dark reaction of photosynthesis takes place in
    (A) thylakoids.
    (B) cytoplasm.
    (C) stroma.
    (D) grana.

QUESTIONS 12 AND 13 REFER TO THE FOLLOWING ECOLOGICAL PYRAMID OF BIOMASS AND ENERGY.

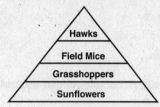

12. Select the correct population changes resulting from hunters reducing the hawk population.
    (A) Grasshoppers increase ÷ Field mice decrease ÷ Sunflowers increase
    (B) Field mice increase ÷ Grasshoppers increase ÷ Sunflowers increase
    (C) Field mice increase ÷ Grasshoppers decrease ÷ Sunflowers increase
    (D) Sunflowers decrease ÷ Grasshoppers decrease ÷ Field mice decrease

13. The second law of thermodynamics would suggest that the most energy-efficient feeding pattern would be if
    (A) field mice ate grasshoppers.
    (B) hawks ate sunflowers.
    (C) hawks ate field mice.
    (D) grasshoppers ate field mice.

14. Aerobic cellular respiration is more important to sustaining life than anaerobic because it produces more
    (A) pyruvic acid.
    (B) sugar.
    (C) energy.
    (D) lactic acid.

15. Which organelle is responsible for oxygen production?
    (A) Mitochondria
    (B) Cilia
    (C) Golgi body
    (D) Chloroplasts

16. An organic catalyst that enhances the chemical reaction is called a(n)

    (A) fat.

    (B) lactic acid.

    (C) polysaccharide.

    (D) enzyme.

17. The first stage of aerobic cellular respiration is

    (A) electron transport chain.

    (B) Krebs cycle.

    (C) glycolysis.

    (D) light reaction.

18. Glycolysis occurs in the

    (A) nucleus.

    (B) mitochondrion.

    (C) plasma membrane.

    (D) cytoplasm.

19. For the aerobic pathway, electron transport systems are located in the

    (A) cytoplasm.

    (B) Golgi bodies.

    (C) lysosomes.

    (D) mitochondrion.

STOP

IF YOU FINISH BEFORE TIME IS CALLED, YOU MAY CHECK YOUR WORK ON THIS SECTION ONLY. DO NOT TURN TO ANY OTHER SECTION IN THE TEST.

BIOLOGY TEST 3

20 Questions • 15 Minutes

Directions: Read each question carefully and consider all possible answers. When you have decided which choice is best, fill in the corresponding space on your answer sheet. There is only one best answer for each question.

1. If body cells of cows contain a total of 40 chromosomes, sperm and egg cells of cows contain how many chromosomes total?
   (A) 10
   (B) 20
   (C) 25
   (D) 40

2. Codominance occurs when
   (A) both the alleles in a heterozygote are expressed phenotypically in an individual.
   (B) expression of 2 different alleles alternates from one generation to the next.
   (C) a heterozygote expresses an intermediate phenotype.
   (D) offspring exhibit several different phenotypic expressions of a single trait.

3. Mitosis in a single human cell usually results in the formation of
   (A) 2 diploid cells.
   (B) 2 haploid cells.
   (C) 4 diploid cells.
   (D) 4 haploid cells.

4. Meiosis in a single human cell usually results in the formation of
   (A) 2 diploid cells.
   (B) 2 haploid cells.
   (C) 4 diploid cells.
   (D) 4 haploid cells.

5. If you reproduce sexually, you produce gametes via
   (A) fertilization.
   (B) mitosis.
   (C) meiosis.
   (D) recombination.

6. If you reproduce asexually, you produce offspring via
   (A) fertilization.
   (B) mitosis.
   (C) meiosis.
   (D) recombination.

7. According to Mendel's Law of Segregation, an organism with the genotype Aa
   (A) produces only gametes containing the A allele.
   (B) produces only gametes containing the a allele.
   (C) half the time produces gametes containing A, and half the time, a.
   (D) three quarters of the time produces gametes containing A, and one quarter of the time, a.

8. What type of allele is expressed in the phenotype of only a homozygous individual?
   (A) Incompletely dominant
   (B) Haploid
   (C) Recessive
   (D) Dominant

9. The sex of a human child is determined by the sex chromosome from
   (A) the mother.
   (B) the father.
   (C) both parents.
   (D) neither parents.

10. Cell division occurs most rapidly in
    (A) heart tissue.
    (B) muscle tissue.
    (C) nervous tissue.
    (D) cancerous tissue.

11. If the sperm cells of a fish have 30 chromosomes, the body cell of the fish has
    (A) 80 chromosomes.
    (B) 60 chromosomes.
    (C) 120 chromosomes.
    (D) None of the above

12. A condition resulting from the presence of an extra twenty-first chromosome is
    (A) hemophilia.
    (B) the Rh-positive condition.
    (C) phenylketonuria.
    (D) Down syndrome.

13. A woman who is a heterozygous carrier for a sex-linked recessive gene will pass it to
    (A) all of her sons.
    (B) all of her daughters.
    (C) all children.
    (D) one half of her sons and one half of her daughters.

14. Persons who have hemophilia cannot produce
    (A) new red blood cells.
    (B) normally shaped red blood cells.
    (C) functional blood clotting factors.
    (D) white blood cells.

15. Which of the following is an example of a sex-linked genetic disorder?
    (A) Tay-Sachs disease
    (B) Cystic fibrosis
    (C) Turner's syndrome
    (D) Hemophilia

16. In the case of the sex-linked trait red-green color-blindness, which one of the following CANNOT occur?
    (A) A carrier mother passing the gene on to her son
    (B) A carrier mother passing the gene on to her daughter
    (C) A color-blind father passing the gene on to his son
    (D) A color-blind father passing the gene on to his daughter

17. The genotype for a man who has blue eyes and hemophilia is
    (A) $x^b y \; x^h y$
    (B) bb hh
    (C) bb $x^h y$
    (D) Bbh

18. If both parents have blood type AB, what will be the blood types of offspring?
    (A) A
    (B) AB
    (C) A, AB, and B
    (D) O

19. Which blood type would be a universal donor?
    (A) A
    (B) AB
    (C) B
    (D) O

20. Males who tend to be tall and have strong criminal records have which of the following sex chromosomes?
   (A) XXY
   (B) XY
   (C) XYY
   (D) XYXY

STOP

IF YOU FINISH BEFORE TIME IS CALLED, YOU MAY CHECK YOUR WORK ON THIS SECTION ONLY. DO NOT TURN TO ANY OTHER SECTION IN THE TEST.

HUMAN ANATOMY AND PHYSIOLOGY TEST 4

100 Questions • 75 Minutes

Directions: Read each question carefully and consider all possible answers. When you have decided which choice is best, fill in the corresponding space on your answer sheet. There is only one best answer for each question.

1. The _____ system picks up fluid leaked from blood vessels, houses white blood cells, and is highly involved in mechanisms of immunity.
   (A) urinary
   (B) endocrine
   (C) integumentary
   (D) lymphatic

2. The major muscle component of inspiration is the
   (A) diaphragm.
   (B) external intercostal muscles.
   (C) internal intercostal muscles.
   (D) abdominal muscles.

3. Skin, nails, and hair are components of the _____ system.
   (A) integumentary
   (B) lymphatic
   (C) skeletal
   (D) endocrine

4. Water reabsorption in the collecting duct of the kidneys is controlled by _____ from the posterior pituitary.
   (A) oxytocin
   (B) ADH
   (C) epinephrine
   (D) aldosterone

5. Most homeostatic control mechanisms are
   (A) positive feedback mechanisms.
   (B) negative feedback mechanisms.
   (C) neural mechanisms.
   (D) endocrine mechanisms.

6. The most important structure(s) in the routine control of respiration is(are) the
   (A) trachea.
   (B) irritant receptors.
   (C) peripheral chemoreceptors.
   (D) central chemoreceptors.

7. A _____ plane is a vertical plane that divides the body into left and right parts.
   (A) frontal
   (B) transverse
   (C) sagittal
   (D) coronal

8. Cardiac output is equal to
   (A) heart rate.
   (B) stroke volume.
   (C) the product of stroke volume and heart rate.
   (D) stroke volume divided by heart rate.

9. Movement of a solute across a biological membrane from an area of high concentration to an area of low concentration occurs via
   (A) osmosis.
   (B) diffusion.
   (C) active transport.
   (D) inertia.

10. The right ventricle pumps blood through the _____ valve into the _____.
    (A) atrioventricular; pulmonary veins
    (B) pulmonary semilunar; pulmonary veins
    (C) atrioventricular; pulmonary arteries
    (D) pulmonary semilunar; pulmonary arteries

11. The primary Beta-2 catechol amine agonist is
    (A) acetylcholine.
    (B) epinephrine.
    (C) norepinephrine.
    (D) nicotine.

12. Action potentials result from an increased membrane permeability to
    (A) calcium.
    (B) sodium.
    (C) potassium.
    (D) chloride.

13. Food is prevented from entering the trachea during swallowing by the
    (A) glottis.
    (B) esophageal sphincter.
    (C) cardiac sphincter.
    (D) epiglottis.

14. Oxygen transported in blood is mainly
    (A) dissolved in plasma.
    (B) combined with hemoglobin.
    (C) CO_2.
    (D) carried as bicarbonate.

15. Pyramidal tract fibers originate in the
    (A) precentral gyrus.
    (B) postcentral gyrus.
    (C) thalamus.
    (D) spinal cord.

16. The transmitter substance at the neuro-muscular junction is
    (A) acetylcholinesterase.
    (B) norepinephrine.
    (C) acetylcholine.
    (D) epinephrine.

17. _____ dilate or constrict to control the flow of blood into a particular capillary bed.
    (A) Arteries
    (B) Arterioles
    (C) Capillaries
    (D) Veins

18. Hormone secretion and neurotransmitter release use the process of _____ to move substances from the cell interior into the extracellular space.
    (A) phagocytosis
    (B) endocytosis
    (C) exocytosis
    (D) pinocytosis

19. The area innervated by all the axons in a single dorsal root is a
    (A) receptive field.
    (B) dermatome.
    (C) sensory unit.
    (D) motor unit.

20. Stratified squamous anatomically describes a form of _____ tissue.
    (A) muscle
    (B) nerve
    (C) connective
    (D) epithelial

21. _____ forms most of the embryonic skeleton, connects the ribs of the sternum, and comprises the solid supportive structures of the nose and trachea.
    (A) Bone
    (B) Areolar connective tissue
    (C) Adipose tissue
    (D) Cartilage

22. _____ is the fibrous protein found in the stratum corneum that helps give the epidermis its protective properties.
    (A) Keratin
    (B) Melanin
    (C) Carotene
    (D) Hemoglobin

23. Pain information is carried by _____ afferents.
    (A) A Delta
    (B) C
    (C) A Alpha
    (D) A Delta and C

24. Increased parasympathetic activity will result in
    (A) increased heart rate.
    (B) increased cardiac output.
    (C) vasoconstriction.
    (D) decreased heart rate.

25. The receptor for the stretch reflex is the
    (A) Golgi tendon organ.
    (B) free nerve ending.
    (C) hair cell.
    (D) muscle spindle.

26. The glomerular membrane is
    (A) more permeable than most other capillaries.
    (B) less permeable than most other capillaries.
    (C) highly permeable to proteins.
    (D) highly permeable to erythrocytes.

27. CO_2 in blood is mainly
    (A) dissolved in plasma.
    (B) carried as bicarbonate.
    (C) dissolved in RBCs.
    (D) combined with hemoglobin.

28. Glucose is returned in blood in the kidneys by
    (A) glomerular filtration.
    (B) tubular reabsorption.
    (C) tubular secretion.
    (D) reabsorption in the collection duct.

29. The outer surface of the diaphysis of a long bone is covered with a double-layered membrane called the _____. The inner layer of that membrane contains bone-forming cells called _____.
    (A) endosteum; osteoblasts
    (B) endosteum; osteoclasts
    (C) periosteum; osteoclasts
    (D) periosteum; osteoblasts

30. Atrial contraction is
    (A) initiated by the AV node.
    (B) most important in a resting subject.
    (C) initiated by the SA node.
    (D) responsible for most of the ventricular filling.

31. The first heart sound is a result of
    (A) closing of the pulmonary valve.
    (B) closing of the AV valves.
    (C) closing of the aortic valve.
    (D) contraction of the atria.

32. The portion of the skull overlying the region of the cerebral cortex primarily involved with visual process is the _____ bone.
    (A) frontal
    (B) parietal
    (C) occipital
    (D) temporal

33. Normally, most of the body's total blood is found in the
    (A) veins.
    (B) arteries.
    (C) capillaries.
    (D) heart.

34. The kneecap, or patella, is an example of a(n) _____ bone.
    (A) long
    (B) short
    (C) flat
    (D) irregular

35. The normal pacemaker of the heart is the
    (A) SA node.
    (B) AV node.
    (C) atria.
    (D) ventricle.

36. Blood pressure is highest in
    (A) arteries.
    (B) arterioles.
    (C) capillaries.
    (D) veins.

37. Water permeability is greatest in the _____ of the nephron.
    (A) collecting duct
    (B) distal convoluted tubule
    (C) loop of Henle
    (D) proximal convoluted tubule

38. Movement of particles across a biological membrane is enhanced by
    (A) large particle size.
    (B) lipid solubility.
    (C) particle charge.
    (D) lipophobic properties.

39. The division of the autonomic nervous system that functions during emergencies is the
    (A) sympathetic.
    (B) parasympathetic.
    (C) craniosacral.
    (D) somatic.

40. Sympathetic preganglionic neurons originate in the
    (A) cervical spinal cord.
    (B) thoracic spinal cord.
    (C) sacral spinal cord.
    (D) coccygeal spinal cord.

41. Cellular energy production takes place within
    (A) rough endoplasmic reticulum.
    (B) smooth endoplasmic reticulum.
    (C) mitochondria.
    (D) Golgi apparatus.

42. _____ is a bending movement that decreases the angle of a joint and brings two articulating bones closer together.
    (A) Retraction
    (B) Flexion
    (C) Extension
    (D) Rotation

43. New epidermal cells are formed in the stratum
    (A) germinativum.
    (B) corneum.
    (C) spinosum.
    (D) lucidum.

44. Women have a larger percentage of adipose tissue than men; this tissue is mainly found in the
    (A) epidermis.
    (B) dermis.
    (C) subcutaneous layer.
    (D) muscle.

45. Membranes that line body cavities that open to the outside are
    (A) mucous.
    (B) serous.
    (C) synovial.
    (D) cutaneous.

46. Epidermal cells are supplied with nutrition from blood vessels located within the
    (A) epidermis.
    (B) dermis.
    (C) subcutaneous layer.
    (D) All of the above

47. The terms visceral, nonstriated, and involuntary are descriptive of _____ muscle.
    (A) skeletal
    (B) smooth
    (C) cardiac
    (D) postural

48. Blood cell formation is a function of the
   _____ system.
   (A) circulatory
   (B) skeletal
   (C) endocrine
   (D) muscular

49. Blood calcium is elevated by
   (A) calcitonin.
   (B) parathyroid hormone.
   (C) growth hormone.
   (D) thyroxine.

50. A 7-year-old patient is perspiring freely on
   the forehead, palms, and soles, indicating
   activity of the
   (A) eccrine glands.
   (B) apocrine glands.
   (C) sebaceous glands.
   (D) ceruminous glands.

51. Flexion of the elbow results from contrac-
   tion of the _____ muscle, and flexion of
   the knee involves contraction of the _____
   muscle.
   (A) biceps brachii; biceps femoris
   (B) triceps brachii; triceps femoris
   (C) biceps femoris; biceps brachii
   (D) triceps femoris; triceps brachii

52. Sweat glands that become functional at
   puberty are
   (A) apocrine.
   (B) eccrine.
   (C) sebaceous.
   (D) ceruminous.

53. An individual with higher than normal
   blood calcium (hypercalcemia) will com-
   pensate by elevating levels of
   (A) parathyroid hormone.
   (B) calcitonin.
   (C) Both (A) and (B)
   (D) Neither (A) nor (B)

54. The _____ system carries hormones to
   their sites of action.
   (A) endocrine
   (B) cardiovascular
   (C) respiratory
   (D) skeletal

55. The most rapidly conducting axons within
   the human nervous system are _____ and
   _____.
   (A) unmyelinated; small diameter
   (B) unmyelinated; large diameter
   (C) myelinated; small diameter
   (D) myelinated; large diameter

56. The basic unit of structure and function
   within the kidneys is the
   (A) glomerulus.
   (B) nephron.
   (C) ureter.
   (D) urethra.

57. The esophagus enters the stomach at the
   _____ region.
   (A) fundus
   (B) cardiac
   (C) body
   (D) pyloric

58. Release of _____ by the posterior pituitary
   will lead to contractions of the smooth
   muscle of the uterus.
   (A) ADH
   (B) ACTH
   (C) oxytocin
   (D) prolactin

59. Inhibition of ADH release will result in
   (A) high blood pressure.
   (B) increased urine output.
   (C) uterine contractions.
   (D) decreased urine output.

60. Ovulation occurs in response to
    (A) FSH.
    (B) ADH.
    (C) prolactin.
    (D) LH.

61. Heartburn results from reflux of gastric fluids into the esophagus. The structure that normally prevents this is the
    (A) pyloric sphincter.
    (B) cardiac spincter.
    (C) ileocecal valve.
    (D) epiglottis.

62. Fat is broken down in the duodenum by _____ from the gallbladder.
    (A) lipase
    (B) amylase
    (C) bile
    (D) HCl

63. Most digestion takes place in the
    (A) stomach.
    (B) duodenum.
    (C) ileum.
    (D) jejunum.

64. Visual receptors are located on the
    (A) lens.
    (B) cornea.
    (C) retina.
    (D) optic tract.

65. Most food absorption takes place in the
    (A) duodenum.
    (B) colon.
    (C) ileum.
    (D) stomach.

66. Centers for cardiovascular and respiratory control, vomiting, and coughing are found within the _____, the most inferior part of the brain stem.
    (A) midbrain
    (B) pons
    (C) medulla
    (D) thalamus

67. Bile is manufactured in the
    (A) duodenum.
    (B) liver.
    (C) gallbladder.
    (D) pancreas.

68. A patient who is abnormally short and developmentally disabled suggests that the patient
    (A) had hyperthyroidism as an infant.
    (B) had hypothyroidism as an infant.
    (C) has adult hyperthyroidism.
    (D) has adult hypothyroidism.

69. Receptors used for color vision are
    (A) hair cells.
    (B) rods.
    (C) cones.
    (D) retinae.

70. The inner lining of the digestive system is the _____ layer.
    (A) mucosal
    (B) submucosal
    (C) muscular
    (D) serosal

71. The _____ has both endocrine and exocrine functions.
    (A) adrenal cortex
    (B) pancreas
    (C) parathyroid
    (D) thyroid

72. Lacrimation refers to the production of
   (A) salvia.
   (B) mucous.
   (C) tears.
   (D) urine.

73. The sense of smell travels over cranial nerve number
   (A) I.
   (B) II.
   (C) III.
   (D) IV.

74. The gland adjacent to the urethra that enlarges in older males is the
   (A) testes.
   (B) seminal vesicle.
   (C) bulbourethral gland.
   (D) prostate.

75. Linear acceleration of the head is detected by receptors within the
   (A) semicircular canals.
   (B) utricles and saccules.
   (C) cochlea.
   (D) middle ear.

76. The most abundant protein in blood is
   (A) alpha globulin.
   (B) albumin.
   (C) gamma globulin.
   (D) fibrin.

77. Fertilization normally occurs within the
   (A) fallopian tube.
   (B) ovary.
   (C) uterus.
   (D) vagina.

78. Depression is characterized by
   (A) high levels of norepinephrine.
   (B) low levels of serotonin.
   (C) high levels of serotonin.
   (D) low levels of norepinephrine.

79. Lymphatic vessels originate at
   (A) vascular capillaries.
   (B) lymphatic capillaries.
   (C) lymph nodes.
   (D) lymphocytes.

80. Human chorionic gonadotropin (HCG) is responsible for
   (A) maintaining the corpus luteum.
   (B) lowering estrogen levels.
   (C) lowering progesterone levels.
   (D) initiating menstruation.

81. Loss of the sense of sweet and sour tastes from the tongue indicate damage to the _____ nerve.
   (A) first
   (B) fifth
   (C) seventh
   (D) tenth

82. Salivation, lacrimation, urination, and defecation are primarily under control of the _____ division of the autonomic nervous system.
   (A) sympathetic
   (B) parasympathetic
   (C) somatic
   (D) voluntary

83. Sperm cells are stored in the _____ after leaving the seminiferous tubules.
   (A) epididymis
   (B) vas deferens
   (C) seminal vesicle
   (D) prostate

84. The hormone from the pancreas that is responsible for elevating blood glucose levels between meals is
   (A) insulin.
   (B) glucagon.
   (C) somatostatin.
   (D) epinephrine.

85. The most abundantly formed elements in blood are
    (A) white blood cells.
    (B) red blood cells.
    (C) globulins.
    (D) albumins.

86. The most rapid mechanism of pH adjustment involves
    (A) buffers.
    (B) the respiratory system.
    (C) the kidneys.
    (D) the liver.

87. Normal pH of blood is
    (A) 6
    (B) 7.4
    (C) 8
    (D) 1.0

88. Hematocrit is a measure of _____ levels.
    (A) white cell
    (B) plasma
    (C) blood
    (D) erythrocyte

89. Cardiac muscle, because of its constant activity, has a high oxygen demand, which must be met without interruption. Oxygen is supplied to cardiac muscle by
    (A) the blood being pumped through the chambers of the heart.
    (B) coronary arteries.
    (C) coronary veins.
    (D) pulmonary arteries.

90. Auditory receptors are
    (A) rods.
    (B) hair cells.
    (C) cones.
    (D) muscle spindles.

91. Blood containing the A antigen and the B antibody is type
    (A) A
    (B) B
    (C) AB
    (D) O

92. Hemoglobin forms abnormal long chains in
    (A) pernicious anemia.
    (B) iron deficiency anemia.
    (C) aplastic anemia.
    (D) sickle cell anemia.

93. Auditory receptors are found within the
    (A) outer ear.
    (B) middle ear.
    (C) auditory ossicles.
    (D) cochlea.

94. Female menopause is characterized by low levels of
    (A) GnRH.
    (B) LH.
    (C) FSH.
    (D) estrogen.

95. Hyperventilation resulting from hysteria may cause
    (A) respiratory acidosis.
    (B) respiratory alkalosis.
    (C) metabolic acidosis.
    (D) metabolic alkalosis.

96. The major component of plasma is
    (A) ions.
    (B) proteins.
    (C) water.
    (D) gases.

97. _____ acts as a contraceptive agent by inhibiting release of GnRH.
    (A) Sperm
    (B) Estrogen
    (C) Testosterone
    (D) LH

facebook.com/petersonspublishing

98. Coagulation is inhibited by

(A) fibrin.

(B) calcium.

(C) thrombin.

(D) heparin.

99. Ovulation is triggered by the release of

(A) FSH.

(B) LH.

(C) GnRH.

(D) estrogen.

100. Testosterone is produced by _____ cells.

(A) prostate

(B) seminiferous

(C) epididymis

(D) interstitial

STOP

IF YOU FINISH BEFORE TIME IS CALLED, YOU MAY CHECK YOUR WORK ON THIS SECTION ONLY. DO NOT TURN TO ANY OTHER SECTION IN THE TEST.

CHEMISTRY TEST 5

21 Questions • 20 Minutes

Directions: Read each question carefully and consider all possible answers. When you have decided which choice is best, fill in the corresponding space on your answer sheet. There is only one best answer for each question.

1. A high concentration of H^+ ions is characteristic of
   (A) high pH.
   (B) strong acid.
   (C) alkaline base.
   (D) Both (A) and (C)

2. Long chains of glucose molecules are involved in the structure of
   (A) proteins.
   (B) fats.
   (C) cholesterol.
   (D) polysaccharides.

3. When a solution has a pH of 7, it is
   (A) a strong base.
   (B) a strong acid.
   (C) a weak base.
   (D) neutral.

4. Which one of the following is NOT a carbohydrate?
   (A) Maltose
   (B) Cellulose
   (C) Glycogen
   (D) Cholesterol

5. An example of an organic compound is
   (A) water (H_2O).
   (B) ammonia (NH_3).
   (C) salt (NaCl).
   (D) glucose ($C_6H_{12}O_6$).

6. A covalent bond is believed to be caused by
   (A) transfer of electrons.
   (B) sharing of electrons.

   (C) release of energy.
   (D) None of the above

7. An atom has the electron configuration (2-8-8-2). This atom would tend to
   (A) gain electrons.
   (B) loose 2 electrons.
   (C) be inert.
   (D) None of the above

8. Which of the following is a dissaccharide?
   (A) Glucose
   (B) Maltose
   (C) Fructose
   (D) Chilin

9. Which one of the following is NOT a carbohydrate?
   (A) Maltose
   (B) Cellulose
   (C) Glycogen
   (D) Wax

10. The basic building blocks of proteins are
    (A) polypeptides.
    (B) glucose.
    (C) amino acids.
    (D) None of the above

11. If the atomic number of magnesium is 12, what will be the number of protons?
    (A) 6
    (B) 10
    (C) 14
    (D) 12

12. Which is NOT an inert element?

   (A) Hydrogen

   (B) Neon

   (C) Oxygen

   (D) Nitrogen

13. Atoms are electrically neutral. This means that an atom will contain

   (A) more protons than neutrons.

   (B) more electrons than protons.

   (C) an equal number of protons and electrons.

   (D) None of the above

14. Which is true of alkaline solutions?

   (A) More H^+ ion than OH ion

   (B) Same amount of H^+ ion + OH^- ion

   (C) More OH^- ion than H^+ ion

   (D) None of the above

15. A common detergent has pH 11.0, so the detergent is

   (A) neutral.

   (B) acidic.

   (C) alkaline.

   (D) None of the above

16. The basic building block of carbohydrate is

   (A) starch.

   (B) chitin.

   (C) sucrose.

   (D) glucose.

17. The number of different amino acids in proteins is

   (A) 20

   (B) 26

   (C) 50

   (D) 92

18. A nucleotide is

   (A) phospholipid, sugar, and base.

   (B) phosphate, sugar, and base.

   (C) phosphate, protein, and base.

   (D) phospholipid, sugar, and protein.

19. Polar bonds form when

   (A) electrons are shared unequally between atoms.

   (B) more than one pair of electrons is shared.

   (C) ions are formed.

   (D) an acid and base are combined.

20. Which of the following is an example of hydrogen bonding?

   (A) The bond between O and H in a single molecule of water

   (B) The bond between O of one water molecule and H of a second water molecule

   (C) The bond between O of one water molecule and O of a second water molecule

   (D) The bond between H of one water molecule and H of a second water molecule

21. The Central Dogma of Information Transfer states that information is passed in what sequence?

   (A) RNA to proteins to DNA

   (B) DNA to RNA to proteins

   (C) Proteins to RNA to DNA

   (D) RNA to DNA to proteins

STOP

IF YOU FINISH BEFORE TIME IS CALLED, YOU MAY CHECK YOUR WORK ON THIS SECTION ONLY. DO NOT TURN TO ANY OTHER SECTION IN THE TEST.

CHEMISTRY AND PHYSICAL SCIENCE TEST 6

50 Questions • 45 Minutes

Directions: Read each question carefully and consider all possible answers. When you have decided which choice is best, fill in the corresponding space on your answer sheet. There is only one best answer for each question. You may use the periodic table on page 312 if needed.

1. The compound that has the greatest polarity is
   (A) CH_3—CH_2—O—CH_2—CH_3.
   (B) CH_3—$CH_2CH_2CH_2$—CH_3.
   (C) CH_3—CH_2—CH_2—CH_2—CH_2—Cl.
   (D) CH_3—CH_2—CH_2—CH_2—CH_2—OH.

2. The formula that represents the strongest acid in the following group is
   (A) HCl.
   (B) HCN.
   (C) HNO_3.
   (D) HCOOH.

3. The sugar with the highest molecular weight of those listed here is
   (A) fructose.
   (B) sucrose.
   (C) glucose.
   (D) None of the above; all have the same molecular weight.

4. A hydride ion and a hydrogen atom both have
   (A) the same number of electrons.
   (B) the same charge.
   (C) the same number of protons.
   (D) equal atomic radii.

5. The general formula for an aldehyde is
   (A) RCOOH.
   (B) RCOOR.
   (C) ROH.
   (D) RCHO.

6. The compound that will not be acidic when dissolved in water is
   (A) HBr.
   (B) N_2O_5.
   (C) CaO.
   (D) NH_4Cl.

7. Atoms that have the same atomic number but different atomic masses
   (A) are from different elements.
   (B) are isobars.
   (C) have different numbers of electrons.
   (D) are isotopes.

8. When electrolysis is done with molten NaCl, the substance produced at the anode is
   (A) chlorine.
   (B) hydrogen.
   (C) sodium.
   (D) oxygen.

9. The non-electrolyte in the following group is
   (A) acetic acid.
   (B) calcium chloride.
   (C) sodium bromide.
   (D) sugar.

10. Rubbing alcohol is
    (A) methyl alcohol.
    (B) ethyl alcohol.
    (C) phenol.
    (D) isopropyl alcohol.

11. Which of the following elements is a transition element?
    (A) Argon
    (B) Copper
    (C) Barium
    (D) Aluminum

12. When calcium reacts with chlorine to form calcium chloride, it
    (A) shares two electrons.
    (B) gains two electrons.
    (C) loses two electrons.
    (D) gains one electron.

13. The compound NaClO is called
    (A) sodium perchlorate.
    (B) sodium oxychloride.
    (C) sodium chlorate.
    (D) sodium hypochlorite.

14. Reaction kinetics deals with
    (A) equilibrium position.
    (B) reaction rates.
    (C) molecular reactant size.
    (D) None of the above

15. A 1-molar solution of K_3PO_4, potassium phosphate, contains in 1 liter
    (A) one mole of potassium ions.
    (B) one mole of oxygen atoms.
    (C) one mole of phosphorus atoms.
    (D) no ions.

16. In the compound propene, $H_2C=CH$ — CH_3, the single bond between two carbon atoms is
    (A) stronger than the double bond.
    (B) shorter than the double bond.
    (C) equal to the double bond in bond strength.
    (D) longer than the double bond.

17. Of the following groups, the least reactive are
    (A) the halogens.
    (B) the inert gases.
    (C) group IIA metals.
    (D) precious metals of group IB.

18. Per liter, compared with a 3-molar aqueous solution, a 3-molal aqueous solution contains
    (A) the same amount of solute.
    (B) more solute.
    (C) less solute.
    (D) a variable amount of solute.

19. For a molecular substance, a gram formula weight
    (A) is unrelated to the gram molecular weight.
    (B) is always equal to the mass corresponding to its empirical formula.
    (C) can always be calculated from its empirical formula alone.
    (D) is identical to its gram molecular weight.

20. If gas A has a molecular weight four times that of gas B, the average speed of gas
    (A) A is about four times that of gas B.
    (B) B is about four times that of gas A.
    (C) A is about twice that of gas B.
    (D) B is about twice that of gas A.

21. Ice can be melted most effectively by _____ if 1 mole is used.
    (A) sucrose
    (B) calcium chloride
    (C) sodium chloride
    (D) methanol

22. Per atom, an element that has an atomic number of 19 contains
    (A) 19 electrons and 19 neutrons.
    (B) 19 electrons and 19 protons.
    (C) 19 protons and 19 neutrons.
    (D) a total of 19 protons and neutrons.

23. In a volume of air at one atmosphere pressure at sea level, the partial pressure of nitrogen will be about
    (A) 490 mm of mercury.
    (B) 760 mm of mercury.
    (C) 106 mm of mercury.
    (D) 608 mm of mercury.

24. If the stirring of a solution results in precipitation of solute with no change in temperature, the solution must have been
    (A) saturated.
    (B) concentrated.
    (C) dilute.
    (D) supersaturated.

25. If the reaction : $A + B \rightarrow C + D$ is designated as first order, the rate depends on
    (A) the concentration of only one reactant.
    (B) the concentration of each reactant.
    (C) no specific concentration.
    (D) the temperature only.

26. The loss of an alpha particle from the radioactive atom $\frac{228}{88}$ would leave

    (A) $\frac{224}{86}$ Rn

    (B) $\frac{222}{86}$ Rn

    (C) $\frac{224}{88}$ Ra

    (D) $\frac{230}{90}$ Th

27. Which of the following is NOT a form of radioactive decay?
    (A) Electron capture
    (B) Beta emission
    (C) Alpha emission
    (D) Proton emission

28. The greatest amount of energy would be produced by the burning of 1 gram of
    (A) fat.
    (B) carbohydrate.
    (C) protein.
    (D) ribonucleic acid.

29. For the reaction: $H_2(g) + Br_2(g) \rightarrow 2HBr(g)$, the reaction can be driven to the left by
    (A) increasing the pressure.
    (B) increasing the hydrogen.
    (C) increasing hydrogen bromide.
    (D) decreasing hydrogen bromide.

30. Carbon-14 has a half life of 5.73×10 years. If a sample contained 1 gram of C-14, the time required to decay to only 0.0625 g would be
    (A) 11.46×10 years.
    (B) 5.73×10 years.
    (C) 22.92×10 years.
    (D) None of the above

31. The oxidation number of Mn in the compound K_2MnO_4 is
    (A) +7.
    (B) +2.
    (C) 0.
    (D) +6.

32. The element with the highest ionization energy of those following is
    (A) Mg.
    (B) Sr.
    (C) Ca.
    (D) Ba.

33. The least electronegative of the following elements is
    (A) Cl.
    (B) F.
    (C) Br.
    (D) I.

34. The element with the smallest atomic radius of the following is
    (A) Sr.
    (B) Mg.
    (C) Ba.
    (D) Ra.

35. Which of the following salts would be more soluble in 1.0 M acid than in pure water?
    (A) KCl
    (B) $CaCO_3$
    (C) $CaCl_2$
    (D) KNO_3

36. Which of the following is NOT an acid/conjugate base pair?
    (A) HCN/CN
    (B) H_2CO_3/OH^-
    (C) H_2SO_4/HSO_4^-
    (D) $H_3PO_4/H_2PO_4^-$

37. In a titration of 40.0 ml of 0.20 M NaOH with 0.4 M HCl, what will be the final volume of the solution when the sodium hydroxide is completely neutralized?
    (A) 42 ml
    (B) 20 ml
    (C) 60 ml
    (D) 80 ml

38. When dissolved in water to form 0.2 M solutions, which of the following would have the highest pH?
    (A) The salt of a strong acid
    (B) A weak acid
    (C) The ammonium salt of a strong acid
    (D) The sodium salt of a weak acid

39. Consider the reaction $N_2(g) + 3H_2(g) \rightarrow 2NH_3$ (g) + heat. Indicate the incorrect statement.
    (A) An increase in temperature will shift the equilibrium to the right.
    (B) An increase in pressure applied will shift the equilibrium to the right.
    (C) The addition of ammonia will shift the equilibrium to the left.
    (D) The addition of H_2 will shift the equilibrium to the right.

40. All of the following are colligative properties of solutions EXCEPT
    (A) vapor pressure.
    (B) osmotic pressure.
    (C) density.
    (D) boiling point elevation.

41. What statement is incorrect?
    (A) London dispersion forces are among those binding the units of molecular solids.
    (B) Molten ionic compounds are conductors of electricity.
    (C) Molecular solids have high melting points.
    (D) Molecular solids are non-conductors.

42. Which of the following groups contain no ionic compounds?
    (A) HCN, NO, $Ca(NO_3)_2$
    (B) KOH, CCL_4, SF_6
    (C) NaH, CaF_2, $NaNH_2$
    (D) CH_2O, H_2S, NH_3

43. In a cubic lattice, an atom lying at the corner of a unit cell is shared by how many unit cells?
    (A) 2
    (B) 4
    (C) 8
    (D) 12

44. On the basis of the following boiling point data, which of the following liquids would be expected to have the highest vapor pressure at room temperature?

SUBSTANCE	BOILING POINT
(A) acetone	56.2°C
(B) ethanol	78.5°C
(C) water	100°C
(D) ethylene glycol	198°C

45. $\frac{34}{17}$ Cl has

   (A) 17 protons, 17 electrons, and 17 neutrons.

   (B) 17 protons, 19 electrons, and 17 neutrons.

   (C) 17 protons, 18 electrons, and 17 neutrons.

   (D) 34 protons, 34 electrons, and 17 neutrons.

46. Which of the following arrangements gives the correct trend of electronegativitism?

   (A) I<Br<Cl<F

   (B) Sr<Ca<Ra<Mg

   (C) Al>Si>P>S

   (D) Na<K<Li<H

47. The number of unpaired electrons in the outer subshell of a phosphorus atom (atomic number: 15) is

   (A) 2.

   (B) 0.

   (C) 3.

   (D) 1.

48. An atom that has five 3 p electrons in its ground state is

   (A) Si.

   (B) P.

   (C) Cl.

   (D) O.

49. How many valence electrons are needed to complete the outer valence shell of sulfur?

   (A) 1

   (B) 2

   (C) 3

   (D) 4

50. Consider three 1-liter flasks at STP. Flask A contains NO gas; Flask B contains NH^3 gas; and Flask C contains N_2 gas. Which flask contains the greatest number of atoms?

   (A) Flask A

   (B) Flask B

   (C) Flask C

   (D) All contain the same number of atoms.

STOP

IF YOU FINISH BEFORE TIME IS CALLED, YOU MAY CHECK YOUR WORK ON THIS SECTION ONLY. DO NOT TURN TO ANY OTHER SECTION IN THE TEST.

ANSWER KEY AND EXPLANATIONS

Cells, Structure, and Function Test 1

1. D	9. D	17. B	25. D	33. B
2. B	10. C	18. B	26. C	34. C
3. D	11. C	19. D	27. B	35. A
4. A	12. C	20. D	28. B	36. B
5. D	13. D	21. B	29. D	37. C
6. B	14. A	22. A	30. B	38. A
7. D	15. B	23. C	31. A	39. C
8. D	16. B	24. D	32. B	40. A

1. **The correct answer is (D).** In facilitated diffusion, large molecules and ions diffuse through channels within membrane proteins. The process requires no input of energy on the part of the cell, since materials move down a concentration gradient. Facilitated diffusion occurs more rapidly when the temperature is higher, and when the concentration gradient is steeper.

2. **The correct answer is (B).** The polymerase chain reaction (PCR) is an in vitro technique.

3. **The correct answer is (D).** In active transport, the transport proteins move a solute against its concentration gradient. Active transport does not proceed spontaneously. It requires an energy (ATP) input.

4. **The correct answer is (A).** A cell immersed in a solution with a lower concentration of dissolved materials (solutes) is in a hypotonic environment. The concentration of water is higher outside of the cell than inside. Under these conditions, water diffuses into the cell.

5. **The correct answer is (D).** Substance x is hydrophobic and nonpolar, so it can easily pass through the membrane due to the phospholipid structure of the membrane.

6. **The correct answer is (B).** A cell is hypertonic when it has higher solute concentration and less water concentration compared to the outside solution, which has more water and less solute (hypotonic), so the water will diffuse inside the cell.

7. **The correct answer is (D).** Oxidation is the loss of electrons or the loss of hydrogen from a substance. Therefore, the carbon-carbon double bonds of unsaturated fats are oxidized more easily than the simple bonds of saturated fats.

8. **The correct answer is (D).** Macromolecules and fluid cross cellular membranes by bulk transport, in which the transported materials are contained within vesicles and do not mix with other materials of the cytoplasm. There are two forms of bulk transport: endocytosis and exocytosis. Endocytosis of a solid is known as phagocytosis.

9. **The correct answer is (D).** In active transport, energy (ATP) is needed. Mitochondria is the main organelle for ATP synthesis.

10. **The correct answer is (C).** Red blood cells have 0.9 percent salt solution whereas sea water has more solute than red blood cells, so it is a hypertonic solution compared to red blood cells.

11. **The correct answer is (C).** If any cell is placed in a hypertonic solution, the cell loses its water, dehydrates, and dies because the cell is hypotonic (more water) compared to outside solutions.

12. **The correct answer is (C).** The movement of materials against a concentration gradient needs energy. (See question answer 3.)

13. **The correct answer is (D).** Every living organism is covered by a cell membrane.

14. **The correct answer is (A).**

15. **The correct answer is (B).** Prokaryote cells do not have membrane-bound organelles.

16. **The correct answer is (B).** The half-life indicates that 100 years are required for ½ of the sample to decay. Therefore, the 31.5 kg should be doubled 4 times.

17. **The correct answer is (B).** Water is a polar molecule whereas oil is a nonpolar molecule. Water molecules have a slightly negative charge in one side and a slightly positive charge in the other side, but lipid molecules do not have any charges.

18. **The correct answer is (B).** All plant cells have an outer rigid covering called a cell wall made up of polysaccharide cellulose; animals do not have cell walls, only cell membranes.

19. **The correct answer is (D).** Prokaryote cells (example bacteria and blue-green algae) do not have a membrane-bound nucleus, but they have naked DNA in the cytoplasm.

20. **The correct answer is (D).** The cytoskeleton is a web of fibrous protein that extends throughout the cell. It alters the shape of a cell, moves the whole cell from one place to another, and pushes or pulls organelles.

21. **The correct answer is (B).** Lysosomes are essentially membrane bags that enclose hydrolytic enzymes, which are involved in breaking down proteins, polysaccharides, and lipids. If the lysosomes break open, the cell itself will be destroyed, because the enzymes they carry are capable of hydrolyzing all the major types of molecules found in a living cell.

22. **The correct answer is (A).** Note the R–COOH group, which makes the compound an acid, with the R–NH$_2$ (amino group) in the alpha position.

23. **The correct answer is (C).** Proteins are composed of chains of amino acids linked by peptide bonds, with primary, secondary, and tertiary structure.

24. **The correct answer is (D).** A virus is not a living cell; it is a submicroscopic, non-cellular particle composed of a nucleic acid core and a protein coat, reproducing only within a host. Therefore, it does not belong to any living kingdom.

25. **The correct answer is (D).** Some bacteria and fungi feed on dead organic matter to get their energy (*saphros* means rotten, putrid).

26. **The correct answer is (C).** Parallel circuits enable electrical currents to take separate paths through individual resistors as shown in circuit II.

27. **The correct answer is (B).** All circuits in a series circuit, as shown in circuit I, must travel through all resistors.

28. **The correct answer is (B).** There are two forms of endocytosis, depending on the kind of material brought into the cell. Endocytosis of fluid is known as pinocytosis.

29. **The correct answer is (D).** All cells can exist as distinct entities because of the cell membrane, which regulates the passage of materials into and out of the cell. Latex membrane does not allow the HIV virus to pass through the membrane, preventing HIV infection.

30. **The correct answer is (B).** Membranes control the types of molecules that can pass in and out of the cell and organelles. Cell membranes are permeable to certain molecules and impermeable to others—a phenomenon known as selectively permeable.

31. **The correct answer is (A).** Three different types of filaments have been identified as major participants in the cytoskeletons: microtubules, microfilaments, and intermediate filaments. They maintain the shape of the cell, enable it to move, anchor its organelles, and direct its traffic.

32. **The correct answer is (B).** Both mitochondria and chloroplasts are energy-producing organelles. Mitochondria release the energy from food as a form of ATP, and the chloroplasts pick up the solar energy and convert it to chemical energy (ATP).

33. **The correct answer is (B).** The slope (m) is 10.

34. **The correct answer is (C).** In enzyme-catalyzed reactions, substrate molecules generally outnumber enzyme molecules, which allow the enzyme to become saturated and the reaction to proceed at maximum velocity.

35. **The correct answer is (A).** Autotrophic organisms, such as plants, all algae, and some bacteria, are able to synthesize their own organic food by using CO_2, H_2O, and sunlight.

36. **The correct answer is (B).** The liquid part of the solution is called solvent.

37. **The correct answer is (C).** With limited resources, as the numbers of individuals produced approach the environmental capacity, reproduction declines and eventually stops.

38. **The correct answer is (A).** The assumption of unlimited resources suggests the absence of a K value.

39. **The correct answer is (C).** Mitochondrion is the powerhouse of the cell. It produces maximum amounts of chemical energy (ATP) for sustaining life.

40. **The correct answer is (A).** Membranes are composed of a phospholipid bilayer of molecules interspersed with protein molecules. Any kind of nonpolar molecule, such as lipids or some other organic solvents (ether, acetone, etc.), can easily pass through the lipid layer of membrane.

Biology Test 2

1. C	5. C	9. C	13. B	17. C
2. D	6. C	10. B	14. C	18. D
3. D	7. C	11. C	15. D	19. D
4. C	8. C	12. C	16. D	

1. **The correct answer is (C).** This is the process by which a glucose molecule is changed to two molecules of pyruvic acid with the liberation of a small amount of energy. In the absence of oxygen, pyruvic acid can be converted to ethanol or to one of several organic acids, of which lactic is the most common. This process is called fermentation.

2. **The correct answer is (D).** In the first stage, aerobic respiration (glycolysis) produces 2 ATP. In the second stage (Krebs cycle), it produces 2 ATP. During the final stage (electron transport chain), it produces 32 ATP.

3. **The correct answer is (D).** Reaction I is an uphill process that takes in radiant energy from the sun and converts it to chemical energy to combine CO_2 and H_2O to produce $C_6H_{12}O_6$ and O_2—which have additional energy.

4. **The correct answer is (C).** The reaction in II is downhill, with energy being released from $C_6H_{12}O_6$, generating CO_2 and H_2O with less energy.

5. **The correct answer is (C).** The reactants of some reactions have more energy than the products. Many such reactions release energy that cells can use, which is what happens during aerobic respiration.

6. **The correct answer is (C).** Each type of enzyme functions best within a certain temperature range. The chemical reaction rates decrease sharply when the temperature becomes too high. Humans usually die when their internal body temperature reaches 44°C (112°F) because it destroys the shape of the enzyme and thereby stops the metabolism.

7. **The correct answer is (C).** The enzyme helpers called co-enzymes are complex organic molecules, many of which are derived from vitamins. These co-enzymes can pick up hydrogen atoms that are liberated during glucose breakdown.

8. **The correct answer is (C).** The stored form of energy is called potential energy. An example is the glucose molecule; when it breaks down, it releases a large quantity of chemical energy to do work.

9. **The correct answer is (C).** All the pigments are present inside the thylakoids; therefore, the chlorophyll molecules and other pigments pick up the solar energy, convert it to chemical energy as a form of ATP and NADPH, and release oxygen during the non-cyclic light reaction.

10. **The correct answer is (B).** During non-cyclic light reactions, energy from the sun drives the formation of ATP (which carries energy) and NADPH (which carries hydrogen and electrons). Oxygen is a by-product of photosynthesis.

11. **The correct answer is (C).** The light independent reactions are the "synthesis" part of photosynthesis. ATP molecules deliver the required energy for the reaction. NADPH molecules deliver the required hydrogen and electrons, and carbon dioxide diffuses inside the stronin. It then forms the energy-rich molecule glucose (the process is called dark reaction).

12. **The correct answer is (C).** Reduction in the hawk population reduced the pressure

on the mouse population, which increased and thus suppressed the grasshopper numbers, which allowed the sunflower population to increase.

13. **The correct answer is (B).** The highest concentration of energy in a ecological pyramid is at the base (producers). Energy is lost as heat at the successive trophic levels.

14. **The correct answer is (C).** Aerobic cellular respiration is more important to sustaining life because it produces 36 ATP compared to anaerobic, which only releases 2 ATP.

15. **The correct answer is (D).** The organelle chloroplast is responsible for photosynthesis, which produces O_2 and the energy-rich molecule carbohydrate.

16. **The correct answer is (D).** All enzymes are protein molecules, and protein is one of the organic molecules necessary for sustaining life.

17. **The correct answer is (C).** Glycolysis is the first stage of cellular respiration in which glucose is broken down step by step to form 2 pyruvic acid inside the cytoplasm.

18. **The correct answer is (D).** The first stage of respiration, the breaking down of the glucose molecules, always takes place inside the cytoplasm because all the enzymes are there for the reaction.

19. **The correct answer is (D).** Electron transport systems and neighboring channel proteins are the machinery embedded in the inner membrane that divides mitochondrion into two compartments.

Biology Test 3

1. B	5. C	9. B	13. D	17. C
2. A	6. B	10. D	14. C	18. C
3. A	7. C	11. B	15. D	19. D
4. D	8. D	12. D	16. C	20. C

1. **The correct answer is (B).** The adult bodies of most plants and animals consist of diploid (2n) rather than haploid (n) cells. A gamete (male sperm and female egg) is always a haploid cell, which means it has one set of chromosomes formed by meiosis of germ cells (2n). So if the germ cell is 40, the gamete will be 20.

2. **The correct answer is (A).** When two alternative alleles are fully apparent in a hybrid, with both phenotypes showing in the organism, we say that the hybrids exhibit codominance. Blood typing of humans provides an excellent example of codominance. The AB blood type inherits an A allele and a B allele. Neither allele is dominant over the other; therefore, codominance causes a new blood type, AB.

3. **The correct answer is (A).** The blood cells of humans divide by mitosis. In mitosis, the diploid number of chromosomes is maintained and the resulting daughter cells are identical to the parent cell.

4. **The correct answer is (D).** Meiosis is the nuclear division that reduces the number of chromosomes in the resulting cells by half. Meiosis is necessary for the production of gametes or sex cells and results in 4 non-identical haploid cells (sperms and eggs).

5. **The correct answer is (C).** The first part of sexual reproduction is meiosis, where the germ cells divide and produce 4 haploid gametes.

6. **The correct answer is (B).** Asexual reproduction occurs without sex and transfers the genes of just one parent to each offspring; it produces offspring that are genetically identical to one another and to their single parent by the process of mitosis.

7. **The correct answer is (C).** The first pattern of inheritance discovered by Mendel was the Law of Segregation. This law describes how the two copies of each gene segregate (separate) during meiosis so that just one copy ends up in each gamete (sperm and egg).

8. **The correct answer is (D).** The dominant will always show the dominant characteristic in their phenotype.

9. **The correct answer is (B).** The sex chromosome of a mother is always XX and the father XY. So, the sex of the child depends on whether he or she gets X or Y from the father. If the child gets X from the father and X from the mother, the child will be a female. If the child gets Y from the father and X from the mother, the child will be a male.

10. **The correct answer is (D).** In normal cells, the cell division is controlled by two sets of genes: one set stimulates and the other set suppresses. In cancer, defective genes may overstimulate cell division or fail to halt cell division.

11. **The correct answer is (B).** Sperm cells are haploid (N), which are formed by meiosis of germ cells (2N); therefore, if the haploid is 30, then germ cells should be 60.

12. **The correct answer is (D).** A person with Down Syndrome has three copies in chromosome 21 rather than two copies. The extra chromosome affects practically every part of the body.

13. **The correct answer is (D).** If we do the Punnet square for a woman who is a heterozygous carrier for sex-linked recessive gene and married to a normal man, half of her sons and half of her daughters will receive this gene.

$X^C X$—girl with recessive gene

$X^C Y$—boy with recessive gene

XY—normal boy

XX—normal girl

14. **The correct answer is (C).** Hemophilia is one of the disorders caused by a Y-linked recessive allele. Many genes in many chromosomes contribute to normal blood clotting, but two gene loci in the Y chromosome are responsible for the two most common clotting disorders—hemophilia A and hemophilia B.

15. **The correct answer is (D).** Hemophilia is a sex-linked disorder because the defective gene is present in the Y sex chromosome.

16. **The correct answer is (C).** The sex-linked trait is present in the X chromosome; therefore, the father cannot pass the gene to his son because the son always receives the Y chromosome, not the X chromosome, from his father.

17. **The correct answer is (C).** The blue gene is the autosomal recessive trait, whereas hemophilia is the sex-linked recessive trait. To get the blue eyes, the person should have two blue-eyes recessive genes. If the person is male, he needs only one recessive gene for hemophilia.

18. **The correct answer is (C).** If both parents are AB, they can only produce two different kinds of gametes (sperm and eggs), A and B. So the blood types of children will be A, AB, and B.

19. **The correct answer is (D).** Blood type O has neither A nor B polysaccharides (antigen) for antibodies to attack.

20. **The correct answer is (C).** Non-disjunction of sex chromosomes (XY) in a man produces four types of abnormal sperms. When these abnormal sperm (YY) fertilize normal X carrying chromosomes, they produce abnormal genotypes (XYY).

Human Anatomy and Physiology Test 4

1. D	21. D	41. C	61. B	81. C
2. A	22. A	42. B	62. C	82. B
3. A	23. D	43. A	63. B	83. A
4. B	24. D	44. C	64. C	84. B
5. B	25. D	45. A	65. C	85. B
6. D	26. A	46. B	66. C	86. A
7. C	27. B	47. B	67. B	87. B
8. C	28. B	48. B	68. B	88. B
9. B	29. D	49. B	69. C	89. B
10. D	30. C	50. A	70. A	90. B
11. B	31. B	51. A	71. B	91. A
12. B	32. C	52. A	72. C	92. D
13. D	33. A	53. B	73. A	93. D
14. B	34. B	54. B	74. D	94. D
15. A	35. A	55. D	75. B	95. B
16. C	36. A	56. B	76. B	96. C
17. B	37. D	57. B	77. A	97. B
18. C	38. B	58. C	78. B	98. D
19. B	39. A	59. B	79. B	99. B
20. D	40. B	60. D	80. A	100. D

1. **The correct answer is (D).** Only the lymphatic system is involved in all three of these processes, although the urinary system does receive fluid from blood vessels.

2. **The correct answer is (A).** Internal and abdominal muscles aid expiration. The external intercostal aid inspiration, but the diaphragm is the major muscle.

3. **The correct answer is (A).** The integument is comprised of skin, hair, nails, and associated structures, such as sweat and sebaceous glands.

4. **The correct answer is (B).** Oxytocin and antidiuretic hormone (ADH) are both products of the posterior pituitary. Oxytocin acts on uterine smooth muscle and mammary tissue, whereas ADH acts within the kidneys to promote water reabsorption. ADH is also a vasoconstriction, and these two actions combine to elevate blood pressure.

5. **The correct answer is (B).** Homeostasis, the tendency to maintain a constant internal environment, most commonly depends upon negative feedback processes, which tend to counter the effects of change.

Positive feedback mechanisms enhance the effects of change, and they generally have a beneficial effect on homeostasis.

6. **The correct answer is (D).** Central chemoreceptors respond to changes in CO_2, which is the most important factor in the control of minute-to-minute respiration.

7. **The correct answer is (C).** Sagittal planes divide the body into left and right parts. Frontal (coronal) planes vertically divide the body into anterior and posterior segments. A transverse section divides the body into superior and inferior parts.

8. **The correct answer is (C).** Cardiac output, the volume of blood by the heart per minute, is equal to the product of stroke volume (L./beat) and heart rate (beats/minute).

9. **The correct answer is (B).** Diffusion is the process by which solutes move from an area of high concentration to an area of low concentration. Osmosis is the movement of water down a concentration gradient. Movement of solute against a concentration gradient requires active transport processes and energy.

10. **The correct answer is (D).** Blood exits the right ventricle through the pulmonary semilunar (pulmonic) valve and enters the pulmonary arteries, which lead to the lungs. Atrioventricular valves (bicuspid and tricuspid) are situated between atria and ventricles. Pulmonary veins come from the lungs back to the heart.

11. **The correct answer is (B).** While both norepinephrine and epinephrine act at Alpha and Beta-1 receptors, epinephrine is the primary agonist at the Beta-2 sites, where it leads to pronounced bronchodilation. Acetylcholine and nicotine are not catechol amines.

12. **The correct answer is (B).** The resting membrane is relatively impermeable to sodium, which is in a high concentration in the extracellular space relative to the intracellular space. An action potential results from the opening of sodium channels, allowing sodium to diffuse into the intracellular space and making that region positive relative to the outside of the cell.

13. **The correct answer is (D).** During swallowing, the epiglottis covers the trachea to prevent ingested material from entering the respiratory tract.

14. **The correct answer is (B).** The amount of dissolved oxygen in blood is minimal compared to the amount carried as oxyhemoglobin. Carbon dioxide and bicarbonate are not physiologic oxygen transporters.

15. **The correct answer is (A).** Pyramidal tract fibers are motor in function and originate in the primary motor cortex, which is directly anterior to the central sulcus, the precentral gyrus. The postcentral gyms is part of the somatosensory system.

16. **The correct answer is (C).** Epinephrine and norepinephrine are catechol amine transmitters in the autonomic and central nervous systems. Acetylcholinesterase is the enzyme that metabolizes acetylcholine at autonomic and neuromuscular sites.

17. **The correct answer is (B).** Arterioles are located between arteries and capillaries. Dilation or constriction of arterioles regulates the flow of blood into capillary beds and provides adjustment of arterial blood pressure.

18. **The correct answer is (C).** Exocytosis moves substances from the intracellular space into extracellular fluid. Endocytosis is a mechanism for moving large particles into cells. Phagocytosis is a type of endocytosis by which solid particles are engulfed. Pinocytosis is endocytosis of fluids.

19. **The correct answer is (B).** Dermatomes are body regions innervated by individual dorsal roots and can be related to segmental spinal levels. Receptive fields, sensory units, and motor units related to innervation are characteristics of individual neurons rather than nerve trunks.

20. **The correct answer is (D).** Epithelial tissue is characterized by cell shape

(squamous, cuboidal, columnar) and cell layering (simple or compound).

21. **The correct answer is (D).** Cartilage forms the skeleton of the embryo and is subsequently converted to bone. Cartilage also forms the nasal septum and the rings of the trachea. Its flexibility makes it an appropriate material to join the ribs to the sternum.

22. **The correct answer is (A).** Keratin is a protein that waterproofs and adds structural strength to skin. It is formed in the deepest layer of the epidermis and migrates to the surface with time. Melanin, carotene, and hemoglobin are pigments in the skin.

23. **The correct answer is (D).** Sharp "pricking" pain information is carried over the small, slowly conducting myelinated A Delta fibers, while burning and aching pain information is transmitted over the even more slowly conducted unmyelinated C fibers. A Alpha fibers, with their high conduction velocity, are involved in other areas, such as proprioception.

24. **The correct answer is (D).** Activation of the parasympathetic division will lead directly to a slowing of the heart through activity of the vagus nerve. Vasoconstriction, increased heart rate and cardiac output, and inhibition of digestion are within the domain of the sympathetic division.

25. **The correct answer is (D).** Muscle spindles respond to moderate muscle stretch. The Golgi tendon organ is the receptor for the inverse stretch reflex, free nerve endings are involved in pain reception, and hair cells are receptors within the auditory and vestibular systems.

26. **The correct answer is (A).** Although the glomerulus is more permeable than most membranes, it still restricts the passage of proteins, blood cells, and other large particles. Damage to the glomerulus can produce filtration disorders such as glomerulonephritis, and substances such as blood and protein may appear in the urine.

27. **The correct answer is (B).** Some CO_2 is carried in a dissolved form obeying Henry's Law, and some is carried by hemoglobin. Most CO_2, however, is carried as bicarbonate.

28. **The correct answer is (B).** Tubular reabsorption is the process by which the kidneys return water and solutes, including glucose, vitamins, and amino acids, to blood. Filtration and secretion involve movement of substances from blood into urine. Glucose is not reabsorbed from the collecting duct.

29. **The correct answer is (D).** Periosteum covers the outer surface of long bones. It contains osteoblasts, cells that form new bone cells. Endosteum lines the hollow inner surface of a long bone. Osteoclasts break down bone cells.

30. **The correct answer is (C).** Activity in the sinoatrial node is responsible for initiating the cardiac cycle, beginning with atrial depolarization and contraction. In a resting subject, the contribution of atrial contraction to ventricular filling is relatively minimal. The AV node is below the atria.

31. **The correct answer is (B).** The first heart sound ("lub") is the atrioventricular valves (tricuspid and bicuspid) closing in response to the ventricles contracting and increasing intraventricular pressure.

32. **The correct answer is (C).** Visual processing occurs within the occipital lobe of the cerebral cortex, which is protected by the occipital bone. Frontal bone covers the frontal cortex, which is involved in, among other things, behavioral and motor events. Parietal bone covers the parietal cortex, which is involved in sensory integration processes, while temporal bone protects the temporal lobe, which is involved in audition.

33. **The correct answer is (A).** Veins have large lumens and thin, distensible walls; they contain up to 65 percent of the body's total blood supply at any time.

34. **The correct answer is (B).** The patella is a sesamoid bone, a special type of short bone.

35. **The correct answer is (A).** The automaticity of the heart is normally a function of the sinoatrial (SA) node, which leads to atrial depolarization. The atrioventricular (AV) node may become a pacemaker under certain pathological conditions.

36. **The correct answer is (A).** Arteries are under the greatest pressure due to the force from the contraction of the heart and the elastic properties of arterial walls.

37. **The correct answer is (D).** Ninety-nine percent of the water filtered at the glomerulus is returned by osmosis, most of which occurs within the proximal convoluted tubule.

38. **The correct answer is (B).** Small, uncharged lipid soluble molecules cross biological membranes more readily than other species. Water-soluble molecules cross if they are sufficiently small.

39. **The correct answer is (A).** The sympathetic division of the autonomic nervous system is involved in dealing with emergencies and stress. Parasympathetic (craniosacral) activity is primarily involved with energy conservation and "vegetative" functions.

40. **The correct answer is (B).** The sympathetic division of the autonomic nervous system is anatomically the thoricolumbar division because of its spinal levels of origin. The parasympathetic division is, anatomically, the craniosacral division.

41. **The correct answer is (C).** Cellular respiration, the utilization of oxygen and glucose, occurs within mitochondria. Rough endoplasmic reticulum is involved in protein synthesis and smooth endoplasmic reticulum is involved in synthesis of lipid materials. Golgi apparatus are involved in cellular packaging and delivery.

42. **The correct answer is (B).** Flexion decreases the angle of a joint, bringing the two bones closer together. Extension increases the angle of a joint, moving the bones farther apart. Retraction and rotation are not joint "bending" in nature.

43. **The correct answer is (A).** Mitosis leading to the formation of new epidermal cells occurs within the stratum germinativum basale, the deepest layer of the epidermis, which has the advantage of being near the blood supply of the underlying dermis.

44. **The correct answer is (C).** Compared to males, females have a larger percentage of fat (and a lower content of water), which is deposited within the subcutaneous layer under the influence of estrogen.

45. **The correct answer is (A).** Mucosal membranes line structures such as components of the digestive, respiratory, and reproductive tracts, which access the outside world. Serous membranes line cavities that do not access the external environment, such as the pleural cavities. Synovial membranes line joint cavities, and cutaneous membranes comprise the skin.

46. **The correct answer is (B).** The epidermis does not contain blood vessels and depends upon the vascular supply of the underlying dermis for its needs.

47. **The correct answer is (B).** Smooth muscle is found within visceral structures (e.g., digestive, reproductive), does not have a striated histological appearance, and is generally under autonomic (involuntary) control. Skeletal muscle is striated and voluntary. Cardiac muscle is striated but involuntary. Postural muscles are skeletal muscles.

48. **The correct answer is (B).** Although carried by the circulatory system and influenced by the endocrine systems, blood cell formation is largely a function of spongy bone within the skeletal system.

49. **The correct answer is (B).** Parathyroid hormone elevates serum calcium levels by initiating mobilization of calcium from the digestive system. Calcitonin lowers blood

calcium and leads to deposition of calcium within bone.

50. **The correct answer is (A).** Eccrine sweat glands of the face, palms, and soles are active in children. Apocrine sweat glands become active at puberty. Sebaceous glands produce sebum and are not found on the soles or palms. Ceruminous glands are found within the external auditory meatus.

51. **The correct answer is (A).** The biceps brachii is a flexor of the elbow, and the triceps femoris is a flexor of the knee.

52. **The correct answer is (A).** Apocrine sweat glands become active at puberty under the influence of sex hormones. Eccrine, sebaceous, and ceruminous glands are active in children.

53. **The correct answer is (B).** Calcitonin is responsible for lowering an elevated serum calcium, partially by depositing the excess mineral in bone. Parathormone will elevate serum calcium levels.

54. **The correct answer is (B).** Although hormones are produced by endocrine glands, their delivery to target organs is primarily via the cardiovascular system.

55. **The correct answer is (D).** Myelin, an "insulating" substance, is responsible for saltatory conduction in which the impulse "skips" from one Node of Ranvier to the next and is rapidly conducted to the end of the cell. The larger the diameter of an axon, the less resistance present and the faster the axon can conduct. Myelinated, large diameter axons comprise the axons with the fastest conduction velocities.

56. **The correct answer is (B).** The nephron is the basic functional unit of kidneys. Nephrons include Bowman's capsule, the proximal convoluted tubule, the loop of Henle, the distal convoluted tubule, and the collecting duct. The glomerulus is part of the circulatory system, the ureters convey urine from the kidneys to the bladder, and the urethra carries urine out from the bladder.

57. **The correct answer is (B).** The esophagus enters the stomach below the fundus at the cardiac region, which contains the cardiac sphincter. The body of the stomach is below and the pyloric region marks the most distal portion of the stomach adjacent to the duodenum of the small intestine.

58. **The correct answer is (C).** Oxytocin, produced by the hypothalamus and released by the posterior pituitary, causes contraction of uterine smooth muscle and plays a role in labor and delivery. ADH is also released by the posterior pituitary, but its role is in water conservation within the kidneys.

59. **The correct answer is (B).** ADH, antidiuretic hormone, when released from the posterior pituitary, causes an increased permeability of the collecting duct of the kidneys to water and leads to water reabsorption and conservation. Inhibition of ADH release, produced for example by the ingestion of alcohol, leads to an increase in urine output.

60. **The correct answer is (D).** FSH begins the maturation process of follicles, but it is the elevation of LH levels that leads to the release of mature egg cells (ovulation). ADH and prolactin do not participate in the process.

61. **The correct answer is (B).** The cardiac sphincter is located at the junction of the esophagus and the stomach and is responsible for preventing gastric reflux. The pyloric sphincter is at the junction of the stomach and the small intestine, the ileocecal valve is at the junction of the small and large intestines, and the epiglottis prevents solids and liquids from entering the trachea.

62. **The correct answer is (C).** Bile, produced in the liver and released from the gall bladder, is involved in fat metabolism in the small intestine. Lipase is also involved in fat metabolism, but it is from the pancreas.

63. **The correct answer is (B).** Although some digestion takes place within all of the

structures listed, the majority of digestive processes take place within the duodenum.

64. The correct answer is (C). Visual receptors, rods and cones, are located at the back of the eye on the retina. The lens and cornea are involved in transmission of light rays from the environment on to the retina; the optic tract is part of the optic neural pathway.

65. The correct answer is (C). Food absorption takes place primarily within the ileum and jejunum. Functions of the stomach and duodenum are primarily digestive, while the colon is principally involved in water reabsorption, some digestion, and vitamin synthesis.

66. The correct answer is (C). The medulla begins at, and is indistinguishable from, the rostral end of the spinal cord, forming the lowest portion of the brain stem, which also includes the pons and the midbrain, both superior. The thalamus, part of the diencephalon, is yet further rostral.

67. The correct answer is (B). Although stored and delivered by the gallbladder, bile is manufactured within the liver. The duodenum is the major site of digestion, where it receives digestive materials from the pancreas.

68. The correct answer is (B). Thyroid hormone contributes to growth and maturation of the nervous system. A hypothyroid infant will show both physical and mental deficits not seen in the adult, since skeletal and brain development have been completed.

69. The correct answer is (C). Rods, which provide vision in black and white, and cones, which provide color vision, are located on the retina at the back of the eye. Hair cells are receptors within the auditory and vestibular systems.

70. The correct answer is (A). Lining the inside of the digestive system is the epithelial mucosal layer, which provides an appropriate setting for absorption of materials into the submucosal layer that contains blood vessels, lymphatics, and

nerves. Serosal membranes surround the digestive tract to form a protective layer.

71. The correct answer is (B). The pancreas is classed as an endocrine gland because of its production of insulin and glucagon, which are secreted directly into blood. As an exocrine gland, the pancreas produces a series of enzymes contained in pancreatic juice, carried by the pancreatic duct.

72. The correct answer is (C). Lacrimation is the activity of the lacrimal glands, which produce lacrimal fluid or tears.

73. The correct answer is (A). Olfaction, the sense of smell, is the domain of the first cranial nerve, the olfactory nerve. Nerves II, III, and IV are involved in the sensory and motor functions of the head and face but not the sense of smell.

74. The correct answer is (D). Immediately distal to the neck of the bladder is the prostate gland. Its enlargement, common in males beginning at about the age of 40, interferes with urine outflow. Benign hyperplasia prostate (BHP) is a non-malignant enlargement of the gland, which is also a common site for cancer in males. Although located in the same general area, the seminal vesicles and bulbourethral (Cowper's) glands do not normally hypertrophy with aging.

75. The correct answer is (B). Linear (vertical and horizontal) acceleration is sensed by receptors within the utricles and saccules; the semicircular canals contain receptors activated by rotational movement. Receptors within the cochlea detect sound, and the middle ear does not contain auditory or vestibular receptor devices.

76. The correct answer is (B). Although the globulins and fibrin are blood proteins, albumin is the protein in the highest plasma concentration.

77. The correct answer is (A). Union of sperm and egg normally occurs within the fallopian (uterine) tubes prior to implantation within the uterus. Implantation at non-uterine sites is termed an ectopic pregnancy.

78. **The correct answer is (B).** Depression may result from low levels of serotonin or decreased responsiveness of sertotonergic receptors in the brain, and this is the basis for the use of serotonin reuptake inhibitors in the treatment of clinical depression. High levels of catechol amines may contribute to clinical anxiety.

79. **The correct answer is (B).** Lymphatic vessels begin as lymphatic capillaries, blind pouches found in peripheral tissue. Lymph nodes are more proximal structures, and lymphocytes are forms of white blood cells.

80. **The correct answer is (A).** HCG rises to detectable levels following egg fertilization, and its presence in blood and urine forms the basis of pregnancy testing. The function of HCG is to maintain the corpus luteum, which is responsible for maintaining estrogen and progesterone levels, and their effects on the endometrium, during early and middle pregnancy.

81. **The correct answer is (C).** Sweet, sour, and salty taste sensations result from activity in the facial nerve, the seventh cranial nerve. The first cranial nerve is involved in olfaction; the fifth is involved in motor and sensory mechanisms of the head and face. Nerve x, the vagus, is not involved in taste from the tongue.

82. **The correct answer is (B).** The parasympathetic division of the autonomic nervous system is primarily involved with energy production and conservation. Its outward effects can be remembered by the acronym, SLUD, salivation, lacrimation, urination, and defecation.

83. **The correct answer is (A).** After their formation within the seminiferous tubules, sperm are stored within the epididymis lying alongside the testes. The epididymis leads to the vas deferens, which ultimately empties into the urethra, which receives material from the seminal vesicles.

84. **The correct answer is (B).** Glucagon elevates blood glucose by (1) promoting the breakdown of glycogen to glucose (glycogenolysis), (2) promoting glucose synthesis (gluconeogenesis), and (3) promoting the release of glucose from liver.

85. **The correct answer is (B).** Erythrocytes (red blood cells) are much more numerous than white cells in blood. Globulins and albumin are proteins, not formed elements.

86. **The correct answer is (A).** Although not as powerful as pH-regulating mechanisms in the respiratory or renal systems, buffer systems essentially act at the rate of chemical reactions. The liver is not involved in the normal control of blood pH.

87. **The correct answer is (B).** Arterial blood pH is critically maintained between 7.35 and 7.45. Either a decline of pH (acidosis) to a level of 7.0 or an increase in pH (alkalosis) to 8.0 is potentially fatal.

88. **The correct answer is (B).** While the hematocrit reveals the level of plasma, it is intended to evaluate the percentage of erythrocytes (red blood cells) in whole blood and subsequently the oxygen-carrying capacity of blood. Normal hematocrit values for females are 37–47 percent, 42–54 percent for males. Platelet and white cell enumerations are also useful diagnostics but do not involve the hematocrit.

89. **The correct answer is (B).** Although about 5 liters of blood are pumped through the heart per minute, the myocardial muscle is dependent upon the coronary arteries for delivery of oxygen.

90. **The correct answer is (B).** The term hair cell is applied to receptors within the auditory and vestibular systems. Rods and cones are visual receptors, and muscle spindles are the receptors for stretch reflexes.

91. **The correct answer is (A).** Blood typing is based on determining the antigen(s) located on the surfaces of erythrocytes; the "opposite" antibody is located within the individual's plasma. A type A patient

therefore has the A antigen and the anti-B antibody. Rh antigens are also located on erythrocyte surfaces leading to an individual being typed as Rh positive (antibody present) or Rh negative (no Rh antigen).

92. **The correct answer is (D).** Sickle cell anemia develops when hemoglobin forms long crystalline chains within erythrocytes, forcing the cells into their bizarre shapes. Pernicious anemia refers to abnormal destruction of red blood cells; iron-deficiency and aplastic anemias involve abnormal blood cell formation.

93. **The correct answer is (D).** Hair cells are the auditory receptors located within the cochlea, part of the inner ear. Auditory ossicles are small bones involved in conduction of vibration through the middle ear.

94. **The correct answer is (D).** Female menopause follows aging of the ovaries and is characterized by low estrogen levels, which, in turn, result in high levels of GnRH, FSH, and LH. The latter two appear to be correlated with the "hot flashes" of menopause.

95. **The correct answer is (B).** Hyperventilation can lead to a decreased arterial CO_2 level, which may result in alkalosis of respiratory origin. Extreme alkalosis may lead to convulsions and may produce seizure activity in epileptic patients.

96. **The correct answer is (C).** Plasma is approximately 90 percent water, with the rest being comprised of numerous solutes, including proteins, nutrients, gases, hormones, ions, and products of cell activity.

97. **The correct answer is (B).** Estrogen is involved in a feedback loop to the hypothalamus such that high levels of estrogen inhibit the release of GnRH, which reduces levels of LH and prevents ovulation.

98. **The correct answer is (D).** Heparin is an endogenous anticoagulant produced by basophils. Fibrin, calcium, and thrombin are all promoters of the coagulation process.

99. **The correct answer is (B).** GnRH from the hypothalamus controls the release of FSH and LH from the anterior pituitary. FSH initiates follicle development, and LH leads directly to ovulation, the release of a mature egg.

100. **The correct answer is (D).** Testosterone is produced by interstitial (Leydig) cells under the influence of ICSH, interstitial cell stimulating hormone. The epididymis and prostate gland are not involved in testosterone synthesis.

Chemistry Test 5

1. B	6. B	10. C	14. C	18. B
2. D	7. B	11. D	15. C	19. A
3. D	8. B	12. B	16. D	20. B
4. D	9. D	13. C	17. A	21. B
5. D				

1. **The correct answer is (B).** Acidic solutions contain hydrogen (H$^+$) ions, while basic (or alkaline) solution contain a basic ion, such as the hydroxyl ion (OH$^-$).

2. **The correct answer is (D).** Carbohydrates consist of molecules made up of C, H, and O in a ratio of 1:2:1 (e.g., glucose is C$_6$H$_{12}$O$_6$). Polysaccharides are chains of three or more simple sugars (e.g., glucose).

3. **The correct answer is (D).** Whether a watery solution is acidic or alkaline depends on its concentration of hydrogen ions (H$^+$) in relation to hydroxyl ions (OH$^-$). The ratio is expressed as the solution pH (the letters stand for potential of hydrogen). The pH scale ranges from 0 (most acidic) to 14 (most alkaline). Pure water is neutral with a pH of 7 because it has equal amounts of hydrogen and hydroxyl ions.

4. **The correct answer is (D).** Carbohydrates consist of molecules made up of C, H, and O in a ratio of 1:2:1, whereas cholesterol is a lipid (steroid) formed of four carbon rings.

5. **The correct answer is (D).** Organic molecules are molecules that contain carbon; they are found in living things.

6. **The correct answer is (B).** Covalence is the mutual attraction between two atoms that share a pair of electrons. It is the strongest type of chemical bond.

$$H^+ = H^+ \rightarrow H^2$$

7. **The correct answer is (B).** For many atoms, the simplest way to attain a completely filled outer energy level is either to gain or to lose 1 or 2 electrons.

8. **The correct answer is (B).** Dissaccharides are double sugars and are formed by linking two simple sugars. For example, glucose and fructose form sucrose, a disaccharide (table sugar).

9. **The correct answer is (D).** Wax is made of glycerol and fatty acids. It is nonpolar and insoluble in water. It is a lipid molecule.

10. **The correct answer is (C).** Proteins are made up of units called amino acids. Amino acids join together by a covalent bond and form polypeptide chains (the primary structure of proteins).

11. **The correct answer is (D).** The nucleus of an atom consists of protons and neutrons. A proton is a subatomic particle with positive electric charge. The number of protons in the nucleus of an atom is equal to the atomic number.

12. **The correct answer is (B).** The chemical activity of an atom is how it reacts with other atoms. Atoms are governed by the number of electrons in their outermost shell. Helium, neon, and other atoms with no electron vacancies in their outermost shell are inert; they tend not to enter into chemical reactions. Hydrogen, oxygen, and other atoms with electron vacancies in their outermost shell tend to interact with other atoms.

13. **The correct answer is (C).** Regardless of the element, atoms have just as many

electrons as protons. This means that they carry no net charge, overall. A proton is always positively charged, and an electron is negatively charged.

14. **The correct answer is (C).** Basic or alkaline solutions have fewer H^+ than OH^- ions; their pH is above 7.

15. **The correct answer is (C).** Alkaline solutions always have a higher pH and more OH^- ions.

16. **The correct answer is (D).** Glucose is a 6-carbon simple sugar and serves as a precursor of many complex compounds and as a building block for larger carbohydrates.

17. **The correct answer is (A).** The basic building block of protein is the amino acid. Each amino acid is a small organic compound with an amino group, a carboxyl group (an acid), a hydrogen atom, and one or more atoms, called its R group. Total amino acids are 20. Examples of amino acids are tryptophane, alanine, glycine, aspartic acid, lysine, proline, etc.

18. **The correct answer is (B).** The small organic compounds called nucleotides have three components: a 5-carbon sugar, a phosphate group, and a nitrogen-containing base. Nucleotides are the basic building blocks of DNA and RNA.

19. **The correct answer is (A).** In polar covalent bonds, atoms of different elements, which have a different number of protons, do not exert the same pull in shared electrons. The more attractive atom ends up with a slight negative charge; the atom is "electronegative." Its effect is balanced out by the other atoms, resulting in a slight positive charge. In simple words, a polar covalent bond has no net charge—but the charge is distributed unevenly between the bond's two ends.

20. **The correct answer is (B).** In a hydrogen bond, a small, highly electronegative atom of a molecule interacts weakly with a hydrogen atom that is already participating in a polar covalent bond.

21. **The correct answer is (B).** Genetic information is encoded in the particular order of nucleotides bases, which follow one another in DNA. RNA molecules function in the processes by which the genetic information in DNA is used to build proteins.

Chemistry and Physical Science Test 6

1. D	11. B	21. B	31. D	41. C
2. A	12. C	22. B	32. A	42. D
3. B	13. D	23. D	33. D	43. C
4. C	14. B	24. D	34. B	44. A
5. D	15. C	25. A	35. B	45. A
6. C	16. D	26. A	36. B	46. A
7. D	17. B	27. D	37. C	47. D
8. A	18. C	28. A	38. D	48. C
9. D	19. D	29. C	39. A	49. B
10. D	20. D	30. C	40. C	50. B

1. **The correct answer is (D).** Polarity is determined by differences in electronegativities between atoms involved in a bond. The difference in electronegativities between hydrogen and oxygen on a scale devised by Linus Pauling is 1.4, and between carbon and oxygen, it is 1.0. Carbon and hydrogen differ by only 0.4 and consequently form nonpolar bonds.

2. **The correct answer is (A).** Hydrochloric acid has the weakest conjugate base (Cl) and therefore dissociates most thoroughly (virtually completely in water) and yields hydrogen ions in high concentration. The other compounds shown dissociate less completely because of their stronger conjugate bases.

3. **The correct answer is (B).** Sucrose is a disaccharide that has nearly twice the molar mass of the other two sugars, which are monosaccharides.

4. **The correct answer is (C).** A hydrogen atom must accept an electron in order to form a hydride ion. No other changes occur. The hydride therefore has a single negative charge, whereas the hydrogen atom is neutral. An extra negative charge with no change in positive charge expands the radius.

5. **The correct answer is (D).** The functional group contains carbonyl plus a hydrogen linked to the carbon (—C—H). The other connection of the carbonyl group is to another carbon atom. The groups COOH, —OH, and —COOR are found in carboxylic acids, alcohols, and esters, respectively.

6. **The correct answer is (C).** Calcium oxide is the only compound in the four that is a metal oxide. Metal oxides form hydroxides (bases) when dissolved in water, but nonmetal oxides form acids.

7. **The correct answer is (D).** The statement given is the definition of an isotope, a form of an atom of an element that differs from other atoms of the same element by the number of neutrons.

8. **The correct answer is (A).** Oxidation, the loss of electrons, occurs at the anode. Molten sodium chloride has only sodium ($Na+$) and chloride ($Cl-$) ions, the latter of which each have a single electron to donate to achieve neutrality. Loss of one electron each yields chlorine atoms, which stabilize by forming diatomic molecules of chlorine gas.

9. **The correct answer is (D).** Sugar alone is the only molecular compound of this

group. The others readily dissociate as ions in polar solvents, such as water.

10. **The correct answer is (D).** Isopropyl alcohol has a low enough molecular weight to make it volatile and thus capable of giving a noticeable cooling effect during evaporation. It is unsuitable for internal consumption, but it is relatively inexpensive. There are disadvantages for the use of any of the others as rubbing alcohol. Methyl alcohol is toxic, phenol causes skin burns, and ethyl alcohol is too valuable for internal consumption and other commercial purposes.

11. **The correct answer is (B).** Argon, barium, and aluminum are in groups VIIIA, IIA, and IIIA, respectively. Copper is the only element that is in the transition area of the periodic table (group IB).

12. **The correct answer is (C).** Calcium and the other metals of the group IIA ionize by losing two electrons. It achieves the stable electron structure of argon, with eight electrons in the outer shell.

13. **The correct answer is (D).** In the series for the oxyhalogen ions (e.g., ClO_4^-, ClO_3^-, ClO^-), the one with the least amount of oxygen is designated hypochlorite.

14. **The correct answer is (B).** Chemical kinetics is the study of reaction rates and how these change with variation of conditions along with the various molecular events that transpire during the overall reaction.

15. **The correct answer is (C).** There is one phosphorus in the formula, but there are three potassiums and four oxygens. The number of atoms or ions present per formula unit equals the corresponding number of moles of each type in one molecule of the compound (the amount present in a liter of a 1-molar solution). In solution, potassium phosphate would separate as potassium ions and phosphate ions.

16. **The correct answer is (D).** Single bonds between carbon atoms are longer but weaker than double bonds between carbon atoms.

17. **The correct answer is (B).** The rare gases have stable electronic structures with eight outer "valence" electrons (2 S and 6 P) and therefore have no compulsion to seek means of donating, accepting, or sharing electrons. The halogens need an electron to achieve stability, whereas group IIA need to donate two electrons to form stable ions with eight electrons on the outermost shell. Group IB metals react but show a high resistance to oxidation.

18. **The correct answer is (C).** A molar solution contains 1 mole of solute per liter of solution. Therefore, 1 mole of solute is combined with less than 1 kilogram (1 liter) of water. In a 1-molal solution, which contains 1 mole of solute per kilogram of water, the total volume for a solution of 1 mole exceeds 1 liter. Therefore, 1 liter of a 1-molal solution contains less than 1 mole.

19. **The correct answer is (D).** For a molecular compound, the gram formula weight is the same as the gram molecular weight. The empirical formula represents the smallest ratio of the different atoms possible in the compound. The molecular formula may be a multiple of the empirical formulas (e.g., twice).

20. **The correct answer is (D).** The ratio of the rates of effusion of two gases (proportional to the speeds of the gas molecules) is inversely proportional to the square roots of their molecular weights; consequently, rate of effusion of A/rate of effusion of

$$B = \sqrt{\frac{1}{4}} = \frac{1}{2}.$$

21. **The correct answer is (B).** The greater the concentration of soluble particles, the greater the lowering of the freezing point of the solvent. A mole of calcium chloride contains 1 mole of calcium ions and 2 moles of chloride ions. A mole of sodium chloride contains only 2 moles of ions, and sucrose and methanol have only 1 mole of particles each per liter of 1-molar solution.

22. **The correct answer is (B).** If the atomic mass of an isotope is unknown, the number

of neutrons cannot be determined. However, if the atomic number is known, the number of protons is known. In an atom, there is no charge, so the number of electrons must equal the number of protons and the atomic number.

23. **The correct answer is (D).** Nitrogen makes up about 80 percent of the air and therefore contributes about 80 percent of the total atmospheric pressure—$0.80 \times 760mm = 608mm$.

24. **The correct answer is (D).** A supersaturated solution contains more dissolved solute than is normal at a given temperature. A disturbance will cause the solution to adjust to the normal concentration with the concurrent expulsion of the excess solute. A saturated solution will remain stable.

25. **The correct answer is (A).** A first-order reaction has a rate that is proportional to the concentration of only one reactant.

26. **The correct answer is (A).** The loss of an alpha particle reduces the number of positive charges by 2 and the atomic mass by 4.

27. **The correct answer is (D).** Positron (with the mass of an electron) emission can occur, but protons are never expelled from the nucleus during radioactive decay.

28. **The correct answer is (A).** Fat yields the highest amount of energy per gram of any of the foods consumed.

29. **The correct answer is (C).** The total number of moles of reactants and products are equal; therefore, a change of pressure has no effect in the equilibrium. Increasing hydrogen or reducing hydrogen bromide drives the reaction to the right. Only increasing hydrogen bromide shifts the equilibrium to the left.

30. **The correct answer is (C).** One gram of carbon-14 must go through 4 half lives to be reduced to 0.0625 grams. $4 \times 5.73 \times 10$ years equal 22.92×10 years.

31. **The correct answer is (D).** Since the oxidation number of a compound is 0, the total positive values must equal the total negative values. Consequently, four times the value for oxygen (–2) must equal the positive values due to potassium (+1 each) and manganese (Mn).

1 (Oxidation number of Mn) +
2 (Oxidation number of K) +
4 (Oxidation number of 0) = 0

Oxidation number of Mn + 2(+1) + 4(–2) = 0

Oxidation number of Mn = +8 – 2 = +6

32. **The correct answer is (A).** Within a group, the element with the lowest atomic number has the highest ionization energy.

33. **The correct answer is (D).** Within a group of nonmetals such as the halogens, the one with the highest atomic number has the least electronegative value.

34. **The correct answer is (B).** The atomic radii of a group of metals increase as the atomic number increases. Therefore, the element with the lowest atomic number has the smallest atomic radius.

35. **The correct answer is (B).** The salt that would yield a weak acid when mixed with acid would dissolve most readily. Calcium carbonate yields carbonic acid (H_2CO_3) when it is acidified. The other salts yield hydrochloric acid (HC1), nitric acid (HNO_3), or phosphoric acid (H_3PO_4), which are all strong acids.

36. **The correct answer is (B).** The conjugate base is obtained when the acid loses a hydrogen ion. Therefore, the conjugate base of carbonic acid, H_2CO_3, is the hydrogen carbonate ion (HCO_3^-).

37. **The correct answer is (C).** The number of moles of HCl required for the titration must equal the number of moles of NaOH (40 ml × 0.2 m = 8 moles). Therefore, 20 ml of 0.4 ml Cl is required. After titration, the total volume of the mixture is 40 + 20 = 60 ml.

38. **The correct answer is (D).** The salt of a weak acid would hydrolyze in solution to remove hydrogen ions from water and leave an excess of hydroxide ions. $H_2O + A \rightarrow HA + OH$. The salt of a strong acid would hydrolyze by removing hydroxide ions from water.

$NH_4 + H_2O \rightarrow NH_4OH + H^+$.

39. **The correct answer is (A).** Heat is produced by the reaction, and, according to Le Chatalier's Principle, the system will adjust to maintain equilibrium. Heating would force the reaction to the left. A pressure increase shifts the reaction in the direction of smaller volumes (right), and addition of more reactant (N_2 or H_2) also pushes the reaction to the right.

40. **The correct answer is (C).** Colligative properties are based on the number of particles. Vapor pressure, osmotic pressure, boiling point elevation, and freezing point lowering all are colligative properties. Density is not.

41. **The correct answer is (C).** Molecular solids are held together by rather weak London forces, which increase with molecular weight. The melting points of molecular substances are relatively low since there are no strong forces, such as ionic forces, to overcome.

42. **The correct answer is (D).** Ionic compounds form readily between non-metals and metals. The only set that has no such combination is CH_2O, H_2S, and NH_3.

43. **The correct answer is (C).** An atom lying at the corner of a unit cell will touch four corners of cubes below and four corners of cubes above.

44. **The correct answer is (A).** A higher boiling point for a liquid is seen when more energy is needed to separate the gaseous molecules from the liquid. It shows that for the same amount of energy, a higher boiling liquid would expel fewer molecules as vapor at any temperature, resulting in a lower vapor pressure. The lowest boiling substance vaporizes most easily and

therefore would have the highest vapor pressure at a specific temperature.

45. **The correct answer is (A).** The mass number of an isotope is the sum of the protons and neutrons in an atom. 17 protons and 17 neutrons are necessary to give a mass number of 34. The number of electrons equals the number of protons in an atom.

46. **The correct answer is (A).** Electronegativism decreases within a group in the periodic table as the atomic number increases. The example shown is the progression from fluorine to iodine.

47. **The correct answer is (D).** Phosphorus has 15 electrons, all of which are paired except 1.

48. **The correct answer is (C).** Chlorine is in the third period and has 7 electrons in its outermost shell. 2 electrons are in an S orbital, leaving 5 electrons for the P orbitals.

49. **The correct answer is (B).** Sulfur in group VIA needs 2 electrons added to its 6 to achieve a stable outer shell of 8 electrons.

50. **The correct answer is (B).** Since all three gases are in equal size flasks with the same temperature and pressure, the total number of moles (hence, the total number of molecules) is equal in each case. However, a molecule of NH_3 contains 4 atoms, a molecule of NO contains 2 atoms, and a molecule of N_2 contains 2 atoms.

READING COMPREHENSION ANSWER SHEETS

Reading Passage 1

1. Ⓐ Ⓑ Ⓒ Ⓓ   2. Ⓐ Ⓑ Ⓒ Ⓓ   3. Ⓐ Ⓑ Ⓒ Ⓓ   4. Ⓐ Ⓑ Ⓒ Ⓓ

Reading Passage 2

1. Ⓐ Ⓑ Ⓒ Ⓓ   2. Ⓐ Ⓑ Ⓒ Ⓓ   3. Ⓐ Ⓑ Ⓒ Ⓓ   4. Ⓐ Ⓑ Ⓒ Ⓓ

Reading Passage 3

1. Ⓐ Ⓑ Ⓒ Ⓓ   3. Ⓐ Ⓑ Ⓒ Ⓓ   5. Ⓐ Ⓑ Ⓒ Ⓓ   7. Ⓐ Ⓑ Ⓒ Ⓓ   8. Ⓐ Ⓑ Ⓒ Ⓓ
2. Ⓐ Ⓑ Ⓒ Ⓓ   4. Ⓐ Ⓑ Ⓒ Ⓓ   6. Ⓐ Ⓑ Ⓒ Ⓓ

Reading Passage 4

1. Ⓐ Ⓑ Ⓒ Ⓓ   3. Ⓐ Ⓑ Ⓒ Ⓓ   5. Ⓐ Ⓑ Ⓒ Ⓓ   7. Ⓐ Ⓑ Ⓒ Ⓓ   9. Ⓐ Ⓑ Ⓒ Ⓓ
2. Ⓐ Ⓑ Ⓒ Ⓓ   4. Ⓐ Ⓑ Ⓒ Ⓓ   6. Ⓐ Ⓑ Ⓒ Ⓓ   8. Ⓐ Ⓑ Ⓒ Ⓓ

answer sheet

Reading Comprehension

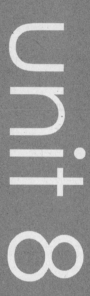

unit 8

OVERVIEW

- **Reading passage 1**
- **Reading passage 2**
- **Reading passage 3**
- **Reading passage 4**
- **Answer key and explanations**

READING PASSAGE 1

4 Questions • 9 Minutes

Directions: Carefully read the following passage and then answer the accompanying questions, basing your answers on what is stated or implied in the passage. When you have decided which choice is best, fill in the corresponding space on your answer sheet. There is only one best answer for each question.

Communicable means "capable of being transmitted or passed through a medium." A communicable disease is an infection that may be transmitted directly or indirectly from one individual to another. The primary objective of programs for the prevention and control of communicable diseases is to prevent the transmission or spreading of the disease by eliminating conditions supportive to infection. Since communicable diseases are caused by microorganisms, the process of infection can be avoided or reversed by eliminating microbial sources, destroying the infectious organisms, creating conditions unfavorable to the growth of infectious microorganisms, and building up the body defenses against microbial attack.

Any measure designed to control or protect anyone from the hazards of the infectious microbes in the environment is called a barrier. The use of barriers is based upon three factors: time, distance, and shielding. "Time" refers to avoiding prolonged exposure; "distance" refers to keeping away from the infectious source; and "shielding" refers to avoiding bodily contact when exposure cannot be avoided (e.g., wearing a mask). The specific plan for selecting barriers in cases where infection exists and for preventing the occurrence of infection is dependent upon the characteristics of the causative microorganism(s). All of these microbes have a certain structure, a specific way of digesting foods, a system for utilizing oxygen or the oxidation-reduction processes, and a technique for reproducing. These microbes are classified by similarities in life characteristics. Therefore, the approach to prevention and control of communicable disease is to eliminate environmental sources or to identify the kind of organisms (by characteristics) and alter their life processes in order to protect human beings from attack.

1. Infectious diseases are "communicable" because they
   (A) attack human beings.
   (B) spread from one source to another.
   (C) cannot be controlled by barriers.
   (D) can cause disease.

2. The goal of programs to control and prevent the spread of communicable diseases is to
   (A) eliminate conditions that support the spread of the disease.
   (B) shield people from the disease.
   (C) avoid contact with people who have the disease.
   (D) find the right barrier to the spread of the disease.

3. A barrier that represents "shielding" would be
   (A) isolating a child with a cold.
   (B) using a stick to pick up infected material.
   (C) short visits with a friend who has pneumonia.
   (D) looking at a baby through a nursery window.

4. Having knowledge of the characteristics of an infectious microorganism helps in the prevention and control of communicable disease in that it
   (A) determines how long the infection will last.
   (B) identifies which methods should be used to counteract the infection.
   (C) establishes whether or not the organism is a hazard.
   (D) relates to the severity of the infection.

STOP

IF YOU FINISH BEFORE TIME IS CALLED, YOU MAY CHECK YOUR WORK ON THIS SECTION ONLY. DO NOT TURN TO ANY OTHER SECTION IN THE TEST.

READING PASSAGE 2

4 Questions • 9 Minutes

Directions: Carefully read the following passage and then answer the accompanying questions, basing your answers on what is stated or implied in the passage. When you have decided which choice is best, fill in the corresponding space on your answer sheet. There is only one best answer for each question.

The "liberated woman" is a phrase that most of us associate with the sixties and seventies. The ERA and NOW's consciousness-raising and bra-burning blitzed the media with a fury. In reality, the American woman had begun to cast off the restraints of feminine suppression long before the seventies, by snipping the strings of her proverbial apron, if not the straps of her bra. We are referring to both the 1920s and the postwar era.

The flood of labor-saving and time-saving devices pouring from the factories freed women of much of the never-ending drudgery that had been the plight of housewives since the beginning of time.

Women also found new freedom outside the home. The vote was finally rendered to women via the Nineteenth Amendment to the Constitution, and the long awaited dream of political equality between the sexes was fulfilled. Members of what was once known as the "gentle sex" cast down their brooms, cast forth their ballots, and fled their kitchens to take part in a social freedom that catapulted their grandmothers right out of their rocking chairs. Chaperones no longer made the scene at young people's parties. Fashion editors reported "the American woman has lifted her skirt far beyond any modest limitation." The hemline was being hoisted nine inches from the ground and was heading for the knee.

The boyish look was in, and women everywhere invaded the strictly male territory known as the barbershop to have their beautiful and once-treasured tresses "bobbed." Breast implants, no way! Damsels of every social station were binding their chests to acquire that fashionable look of masculinity. In contrast to this trend of fashion, beautiful debutantes took heed to the cliche "powder and paint will make you what you ain't" and plastered their faces doll-style with rouge and lipstick.

Young ladies no longer puffed secretly into the fireplaces of their homes to conceal the damnable sin of which they were partaking. Women were smoking in public for the first time.

Extensive vicissitudes in lifestyle and values placed women in the workplace. The "Roaring Twenties" were characterized by women finding new opportunities for employment in the booming cities. Though they were limited to a few low-paying jobs hastily labeled "women's work," such as retail clerking and office typing, they were making an impact on the post-war era. A feisty feminist, Margaret Sanger, led a birth-control movement and openly defended the use of contraceptives. To add insult to injury, the women of the twenties deflated many a male ego with the organization of the National Women's Party in 1923.

"You've Come a Long Way Baby" was putting it mildly in the twenties. In all probability, the women of the 1990s recoined the phrase ". . . and you ain't seen nothin' yet!"

1. This passage would suggest that women of the 1920s were
    (A) docile in their attitudes regarding social change.
    (B) assertive in their views on women's social and political status.
    (C) willing to compromise on political issues concerning women.
    (D) eager to return to life in the kitchen.

2. A fitting title for this passage would be
    (A) "You've Come a Long Way Baby—Twenties Style."
    (B) "Women in the Workplace."
    (C) "Women's Political Advancements in the Twenties."
    (D) "Male Bashing in the Twenties."

3. The tone of this passage would suggest that the author is
    (A) a male chauvinist.
    (B) a product of the seventies.
    (C) a trendy individual.
    (D) a historian of women's changing roles in U.S. society.

4. The message of this passage is that the era known as the "Roaring Twenties" was characterized by
    (A) an increase in women's unemployment.
    (B) marked social change.
    (C) an industrial slump.
    (D) an indifference to fashion and style.

STOP

IF YOU FINISH BEFORE TIME IS CALLED, YOU MAY CHECK YOUR WORK ON THIS SECTION ONLY. DO NOT TURN TO ANY OTHER SECTION IN THE TEST.

READING PASSAGE 3

8 Questions • 10 Minutes

Directions: Carefully read the following passage and then answer the accompanying questions, basing your answers on what is stated or implied in the passage. When you have decided which choice is best, fill in the corresponding space on your answer sheet. There is only one best answer for each question.

Every cell in the body is bathed in water. The substances dissolved in the water provide the immediate environment for the cells' existence, that is, for their respiration, digestion, excretion, and reproduction. This water—70% of our body weight and originally from our food and drink—is carried in the blood and is distributed in three places in the body. In terms of body weight:

- 5% remain in blood
- 15% go to tissue spaces
- 50% go inside the cell

Of course, more water is needed in the cell than elsewhere in the body because there are more solutes to be dissolved and because ionization must take place for anabolism and catabolism—two divisions of metabolism—to function..

All of the substances inside the cell and outside the cell in the tissue spaces were at one time a part of the blood. The blood is the transportation system of the body and, therefore, is the recipient of all substances, which include vitamins, nutrients, hormones, oxygen, and carbon dioxide. Substances are "unloaded" by pushing out those that can filter through the tiny openings of the semipermeable membranes of the capillaries into the tissue spaces. These substances, along with water, are then sucked into the semipermeable membranes of the cells. At the same time, the cell has produced waste substances; it now pushes those out into the tissue fluid so that they can be pushed into the capillaries and thereby excreted by the kidneys, skin, respiratory system, etc.

The pushing and sucking forces are regulated by concentrations. The more concentrated a substance is, the more force it has. What determines whether that force will push or suck is whether the substance is primarily water (solvent) or particles dissolved in water (solute). If water is the primary component of a substance, it will be sucked; that is, it will pass from a lesser to a greater concentration. This is called osmosis. The substance that is sucking in the water has the greater force or pull, called osmotic pressure, because it has the greater concentration. If solutes are the primary component, they can be pushed only by diffusion from a greater to a lesser concentration. The sucking and pushing processes go on simultaneously, and that is why we identify this mechanism as being dynamic. The "equilibrium" of body fluids is explained in terms of a balance of forces. This dynamic factor is controlled by three things:

1. How much of the substance is present (solute/solvent)
2. What kind of substance is present (electrolytes/non-electrolytes)
3. The placement and distribution of the substance (cell/tissue space/blood)

The concentration of a solution is determined by the relationship between the solutes and water. "Solutes" may be electrolytes or non-electrolytes. Non-electrolytes do not ionize and, therefore, they affect the concentration of a solution and its diffusion processes, but they do not affect the osmolarity of a solution. Osmotic pressure is determined by "tonic" relationships. "Tonic" refers to the comparison of the number of specific ions per unit volume in two given solutions—*iso* being "the same as," *hypo* being "less than," and *hyper* being "more than."

Given two solutions of the same solute, the more concentrated solution contains more solute particles, has a higher potential osmotic pressure, and is hypertonic as compared with the less concentrated solution. Given two solutions of different solutes, the solution containing more particles has the greater concentration, but there are no "tonic" relationships.

1. Why is an adequate intake of water essential to life?
   (A) Solutes will dissolve only in water.
   (B) Water is the medium for exchange of solutes.
   (C) Osmosis will take place only in water.
   (D) Water is necessary for metabolism.

2. The blood is described as "the transportation system of the body" because
   (A) blood has the capacity for osmosis and diffusion.
   (B) all nutrients and wastes are received by the blood.
   (C) blood has a higher concentration than any other body fluid.
   (D) all metabolic processes are controlled by the blood.

3. The concentration of a solution is directly determined by
   (A) placement of solutes.
   (B) distribution of water.
   (C) percentage of solute to solvent.
   (D) percentage of electrolytes to non-electrolytes.

4. The largest percentage of H_2O in the body is found
   (A) intracellularly.
   (B) extracelluarly.
   (C) intravascularly.
   (D) interstitially.

5. In the process of osmosis (sucking), the primary factor is
   (A) water.
   (B) solute.
   (C) ionization.
   (D) force.

6. If blood cells were placed in a hypertonic solution of salt, which one of the following blood cell reactions would take place?
   (A) Swelling
   (B) Shrinkage
   (C) Destruction
   (D) No change

7. The primary factor in diffusion (pushing) is
   (A) water.
   (B) solute.
   (C) ionization.
   (D) force.

8. If there are two solutions of sodium chloride, which of the following factors will determine which solution has the highest potential for osmosis?
   (A) Isotonicity
   (B) Hypotonicity
   (C) Hypertonicity
   (D) All of the above

STOP

IF YOU FINISH BEFORE TIME IS CALLED, YOU MAY CHECK YOUR WORK ON THIS SECTION ONLY. DO NOT TURN TO ANY OTHER SECTION IN THE TEST.

READING PASSAGE 4

9 Questions • 17 Minutes

Directions: Carefully read the following passage and then answer the accompanying questions, basing your answers on what is stated or implied in the passage. When you have decided which choice is best, fill in the corresponding space on your answer sheet. There is only one best answer for each question.

As the world's population grows, the part played by humans in influencing plant life becomes increasingly great. In old and densely populated countries, as in western Europe, humans determine almost wholly what shall grow and what shall not grow. In such regions, the influence of humans on plant life is in large measure a beneficial one. Laws, often centuries old, protect plants of economic value and preserve soil fertility. In newly settled countries, the situation is, unfortunately, quite the reverse. The pioneer's life is too strenuous for him to think of posterity.

Some years ago, Mt. Mitchell, the highest summit east of the Mississippi, was covered with a magnificent forest. A lumber company was given full rights to fell the trees. Those not cut down were crushed. The mountain was left a waste area where fire would rage and erosion complete the destruction. There was no stopping the devastating foresting of the company for the contract had been given. Under a more enlightened civilization, this could not have happened. The denuding of Mt. Mitchell is a minor chapter in the destruction of lands in the United States; and this country is by no means the only sufferer. China, India, Egypt, and East Africa all have their thousands of square miles of wasteland, the result of human indifference to the future.

Deforestation, grazing, and poor farming techniques are the chief causes of the destruction of land fertility. Wasteful cutting of timber is the first step. Grazing follows lumbering, often bringing about ruin. The Caribbean slopes of northern Venezuela are barren wastes, owing first to ruthless cutting of forests and then to destructive grazing. Hordes of goats roamed these slopes until only a few thorny acacias and cacti remained. Erosion completed the devastation. What is illustrated there on a small scale is the story of vast areas in China and India, countries where famines occur regularly.

Humans are not wholly to blame, for nature is often merciless. In parts of India and China, plant life, even when left undisturbed, cannot cope with either the disastrous floods of wet seasons or the destructive winds of the dry season. Humans have learned much; prudent land management has been the policy of the Chinese people since 2700 B.C.E., but even they have not learned enough.

When the American forestry service was in its infancy, it met with much opposition from legislators, who loudly claimed that the protected land would in one season yield a crop of cabbages of more value than all the timber on it. Herein lay the fallacy: that one season's crop is all that need be thought of. Nature, through the years, adjusts crops to the soil and to the climate. Forests usually occur where precipitation exceeds evaporation. If the reverse is true, grasslands are found; where evaporation is still greater, desert or scrub vegetation alone survives. The phytogeographic map of a country is very similar to the climatic map based on rainfall, evaporation, and temperature. Humans ignore this natural adjustment of crops and strive for one "bumper" crop in a single season; it may be produced, but "year in and year out, the yield of the grassland is certain; that of the planted fields, never."

Humans are learning; we spray trees with insecticides and fungicides; import ladybugs to destroy aphids; irrigate, fertilize, and rotate crops; but we are still indifferent to many of the consequences of short-sighted policies.

In spite of the evidence from the experience of this country, the people of other countries still in the pioneer stage farm as wastefully as did our own pioneers. In the interiors of Central and South America, natives fell superb forest trees and leave them to rot in order to obtain virgin soil for cultivation. Where the land is hilly, it readily washes, and after one or two seasons, it is unfit for crops. So the frontier farmer pushes back into the primeval forest, moving his hut as he goes, and fells more monarchs to lay bare another patch of ground for his plantings to support his family. Valuable timber that will require a century to replace is destroyed and the land laid waste to produce what could be supplied for a pittance.

How badly humans can err in the handling of land is shown by the draining of extensive swamp areas, which to the uninformed would seem to be a very good thing to do. One of the first effects of the drainage is the lowering of the water table, which may bring about the death of the dominant species and leave to another species the possession of the soil, even when the difference in water level is little more than an inch. Bog country will frequently yield marketable crops of cranberries and blueberries, but, if drained, will grow neither these nor any other economically useful plant on the fallow soil. Swamps and marshes may have their drawbacks, but humans should beware of disturbing the ecosphere. When drained, wetlands may leave waste land, the surface of which can erode rapidly and be blown away in dust blizzards disastrous to both humans and wild beasts.

1. The best title for this passage might be
   (A) "How to Increase Soil Productivity."
   (B) "Conservation of Natural Resources."
   (C) "Humans' Effect on Soil."
   (D) "Soil Conditions and Plant Growth."

2. A policy of good management is sometimes upset by
   (A) the indifference of humans.
   (B) centuries-old laws.
   (C) floods and winds.
   (D) grazing animals.

3. Areas in which the total amounts of rain and snow falling on the ground are greater than the moisture evaporated will support
   (A) forests.
   (B) grasslands.
   (C) scrub vegetation.
   (D) no plants.

4. Pioneers usually do not have a long-range view on soil problems since they
   (A) are not protected by laws.
   (B) live under adverse conditions.
   (C) use poor methods of farming.
   (D) must protect themselves from famine.

5. A *bumper crop* is a crop that
   (A) is harvested from grasslands.
   (B) is protected from pests.
   (C) has to be irrigated.
   (D) is unusually large.

6. What is meant by, "the yield of the grasslands is certain; that of the planted field, never"?
   (A) It is impossible to get good harvests from a field year after year.
   (B) Crops planted in former grasslands will not give good yields.
   (C) Through the indifference of humans, dust blizzards have occurred in former grasslands.
   (D) If humans do not interfere, plants will grow in the most suitable environment.

7. The first act of prudent land management might be to
   (A) prohibit drainage of swamps.
   (B) use irrigation and crop rotation in planted areas.
   (C) increase use of fertilizers.
   (D) prohibit excessive forest lumbering.

8. The results of effective land management may usually be found in
   (A) heavily populated areas.
   (B) areas not given over to grazing.
   (C) underdeveloped areas.
   (D) ancient civilizations.

9. The word *monarchs* (paragraph 7) refers to
   (A) kings and queens.
   (B) forests.
   (C) huge, stately trees.
   (D) a type of butterfly.

STOP

IF YOU FINISH BEFORE TIME IS CALLED, YOU MAY CHECK
YOUR WORK ON THIS SECTION ONLY. DO NOT TURN TO ANY
OTHER SECTION IN THE TEST.

ANSWER KEY AND EXPLANATIONS

Reading Passage 1

| 1. B | 2. A | 3. D | 4. B |

1. **The correct answer is (B).** The answer is stated in sentence 2 of paragraph 1.

2. **The correct answer is (A).** The answer is stated in sentence 3 of paragraph 1. The other answers are specific ways to eliminate conditions that spread communicable diseases, but they are not the goal of the program, only tools or tactics.

3. **The correct answer is (D).** Answering this question requires applying information from sentence 3 in paragraph 2 that defines "shielding."

4. **The correct answer is (B).** The answer is stated in sentence 4 in paragraph 2.

Reading Passage 2

| 1. B | 2. A | 3. D | 4. B |

1. **The correct answer is (B).** This answer can be inferred from information in paragraphs 3, 4, 5, and 6.

2. **The correct answer is (A).** A title should reflect the main idea of a piece, and choice (A) best suggests the contents of the passage. Choices (B) and (C) suggest only specific information discussed in the passage, not the overall theme. Choice (D) isn't discussed in the passage.

3. **The correct answer is (D).** To answer this question, you need to infer the tone based on the information in the piece. The tone is celebratory of the changes in women's lives in the 1920s. Choice (D) is the only answer that fits that description. Choice (A) is incorrect because a male chauvinist would not applaud the changes. Choice (B) is incorrect because the passage is about the 1920s, not the 1970s, and no connection is made between the 1920s and 1970s. Applauding changes to women's lives doesn't mark someone as trendy, so choice (C) doesn't make sense.

4. **The correct answer is (B).** The passage is mainly about social change, so based on that, you can conclude that the "Roaring Twenties" were characterized by social change. Choice (A) is the opposite of what the passage says. Choice (C) is incorrect because the passage doesn't discuss industrial output or employment, either negatively or positively. Choice (D) is the opposite of what paragraphs 3 and 4 say.

Reading Passage 3

| 1. D | 3. C | 5. A | 7. B | 8. C |
| 2. B | 4. A | 6. B | | |

1. **The correct answer is (D).** The answer is found in the final sentence in paragraph 1.

2. **The correct answer is (B).** The answer is stated in sentence 2, paragraph 2.

3. **The correct answer is (C).** The answer is stated in the first sentence after the enumerated list in paragraph 3. Don't be fooled because the sentence says "relationship" instead of "percentage."

4. **The correct answer is (A).** The answer is stated in the list of percentages in paragraph 1. The prefix *intra-* means "within," so the correct answer is "50% go inside the cell."

5. **The correct answer is (A).** The answer is stated in sentence 4 of paragraph 3.

6. **The correct answer is (B).** This answer requires drawing a conclusion. If the cell were placed in a hypertonic solution, the water from the cell would move to the solution of greater concentration via osmosis and the cell would therefore shrink.

7. **The correct answer is (B).** The answer is stated in sentence 7 in paragraph 3.

8. **The correct answer is (C).** This answer requires drawing a conclusion. Based on information in the last sentence in the paragraph 3, hypertonicity would determine which solution has the highest potential for osmosis.

Reading Passage 4

1. C	3. A	5. D	7. D	9. C
2. C	4. B	6. D	8. A	

1. **The correct answer is (C).** The title of a passage should reflect the main idea of the piece. Choices (A), (B), and (D) reflect only parts of the passage, not what the whole piece is about.

2. **The correct answer is (C).** The answer is stated in sentence 2 of paragraph 4.

3. **The correct answer is (A).** The answer is found in sentence 4 of paragraph 5 which discusses precipitation.

4. **The correct answer is (B).** The answer is stated in the final sentence in paragraph 1.

5. **The correct answer is (D).** A bumper crop is one that is unusually large or abundant. This can be inferred from information in paragraph 5, sentences 1, 2, and 6.

6. **The correct answer is (D).** To answer this question, you need to interpret that quotation. The information in paragraph 5 helps determine that only choice (D) is correct. Choice (A) is incorrect; first, because it doesn't deal with the idea of the quotation, and second, because the final sentence says the opposite; bumper crop may be produced in a single season. Choice (B) is incorrect because the final sentence implies the opposite; a good crop may be produced in a field planted in any environment. It doesn't stipulate that a good crop won't be possible if planted in grasslands. Choice (C) is incorrect because the reference in the final sentence in paragraph 8 is to dust blizzards occurring in former wetlands, not former grasslands.

7. **The correct answer is (D).** This answer can be inferred from sentence 1 in paragraph 3. If the first step in destroying land fertility is the "wasteful cutting of timber," then the first step in prudent land management would be to prohibit excessive forest lumbering.

8. **The correct answer is (A).** The answer is found in paragraph 1, sentence 2.

9. **The correct answer is (C).** In paragraph 7, sentence 4, the writer is likening huge and stately trees reaching high in the air to human rulers.

PART V

PRACTICE FOR PRACTICAL/ VOCATIONAL NURSING SCHOOL ENTRANCE EXAMINATIONS

VERBAL ABILITY ANSWER SHEETS

Antonyms Test 1

1. Ⓐ Ⓑ Ⓒ Ⓓ	11. Ⓐ Ⓑ Ⓒ Ⓓ	21. Ⓐ Ⓑ Ⓒ Ⓓ	31. Ⓐ Ⓑ Ⓒ Ⓓ	41. Ⓐ Ⓑ Ⓒ Ⓓ
2. Ⓐ Ⓑ Ⓒ Ⓓ	12. Ⓐ Ⓑ Ⓒ Ⓓ	22. Ⓐ Ⓑ Ⓒ Ⓓ	32. Ⓐ Ⓑ Ⓒ Ⓓ	42. Ⓐ Ⓑ Ⓒ Ⓓ
3. Ⓐ Ⓑ Ⓒ Ⓓ	13. Ⓐ Ⓑ Ⓒ Ⓓ	23. Ⓐ Ⓑ Ⓒ Ⓓ	33. Ⓐ Ⓑ Ⓒ Ⓓ	43. Ⓐ Ⓑ Ⓒ Ⓓ
4. Ⓐ Ⓑ Ⓒ Ⓓ	14. Ⓐ Ⓑ Ⓒ Ⓓ	24. Ⓐ Ⓑ Ⓒ Ⓓ	34. Ⓐ Ⓑ Ⓒ Ⓓ	44. Ⓐ Ⓑ Ⓒ Ⓓ
5. Ⓐ Ⓑ Ⓒ Ⓓ	15. Ⓐ Ⓑ Ⓒ Ⓓ	25. Ⓐ Ⓑ Ⓒ Ⓓ	35. Ⓐ Ⓑ Ⓒ Ⓓ	45. Ⓐ Ⓑ Ⓒ Ⓓ
6. Ⓐ Ⓑ Ⓒ Ⓓ	16. Ⓐ Ⓑ Ⓒ Ⓓ	26. Ⓐ Ⓑ Ⓒ Ⓓ	36. Ⓐ Ⓑ Ⓒ Ⓓ	46. Ⓐ Ⓑ Ⓒ Ⓓ
7. Ⓐ Ⓑ Ⓒ Ⓓ	17. Ⓐ Ⓑ Ⓒ Ⓓ	27. Ⓐ Ⓑ Ⓒ Ⓓ	37. Ⓐ Ⓑ Ⓒ Ⓓ	47. Ⓐ Ⓑ Ⓒ Ⓓ
8. Ⓐ Ⓑ Ⓒ Ⓓ	18. Ⓐ Ⓑ Ⓒ Ⓓ	28. Ⓐ Ⓑ Ⓒ Ⓓ	38. Ⓐ Ⓑ Ⓒ Ⓓ	48. Ⓐ Ⓑ Ⓒ Ⓓ
9. Ⓐ Ⓑ Ⓒ Ⓓ	19. Ⓐ Ⓑ Ⓒ Ⓓ	29. Ⓐ Ⓑ Ⓒ Ⓓ	39. Ⓐ Ⓑ Ⓒ Ⓓ	49. Ⓐ Ⓑ Ⓒ Ⓓ
10. Ⓐ Ⓑ Ⓒ Ⓓ	20. Ⓐ Ⓑ Ⓒ Ⓓ	30. Ⓐ Ⓑ Ⓒ Ⓓ	40. Ⓐ Ⓑ Ⓒ Ⓓ	50. Ⓐ Ⓑ Ⓒ Ⓓ

Antonyms Test 2

1. Ⓐ Ⓑ Ⓒ Ⓓ	5. Ⓐ Ⓑ Ⓒ Ⓓ	9. Ⓐ Ⓑ Ⓒ Ⓓ	13. Ⓐ Ⓑ Ⓒ Ⓓ	17. Ⓐ Ⓑ Ⓒ Ⓓ
2. Ⓐ Ⓑ Ⓒ Ⓓ	6. Ⓐ Ⓑ Ⓒ Ⓓ	10. Ⓐ Ⓑ Ⓒ Ⓓ	14. Ⓐ Ⓑ Ⓒ Ⓓ	18. Ⓐ Ⓑ Ⓒ Ⓓ
3. Ⓐ Ⓑ Ⓒ Ⓓ	7. Ⓐ Ⓑ Ⓒ Ⓓ	11. Ⓐ Ⓑ Ⓒ Ⓓ	15. Ⓐ Ⓑ Ⓒ Ⓓ	19. Ⓐ Ⓑ Ⓒ Ⓓ
4. Ⓐ Ⓑ Ⓒ Ⓓ	8. Ⓐ Ⓑ Ⓒ Ⓓ	12. Ⓐ Ⓑ Ⓒ Ⓓ	16. Ⓐ Ⓑ Ⓒ Ⓓ	20. Ⓐ Ⓑ Ⓒ Ⓓ

Synonyms Test 3

1. Ⓐ Ⓑ Ⓒ Ⓓ	11. Ⓐ Ⓑ Ⓒ Ⓓ	21. Ⓐ Ⓑ Ⓒ Ⓓ	31. Ⓐ Ⓑ Ⓒ Ⓓ	41. Ⓐ Ⓑ Ⓒ Ⓓ
2. Ⓐ Ⓑ Ⓒ Ⓓ	12. Ⓐ Ⓑ Ⓒ Ⓓ	22. Ⓐ Ⓑ Ⓒ Ⓓ	32. Ⓐ Ⓑ Ⓒ Ⓓ	42. Ⓐ Ⓑ Ⓒ Ⓓ
3. Ⓐ Ⓑ Ⓒ Ⓓ	13. Ⓐ Ⓑ Ⓒ Ⓓ	23. Ⓐ Ⓑ Ⓒ Ⓓ	33. Ⓐ Ⓑ Ⓒ Ⓓ	43. Ⓐ Ⓑ Ⓒ Ⓓ
4. Ⓐ Ⓑ Ⓒ Ⓓ	14. Ⓐ Ⓑ Ⓒ Ⓓ	24. Ⓐ Ⓑ Ⓒ Ⓓ	34. Ⓐ Ⓑ Ⓒ Ⓓ	44. Ⓐ Ⓑ Ⓒ Ⓓ
5. Ⓐ Ⓑ Ⓒ Ⓓ	15. Ⓐ Ⓑ Ⓒ Ⓓ	25. Ⓐ Ⓑ Ⓒ Ⓓ	35. Ⓐ Ⓑ Ⓒ Ⓓ	45. Ⓐ Ⓑ Ⓒ Ⓓ
6. Ⓐ Ⓑ Ⓒ Ⓓ	16. Ⓐ Ⓑ Ⓒ Ⓓ	26. Ⓐ Ⓑ Ⓒ Ⓓ	36. Ⓐ Ⓑ Ⓒ Ⓓ	46. Ⓐ Ⓑ Ⓒ Ⓓ
7. Ⓐ Ⓑ Ⓒ Ⓓ	17. Ⓐ Ⓑ Ⓒ Ⓓ	27. Ⓐ Ⓑ Ⓒ Ⓓ	37. Ⓐ Ⓑ Ⓒ Ⓓ	47. Ⓐ Ⓑ Ⓒ Ⓓ
8. Ⓐ Ⓑ Ⓒ Ⓓ	18. Ⓐ Ⓑ Ⓒ Ⓓ	28. Ⓐ Ⓑ Ⓒ Ⓓ	38. Ⓐ Ⓑ Ⓒ Ⓓ	48. Ⓐ Ⓑ Ⓒ Ⓓ
9. Ⓐ Ⓑ Ⓒ Ⓓ	19. Ⓐ Ⓑ Ⓒ Ⓓ	29. Ⓐ Ⓑ Ⓒ Ⓓ	39. Ⓐ Ⓑ Ⓒ Ⓓ	49. Ⓐ Ⓑ Ⓒ Ⓓ
10. Ⓐ Ⓑ Ⓒ Ⓓ	20. Ⓐ Ⓑ Ⓒ Ⓓ	30. Ⓐ Ⓑ Ⓒ Ⓓ	40. Ⓐ Ⓑ Ⓒ Ⓓ	50. Ⓐ Ⓑ Ⓒ Ⓓ

answer sheet

Synonyms Test 4

1. (A) (B) (C) (D)	5. (A) (B) (C) (D)	9. (A) (B) (C) (D)	13. (A) (B) (C) (D)	17. (A) (B) (C) (D)
2. (A) (B) (C) (D)	6. (A) (B) (C) (D)	10. (A) (B) (C) (D)	14. (A) (B) (C) (D)	18. (A) (B) (C) (D)
3. (A) (B) (C) (D)	7. (A) (B) (C) (D)	11. (A) (B) (C) (D)	15. (A) (B) (C) (D)	19. (A) (B) (C) (D)
4. (A) (B) (C) (D)	8. (A) (B) (C) (D)	12. (A) (B) (C) (D)	16. (A) (B) (C) (D)	20. (A) (B) (C) (D)

Spelling Usage Test 5

1. (A) (B) (C) (D)	8. (A) (B) (C) (D)	15. (A) (B) (C) (D)	22. (A) (B) (C) (D)	29. (A) (B) (C) (D)
2. (A) (B) (C) (D)	9. (A) (B) (C) (D)	16. (A) (B) (C) (D)	23. (A) (B) (C) (D)	30. (A) (B) (C) (D)
3. (A) (B) (C) (D)	10. (A) (B) (C) (D)	17. (A) (B) (C) (D)	24. (A) (B) (C) (D)	31. (A) (B) (C) (D)
4. (A) (B) (C) (D)	11. (A) (B) (C) (D)	18. (A) (B) (C) (D)	25. (A) (B) (C) (D)	32. (A) (B) (C) (D)
5. (A) (B) (C) (D)	12. (A) (B) (C) (D)	19. (A) (B) (C) (D)	26. (A) (B) (C) (D)	33. (A) (B) (C) (D)
6. (A) (B) (C) (D)	13. (A) (B) (C) (D)	20. (A) (B) (C) (D)	27. (A) (B) (C) (D)	34. (A) (B) (C) (D)
7. (A) (B) (C) (D)	14. (A) (B) (C) (D)	21. (A) (B) (C) (D)	28. (A) (B) (C) (D)	35. (A) (B) (C) (D)

Verbal Ability

OVERVIEW

- Antonyms test 1
- Antonyms test 2
- Synonyms test 3
- Synonyms test 4
- Spelling usage test 5
- Answer key and explanations

ANTONYMS TEST 1

50 Questions • 30 Minutes

Review Unit 1, Antonyms, before attempting this test.

Directions: For each question, select the word that is opposite in meaning to the capitalized word. Fill in the corresponding space on your answer sheet.

1. GARRULOUS
   - (A) talkative
   - (B) reserved
   - (C) unruly
   - (D) fraternal

2. TRANSLUCENT
   - (A) patent
   - (B) transitory
   - (C) transparent
   - (D) opaque

3. BENEVOLENT
   - (A) generous
   - (B) charitable
   - (C) malevolent
   - (D) good

4. LETHARGIC
   (A) energetic
   (B) sluggish
   (C) apathetic
   (D) fatal

5. AMICABLE
   (A) lonely
   (B) reactionary
   (C) hostile
   (D) laconic

6. TRANQUILITY
   (A) complacency
   (B) tumult
   (C) plagiarism
   (D) prophecy

7. PROCRASTINATE
   (A) elegiac
   (B) mediate
   (C) expedite
   (D) investiture

8. QUIESCENT
   (A) restless
   (B) slow
   (C) mendicant
   (D) malignant

9. DELETERIOUS
   (A) fractious
   (B) pathetic
   (C) salubrious
   (D) gullible

10. COGNIZANCE
    (A) ignorance
    (B) abeyance
    (C) anecdote
    (D) idiom

11. CLEMENCY
    (A) mercy
    (B) indulgence
    (C) kindness
    (D) vindictiveness

12. IGNOBLE
    (A) honorable
    (B) shameful
    (C) disgraceful
    (D) humble

13. CURSORY
    (A) hasty
    (B) superficial
    (C) awful
    (D) thorough

14. ADMONISH
    (A) warn
    (B) praise
    (C) advise
    (D) reprove

15. PHLEGMATIC
    (A) energetic
    (B) dull
    (C) extraordinary
    (D) morbid

16. LAMENTABLE
    (A) laughable
    (B) generous
    (C) emotional
    (D) doleful

17. PERILOUS
    (A) vivacious
    (B) unresponsive
    (C) safe
    (D) hazardous

18. INIQUITOUS
    - **(A)** unequaled
    - **(B)** unfriendly
    - **(C)** righteous
    - **(D)** injurious

19. ASSIDUOUS
    - **(A)** cooperative
    - **(B)** indifferent
    - **(C)** active
    - **(D)** satisfactory

20. CORROBORATE
    - **(A)** fascinate
    - **(B)** corrupt
    - **(C)** confirm
    - **(D)** dispute

21. CONFLUENCE
    - **(A)** convention
    - **(B)** sympathy
    - **(C)** divergence
    - **(D)** concurrence

22. DASTARDLY
    - **(A)** cowardly
    - **(B)** bravely
    - **(C)** friendly
    - **(D)** sinfully

23. ABSTRUSE
    - **(A)** understandable
    - **(B)** hidden
    - **(C)** absurd
    - **(D)** religious

24. ILLUSION
    - **(A)** delusion
    - **(B)** conception
    - **(C)** reality
    - **(D)** dramatization

25. AVARICIOUS
    - **(A)** greedy
    - **(B)** persuasive
    - **(C)** generous
    - **(D)** gracious

26. COERCE
    - **(A)** enforce
    - **(B)** cohere
    - **(C)** forestall
    - **(D)** coax

27. TEMERITY
    - **(A)** recklessness
    - **(B)** prudence
    - **(C)** support
    - **(D)** sanity

28. LACONIC
    - **(A)** verbose
    - **(B)** concise
    - **(C)** serene
    - **(D)** interesting

29. CREDULOUS
    - **(A)** exuberant
    - **(B)** skeptical
    - **(C)** dangerous
    - **(D)** legible

30. INCARCERATE
    - **(A)** immunize
    - **(B)** anesthetize
    - **(C)** transport
    - **(D)** release

31. OBTUSE
    - **(A)** oblique
    - **(B)** obese
    - **(C)** perpendicular
    - **(D)** acute

32. MUNIFICENT
    (A) political
    (B) miserly
    (C) liberal
    (D) educational

33. DERANGED
    (A) unsettled
    (B) paralyzed
    (C) sane
    (D) awkward

34. LEVITY
    (A) flippancy
    (B) peace
    (C) gravity
    (D) trickery

35. EQUANIMITY
    (A) peace
    (B) inflation
    (C) agitation
    (D) tranquility

36. MARAUD
    (A) purchase
    (B) plunder
    (C) masticate
    (D) elevate

37. ENCOMIUM
    (A) immorality
    (B) praise
    (C) egotism
    (D) defamation

38. ABOMINABLE
    (A) delightful
    (B) horrible
    (C) meaningful
    (D) insane

39. ABSTEMIOUS
    (A) frugal
    (B) happy
    (C) greedy
    (D) radiant

40. ADVERTENT
    (A) retentive
    (B) inconsiderate
    (C) empathetic
    (D) abnormal

41. ENIGMATIC
    (A) perplexing
    (B) explicit
    (C) persistent
    (D) officious

42. EXECRABLE
    (A) unusual
    (B) detestable
    (C) fallible
    (D) pleasant

43. IGNOMINIOUS
    (A) reputable
    (B) shameful
    (C) intangible
    (D) irascible

44. SAGACITY
    (A) sorrowfulness
    (B) support
    (C) satisfaction
    (D) stupidity

45. PROVERBIAL
    (A) innovative
    (B) current
    (C) wise
    (D) cautious

46. ANNIHILATE
   (A) advertise
   (B) destroy
   (C) preserve
   (D) announce

47. AFFABLE
   (A) discourteous
   (B) beloved
   (C) sociable
   (D) debonair

48. CAPRICIOUS
   (A) logical
   (B) agreeable
   (C) awkward
   (D) constant

49. CONTINGENT
   (A) conditional
   (B) independent
   (C) confinable
   (D) familiar

50. PRETENTIOUS
   (A) meddling
   (B) modest
   (C) emaciated
   (D) authentic

STOP

IF YOU FINISH BEFORE TIME IS CALLED, YOU MAY CHECK YOUR WORK ON THIS SECTION ONLY. DO NOT TURN TO ANY OTHER SECTION IN THE TEST.

ANTONYMS TEST 2

20 Questions • 10 Minutes

Review Unit 1, Antonyms, before attempting this test.

Directions: For each question, select the word that is opposite in meaning to the capitalized word. Fill in the corresponding space on your answer sheet.

1. DECEIT
   - (A) fraud
   - (B) truthfulness
   - (C) treachery
   - (D) imposition

2. DOCILE
   - (A) teachable
   - (B) compliant
   - (C) tame
   - (D) inflexible

3. HARMLESS
   - (A) safe
   - (B) hurtful
   - (C) innocent
   - (D) innocuous

4. MELANCHOLY
   - (A) jolly
   - (B) low-spirited
   - (C) dreamy
   - (D) sad

5. IMPETUOUS
   - (A) violent
   - (B) furious
   - (C) calm
   - (D) vehement

6. JOY
   - (A) gladness
   - (B) grief
   - (C) mirth
   - (D) delight

7. LUNACY
   - (A) sanity
   - (B) madness
   - (C) derangement
   - (D) mania

8. MOIST
   - (A) dank
   - (B) dry
   - (C) damp
   - (D) humid

9. PUERILE
   - (A) youthful
   - (B) weak
   - (C) silly
   - (D) mature

10. WEIGHT
    - (A) gravity
    - (B) heaviness
    - (C) lightness
    - (D) triviality

11. SUPERFLUOUS
    - (A) necessary
    - (B) excessive
    - (C) unnecessary
    - (D) expanded

12. REFORM
    - (A) amend
    - (B) correct
    - (C) better
    - (D) corrupt

13. SCANTY
    - (A) bare
    - (B) ample
    - (C) insufficient
    - (D) meager

14. MISERY
    - (A) happiness
    - (B) woe
    - (C) privation
    - (D) penury

15. PROPER
    - (A) honest
    - (B) appropriate
    - (C) wrong
    - (D) pertinent

16. INCONGRUOUS
    - (A) compatible
    - (B) absurd
    - (C) contrary
    - (D) incoherent

17. FATIGUE
    - (A) lassitude
    - (B) weariness
    - (C) malaise
    - (D) vigor

18. HASTEN
    - (A) delay
    - (B) accelerate
    - (C) dispatch
    - (D) expedite

19. ABSORB
    - (A) emit
    - (B) engulf
    - (C) engross
    - (D) consume

20. ABUSE
    - (A) ribaldry
    - (B) protection
    - (C) contumely
    - (D) obloquy

STOP

IF YOU FINISH BEFORE TIME IS CALLED, YOU MAY CHECK
YOUR WORK ON THIS SECTION ONLY. DO NOT TURN TO ANY
OTHER SECTION IN THE TEST.

SYNONYMS TEST 3

50 Questions • 30 Minutes

Review Unit 1, Synonyms, before attempting this test.

Directions: In each of the following, choose the word that best corresponds in meaning to the italicized word. Fill in the corresponding space on your answer sheet.

1. Her efforts to revive the child were *futile*.
   (A) strong
   (B) clumsy
   (C) useless
   (D) sincere

2. The supply of pamphlets has been *depleted*.
   (A) exhausted
   (B) delivered
   (C) included
   (D) rejected

3. The *gist* of his speech was that we should strike.
   (A) end
   (B) essence
   (C) strength
   (D) spirit

4. The soldier was decorated for his *valor* in battle in Afghanistan.
   (A) injury
   (B) ability
   (C) cooperation
   (D) courage

5. When Mary arrived in California, her future seemed *auspicious*.
   (A) bleak
   (B) uncertain
   (C) promising
   (D) somber

6. To our *consternation*, the child's bicycle rolled into the busy street.
   (A) dismay
   (B) amazement
   (C) incompetence
   (D) annoyance

7. *Indolence* is a habit that cannot be excused.
   (A) inability
   (B) snoring
   (C) carelessness
   (D) idleness

8. The political candidate made *cogent* remarks.
   (A) pleasing
   (B) convincing
   (C) flattering
   (D) slandering

9. A *prolific* writer is one who is
   (A) productive.
   (B) popular.
   (C) frank.
   (D) effective.

10. He was *meticulous* when performing his work.
    (A) careless
    (B) patient
    (C) scrupulous
    (D) nervous

11. There were *sporadic* outbreaks of food poisoning at the camp.
    (A) epidemic
    (B) widespread
    (C) serious
    (D) scattered

12. The motion passed even though there were three *dissenting* votes.
    (A) annoying
    (B) disagreeing
    (C) abstaining
    (D) approving

13. It is *traditional* for the bride to wear a white gown.
    - (A) normal
    - (B) customary
    - (C) ordinary
    - (D) gracious

14. The company has *rescinded* the order.
    - (A) canceled
    - (B) revised
    - (C) confirmed
    - (D) misinterpreted

15. Although the prisoner was released early, he was *vindictive* toward society.
    - (A) prejudiced
    - (B) impatient
    - (C) revengeful
    - (D) unreasonable

16. The *sedulous* student worked many hours in the laboratory.
    - (A) eager
    - (B) persistent
    - (C) intelligent
    - (D) inexperienced

17. The neighbors were *interrogated* by the police.
    - (A) arrested
    - (B) detained
    - (C) investigated
    - (D) questioned

18. The lifeguard *disparaged* his brave rescue of the child.
    - (A) explained
    - (B) belittled
    - (C) demonstrated
    - (D) elucidated

19. The water could not *permeate* the rubber apron.
    - (A) penetrate
    - (B) wet
    - (C) harm
    - (D) discolor

20. The *docile* dog waited at the gate.
    - (A) mongrel
    - (B) hungry
    - (C) intractable
    - (D) obedient

21. The two hospitals in our town will *amalgamate* next year.
    - (A) close
    - (B) expand
    - (C) relocate
    - (D) merge

22. She wasted her money on *frivolous* things.
    - (A) sweet
    - (B) expensive
    - (C) unimportant
    - (D) cheap

23. The teacher *divulged* the test grades.
    - (A) whispered
    - (B) disregarded
    - (C) revealed
    - (D) averaged

24. The *salary* offered for the job did not match her experience.
    - (A) reimbursement
    - (B) remuneration
    - (C) indemnity
    - (D) reparation

25. The art dealer *scrutinized* the painting to verify its authenticity.
    - (A) touched
    - (B) bought
    - (C) inspected
    - (D) measured

26. The bridge was closed because it was *decrepit*.
    - (A) slippery
    - (B) weak
    - (C) swaying
    - (D) flooded

27. The driver *conceded* that he was at fault.
    (A) denied
    (B) explained
    (C) complained (D) admitted

28. The machinery in the vocational classroom was *obsolete*.
    (A) out-of-date
    (B) new
    (C) reliable
    (D) complicated

29. The speaker made *candid* remarks about the candidate's record.
    (A) biased
    (B) confidential
    (C) frank
    (D) insulting

30. When the hostage was released, he was speaking *incoherently*.
    (A) disconnectedly
    (B) cohesively
    (C) prodigiously
    (D) sluggishly

31. The mother tried to *pacify* the child.
    (A) detain
    (B) restrain
    (C) accompany
    (D) calm

32. The head nurse on 2 West was young and *vivacious*.
    (A) kind
    (B) lively
    (C) short
    (D) talkative

33. The town was *devastated* after the earthquake.
    (A) rebuilt
    (B) deserted
    (C) destroyed
    (D) saved

34. The teacher *digressed* from her custom and didn't give any homework.
    (A) deviated
    (B) reposed
    (C) alighted
    (D) moored

35. The Colonel was a *gallant* man.
    (A) rude
    (B) fastidious
    (C) cowardly
    (D) chivalrous

36. The evening *reflected* the host's interest in good food, good wine, and good company.
    (A) contemplated
    (B) demonstrated
    (C) imitated
    (D) possessed

37. When I visited her in the nursing home, she was *querulous* and unhappy.
    (A) satisfied
    (B) cheerful
    (C) complaining
    (D) painful

38. The FBI agent kept a *vigilant* guard on the suspect.
    (A) careful
    (B) continuous
    (C) observant
    (D) reciprocal

39. The play treated current social issues *satirically*.
    (A) contemptuously
    (B) interminably
    (C) musically
    (D) ironically

40. She felt an *antipathy* for lizards.
    (A) aversion
    (B) fondness
    (C) interest
    (D) fear

41. The hiker had a *premonition* of danger.
  (A) vision
  (B) forewarning
  (C) recurrence
  (D) apprehend

42. The policeofficer *confiscated* the illegal drugs.
  (A) stored
  (B) distributed
  (C) destroyed
  (D) appropriated

43. John was asked to resign because of his *impropriety*.
  (A) age
  (B) tardiness
  (C) dishonesty
  (D) absenteeism

44. There is no *tangible* evidence of damage.
  (A) concrete
  (B) theoretical
  (C) verified
  (D) scientific

45. Her *blithe* spirit made her popular.
  (A) free
  (B) cheerful
  (C) kind
  (D) insolent

46. The jury *deliberated* for 8 hours.
  (A) met
  (B) convened
  (C) considered
  (D) summarized

47. He had a *sinister* motive for entering the building.
  (A) practical
  (B) treacherous
  (C) important
  (D) honest

48. The requirements for admission to the school were *stringent*.
  (A) unusual
  (B) numerous
  (C) rigid
  (D) lax

49. The students refused to give up their *prerogatives*.
  (A) demands
  (B) rights
  (C) ideals
  (D) duties

50. The widow and her children were *destitute*.
  (A) impoverished
  (B) detained
  (C) loathed
  (D) ill

STOP

IF YOU FINISH BEFORE TIME IS CALLED, YOU MAY CHECK YOUR WORK ON THIS SECTION ONLY. DO NOT TURN TO ANY OTHER SECTION IN THE TEST.

SYNONYMS TEST 4

20 Questions • 10 Minutes

Review Unit 1, Synonyms, before attempting this test.

Directions: For each question, select the word that corresponds in meaning to the capitalized word. Fill in the corresponding space on your answer sheet.

1. COMPETENT
   (A) agreeable
   (B) inept
   (C) vigorous
   (D) capable

2. OMNIBUS
   (A) threatening
   (B) all-embracing
   (C) rotund
   (D) slow-moving

3. INGENUITY
   (A) deceitfulness
   (B) appeal
   (C) cleverness
   (D) innocence

4. CONCAVE
   (A) curving inward
   (B) curving outward
   (C) oval-shaped
   (D) rounded

5. CANON
   (A) barrier
   (B) noisy place
   (C) guiding principle
   (D) rigorous

6. PROPITIOUS
   (A) questionable
   (B) well-known
   (C) free
   (D) favorable

7. VACILLATING
   (A) changeable
   (B) decisive
   (C) equalizing
   (D) progressing

8. FORFEIT
   (A) exchange
   (B) relinquish
   (C) protect
   (D) withdraw

9. QUERY
   (A) question
   (B) look over carefully
   (C) follow through
   (D) act peculiarly

10. STEADFAST
    (A) gradual
    (B) strong
    (C) friendly
    (D) unwavering

11. ACCESS
    (A) too much
    (B) extra
    (C) admittance
    (D) arrival

12. PERMUTATION
    (A) alteration
    (B) permission
    (C) combination
    (D) seepage

13. SPRITZ
    (A) spray
    (B) bubble
    (C) protrude
    (D) sail

14. PERSONABLE
    (A) intimate
    (B) cheerful
    (C) attractive
    (D) superficial

15. EXPEDITE
    (A) dismiss
    (B) advise
    (C) accelerate
    (D) demolish

16. COMPULSORY
    (A) imperative
    (B) impossible
    (C) imminent
    (D) logical

17. PRACTICABLE
    (A) lenient
    (B) feasible
    (C) simple
    (D) visible

18. AGREE
    (A) inquire
    (B) acquiesce
    (C) discharge
    (D) endeavor

19. FLORID
    (A) overflowing
    (B) ruddy
    (C) seedy
    (D) flowery

20. NEARNESS
    (A) adherence
    (B) declivity
    (C) worldliness
    (D) proximity

STOP

> IF YOU FINISH BEFORE TIME IS CALLED, YOU MAY CHECK
> YOUR WORK ON THIS SECTION ONLY. DO NOT TURN TO ANY
> OTHER SECTION IN THE TEST.

SPELLING USAGE TEST 5

35 Questions • 20 Minutes

Directions: Select the word that belongs in the blank space in the sentence. Fill in the corresponding space on your answer sheet.

1. The demonstrators were _____ from the property.
   (A) band
   (B) banned

2. The nurse had to _____ the baby.
   (A) weigh
   (B) way

3. She looked on the _____ for the date of the meeting.
   (A) calendar
   (B) calender

4. The perfume had a _____ of roses.
   (A) sent
   (B) scent

5. The injury caused a _____ on her arm.
   (A) bruise
   (B) brews

6. The student received a _____ for passing the test.
   (A) complement
   (B) compliment

7. The _____ gave the faculty members their assignments.
   (A) principal
   (B) principle

8. The ulcer on the patient's foot did not _____.
   (A) heel
   (B) heal

9. A tiny opening in the skin is called a _____.
   (A) pour
   (B) pore

10. The _____ after surgery caused the child to cry.
    (A) pain
    (B) pane

11. A _____ is a sour berry.
    (A) current
    (B) currant

12. It is important to _____ in order to strengthen muscles.
    (A) exercise
    (B) exorcise

13. The administrative assistant purchased new _____ on which to print letters.
    (A) stationery
    (B) stationary

14. They wanted _____ food right away.
    (A) there
    (B) their

15. He was too _____ to climb the stairs.
    (A) week
    (B) weak

16. The _____ is a timid animal.
    (A) dear
    (B) deer

17. I want to _____ the president.
    (A) meat
    (B) meet

18. She wanted a _____ of candy.
    (A) piece
    (B) peace

19. The child did not _____ the vase.
    (A) brake
    (B) break

20. To _____ means to stop living.
    (A) dye
    (B) die

21. She wanted to purchase two _____ of milk.
    (A) quartz
    (B) quarts

22. He could not _____ his book.
    (A) find
    (B) fined

23. The _____ led to a dead-end street.
    (A) rode
    (B) road

24. The telephone was _____.
    (A) ringing
    (B) wringing

25. The _____ was chocolate cake.
    (A) dessert
    (B) desert

26. The thief was going to _____ the money.
    (A) steel
    (B) steal

27. She placed an _____ in the local newspaper.
    (A) ad
    (B) add

28. He turned _____ because he was so afraid.
    (A) pale
    (B) pail

29. The man wanted the bank to _____ him some money.
    (A) lone
    (B) loan

30. The area around the incision was _____.
    (A) sore
    (B) soar

31. The _____ in the paragraph was not clear.
    (A) clause
    (B) claws

32. The passenger had to pay a _____ to ride the bus.
    (A) fair
    (B) fare

33. When her blood pressure dropped, she started to _____.
    (A) feint
    (B) faint

34. He _____ a loud sound.
    (A) heard
    (B) herd

35. We will go _____ or not it rains.
    (A) weather
    (B) whether

STOP

IF YOU FINISH BEFORE TIME IS CALLED, YOU MAY CHECK YOUR WORK ON THIS SECTION ONLY. DO NOT TURN TO ANY OTHER SECTION IN THE TEST.

ANSWER KEY AND EXPLANATIONS

Antonyms Test 1

1. B	11. D	21. C	31. D	41. B
2. D	12. A	22. B	32. B	42. D
3. C	13. D	23. A	33. C	43. A
4. A	14. B	24. C	34. C	44. D
5. C	15. A	25. C	35. C	45. A
6. B	16. A	26. D	36. A	46. C
7. C	17. C	27. B	37. D	47. A
8. A	18. C	28. A	38. A	48. D
9. C	19. B	29. B	39. C	49. B
10. A	20. D	30. D	40. B	50. B

1. **The correct answer is (B).** *Garrulous* means "talkative," so its antonym is choice (B), *reserved,* meaning "marked by self-restraint, silent, formal." Choice (A) is incorrect because *talkative* is a synonym for *garrulous.* Choice (C) is incorrect because *unruly*, means "difficult to control." Choice (D) is incorrect because *fraternal* means both "brotherly" and "relating to a fraternity"

2. **The correct answer is (D).** *Translucent* means "allowing some light to pass through, semitransparent," so *opaque,* meaning "something that does not allow light to pass through," is its antonym. It is also an antonym of *transparent*, choice (C), which is closer to the meaning of *translucent* than to an opposite meaning. Choice (A) is incorrect because *patent* may mean "the grant of sole rights to an inventor of his or her invention" or "obvious, clear." Choice (B) is incorrect because *transitory* means "fleeting, short-lived."

3. **The correct answer is (C).** *Benevolent* means "generous in helping others, showing kindness," whereas choice (C), *malevolent,* means "evil, wicked." Choice (A) is incorrect because *generous* is similar

in meaning to *benevolent.* Choice (B) is incorrect because *charitable* is also similar in meaning to *benevolent.* The same goes for Choice (D), *good.*

4. **The correct answer is (A).** To be lethargic is to be sluggish, so Choice (B) is incorrect. However, choice (A), *energetic,* being full of energy, is the opposite of *lethargic* and the correct answer. Choice (C) is incorrect because *apathetic* means "showing or feeling a lack of interest or little or no emotion; being indifferent," which is not quite the right antonym for *lethargic,* which is lacking in energy. Choice (D) is incorrect because *fatal* means "causing death" or "causing destruction."

5. **The correct answer is (C).** To be *amicable* is "to be friendly," so *hostile* is the correct answer. Choice (A) is incorrect because *lonely* is not an antonym for *amicable,* and neither is choice (B), *reactionary*, meaning "someone opposed to progress or change" or the adjective meaning "characterized by opposition to progress or change." Choice (D) is incorrect because *laconic* means "using few words, terse, to the point."

6. **The correct answer is (B).** *Tranquility* means "a state or condition of peace and calm," so *tumult*, meaning "a great amount of noise and confusion, a violent disturbance," is the opposite and the correct answer. Choice (A) is incorrect because *complacency* means "a feeling of satisfaction, contentment," or "smugness" and is neither the same as nor the opposite of *tranquility.* Choice (C) is incorrect because *plagiarism* is stealing someone else's writing and calling it your own. Choice (D) is incorrect because a *prophecy* is a prediction or knowledge of the future.

7. **The correct answer is (C).** To *procrastinate* is "to put off doing something," whereas to *expedite* is "to speed something up, to do something quickly and efficiently." Choice (A) is incorrect because *elegiac* means "characteristic of an elegy," which is a sad or melancholy poem or song often composed for someone who has died. Choice (B) is incorrect because *mediate* is "to intervene, to work to bring about an agreement between disputing parties." Choice (D) is incorrect because an *investiture* is a formal ceremony presenting certain authority and symbols of that authority to a person.

8. **The correct answer is (A).** *Quiescent* means "being quiet, inactive, or still," so *restless* is an antonym. Choice (B) is incorrect because *slow* is closer in meaning to *quiescent* than to its opposite. Choice (C) is incorrect because a *mendicant* is a beggar. Choice (D) is incorrect because *malignant* means "dangerous to health" or "tending to cause harm."

9. **The correct answer is (C).** *Deleterious* means "having a harmful effect," whereas *salubrious* means "favorable to health." Choice (A) is incorrect because *fractious* means "unruly, inclined to troublemaking." Choice (B) is incorrect because *pathetic* means "deserving of pity" or "inspiring a mix of contempt and pity." Choice (D) is incorrect because *gullible* means "easily taken advantage of, easily tricked."

10. **The correct answer is (A).** *Cognizance* is having knowledge of something, being aware, whereas *ignorance* is the lack of knowledge. Choice (B) is incorrect because to be in *abeyance* is "to temporarily set aside or suspended." Choice (C) is incorrect because an *anecdote* is a short account of something that happened and may be humorous. Choice (D) is incorrect because an *idiom* is an expression the meaning of which can't be predicted from the meanings of the individual words.

11. **The correct answer is (D).** *Clemency* is mercy or leniency, often in a legal sense, whereas *vindictiveness,* seeking revenge, is the opposite. Choice (A) is incorrect because *mercy* is the same as *clemency.* Choice (B) is incorrect because *indulgence* means "extravagance," "yielding to someone else's wishes," or "the act of indulging or gratifying a desire." Choice (C) is incorrect because *kindness* is not the opposite of *clemency.*

12. **The correct answer is (A).** *Ignoble* means "the opposite of noble," that is, "dishonorable, despicable," so *honorable* is an antonym. Choice (B) is incorrect because *shameful* is closer to the meaning of *ignoble* than to an antonym, which is also true for choice (C), *disgraceful.* Choice (D) is incorrect because *humble* means "meek, modest" or "showing deference and respect."

13. **The correct answer is (D).** A *cursory* glance is a quick, superficial or hasty glance, so *thorough* is an appropriate antonym. Choice (A) is incorrect because *hasty* means the same as *cursory.* Choice (B) is incorrect because *superficial* is also a meaning of *cursory.* Choice (C) is incorrect because *awful* doesn't relate to *cursory.*

14. **The correct answer is (B).** *Admonish* means "to reprove firmly, but not harshly," that is, "to express disapproval of." The word can mean also "to counsel or warn against." *Praise* is the opposite of "speaking against." Choices (A) and (D) are incorrect because both *warn* and *reprove* are meanings of *admonish.* Choice (C) is incorrect because *advise* means "to offer advice or counsel," which is similar to one meaning of *admonish.*

15. **The correct answer is (A).** *Phlegmatic* means "not easily excited," "not showing a great amount of emotion, or "a calm, sluggish temperament," so *energetic* is an antonym. Choice (B) is incorrect because *dull* is similar to *phlegmatic*. Choice (C) is incorrect because *extraordinary* does not relate to *phlegmatic*. Choice (D) is incorrect because *morbid* means "having an unusual interest in death" or "gruesome, ghoulish."

16. **The correct answer is (A).** *Lamentable* means "regrettable, unfortunate, sad," whereas *laughable* is the opposite. Choice (B) is incorrect because *generous* has no relation to *lamentable*. Choice (C) is incorrect because *emotional* is not an antonym for *lamentable*. Choice (D) is incorrect because *doleful* means "causing grief" or "filled with sadness."

17. **The correct answer is (C).** *Perilous* means "dangerous, hazardous," so its antonym is *safe*. Choice (A) is incorrect because *vivacious* means "lively, full of life and spirit." Choice (B) is incorrect because *unresponsive* means "not responding or reacting. Choice (D) is incorrect because *hazardous* is a synonym for *perilous*.

18. **The correct answer is (C).** *Iniquitous* means "wicked, evil," so *righteous*, meaning "virtuous, without guilt" is its antonym. Choice (A) is incorrect because *unequaled* has no relation to *iniquitous*, and neither does choice (B), *unfriendly*. Choice (D) is incorrect because *injurious* means "harmful, causing injury."

19. **The correct answer is (B).** *Assiduous* means "diligent, hardworking, persevering," whereas *indifferent* means "apathetic, have no great interest in or for or against something or someone," so it is an antonym of *assiduous*. Choice (A) is incorrect because *cooperative* has no relation to *assiduous*. *Active*, choice (C), is incorrect because it's similar in meaning to *assiduous*. Choice (D) is incorrect because *satisfactory* has no relation to *assiduous*.

20. **The correct answer is (D).** *Corroborate* means "to confirm or support," whereas *dispute* is the opposite—to disagree. Choice (A) is incorrect because *fascinate* has no relation to *corroborate*; neither does choice (B), *corrupt*. Choice (C) is incorrect because *confirm* is a synonym rather than an antonym for *corroborate*.

21. **The correct answer is (C).** *Confluence* means "a point where things merge, often two rivers," whereas a *divergence* is the act or result of diverging, that is, moving apart. Choice (A) is incorrect because a *convention* is a gathering together, so it's close in meaning to *confluence*, rather than being opposite in meaning. Choice (B) is incorrect because *sympathy* means "sharing another's feelings or emotions." Choice (D) is incorrect because *concurrence* means "agreement," "cooperation," or "coincidence."

22. **The correct answer is (B).** *Dastardly* means "cowardly, mean, malicious," whereas *bravely* is the opposite. Choice (A) is incorrect because *cowardly* is one of the definitions of *dastardly*. Choice (C) is incorrect because *friendly* has no relation to *dastardly*. Choice (D) is incorrect because *sinfully* is not the same as *dastardly*, but is close in meaning.

23. **The correct answer is (A).** *Abstruse* means "difficult to understand, incomprehensible to ordinary people," so *understandable* is the opposite. Choice (B) is incorrect because *hidden* is similar in meaning to *abstruse*. Choice (C) is incorrect because *absurd*, ridiculous or completely false, has no relation to *abstruse*. Choice (D) is incorrect because *religious* has no relation to *abstruse*.

24. **The correct answer is (C).** An *illusion* is a false idea or belief, or a false or misleading perception, so *reality* is the opposite. Choice (A) is incorrect because a *delusion* is a false belief that a person holds despite evidence to the contrary, so it is similar to an *illusion*, rather than being an antonym. Choice (B) is incorrect because a *conception* is the creation of something, such as an idea, plan, or design. Choice (D) is incorrect because a *dramatization* is acting out

a scene or play or the conversion of a piece of writing into a dramatic presentation.

25. **The correct answer is (C).** To be *avaricious* is to be greedy, so its antonym is *generous*. Choice (A) is incorrect because *greedy* is a definition of *avaricious*. Choice (B) is incorrect because *persuasive* has no relation to *avaricious*, and neither does choice (D), *gracious*.

26. **The correct answer is (D).** *Coerce* means "to force someone to do or think in a certain way by means of threats or violence," whereas *coax* means "to persuade by pleading or flattering, to manipulate a person." Choice (A) is incorrect because *enforce*, "to compel obedience," is similar to *coerce* rather than being an antonym. Choice (B) is incorrect because *cohere* means "to stick or hold together." Choice (C) is incorrect because *forestall* means "to delay or stop something from happening" or "to anticipate."

27. **The correct answer is (B).** *Temerity* means ""foolhardiness, recklessness, daring," which is the opposite of *prudence*, meaning "caution" and also "care taken in manage one's resources. Choice (A) is incorrect because *recklessness* is a definition of *temerity*. Choice (C) is incorrect because *support* has no relation to *temerity*, nor does Choice (D) *sanity*.

28. **The correct answer is (A).** *Laconic* means "terse, using few words," whereas *verbose*, meaning "wordy," is the opposite. Choice (B) is incorrect because *concise*, meaning "brief, using few words," is a synonym. Choice (C) is incorrect because *serene*, meaning "calm," has no relation to *laconic*. Choice (D) is incorrect because *interesting* has no relation to *laconic*.

29. **The correct answer is (B).** A *credulous* person is someone who believes too easily what people say without evidence, whereas a *skeptical* person is one who tends to doubt what people say. Choice (A) is incorrect because *exuberant* means "full of joy," "full of life or vitality," or "lavish;" none of these definitions bears a relation to *credulous*.

Choices (C) and (D), *dangerous* and *legible*, meaning "apparent" or "able to be read," have no relation to *credulous*.

30. **The correct answer is (D).** To *incarcerate* someone is "to imprison" the person, so to *release* a person is the opposite. Choice (A) is incorrect because *immunize* is either "to grant a person protection from prosecution" or "to vaccinate against disease." Choice (B) is incorrect because *anesthetize* is "to administer anesthesia." Choice (C) is incorrect because *transport* is "to move or carry."

31. **The correct answer is (D).** *Obtuse* means "insensitive emotionally" or "not sharp or pointed," whereas *acute*, meaning "perceptive" or "having a sharp point or end," is the antonym. Choice (A) is incorrect because *oblique* means "slanting, sloping." Choice (B) is incorrect because *obese* means "excessively overweight." Choice (C) is incorrect because *perpendicular* means "being at right angles to a horizontal plane."

32. **The correct answer is (B).** *Munificent* means "very generous," whereas *miserly* means "very stingy." Choice (A) is incorrect because *political* has no relation to *munificent*. Choice (C) is incorrect because *liberal* may mean "generous, munificent," so it is a synonym. Choice (D) is incorrect because *educational* has no relation to *munificent*.

33. **The correct answer is (C).** *Deranged* means "driven insane, insane," whereas *sane* is the opposite. Choice (A) is incorrect because *unsettled*, meaning "disturbed, unpredictable," is closer to the meaning of *deranged* than to its opposite. Choice (B) is incorrect because *paralyzed* has no relation to *deranged*, and neither does *awkward*, choice (D).

34. **The correct answer is (C).** *Levity* means "lack of appropriate seriousness, light-hearted behavior," whereas *gravity*, meaning "seriousness," is the opposite. Choice (A) is incorrect because *flippancy* means "disrespectful and inappropriate levity," so it is a synonym. Choice (B) is incorrect

because *peace* has no relation to *levity*, and neither does choice (D), *trickery*.

35. **The correct answer is (C).** *Equanimity* means "calmness of temperament and/or mind," whereas *agitation*, being in a state of excitement or worry, is the opposite. Choice (A) is incorrect because *peace* is similar to *equanimity*. Choice (B) is incorrect because *inflation* means "being pompous" or "a general increase in prices." Choice (D) is incorrect because *tranquility* means "free from stress or emotion" and so is close in meaning to *equanimity* rather than being an antonym.

36. **The correct answer is (A).** To *maraud* is "to raid and rob, to attack and rob," whereas to *purchase* is the opposite. Choice (B) is incorrect because *plunder*, meaning "to rob, especially in time of war" is a synonym. Choice (C) is incorrect because *masticate* is "to chew." Choice (D) is incorrect because *elevate* is "to raise up."

37. **The correct answer is (D).** An *encomium* is warm praise of someone, a tribute, whereas *defamation* is falsely accusing someone or falsely attacking a person's character. Choice (A) is incorrect because *immorality* is the lack of moral qualities or behaving without morals. While choice (A) may be tempting, *defamation* is a better choice for the answer. Choice (B) is incorrect because *praise* is a synonym for *encomium*. Choice (C) is incorrect because *egotism*, meaning "an inflated sense of self-worth," has no relation to *encomium*.

38. **The correct answer is (A).** *Abominable* means "hateful, detestable" or "very bad or displeasing," so the antonym is *delightful*. Choice (B) is incorrect because *horrible* isn't a synonym for *abominable*, but it means "dreadful" or "very unpleasant, disagreeable." Choice (C) is incorrect because *meaningful* has no relation to *abominable*; neither has choice (D), *insane*.

39. **The correct answer is (C).** *Abstemious* means "moderate or sparing, especially in regard to eating and drinking." *Greedy*, on the other hand, means "excessively desirous of acquiring wealth, avaricious, acquisitive." Choice (A) is incorrect because *frugal* means "thrifty" or "not costly," so it's a synonym of *abstemious*. Choice (B) is incorrect because *happy* has no relation to *abstemious*. Choice (D) is incorrect because *radiant* has no relation to *abstemious*.

40. **The correct answer is (B).** *Advertent* means "paying or giving attention or care to," whereas *inconsiderate* means "lacking in care or thought or others, thoughtless." Choice (A) is incorrect because *retentive*, meaning "having the power or capacity to retain information, good at remembering," is a synonym for *advertent*. Choice (C) is incorrect because *empathetic* means "understanding and identifying with others' feelings." Choice (D) is incorrect because *abnormal* has no relation to *advertent*.

41. **The correct answer is (B).** Something that is *enigmatic* is mysterious or puzzling, whereas something that is *explicit* is clearly expressed, not implied. Choice (A) is incorrect because *perplexing* is similar to *enigmatic*. Choice (C) is incorrect because *persistent* means "refusing to give up" and has no relation to *enigmatic*. Choice (D) is incorrect because *officious* means "unnecessarily or excessively eager" or "intruding in an offensive way."

42. **The correct answer is (D).** *Execrable* means "hateful," "disgusting, unpleasant," or "of very poor quality," whereas *pleasant* is its opposite. Choice (A) is incorrect because *unusual* has no relation to *execrable*. The same goes for choice (C) because *fallible* means "capable of error or mistakes." Choice (B) is incorrect because *detestable* is a synonym for *execrable*, not an antonym.

43. **The correct answer is (A).** *Ignominious* means "shameful or disgraceful" or "deserving of shame or disgrace," whereas *reputable* means "honorable, having a good reputation." Choice (B) is incorrect because *shameful* is a definition of *ignominious*. Choice (C) is incorrect because *intangible* means "not able to be perceived by touch" or "unclear," neither of which relate to *ig-*

nominious. Choice (D) is incorrect because *irascible* means "easily angered."

44. **The correct answer is (D).** *Sagacity* is wisdom, whereas *stupidity* is its opposite. Choice (A) is incorrect because *sorrowfulness* has no relation to sagacity. Choice (B) is incorrect because *support* has not relation to *sagacity,* and neither does choice (C), *satisfaction.*

45. **The correct answer is (A).** *Proverbial* means "widely known" and also "conventional, traditional," so *innovative* is its opposite. Choice (B) is incorrect because *current* means "in the here and now." Choice (C) is incorrect because *wise* has no relation to *proverbial.* Choice (D) is incorrect because *cautious* has no relation to *proverbial.*

46. **The correct answer is (C).** *Annihilate* means "to destroy completely, to wipe out, to abolish," whereas *preserve* is the opposite. Choice (A) is incorrect because *advertise* has no relation to *annihilate.* Choice (B) is incorrect because *destroy* is a synonym for *annihilate.* Choice (D) is incorrect because *announce* has no relation to *annihilate.*

47. **The correct answer is (A).** An *affable* person is kindly, easy to talk to, and approachable. The opposite is *discourteous* person, one lacking in courtesy. Choice (B) is incorrect because *beloved* has no relation to *affable.* Choice (C) is incorrect because *sociable* is a near synonym for *affable.* Choice (D) is incorrect because *debonair* means "refined, urbane" and also "affable," so it also is a synonym.

48. **The correct answer is (D).** *Capricious* means "liable to sudden and unpredictable changes in behavior or attitude," whereas *constant* is the opposite. Choice (A) is incorrect because *logical,* meaning "rational, well thought out, characterized by valid or clear reasoning," is not quite an antonym. Choices (B) (C) are incorrect because *agreeable* and *awkward* have no relation to *capricious.*

49. **The correct answer is (B).** *Contingent* means "dependent on events or circumstances," whereas *independent* is the opposite. Choice (A) is incorrect because *conditional* means "depending on other factors," so it's a synonym. Choice (C) is incorrect because *confinable* means "restricted within certain bounds" or "kept in." Choice (D) is incorrect because *familiar* has no relation to *contingent.*

50. **The correct answer is (B).** *Pretentious* means "trying to be something that one isn't, claiming a distinction or importance that is not deserved," whereas *modest,* or humble, is the opposite. Choice (A) is incorrect because *meddling* means "intruding on others' lives, interfering." Choice (C) is incorrect because *emaciated* means "excessively thin, especially from disease or hunger." Choice (D) is incorrect because *authentic* means "real, genuine."

Antonyms Test 2

1. B	5. C	9. D	13. B	17. D
2. D	6. B	10. D	14. A	18. A
3. B	7. A	11. A	15. C	19. A
4. A	8. B	12. D	16. A	20. B

1. **The correct answer is (B).** *Deceit* means "a trick, fraud" or "misleading someone deliberately, a misrepresentation," whereas *truthfulness* is the opposite. Choice (A) is incorrect because *fraud* is a definition of *deceit.* Choice (C) is incorrect because *treachery* is also a synonym for *deceit.* Choice (D) is incorrect because *imposition* means "something forced on a person," which has no relation to *deceit.*

2. **The correct answer is (D).** *Docile* means "teachable" "or willing to be managed or supervised," so *inflexible*, meaning "unwilling, obstinate" as well as "rigid, stiff," is the opposite. Choice (A) is incorrect because *teachable* is a definition of *docile*. Choice (B) is incorrect because *compliant* means "willing to be managed, to agree to do something as requested or required by someone else," so it's a synonym for *docile.* Choice (C) is incorrect because *tame* means "not afraid or timid."

3. **The correct answer is (B).** *Hurtful* is the opposite of *harmless.* Choice (A) is incorrect because *safe* is not an antonym for *harmless.* Choice (C) is incorrect because *innocent* is not an antonym, and neither is choice (D), *innocuous*, meaning "harmless," making it a synonym instead.

4. **The correct answer is (A).** *Melancholy* means "tendency to depression, gloominess," whereas the opposite is *jolly.* Choice (B) is incorrect because *low-spirited* is similar to *melancholy.* Choice (C) is incorrect because *dreamy* means "impractical, vague," "lacking liveliness," or "gentle, relaxing," none of which fit as opposites of *melancholy.* Choice (D) is incorrect because *sad* is closer in meaning to *melancholy* than to an antonym.

5. **The correct answer is (C).** *Impetuous* means "impulsive, acting quickly without a great amount of thought," whereas *calm* is its opposite. Choice (A) is incorrect because *violent* is not an antonym. *Furious*, choice (B) and *vehement*, choice (D), are incorrect because both have an element of intensity, and neither is an antonym of *impetuous.*

6. **The correct answer is (B).** The opposite of *joy* is *grief.* Choice (A) is incorrect because *gladness* is similar to joy, not the opposite. Choice (C) is incorrect because *mirth,* meaning "gladness and laughter," may express a feeling of joy. Choice (D) is incorrect because *delight* is closer in meaning to *joy* than to an opposite idea.

7. **The correct answer is (A).** *Lunacy* means "insanity," so *sanity* is its opposite. Choices (B), (C), and (D) are all synonyms for *lunacy,* rather than being antonyms.

8. **The correct answer is (B).** *Moist* and *dry* are antonyms. Choice (A) is incorrect because *dank* means "damp or humid," choices (C) and (D).

9. **The correct answer is (D).** *Puerile* means "juvenile" or "immature, childish," so the opposite is *mature.* Choice (A) is incorrect because *youthful* is a synonym for the first meaning. Choice (B) is incorrect because *weak* has no relation to *puerile.* Choice (C) is incorrect because *silly* is closer in meaning to *puerile* than its opposite.

10. **The correct answer is (D).** *Weight* may mean "emphasis, importance" so *triviality,* meaning "something unimportant, frivolous" can be its antonym. Choice (A) is incorrect because *gravity* means "seriousness, importance," so it's a synonym. Choices (B) and (C) are incorrect because

heaviness and *lightness* are qualities of weight.

11. **The correct answer is (A).** *Superfluous* means "beyond what is needed," whereas *necessary* is the opposite. Choice (B) is incorrect because *excessive* is similar in meaning to *superfluous,* as is choice (C), *unnecessary.* Choice (D) is incorrect because *expanded* has no relation to *superfluous.*

12. **The correct answer is (D).** To *reform* is "to improve," so its antonym is to *corrupt,* meaning "to pervert, to cause someone to become dishonest, to destroy someone's integrity." Choices (A), (B), and (C) are incorrect because *amend,* meaning "to improve," *correct,* and *better* as a verb are synonyms.

13. **The correct answer is (B).** *Scanty* means "limited, insufficient, small," whereas *ample* means "large, more than sufficient, abundant." Choices (A), (C), and (D), *bare, insufficient,* and *meager,* are incorrect because they are synonyms.

14. **The correct answer is (A).** *Misery* is the opposite of *happiness.* Choice (B) is incorrect because *woe* is similar in meaning to *misery.* Choice (C) is incorrect *privation* means "lack of the basic necessities of life." Choice (D) is incorrect because *penury* is extreme poverty.

15. **The correct answer is (C).** *Proper,* meaning "correct, appropriate," and *wrong* are antonyms. Choice (A) is incorrect because *honest* is similar in meaning to *proper.* Choice (B) is incorrect because *appropriate* is a definition of *proper.* Choice (D) is incorrect because *pertinent* means "having relevance, being appropriate."

16. **The correct answer is (A).** *Incongruous* means "incompatible, not in agreement with principles, inconsistent with," so *compatible* is its antonym. Choice (B) is incorrect because *absurd* means "ridiculous" or "unreasonable." Choice (C) is incorrect because *contrary* means "obstinate" or "opposed" and is somewhat similar to *incongruous.* Choice (D) is incorrect because

incoherent means "lacking in clarity or organization" or "inarticulate."

17. **The correct answer is (D).** *Vigor,* meaning "mental or physical strength, energy" or "enthusiasm, intensity," is the opposite of *fatigue,* meaning "tiredness, weariness." Choice (A) is incorrect because *lassitude* means "physical or mental weariness." Choice (B) is incorrect because *weariness* is similar in meaning to *fatigue.* Choice (C) is incorrect because *malaise* means "a feeling of depression or general unease."

18. **The correct answer is (A).** To *hasten* is "to hurry," and to *delay* is "to postpone," "to hinder, to cause to be late," or "to linger." Choice (B) is incorrect because *accelerate* is "to speed up, to hurry up." Choice (C) is incorrect because *dispatch* means "to send off promptly, to do something promptly." Choice (D) is incorrect because *expedite* also means "to speed up, to accelerate."

19. **The correct answer is (A).** *Absorb* means "to soak up," "to occupy one's interest or attention," or "to take in, assimilate," whereas *emit* means "to give out or off, to release, to discharge." Choice (B) is incorrect because *engulf* means "to overwhelm, to immerse." Choice (C) is incorrect because one meaning of *engross* is "to absorb," so the word is a synonym. Choice (D) is incorrect because *consume* means "to eat and/or drink," "to use up," or "to obsess over something or someone."

20. **The correct answer is (B).** *Abuse* means "misuse" as well as "maltreatment," whereas *protection* is the opposite. Choice (A) is incorrect because *ribaldry* means "vulgar or obscene language." Choice (C) is incorrect because *contumely* means "rude behavior or language" or "an insult." Choice (D) is incorrect because *obloquy* means "a false accusation."

Synonyms Test 3

1. C	11. D	21. D	31. D	41. B
2. A	12. B	22. C	32. B	42. D
3. B	13. B	23. C	33. C	43. C
4. D	14. A	24. B	34. A	44. A
5. C	15. C	25. C	35. D	45. B
6. A	16. B	26. B	36. B	46. C
7. D	17. D	27. D	37. C	47. B
8. B	18. B	28. A	38. C	48. C
9. A	19. A	29. C	39. D	49. B
10. C	20. D	30. A	40. A	50. A

1. **The correct answer is (C).** *Futile* and *useless* are synonyms. Choices (A), (B), and (D) are incorrect because *strong, clumsy,* and *sincere* have no relation to *usefulness.*

2. **The correct answer is (A).** *Exhausted* may mean "used up," which makes it a synonym for *depleted* in this sentence. Choices (B) and (D), *delivered* and *rejected,* make sense in the sentence, but are not synonyms, so they are incorrect. Choice (C) is incorrect because *included* is not a synonym.

3. **The correct answer is (B).** *Essence* means "essential part, central meaning" and is a synonym for *gist.* Choices (A), (C), and (D) could fit the sense of the sentence, but *end, strength,* and *spirit* are not synonyms for *essence.*

4. **The correct answer is (D).** *Valor* and *courage* are synonyms. Although choices (A) and (B) may fit the sense of the sentence, *injury* and *ability* are not synonyms for *valor. Cooperation,* choice (C), isn't a synonym and doesn't make sense.

5. **The correct answer is (C).** *Auspicious* and *promising* are synonyms. Choice (A) is incorrect because *bleak,* meaning "gloomy, somber, with little hope" or "cold and damp," is an antonym. The same goes for

choice (D), *somber.* Choice (B) is incorrect because *uncertain* is also an antonym.

6. **The correct answer is (A).** *Consternation* and *dismay* are synonyms. Choices (B), (C), (D), *amazement; incompetence,* meaning "lack of physical or intellectual ability; and *annoyance,* all work in the context, but are incorrect because none of them are synonyms for *consternation.*

7. **The correct answer is (D).** *Indolence* and *idleness,* or being inactive, are synonyms. Choice (A) is incorrect because *inability* is not a habit. Choice (B) is incorrect because *snoring* makes no sense. Choice (C) is incorrect because although *carelessness* may be a habit, it's not a synonym for *indolence.*

8. **The correct answer is (B).** *Cogent,* meaning "convincing, persuasive," and *convincing* are synonyms. The other choices fit the sense of the sentence, but *pleasing, flattering,* and *slandering* aren't synonyms for *cogent.*

9. **The correct answer is (A).** *Prolific* means "producing a great amount of work," so *productive* is a synonym. Choices (B), (C), and (D) could all fit the sense of the sentence, but *popular, frank,* and *effective* aren't synonyms.

10. **The correct answer is (C).** *Meticulous* means "very careful" or "excessively concerned with details," so *scrupulous*, meaning "painstaking, conscientious" are synonyms. Choice (A) is incorrect because *careless* is an antonym. Choice (B) is incorrect because *patient*, while tempting, is not a synonym. Choice (D) is incorrect because *nervous* is not a synonym.

11. **The correct answer is (D).** *Sporadic* means "intermittent, occurring at irregular intervals" so *scattered*, meaning "to occur at widely spaced time periods," is a synonym. Choice (A) is incorrect because *epidemic* may mean "spreading an infection rapidly and over a wide area to infect many people" and thus is an antonym. Choice (B) is incorrect because *widespread* has no relation to *sporadic*. Choice (C) is incorrect because *serious* fits the sense, but is not a synonym.

12. **The correct answer is (B).** Even if you didn't know the meaning of *dissent*, the context tells you that you're looking for a negative word. That rules out choice (D), *approving*. You can eliminate choice (A) because *"annoying* votes" doesn't make sense. If you're not sure about the meaning of *abstaining* ("choosing not to vote, refraining from voting"), go on to the next word, *disagreeing*, which does make sense and is the best answer.

13. **The correct answer is (B).** *Traditional* and *customary* are synonyms. Choice (A), *normal*, is tempting, but is incorrect because it means "regular, typical" and doesn't quite have the same connotation as *traditional*, meaning "conventional, standard, what is commonly accepted." Choice (C), *ordinary*, is incorrect for the same reason, although also a tempting choice. Choice (D) is incorrect because *gracious* has no relation to *traditional*.

14. **The correct answer is (A).** *Rescinded* and *canceled* are synonyms. Choice (B) is incorrect because *revised* is "to rework" or "to rewrite," which is not the same as *rescinding* something. Choice (C) is incorrect because *confirmed* is an antonym. Choice (D) is

incorrect because *misinterpreted* has no relation to *rescinded*.

15. **The correct answer is (C).** *Vindictive* and *revengeful* are synonyms. Choice (A) is incorrect because *prejudiced* means "being biased, having an opinion or belief based on emotions." *Vindictive* is a more intense word. Choice (B) is incorrect because *impatient* has no relation to *vindictive*, but the sentence might lead you incorrectly to choose this answer because of the phrase "released early," which is why it's important to read questions quickly, but carefully. Choice (D) is incorrect because *unreasonable* has no relation to *vindictive*.

16. **The correct answer is (B).** *Sedulous* means "persevering, persistent," so *persistent* is a synonym. Choices (A), (C), and (D) are incorrect because *eager, intelligent,* and *inexperienced* are not synonyms.

17. **The correct answer is (D).** To *interrogate* is "to *question*." The other choices, *arrested, detained,* and *investigated,* all make sense in the context, but aren't synonyms for *interrogate*.

18. **The correct answer is (B).** To *disparage* is "to speak in disapproving terms, to belittle," so *belittled* is a synonym. The other choices, *explained, demonstrated,* and *elucidated,* could fit the sentence, but none are synonyms for *disparage*. *Elucidate*, choice (D), means "to explain in order to clarify, to make clear."

19. **The correct answer is (A).** To *permeate* is "to pass through, to penetrate," or ""to spread throughout," so *penetrate* and *permeate* in this sentence are synonyms. The other choices, *wet, harm,* and *discolor,* may seem to make sense, but they're not synonyms.

20. **The correct answer is (D).** *Docile* means "easy to manage, submissive," so *obedient* is a synonym. Choice (A) is incorrect because *mongrel* refers to a type of dog. Choice (B) is incorrect because *hungry* has no relation to *docile*. Choice (C) is incorrect because

intractable means "difficult to manage" and so is an antonym.

21. **The correct answer is (D).** To *amalgamate* is "to combine, unite, merge," so *merge* is a synonym. The other choices, *close, expand,* and *relocate,* make sense in the sentence, but aren't synonyms for *amalgamate.*

22. **The correct answer is (C).** *Frivolous,* meaning "trivial, not serious, silly" and *unimportant* are synonyms. Choice (A) is incorrect because *sweet* has no relation to *frivolous.* Both choices (B) and (D) may be tempting because frivolous things may be cheap, but not necessarily, and they could be expensive though silly. In both cases, however, they are not synonyms for *frivolous.*

23. **The correct answer is (C).** To *divulge* is "to *reveal.*" Choice (A) is incorrect because while the teacher might for some reason *whisper* the grades, it is not a synonym. Choice (B) is incorrect because *disregarded* has no relation to *divulged.* Choice (D) is incorrect because *averaged* has no relation to *divulged,* though it does make sense in the context.

24. **The correct answer is (B).** A *salary* is the same as *remuneration.* Choice (A) is incorrect because a *reimbursement* is a repayment of money spent, not a wage for a job done. Choice (C) is incorrect because *indemnity* means "money compensation for damage, loss, or injury." Choice (D) is incorrect because a *reparation* is money paid to compensate for an injury or insult.

25. **The correct answer is (C).** *Scrutinized* means "to examine closely," so *inspected* is a synonym. Choices (A) and (D), *touched* and *measured,* make sense in the context, but neither is a synonym for *scrutinized.* Choice (B) is incorrect because *bought* has no relation to *scrutinized.*

26. **The correct answer is (B).** *Decrepit* means "weakened, worn out, or broken down," so *weak* is a synonym. The other choices, *slippery, swaying,* and *flooded,* make sense

in context, but are not synonyms and, therefore, are incorrect.

27. **The correct answer is (D).** *Conceded* is the same as *admitted.* Choice (A) is incorrect because *denied* is an antonym. Choice (B) is incorrect because *explained* means merely "to make something understandable"; it doesn't include the idea of admitting something. Choice (C) is incorrect because *complained* has no relation to *conceded.*

28. **The correct answer is (A).** *Obsolete* means "out-of-date." Choice (B) is incorrect because *new* is an antonym. Choices (C) and (D), *reliable* and *complicated,* make sense in context, but are no synonyms.

29. **The correct answer is (C).** *Candid* means "frank, outspoken, open, unreserved," so *frank* is a synonym. The other choices, *biased, confidential,* and *insulting,* make sense in context, but are not synonyms for *candid. Confidential* may tempt you, but it means "something spoken, written, or given in confidence" as well as "secret."

30. **The correct answer is (A).** *Incoherently* means the same as *disconnectedly.* Choice (B) is incorrect because *cohesively* means "sticking together" or "consistent, logically connected," so it's an antonym rather than a synonym. Choice (C) is incorrect because *prodigiously* means "extraordinary" or "huge in size, extent, or force." Choice (D) is incorrect because *sluggishly* means "slowly" or "lacking in energy."

31. **The correct answer is (D).** To *pacify* is "to *calm.*" Choice (A) is incorrect because *detain,* meaning "to stop," is not a synonym. Choice (B) is incorrect because *restrain* is "to hold back, to control." Choice (C) is incorrect because *accompany* has no relation to *pacify.*

32. **The correct answer is (B).** *Vivacious* and *lively* are synonyms. All the other choices, *kind, short,* and *talkative,* work in the sentence, but none are synonyms for *vivacious.*

33. **The correct answer is (C).** *Devastated* means "*destroyed.*" Choice (A) is incorrect because *rebuilt* is an antonym. Choice (B)

is incorrect because a devastated town may be *deserted*, but that is not a synonym. Choice (D) is incorrect because *saved* is not a synonym.

34. **The correct answer is (A).** One meaning of *digress* is "to deviate or depart from a direct course," so *deviated* is a synonym. Choice (B) is incorrect because *repose* means "to put something somewhere" or "to lie down for rest." Choice (C) is incorrect because *alight* means "to come to rest, to settle." Choice (D) is incorrect because *moored* is what one does with a boat, that is, make it fast or tie it up at a dock.

35. **The correct answer is (D).** *Gallant* and *chivalrous*, meaning "gallant, courteous, gentlemanly," are synonyms. Choice (A) is incorrect because *rude* is the opposite. Choice (B) is incorrect because *fastidious* means "showing careful attention to detail," "difficult to please," or "fussy." Choice (C) is incorrect because *cowardly* has no relation to *gallant*.

36. **The correct answer is (B).** *Reflect* can mean the same as *demonstrate*. Choice (A) is incorrect because *contemplate* means "to think about intently." Choice (C) is incorrect because *imitate* means "to use something as a model, to reproduce," and the context doesn't suggest this meaning. Choice (D) is incorrect because *possessed* has no relation to *reflect*.

37. **The correct answer is (C).** *Querulous* means "*complaining,* grumbling." A *satisfied* or *cheerful* person wouldn't be complaining, so choices (A) and (B) are incorrect. Choice (D) is incorrect because pain might make a person complain, but *painful* is not a synonym.

38. **The correct answer is (C).** To be *vigilant* is "to be watchful, *observant.*" Choice (A) is incorrect because *careful* may tempt you, but it is not as close a synonym as *observant* is. Choice (B) is incorrect because *continuous* is not a synonym. Choice (D) is incorrect because *reciprocal* means "something concerning two or more people or things."

39. **The correct answer is (D).** *Satirically* and *ironically* are synonyms when they mean "witty, humorous language used to convey insults or ridicule." Choice (A) is incorrect because *contemptuously* means "without respect, scornfully," and while close in meaning to *satirically*, *ironically* is the closer match. Choice (B) is incorrect because *interminably* means "seemingly endless" or "tedious." Choice (C) is incorrect because *musically* is not a synonym.

40. **The correct answer is (A).** An *antipathy* is an *aversion,* or strong dislike, disgust, loathing. Choice (B) is incorrect because *fondness* is the opposite. Choice (C) is incorrect because an *interest* implies a positive feeling, which makes it closer to an antonym than a synonym. Choice (D) is incorrect because *fear* may tempt you, but that is not a synonym.

41. **The correct answer is (B).** A *premonition* is a *forewarning,* a sense or feeling of evil about the future. Choice (A) is incorrect because a premonition is a feeling, not a *vision.* Choice (C) is incorrect because *recurrence* means "something that happens again" or "a returning thought or memory." Choice (D) is incorrect because *apprehend* means "to understand" as well as "to arrest."

42. **The correct answer is (D).** To *appropriate* means "to seize, to confiscate." Choice (A) is incorrect because *stored* has no relation to *confiscated.* Choice (B) is incorrect because *distributed* is an antonym for *confiscated.* Choice (C) is incorrect because *destroyed* makes sense in the context, but is not a synonym for confiscated.

43. **The correct answer is (C).** *Impropriety* means "an improper act or behavior," so *dishonesty* is its synonym. Choice (A) is incorrect because *age* has no relation to *impropriety.* Choices (B) and (D) are incorrect because *tardiness* and *absenteeism* may be improper, but being late or absent is not a synonym for *impropriety.*

44. **The correct answer is (A).** *Tangible,* meaning "possible to touch" or "real and concrete," and *concrete,* meaning "able to

be perceived, real," are synonyms. Choice (B) is incorrect because *theoretical* is an antonym. Choice (C) is incorrect because *verified* means "having determined the truth of something." Choice (D) is incorrect because *scientific* might work in the context, but is not a synonym.

45. **The correct answer is (B).** *Blithe* means "happy, *cheerful,*" as well as "carefree." Choice (A) is incorrect because *free* is not the same as *carefree,* meaning "without any worries or responsibilities." Choice (C) is incorrect because *kind* has no direct relation with *blithe.* Choice (D) is incorrect because *insolent* means "arrogant, disrespectful."

46. **The correct answer is (C).** To *deliberate* is "to think carefully, often with a group," that is, "to *consider.*" All the other choices, *met, convened,* and *summarized,* make sense in context, but they are not synonyms for deliberated.

47. **The correct answer is (B).** *Sinister* means "ominous," "threatening," or "*treacherous.*" All the other choices, *practical, important,* and *honest,* make sense in the context, but are not synonyms.

48. **The correct answer is (C).** *Stringent* means "severe," "tight," or "*rigid.*" All the other choices, *unusual, numerous,* and *lax,* work in the sentence, but they are not synonyms.

49. **The correct answer is (B).** *Prerogative* means "exclusive *right* or privilege." Choices (A) and (C), *demands* and *ideals,* make sense in the context, but they are not synonyms. Choice (D) can be eliminated because it doesn't make sense in this sentence.

50. **The correct answer is (A).** *Destitute* is extreme poverty, in other words, *impoverished.* Choice (B) is incorrect because *detained* means "stopped, not allowed to leave" or "confined in custody." Choice (C) is incorrect because *loathed* means "hated." Choice (D) is incorrect because *ill* is not a synonym for *destitute.*

Synonyms Test 4

1. D	5. C	9. A	13. A	17. B
2. B	6. D	10. D	14. C	18. B
3. C	7. A	11. C	15. C	19. B
4. A	8. B	12. A	16. A	20. D

1. **The correct answer is (D).** A *competent* person is a *capable* person. Choice (A) is incorrect because being *agreeable* has no relation to being competent. Choice (B) is incorrect because *inept* is an antonym. Choice (C) is incorrect because *vigorous* has nothing to do with competence.

2. **The correct answer is (B).** *Omnibus* means "providing for many things at once, comprehensive," so *all-embracing* is a synonym. Choice (A) is incorrect because *threatening* has no relation to *omnibus*, and neither do choice (C), *rotund*, meaning "round," and choice (D), *slow-moving*.

3. **The correct answer is (C).** *Ingenuity* means "*cleverness,* inventiveness." None of the other choices, *deceitfulness, appeal,* or *innocence* are synonyms.

4. **The correct answer is (A).** *Concave* means "*curving inward*." Choice (B) is incorrect because it's the reverse of *concave*. Choices (C) and (D) are incorrect because they do not describe the shape correctly.

5. **The correct answer is (C).** *Canon* means "a *guiding principle,* a collection of such rules or laws." None of the other choices, *barrier, noisy place,* or *rigorous,* are synonyms.

6. **The correct answer is (D).** *Propitious* means "*favorable,* auspicious." The other choices, *questionable, well-known,* and *free,* do not have any relation to *propitious*.

7. **The correct answer is (A).** *Vacillating* means "indecisive, uncertain, moving back and forth from one opinion or course of action to another," so *changeable* is a synonym. Choice (B) is incorrect because *decisive* is an antonym. Choice (C) is incorrect because *equalizing,* "making things equal,"

is not a synonym. Choice (D) is incorrect because *progressing* may be movement, but it's not a synonym.

8. **The correct answer is (B).** To *forfeit* is "to give up something as a penalty, to surrender something," in other words, to *relinquish* something. Choice (A) is incorrect because an *exchange* is not a synonym. Neither *protect* nor *withdraw,* hoices (C) and Choice (D), is a synonym.

9. **The correct answer is (A).** To *query* is "to *question*." Choice (B) is incorrect because you might come up with a query after *looking over something carefully,* but choice (B) is not a synonym. Choice (C) is incorrect because *following through* is not a synonym, and neiter is choice (D), *acting peculiarly*.

10. **The correct answer is (D).** *Steadfast* means "dependable, especially in terms of loyalty" or "determined, resolute," so *unwavering,* meaning "resolute, determined," is a synonym. Choice (B), *strong,* may be tempting, but it is not as close in meaning as *unwavering*. Choices (A) and (C) are incorrect because *gradual* and *friendly* have no relation to *steadfast*.

11. **The correct answer is (C).** *Access* is *admittance*. Choice (A) is incorrect because *too much* is not a synonym, but on a quick read you might think that *access* was *excess*. Read quickly, but with concentration so you don't fall into a trap like this. Choice (B) is incorrect because *extra* is not a synonym, and neither is choice (D), *arrival*.

12. **The correct answer is (A).** *Permutation* means "a complete change," or "one thing is substituted for another," so the word that is the closest in meaning is *alteration,* meaning "a change, a modification." Choice

(B) is incorrect because *permission* is not the same. Choice (C) is incorrect because *combination* is not a synonym either. Choice (D) is incorrect because *seepage* means "process of leaking or oozing."

13. **The correct answer is (A).** To *spritz* is "to spray." None of the other choices, *bubble, protrude,* or *sail,* have any relation to *spritz.* Choice (C), *protrude,* means "to stick out."

14. **The correct answer is (C).** *Personable* means "*attractive,* pleasing." Choice (A) is incorrect because *intimate* means "deeply personal," or "characteristic of a close or warm personal relationship." Choice (B) is incorrect because *cheerful* is not a synonym. Choice (D) is incorrect because *superficial* means "on the surface, insignificant" and is closer to being an antonym than a synonym.

15. **The correct answer is (C).** *Expedite* means "to hurry up something, to speed up," so *accelerate* is its synonym. Choice (A) is incorrect because *dismiss* is not a synonym, and neither is *advise,* choice (B). Choice (C) is incorrect because *demolish* means "to tear down, to destroy."

16. **The correct answer is (A).** *Compulsory* means "required, obligatory" and *imperative* means "obligatory" as well as "urgent." Choice (B) is incorrect because *impossible* has no relation to *compulsory.* Choice (C) is incorrect because *imminent* means "about to occur." Choice (D) is incorrect because *logical* has no relation to *compulsory.*

17. **The correct answer is (B).** *Practicable* means "*feasible,* able to happen." Choice (A) is incorrect because *lenient* means "generous, not harsh." Choice (C) is incorrect because *simple* has no relation to *practicable,* and neither does choice (D), *visible.*

18. **The correct answer is (B).** *Agree* and *acquiesce* are synonyms. *Inquire, discharge,* and *endeavor* have no relation to *agree* and are, therefore, incorrect answers. *Endeavor,* Choice (D), means "to attempt to do something by great effort" or "an activity undertaken with great purpose and industry, that is, hard work."

19. **The correct answer is (B).** *Florid* is similar to *ruddy,* meaning "flushed, rosy colored." None of the other choices, *overflowing, seedy,* and *flowery,* are synonyms.

20. **The correct answer is (D).** *Nearness* and *proximity* are synonyms. Choice (A) is incorrect because *adherence* means "attachment to something, loyal support." Choice (B) is incorrect because *declivity* means "downward slope." Choice (C) is incorrect because *worldliness* has no relation to *nearness.*

Spelling Usage Test 5

1. B	8. B	15. B	22. A	29. B
2. A	9. B	16. B	23. B	30. A
3. A	10. A	17. B	24. A	31. A
4. B	11. B	18. A	25. A	32. B
5. A	12. A	19. B	26. B	33. B
6. B	13. A	20. B	27. A	34. A
7. A	14. B	21. B	28. A	35. B

1. **The correct answer is (B).** *Banned* means "prohibited," whereas a *band* plays music.

2. **The correct answer is (A).** To *weigh* is "to find the weight of something," and *way* is "a road, path, highway" or "the usual method or manner of doing something."

3. **The correct answer is (A).** *Calendar* is spelled with *–dar* as the last syllable.

4. **The correct answer is (B).** *Scent* is an odor or aroma, where *sent* is the past participle of *to send*.

5. **The correct answer is (A).** A *bruise* is a discoloration because of trauma to a part of the body, whereas *brews* are sold in bars, pubs, and taverns.

6. **The correct answer is (B).** *Compliment* is the spelling of the word that means "an expression of praise or admiration," whereas *complement* is something that "completes" or "makes up a whole." An easy way to remember the difference is that *complEment* and *complEte* both have "e."

7. **The correct answer is (A).** A *principal* is a person, and a *principle* is a rule. To remember, think princi*pal* is a *pal* and princip*le* is a ru*le*.

8. **The correct answer is (B).** A *heel* is a part of a foot, and in this case, it needs to *heal*, or get better.

9. **The correct answer is (B).** Remember that sweat may *pour* out of *pores* on the skin, not the other way around.

10. **The correct answer is (A).** A *pane* is a sheet of glass on a window or door, or a panel on a wall, window, or door, and has no relation to the suffering of *pain*.

11. **The correct answer is (B).** A *currant* is a berry, and to be *current* is "to be in the here-and-now, the immediate present."

12. **The correct answer is (A).** To *exercise* is to be physically active, whereas to *exorcise* is to expel or drive out an evil spirit.

13. **The correct answer is (A).** The "e" in *statio-nEry* is a handy reminder that this spelling means "envelopes and sheets of paper for lettErs." *StationAry* means *immovAble*.

14. **The correct answer is (B).** *Their* is a possessive adjective, and *there* is a pronoun, or in simpler terms, *their* needs to have a noun to modify and *there* usually stands alone as the subject of a sentence. (To add to this, remember that "they're" is a contraction standing for "they are.")

15. **The correct answer is (B).** *Weak* means "frail, lacking in strength," and *week* is seven days.

16. **The correct answer is (B).** *Deer* is the animal, and *dear* is someone who is loved and valued.

17. **The correct answer is (B).** To *meet* is "to be introduced to, to come into the presence of," whereas *meat* is the flesh of animals that can be eaten." *Meat* can also mean "the substance of something such as an argument."

18. **The correct answer is (A).** A *piece* is part of something, and *peace* means "calm," "the absence of war," or "an agreement to end war."

19. **The correct answer is (B).** The child may have *braked* in time so as not to *break* the vase. To *brake* is "to reduce speed."

20. **The correct answer is (B).** To *die* is "to stop living," whereas to *dye* is "to give color to something."

21. **The correct answer is (B).** *Quarts* is the plural of *quart*, a way to measure volume or capacity. *Quartz* is a hard glossy mineral, often with color in it.

22. **The correct answer is (A).** To *find* is "to locate something," whereas to be *fined* is "to pay money as a penalty for a violation of a law."

23. **The correct answer is (B).** Think "He rode his motorbike on the road" to help you remember the difference between a way for travelers (*road*) and the past tense of *ride*, *rode*.

24. **The correct answer is (A).** A telephone *rings*, but someone who is afraid or in trouble may *wring* his or her hands, that is, twist, squeeze, and clasp and unclasp hands. Someone can also *wring* clothes to get the water out.

25. **The correct answer is (A).** You might like to eat chocolate cake in the *desert*, but the cake is *dessert*. A *desert* is a dry, often sandy stretch of land that gets little or no precipitation.

26. **The correct answer is (B).** The thief might have a problem *steal*ing money in a *steel* safe. To *steal* is "to rob," but *steel* is a hard, durable, strong combination of iron and carbon. As a verb, to *steel* means "to strengthen, to make strong or hard;" for example, "he steeled himself to face his wife after his diagnosis."

27. **The correct answer is (A).** The word *ad* is short for *advertisement*; note that it has only one "d." This is way one to remember the difference to *add*.

28. **The correct answer is (A).** To turn *pale* is "to lose color," usually because of fear or a shock. A *pail* is a bucket.

29. **The correct answer is (B).** To *loan* is "to lend," whereas *lone* means "only one, alone, solitary."

30. **The correct answer is (A).** If something is *sore,* it is painful. To *soar* is "to rise, to fly, to climb swifly."

31. **The correct answer is (A).** A *clause* may be "a group of words in a sentence," but in this particular case, it is a section in a legal document. *Claws* are what cats have on their paws.

32. **The correct answer is (B).** A *fare* is money paid to ride a bus, train, or airplane, whereas a *fair* is an outdoor event with rides and games. It's sometimes called a carnival.

33. **The correct answer is (B).** To *faint* is "to lose consciousness, to pass out from weakness." A *feint* is "to deceive by making a misleading move"; for example, "the center feinted to the left and then abruptly swiveled to her right and made a shot at the basket."

34. **The correct answer is (A).** The loud sound he *heard* may have been a *herd* of cattle. To help you remember the difference between *heard* and *herd*—a group of cattle, sheep, or other domestic animals—think of the *ear* in h*EAR*d.

35. **The correct answer is (B).** *Weather* is the day-to-day temperature, cloudiness, and precipitation of a particular place over time. *Whether* is a conjunction that sets up a choice or alternative as this question does: We will go *whether* or not it rains.

Arithmetic and Mathematics

OVERVIEW

- Review of basic operations
- Decimals, ratios and proportions, and percent decimals
- Ratios and proportions
- Solutions to practice exercises
- Arithmetic test 1
- Arithmetic test 2
- Answer key and explanations
- Final arithmetic and mathematics test
- Answer key and explanations

Arithmetic is an important part of the study of pharmacology and the related sciences. In this section, practice problems on fractions, decimals, ratio, proportion, and percent are included with a review of the appropriate processes. The problem solutions are presented after each set of exercises. If you have made errors, go back to the explanation for that kind of problem. After you have completed all practice tests, take the final test.

REVIEW OF BASIC OPERATIONS

Fractions

Reduction of Fractions

To reduce fractions to lowest terms, divide both the numerator and the denominator by the same number.

Example:

$$\frac{4}{8} = \frac{4 \div 4}{8 \div 4} = \frac{1}{2}$$

PRACTICE EXERCISE A

Reduce the following fractions to their lowest terms.

1. $\frac{8}{16} =$ _____   2. $\frac{3}{12} =$ _____

569

3. $\frac{5}{10} =$ _____

4. $\frac{25}{100} =$ _____

5. $\frac{18}{72} =$ _____

6. $\frac{50}{60} =$ _____

7. $\frac{27}{54} =$ _____

8. $\frac{4}{64} =$ _____

9. $\frac{12}{144} =$ _____

10. $\frac{25}{150} =$ _____

Improper Fractions

To change an improper fraction to a mixed number, divide the numerator by the denominator and show the remainder, if any, over the denominator. Reduce to the lowest terms.

Examples:

$$\frac{15}{9} = 1\frac{6}{9} = 1\frac{2}{3}$$

$$\frac{21}{7} = 7\overline{)21} \begin{array}{r} 3 \\ \underline{21} \\ 0 \end{array} \qquad 9\overline{)15} \begin{array}{r} 1 \\ \underline{9} \\ 6 \end{array}$$

To change a mixed number to an improper fraction, add the numerator of the fraction to the product of the whole number and the denominator of the fraction. Show the total over the denominator of the fraction.

Example:

$$4\frac{3}{8} = \frac{(4 \times 8) + 3}{8} = \frac{32 + 3}{8} = \frac{35}{8}$$

PRACTICE EXERCISE B

Change the following improper fractions to mixed numbers and vice versa.

1. $\frac{15}{4} =$ _____

2. $\frac{13}{6} =$ _____

3. $\frac{27}{5} =$ _____

4. $\frac{17}{3} =$ _____

5. $\frac{99}{10} =$ _____

6. $2\frac{1}{9} =$ _____

7. $6\frac{4}{5} =$ _____

8. $8\frac{3}{4} =$ _____

9. $3\frac{7}{8} =$ _____

10. $2\frac{1}{6} =$ _____

Addition of Fractions

To add two or more fractions, the denominators must be the same. Rewrite each fraction as an equivalent fraction with the Least (smallest) Common Multiple (LCM) as the common denominator. Then add the numerators and reduce the answer to lowest terms.

Example:

Add $\frac{2}{3} + \frac{3}{4}$

Multiples of 3 = 3, 6, 9, 12, 15, 18, 21, 24, . . .

Multiples of 4 = 4, 8, 12, 16, 20, 24, . . .

Common multiples are 12 and 24

LCM = 12 (the common denominator)

To make an equivalent fraction, divide the common denominator by the original denominator and multiply the original numerator by the result.

$12 \div 3 = 4; 2 \times 4 = 8$

$12 \div 4 = 3; 3 \times 3 = 9$

Add and reduce to lowest terms. $\frac{2}{3} + \frac{3}{4} = \frac{8}{12} + \frac{9}{12} = \frac{17}{12} = 1\frac{5}{12}$

PRACTICE EXERCISE C

Add the following fractions.

1. $\frac{1}{2}$
    $\frac{1}{3}$
    $+\frac{1}{6}$

2. $\frac{3}{4}$
    $\frac{1}{12}$
    $+\frac{2}{3}$

3. $7\frac{2}{3}$
    $3\frac{5}{24}$
    $+\frac{5}{12}$

4. $1\frac{1}{4}$
    $5\frac{3}{16}$
    $+2\frac{5}{12}$

5. $26\frac{3}{5}$
    $14\frac{1}{5}$
    $+5\frac{7}{8}$

6. $7\frac{5}{8}$
    $\frac{1}{32}$
    $+3\frac{1}{10}$

7. $4\dfrac{1}{2}$

        $3\dfrac{1}{4}$

      $+9\dfrac{3}{8}$

9. $1\dfrac{3}{24}$

        $8\dfrac{1}{3}$

      $+3\dfrac{5}{6}$

8. $7\dfrac{11}{12}$

      $16\dfrac{3}{4}$

      $+2\dfrac{4}{18}$

10. $5\dfrac{5}{6}$

        $7\dfrac{3}{8}$

      $+2\dfrac{3}{10}$

Subtraction of Fractions

Rewrite each fraction as an equivalent fraction with the LCM as the common denominator. If the fraction of the mixed number to be subtracted is larger than the one from which it is to be subtracted, you must borrow 1 from the whole number of the larger mixed number. Add the numerator and denominator of the larger mixed number to make a new numerator. Subtract and reduce to lowest terms.

Example:

$9\dfrac{1}{2} = 9\dfrac{3}{6} = 8\dfrac{9}{6}$ Find the common denominator and make equivalent fractions. Borrow from the whole number of the larger mixed number $(9 - 1 = 8)$

$-1\dfrac{2}{3} = 1\dfrac{4}{6} = 1\dfrac{4}{6}$ Add the numerator and denominator to make a new numerator $(3 + 6 = 9)$.

$\rule{3cm}{0.4pt}$

    $7\dfrac{5}{6}$ Subtract and reduce to lowest terms.

PRACTICE EXERCISE D

Subtract the following fractions.

1. $\dfrac{5}{8}$

      $-\dfrac{3}{16}$

4. $3\dfrac{1}{8}$

      $-1\dfrac{3}{4}$

2. $7\dfrac{5}{12}$

      $-3\dfrac{1}{4}$

5. $\dfrac{7}{9}$

      $-\dfrac{1}{6}$

6. $\dfrac{17}{20}$

      $-\dfrac{3}{4}$

3. $\dfrac{1}{2}$

      $-\dfrac{1}{8}$

7. $5\dfrac{3}{8}$

$-1\dfrac{7}{16}$

9. $4\dfrac{3}{4}$

$-2\dfrac{2}{3}$

8. $\dfrac{2}{5}$

$-\dfrac{2}{9}$

10. $11\dfrac{7}{8}$

$-1\dfrac{3}{4}$

Multiplication of Fractions

To multiply fractions, multiply the numerators, then multiply the denominators. You may be able to simplify the fractions before multiplying, which allows you to work with smaller numbers. To simplify, divide the numerator of one fraction and the denominator of another fraction by the same number. Multiply and reduce to lowest terms.

Example:

$$\dfrac{12}{25} \times \dfrac{5}{9} = \dfrac{\overset{4}{\cancel{12}}}{\underset{5}{\cancel{25}}} \times \dfrac{\overset{1}{\cancel{5}}}{\underset{3}{\cancel{9}}} = \dfrac{4}{15}$$

To multiply a fraction by a whole number, change the whole number to a fraction by placing the whole number over 1. Multiply, simplify, if possible, and reduce to lowest terms.

Example:

$$4 \times \dfrac{1}{12} = \dfrac{4}{1} \times \dfrac{1}{12} = \dfrac{\overset{1}{\cancel{4}}}{1} \times \dfrac{1}{\underset{3}{\cancel{12}}} = \dfrac{1}{3}$$

To multiply mixed numbers, change the mixed number to an improper fraction. Simplify, if possible, and then multiply. Reduce answer to lowest terms.

Example:

$$3\dfrac{1}{2} \times \dfrac{6}{21} = \dfrac{7}{2} \times \dfrac{6}{21} = \dfrac{\overset{1}{\cancel{7}}}{\underset{1}{\cancel{2}}} \times \dfrac{\overset{3}{\cancel{6}}}{\underset{3}{\cancel{21}}} = \dfrac{3}{3} = 1$$

PRACTICE EXERCISE E

Multiply the following fractions.

1. $\dfrac{2}{3} \times \dfrac{1}{8} =$ _____

2. $\dfrac{2}{5} \times \dfrac{5}{12} =$ _____

3. $\dfrac{4}{21} \times \dfrac{7}{8} =$ _____

4. $\dfrac{15}{16} \times \dfrac{9}{10} =$ _____

5. $\dfrac{4}{6} \times \dfrac{2}{4} =$ _____

6. $3\dfrac{3}{8} \times \dfrac{27}{8} =$ _____

7. $\dfrac{1}{2} \times 8 =$ _____

8. $6\dfrac{1}{2} \times 5\dfrac{4}{8} =$ _____

9. $3\dfrac{2}{3} \times \dfrac{3}{4} =$ _____

10. $9 \times 3\dfrac{1}{3} =$ _____

Division of Fractions

To divide fractions, invert the divisor (the second fraction) and change the sign from division ($\div$) to multiplication ($\times$). Then follow the rules for multiplication. Whole numbers are written as fractions with denominator of 1. Mixed numbers are written as improper fractions.

Example:

$$\frac{2}{3} \div \frac{3}{4} = \frac{2}{3} \times \frac{4}{3} = \frac{8}{9}$$

$$5 \div 6\frac{2}{3} = \frac{5}{1} \div \frac{20}{3} = \frac{\overset{1}{\cancel{5}}}{1} \times \frac{3}{\underset{4}{\cancel{20}}} = \frac{3}{4}$$

PRACTICE EXERCISE F

Divide the following fractions.

1. $2\dfrac{1}{5} \div 11 =$ _____

2. $\dfrac{1}{50} \div \dfrac{1}{200} =$ _____

3. $6\dfrac{3}{5} \div 8\dfrac{3}{10} =$ _____

4. $\dfrac{3}{4} \div \dfrac{1}{8} =$ _____

5. $\dfrac{5}{12} \div \dfrac{5}{60} =$ _____

6. $10\dfrac{1}{2} \div \dfrac{1}{3} =$ _____

7. $\dfrac{1}{60} \div \dfrac{1}{2} =$ _____

8. $8 \div \dfrac{2}{3} =$ _____

9. $\dfrac{1}{6} \div \dfrac{1}{3} =$ _____

10. $\dfrac{7}{8} \div \dfrac{3}{4} =$ _____

DECIMALS, RATIOS AND PROPORTIONS, AND PERCENT

DECIMALS

The decimal system is based on the number 10. All numbers to the right of the decimal point are decimal fractions whose denominator is 10 or a multiple of 10. *Tenths* are directly after the decimal point, *hundredths* two places after, *thousandths* three places after, *ten-thousandths* four places after, etc. Whole numbers are written to the left of the decimal point, and the decimal point is read as "and."

Changing Fractions to Decimals

To change a fraction to a decimal, divide the numerator by the denominator. Write a decimal after the numerator and add as many zeros as needed. The division ends when the remainder is zero.

Example:

$$\frac{3}{4} = 4\overline{)3.00}$$

```
      .75
4)3.00
  28
  20
  20
   0
```

Sometimes, the division is not exact and a remainder may repeat itself. Draw a bar over the number in the answer that repeats.

$$\frac{1}{12} = 12\overline{)1.0000} = .08\overline{3}$$

```
        .0833
12)1.0000
   96
   40
   36
    40
    36
     4
```

PRACTICE EXERCISE G

Change the following fractions to decimals.

1. $\frac{1}{4}$ = _____

2. $\frac{7}{8}$ = _____

3. $\frac{5}{6}$ = _____

4. $\frac{5}{125}$ = _____

5. $\frac{5}{16}$ = _____

6. $\frac{3}{25}$ = _____

7. $\frac{9}{20}$ = _____

8. $\frac{1}{75}$ = _____

9. $\frac{3}{8}$ = _____

10. $\frac{3}{10}$ = _____

Changing Decimals to Fractions

Decimals may be changed to fractions by dropping the decimal point and using the proper denominator. The number of decimal places to the right of the decimal point represents the number of zeros to be used in the denominator preceded by the number 1. Remove the decimal point from the number that you are converting and this becomes the numerator.

Example:

Change 0.025 to a fraction. There are 3 places to the right of the decimal point. Therefore, the denominator is 1 followed by 3 zeros (1,000). Next, remove the decimal point from 0.025; this number (25) becomes the numerator.

$$0.025 = \frac{25}{1,000}$$

PRACTICE EXERCISE H

Change the following decimals to fractions and reduce to lowest terms.

1. $0.16 =$ _____

2. $0.04 =$ _____

3. $0.125 =$ _____

4. $0.06 =$ _____

5. $0.257 =$ _____

6. $0.75 =$ _____

7. $0.250 =$ _____

8. $0.525 =$ _____

9. $0.2 =$ _____

10. $4.75 =$ _____

Adding Decimals

To add decimals, place the numbers in columns so that the decimal points are directly under one another. Then add in the same manner that you would add columns of whole numbers. Place a decimal point in your answer directly under the others.

Example:

Add $22.05 + 1.375 + 10.2$

```
 22.05
  1.375
 10.2
 ─────
 33.625
```

PRACTICE EXERCISE I

Add the following decimals.

1. $7.2 + 3.57 + 10.8 =$ _____

2. $48.3 + 18.25 + 4.002 =$ _____

3. $6.3 + 0.005 + 2.67 =$ _____

4. $25.4 + 37.06 + 41 =$ _____

5. $8.50 + 19.625 + 0.17 =$ _____

6. $29.042 + 2.6 + 3.120 =$ _____

7. $5.4 + 8.62 + 0.95 =$ _____

8. $2.246 + 16.8 + 4.26 =$ _____

9. $16.1 + 1.12 + 3.525 =$ _____

10. $30.7 + 4.05 + 20.5 =$ _____

Subtracting Decimals

To subtract decimals, use the same rule as for adding decimals: place decimal points directly under one another. Then subtract in the same manner you would subtract whole numbers, placing the decimal point in your answer directly under the others.

Example:

$$
\begin{array}{r}
50.789 \\
-24.19 \\
\hline
26.599
\end{array}
$$

PRACTICE EXERCISE J

Subtract the following decimals.

1. $5.67 - 3.9 =$ _____
2. $37.2 - 25.37 =$ _____
3. $17.4 - 13.262 =$ _____
4. $58.94 - 27.363 =$ _____
5. $2.425 - 0.675 =$ _____

6. $15 - 7.82 =$ _____
7. $205.6 - 105.23 =$ _____
8. $246.52 - 107.988 =$ _____
9. $35.25 - 17.0 =$ _____
10. $1,725.5 - 50.6325 =$ _____

Multiplying Decimals

To multiply decimals, multiply the numbers as if they were whole numbers. Then place the decimal point in the answer by counting from the right the combined number of decimal places in the multiplier and the multiplicand.

Example:

$$
\begin{array}{r}
2.56 \quad \text{(2 decimal places)} \\
\times \quad 0.6 \quad \text{(1 decimal place)} \\
\hline
1.536 \quad \text{(2 + 1 = 3 decimal places)}
\end{array}
$$

PRACTICE EXERCISE K

Multiply the following decimals.

1. $5.64 \times 1.2 =$ _____
2. $4.25 \times 12 =$ _____
3. $35.6 \times 2.5 =$ _____
4. $4.92 \times 9.5 =$ _____
5. $51 \times 0.92 =$ _____

6. $28.6 \times 8.16 =$ _____
7. $50.06 \times 2.15 =$ _____
8. $32.2 \times 3.15 =$ _____
9. $21.0 \times 41.6 =$ _____
10. $8.06 \times 3.654 =$ _____

Dividing Decimals

To divide decimals, the divisor must always be a whole number. If the divisor is a decimal, move the decimal to the right as many places as necessary to make the decimal a whole number. Then move the decimal point in the dividend the same number of places to the right to avoid changing the value of the quotient. The decimal point in the quotient is placed directly above the decimal point in the dividend.

Example:

$$.25\overline{)28} = .25\overline{)28.00}$$

$$\begin{array}{r} 112 \\ \hline 25 \\ \hline 30 \\ 25 \\ \hline 50 \\ 50 \\ \hline 0 \end{array}$$

PRACTICE EXERCISE L

Divide the following decimals.

1. $100 \div 2.5 =$ _____

2. $0.9 \div 0.3 =$ _____

3. $38.59 \div 1.7 =$ _____

4. $115 \div 1.5 =$ _____

5. $5.5 \div 2.5 =$ _____

6. $3.22 \div 0.46 =$ _____

7. $4.65 \div 1.5 =$ _____

8. $15 \div 7.5 =$ _____

9. $0.042 \div 0.3 =$ _____

10. $0.006 \div 0.05 =$ _____

RATIOS AND PROPORTIONS

Ratio

A ratio is the comparison of two numbers by division. A ratio can be written using the symbol (:) or can be written as a fraction. The ratio 1 : 8 shows the relationship between 1 and 8. The ratio 1 : 8 can be written as the fraction $\frac{1}{8}$.

Example:

$$2 : 50 = 1 : 25$$

$$2 : 50 = \frac{2}{50} = \frac{1}{25}$$

$$\therefore 2 : 50 = 1 : 25$$

PRACTICE EXERCISE M

Write the following fractions as ratios and reduce to lowest terms.

1. $\dfrac{4}{5} =$ _____

2. $\dfrac{1}{3} =$ _____

3. $\dfrac{3}{4} =$ _____

4. $\dfrac{3}{8} =$ _____

5. $\dfrac{1}{10} =$ _____

6. $\dfrac{2}{3} =$ _____

7. $\dfrac{1}{2} =$ _____

8. $\dfrac{25}{50} =$ _____

9. $\dfrac{3}{9} =$ _____

10. $\dfrac{2}{5} =$ _____

Proportion

A proportion states that two ratios are equal. Proportions may be expressed in two ways:

Example:

$$\frac{1}{2} = \frac{50}{100} \text{ or } 1:2::50:100$$

Both are read: *One is to two as fifty is to one hundred.* The product of the means equals the product of the extremes.

Example:

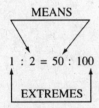

$$1:2 = 50:100$$

If one number is not known, substitute an alphabet letter and solve for the unknown number by multiplying the means and the extremes, or multiplying the diagonals.

Example:

$$5:y = 25:125$$

$$\frac{5}{y} = \frac{25}{125}$$

$$25 \times y = 5 \times 125$$

$$25y = 625$$

$$y = 25$$

PRACTICE EXERCISE N

Solve for x in the following proportions.

1. $8 : 10 = x : 30$ _____

2. $\dfrac{9}{15} = \dfrac{x}{5}$ _____

3. $x : 80 = 3 : 12$ _____

4. $\dfrac{3}{x} = \dfrac{8}{24}$ _____

5. $2 : 3 = x : 63$ _____

6. $5 : 15 = x : 60$ _____

7. $\dfrac{7}{x} = \dfrac{4}{28}$ _____

8. $0.2 : 8 = 25 : x$ _____

9. $\dfrac{5}{7} = \dfrac{x}{28}$ _____

10. $\dfrac{1}{10}x : 2,000 = 1 : 100$ _____

Percentages

To change a decimal to a percent, multiply the decimal by 100 (move the decimal point two places to the right), and then add the percent sign.

Example:

$$0.25 = .25$$
$$= 25\%$$

To find the percent of a number, change the percent to its decimal equivalent, or to a fraction, and multiply.

Example:

Find 7% of 40. (Note: "of" means multiply.)

$$\begin{array}{r} 40 \\ \times .07 \\ \hline 2.80 \end{array} \quad \text{or} \quad \frac{7}{\cancel{100}_{10}} \times \frac{\cancel{40}^{4}}{1} = \frac{28}{10} = 2.8$$

To find the percent one number is of another, use the is/of method. The "is" number is the numerator, and the "of" number is the denominator.

Example:

18 is what percent of 24?

$$\frac{18}{24} = \frac{3}{4} \qquad 4\overline{)3.00}^{.75} = 75\%$$
$$\begin{array}{r} \underline{28} \\ 20 \\ \underline{20} \\ 0 \end{array}$$

Example:

What percent of 500 is 125?

$$\frac{125}{500} = \frac{1}{4}$$

$$4\overline{)1.00} = 25\%$$
$$\underline{8}$$
$$20$$
$$\underline{20}$$
$$0$$

To find the percent of change, subtract to find the amount of change. Then find what the percent is of the original amount using the is/of method.

Example:

A sweater is on sale for $42. The original price was $56. What is the percent of change?

$$\begin{array}{r} \$56 \\ -\ 42 \\ \hline \$14 \end{array}$$

$$\frac{14}{56} = \frac{1}{4} = 4\overline{)1.00} = 25\%$$
$$\underline{8}$$
$$20$$
$$\underline{20}$$
$$0$$

PRACTICE EXERCISE O

Solve the following percentage problems.

1. 0.225 = _____%

2. 3.45 = _____%

3. 0.7 = _____%

4. 0.14 = _____%

5. 4.5 = _____%

6. 24 percent of 72 = _____

7. 5 percent of 12 = _____

8. 225 is what percent of 300? _____

9. What percent of 60 is 24? _____

10. What percent of 45 is 135? _____

Roman Numerals

Roman numerals are written using letters of the alphabet. The letters used to designate arabic numbers are:

Roman	Arabic Equivalent
I	1
V	5
X	10
L	50
C	100
D	500
M	1,000

Rules Governing the Use of Roman Numerals

Addition—placing one or more Roman numerals after the basic numeral adds to its value.

VII = 7

The same numeral cannot be repeated more than three times in succession. If this seems necessary, the rule for subtraction is used.

XXX = 30; XXXX—not allowed, so use XL = 40.

Subtraction—placing one or more Roman numerals in front of the basic numeral removes value from it.

IV = 4

The symbols, V, D, and L are never used in subtraction.

PRACTICE EXERCISE P

Convert the following to Roman numerals.

1. 8 _____	**8.** 36 _____	**15.** 18 _____
2. 15 _____	**9.** 56 _____	**16.** 526 _____
3. 50 _____	**10.** 19 _____	**17.** 94 _____
4. 4 _____	**11.** 25 _____	**18.** 39 _____
5. 23 _____	**12.** 100 _____	**19.** 62 _____
6. 44 _____	**13.** 37 _____	**20.** 1,980 _____
7. 93 _____	**14.** 7 _____	

PRACTICE EXERCISE Q

Convert the following to Arabic numbers.

1. XXIV _____	**8.** XIX _____	**15.** LXIX _____
2. XVII _____	**9.** XXX _____	**16.** XVII _____
3. L _____	**10.** XXIX _____	**17.** XXII _____
4. XL _____	**11.** VI _____	**18.** XI _____
5. V _____	**12.** LXX _____	**19.** CCIV _____
6. III _____	**13.** C _____	**20.** MCXV _____
7. M _____	**14.** XCII _____	

SOLUTIONS TO PRACTICE EXERCISES

Practice Exercise A

1. $\frac{8}{16} = \frac{1}{2}$

2. $\frac{3}{12} = \frac{1}{4}$

3. $\frac{5}{10} = \frac{1}{2}$

4. $\frac{25}{100} = \frac{1}{4}$

5. $\frac{18}{72} = \frac{1}{4}$

6. $\frac{50}{60} = \frac{5}{6}$

7. $\frac{27}{54} = \frac{1}{2}$

8. $\frac{4}{64} = \frac{1}{16}$

9. $\frac{12}{144} = \frac{1}{12}$

10. $\frac{25}{150} = \frac{1}{6}$

Practice Exercise B

1. $\frac{15}{4} = 3\frac{3}{4}$

2. $\frac{13}{6} = 2\frac{1}{6}$

3. $\frac{27}{5} = 5\frac{2}{5}$

4. $\frac{17}{3} = 5\frac{2}{3}$

5. $\frac{99}{10} = 9\frac{9}{10}$

6. $2\frac{1}{9} = \frac{19}{9}$

7. $6\frac{4}{5} = \frac{34}{5}$

8. $8\frac{3}{4} = \frac{35}{4}$

9. $3\frac{7}{8} = \frac{31}{8}$

10. $2\frac{1}{6} = \frac{13}{6}$

Practice Exercise C

1.
$$\frac{1}{2} = \frac{3}{6}$$
$$\frac{1}{3} = \frac{2}{6}$$
$$\frac{1}{6} = \frac{1}{6}$$
$$\overline{\frac{6}{6} = 1}$$

2.
$$\frac{3}{4} = \frac{9}{12}$$
$$\frac{1}{12} = \frac{1}{12}$$
$$\frac{2}{3} = \frac{8}{12}$$
$$\overline{\frac{18}{12} = 1\frac{6}{12} = 1\frac{1}{2}}$$

3.
$$7\frac{2}{3} = 7\frac{16}{24}$$
$$3\frac{5}{24} = 3\frac{5}{24}$$
$$\frac{5}{12} = \frac{10}{24}$$
$$\overline{10\frac{31}{24} = 11\frac{7}{24}}$$

4.
$$1\frac{1}{4} = 1\frac{12}{48}$$
$$5\frac{3}{16} = 5\frac{9}{48}$$
$$2\frac{5}{12} = 2\frac{20}{48}$$
$$\overline{8\frac{41}{48}}$$

5.
$$26\frac{3}{5} = 26\frac{24}{40}$$
$$14\frac{1}{5} = 14\frac{8}{40}$$
$$5\frac{7}{8} = 5\frac{35}{40}$$
$$45\frac{67}{40} = 46\frac{27}{40}$$

6.
$$7\frac{5}{8} = 7\frac{100}{160}$$
$$\frac{1}{32} = \frac{5}{160}$$
$$3\frac{1}{10} = 3\frac{16}{160}$$
$$10\frac{121}{160}$$

7.
$$4\frac{1}{2} = 4\frac{4}{8}$$
$$3\frac{1}{4} = 3\frac{2}{8}$$
$$9\frac{3}{8} = 9\frac{3}{8}$$
$$16\frac{9}{8} = 17\frac{1}{8}$$

8.
$$7\frac{11}{12} = 7\frac{33}{36}$$
$$16\frac{3}{4} = 16\frac{27}{36}$$
$$2\frac{4}{18} = 2\frac{8}{36}$$
$$25\frac{68}{36} = 26\frac{32}{36} = 26\frac{8}{9}$$

9.
$$1\frac{3}{24} = 1\frac{3}{24}$$
$$8\frac{1}{3} = 8\frac{8}{24}$$
$$3\frac{5}{6} = 3\frac{20}{24}$$
$$12\frac{31}{24} = 13\frac{7}{24}$$

10.
$$5\frac{5}{6} = 5\frac{100}{120}$$
$$7\frac{3}{8} = 7\frac{45}{120}$$
$$2\frac{3}{10} = 2\frac{36}{120}$$
$$14\frac{181}{120} = 15\frac{61}{120}$$

Practice Exercise D

1.
$$\frac{5}{8} = \frac{10}{16}$$
$$-\frac{3}{16} = \frac{3}{16}$$
$$\frac{7}{16}$$

2.
$$7\frac{5}{12} = 7\frac{5}{12}$$
$$-3\frac{1}{4} = 3\frac{3}{12}$$
$$4\frac{2}{12} = 4\frac{1}{6}$$

3.
$$\frac{1}{2} = \frac{4}{8}$$
$$-\frac{1}{8} = \frac{1}{8}$$
$$\frac{3}{8}$$

4.
$$3\frac{1}{8} = 3\frac{1}{8} = 2\frac{9}{8}$$
$$-1\frac{3}{4} = 1\frac{6}{8} = 1\frac{6}{8}$$
$$1\frac{3}{8}$$

5.
$$\frac{7}{9} = \frac{14}{18}$$
$$-\frac{1}{6} = \frac{3}{18}$$
$$\frac{11}{18}$$

6.
$$\frac{17}{20} = \frac{17}{20}$$
$$-\frac{3}{4} = \frac{15}{20}$$
$$\frac{2}{20} = \frac{1}{10}$$

7.
$$5\frac{3}{8} = 5\frac{6}{16} = 4\frac{22}{16}$$
$$-1\frac{7}{16} = 1\frac{7}{16} = 1\frac{7}{16}$$
$$\overline{\hspace{2cm}3\frac{15}{16}}$$

9.
$$4\frac{3}{4} = 4\frac{9}{12}$$
$$-2\frac{2}{3} = 2\frac{8}{12}$$
$$\overline{\hspace{2cm}2\frac{1}{12}}$$

8.
$$\frac{2}{5} = \frac{18}{45}$$
$$-\frac{2}{9} = \frac{10}{45}$$
$$\overline{\hspace{2cm}\frac{8}{45}}$$

10.
$$11\frac{7}{8} = 11\frac{7}{8}$$
$$-1\frac{3}{4} = 1\frac{6}{8}$$
$$\overline{\hspace{2cm}10\frac{1}{8}}$$

Practice Exercise E

1. $\dfrac{\overset{1}{\cancel{2}}}{3} \times \dfrac{1}{\underset{4}{\cancel{8}}} = \dfrac{1}{12}$

2. $\dfrac{\overset{1}{\cancel{2}}}{\underset{1}{\cancel{3}}} \times \dfrac{\overset{1}{\cancel{3}}}{\underset{6}{\cancel{12}}} = \dfrac{1}{6}$

3. $\dfrac{\overset{1}{\cancel{4}}}{21} \times \dfrac{\overset{1}{\cancel{7}}}{\underset{2}{\cancel{8}}} = \dfrac{1}{6}$

4. $\dfrac{\overset{3}{\cancel{15}}}{16} \times \dfrac{9}{\underset{2}{\cancel{10}}} = \dfrac{27}{32}$

5. $\dfrac{\overset{1}{\cancel{4}}}{\underset{3}{\cancel{6}}} \times \dfrac{\overset{1}{\cancel{2}}}{\underset{1}{\cancel{4}}} = \dfrac{1}{3}$

6. $3\frac{3}{8} \times \frac{27}{8} = \frac{27}{8} \times \frac{27}{8} = \frac{729}{64} = 11\frac{25}{64}$

7. $\dfrac{1}{2} \times 8 = \dfrac{1}{\underset{1}{\cancel{2}}} \times \dfrac{\overset{4}{\cancel{8}}}{1} = 4$

8. $6\frac{1}{2} \times 5\frac{4}{8} = \dfrac{13}{2} \times \dfrac{\overset{11}{\cancel{44}}}{\underset{2}{\cancel{8}}} = \dfrac{143}{4} = 35\frac{3}{4}$

9. $3\frac{2}{3} \times \dfrac{3}{4} = \dfrac{11}{\underset{1}{\cancel{3}}} \times \dfrac{\overset{1}{\cancel{3}}}{4} = \dfrac{11}{4} = 2\frac{3}{4}$

10. $9 \times 3\frac{1}{3} = \dfrac{\overset{3}{\cancel{9}}}{1} \times \dfrac{10}{\underset{1}{\cancel{3}}} = 30$

Practice Exercise F

1. $2\dfrac{1}{5} \div 11 = \dfrac{11}{5} \div \dfrac{11}{1} = \dfrac{\cancel{11}^{1}}{5} \times \dfrac{1}{\cancel{11}_{1}} = \dfrac{1}{5}$

2. $\dfrac{1}{50} \div \dfrac{1}{200} = \dfrac{1}{\cancel{50}_{1}} \times \dfrac{\cancel{200}^{4}}{1} = \dfrac{4}{1} = 4$

3. $6\dfrac{3}{5} \div 8\dfrac{3}{10} = \dfrac{33}{5} \div \dfrac{83}{10} = \dfrac{33}{\cancel{5}_{1}} \times \dfrac{\cancel{10}^{2}}{83} = \dfrac{66}{83}$

4. $\dfrac{3}{4} \div \dfrac{1}{8} = \dfrac{3}{\cancel{4}_{1}} \times \dfrac{\cancel{8}^{2}}{1} = \dfrac{6}{1} = 6$

5. $\dfrac{5}{12} \div \dfrac{5}{60} = \dfrac{\cancel{5}^{1}}{\cancel{12}_{1}} \times \dfrac{\cancel{60}^{5}}{\cancel{5}_{1}} = \dfrac{5}{1} = 5$

6. $10\dfrac{1}{2} \div \dfrac{1}{3} = \dfrac{21}{2} \times \dfrac{3}{1} = \dfrac{63}{2} = 31\dfrac{1}{2}$

7. $\dfrac{1}{60} \div \dfrac{1}{2} = \dfrac{1}{\cancel{60}_{30}} \times \dfrac{\cancel{2}^{1}}{1} = \dfrac{1}{30}$

8. $8 \div \dfrac{2}{3} = \dfrac{\cancel{8}^{4}}{1} \times \dfrac{3}{\cancel{2}_{1}} = \dfrac{12}{1} = 12$

9. $\dfrac{1}{6} \div \dfrac{1}{3} = \dfrac{1}{\cancel{6}_{2}} \times \dfrac{\cancel{3}^{1}}{1} = \dfrac{1}{2}$

10. $\dfrac{7}{8} \div \dfrac{3}{4} = \dfrac{7}{\cancel{8}_{2}} \times \dfrac{\cancel{4}^{1}}{3} = \dfrac{7}{6} = 1\dfrac{1}{6}$

Practice Exercise G

1. **The correct answer is 0.25.**

$$\dfrac{1}{4} = 4\overline{)1.00}^{.25}$$

2. **The correct answer is 0.875.**

$$\dfrac{7}{8} = 8\overline{)7.000}^{.875}$$
$$\underline{64}$$
$$60$$
$$\underline{56}$$
$$40$$
$$\underline{40}$$
$$0$$

3. **The correct answer is $0.8\overline{3}$.**

$$\dfrac{5}{6} = 6\overline{)5.00}^{.083\overline{3}}$$
$$\underline{48}$$
$$20$$
$$\underline{18}$$
$$2$$

4. **The correct answer is 0.04.**

$$\dfrac{5}{125} = 125\overline{)5.00}^{.04}$$
$$\underline{500}$$
$$0$$

5. **The correct answer is 0.3125.**

$$\dfrac{5}{16} = 16\overline{)5.000}^{.3125}$$
$$\underline{48}$$
$$20$$
$$\underline{16}$$
$$40$$
$$\underline{32}$$
$$80$$
$$\underline{80}$$
$$0$$

6. **The correct answer is 0.12.**

$$\dfrac{3}{25} = 25\overline{)3.00}^{.12}$$
$$\underline{25}$$
$$50$$
$$\underline{50}$$
$$0$$

7. The correct answer is 0.45.

$$\frac{9}{20} = 20\overline{)9.00}^{.45}$$
$$\underline{80}$$
$$100$$
$$\underline{100}$$
$$0$$

8. The correct answer is $0.01\overline{3}$.

$$\frac{1}{75} = 75\overline{)1.000}^{.01\overline{3}}$$
$$\underline{75}$$
$$250$$
$$\underline{225}$$
$$25$$

9. The correct answer is 0.375.

$$\frac{3}{8} = 8\overline{)3.000}^{.375}$$
$$\underline{24}$$
$$60$$
$$\underline{56}$$
$$40$$
$$\underline{40}$$
$$0$$

10. The correct answer is 0.3.

$$\frac{3}{10} = 10\overline{)3.00}^{.30}$$
$$\underline{30}$$
$$00$$

Practice Exercise H

1. $0.16 = \frac{16}{100} = \frac{4}{25}$

2. $0.04 = \frac{4}{100} = \frac{1}{25}$

3. $0.125 = \frac{125}{1,000} = \frac{1}{8}$

4. $0.06 = \frac{6}{100} = \frac{3}{50}$

5. $0.257 = \frac{257}{1,000}$

6. $0.75 = \frac{75}{100} = \frac{3}{4}$

7. $0.250 = \frac{250}{1,000} = \frac{1}{4}$

8. $0.525 = \frac{525}{1,000} = \frac{21}{40}$

9. $0.2 = \frac{2}{10} = \frac{1}{5}$

10. $4.75 = 4\frac{75}{100} = 4\frac{3}{4}$

Practice Exercise I

1.
$$\begin{array}{r} 7.2 \\ 3.57 \\ +\ 10.8 \\ \hline 21.57 \end{array}$$

2.
$$\begin{array}{r} 48.3 \\ 18.25 \\ +\ 4.002 \\ \hline 70.552 \end{array}$$

3.
$$\begin{array}{r} 6.3 \\ 0.005 \\ +\ 2.67 \\ \hline 8.975 \end{array}$$

4.
$$\begin{array}{r} 25.4 \\ 37.06 \\ +\ 41.0 \\ \hline 103.46 \end{array}$$

5.
$$\begin{array}{r} 8.50 \\ 19.625 \\ +\ 0.17 \\ \hline 28.295 \end{array}$$

6.
$$\begin{array}{r} 29.042 \\ 2.6 \\ +\ 3.12 \\ \hline 34.762 \end{array}$$

7.
```
    5.4
    8.62
  + 0.95
   14.97
```

8.
```
    2.246
   16.8
  + 4.26
   23.306
```

9.
```
   16.1
    1.12
  + 3.525
   20.745
```

10.
```
   30.7
    4.05
  + 20.5
   55.25
```

Practice Exercise J

1.
```
    5.67
  − 3.90
    1.77
```

2.
```
   37.20
  − 25.37
   11.83
```

3.
```
   17.400
  − 13.262
    4.138
```

4.
```
   58.940
  − 27.363
   31.577
```

5.
```
    2.425
  − 0.675
    1.750
```

6.
```
   15.00
  − 7.82
    7.18
```

7.
```
   205.60
  − 105.23
   100.37
```

8.
```
   246.520
  − 107.988
   138.532
```

9.
```
   35.25
  − 17.00
   18.25
```

10.
```
   1725.5000
  − 50.6325
   1674.8675
```

Practice Exercise K

1.
```
    5.64
  ×  1.2
    1128
     564
    6.768
```

2.
```
    4.25
  ×  12
     850
     425
   51.00
```

3.
```
   35.6
  ×  2.5
    1780
     712
   89.00
```

4.
```
    4.92
  ×  9.5
    2460
    4428
   46.740
```

facebook.com/petersonspublishing

5.
```
      51
  × 0.92
     102
    459
   46.92
```

8.
```
     32.2
   × 3.15
    1610
     322
     966
  101.430
```

6.
```
     28.6
   × 8.16
    1716
     286
    2288
  233.376
```

9.
```
     21.0
   × 41.6
    1260
     210
     840
   873.60
```

7.
```
     50.06
   ×  2.15
    25030
     5006
    10012
   107.6290
```

10.
```
      8.06
   × 3.654
     3224
     4030
     4839
     2418
   29.45124
```

Practice Exercise L

1. The correct answer is 40.

$$
2.5\overline{)100.0} \quad \begin{array}{c} 40. \end{array}
$$

2. The correct answer is 3.

$$
.3\overline{).9} \quad \begin{array}{c} 3. \end{array}
$$

3. The correct answer is 22.7.

```
         22.7
  1.7)38.59
     34
      45
      34
     119
     119
       0
```

4. The correct answer is $76.\overline{6}$.

```
        76.66
  1.5)115.000
     105
     100
      90
     100
      90
      10
```

5. The correct answer is 2.2.

```
        2.2
  2.5)5.50
     50
     50
     50
```

6. The correct answer is 7.

$$.46\overline{)3.22}$$
$$\underline{322}$$
$$0$$

7. The correct answer is 3.1.

$$1.5\overline{)4.65}$$
$$\underline{4.5}$$
$$15$$
$$\underline{15}$$

8. The correct answer is 2.

$$7.5\overline{)15.0}$$
$$\underline{150}$$
$$0$$

9. The correct answer is 0.14.

$$.3\overline{).042}$$
$$\underline{3}$$
$$12$$
$$\underline{12}$$

10. The correct answer is 0.12.

$$.05\overline{).0060}$$
$$\underline{5}$$
$$10$$

Practice Exercise M

1. $\frac{4}{5} = 4:5$

2. $\frac{1}{3} = 1:3$

3. $\frac{3}{4} = 3:4$

4. $\frac{3}{8} = 3:8$

5. $\frac{1}{10} = 1:10$

6. $\frac{2}{3} = 2:3$

7. $\frac{1}{2} = 1:2$

8. $\frac{25}{50} = 25:50 = 1:2$

9. $\frac{3}{9} = 3:9 = 1:3$

10. $\frac{2}{5} = 2:5$

Practice Exercise N

1. $8:10 = x:30$
$10x = 240$
$x = 24$

2. $9:15 = x:5$
$15x = 45$
$x = 3$

3. $x:80 = 3:12$
$12x = 240$
$x = 20$

4. $3:x = 8:24$
$8x = 72$
$x = 9$

5. $2:3 = x:63$
$3x = 126$
$x = 42$

6. $5:15 = x:60$
$15x = 300$
$x = 20$

7. $7 : x = 4 : 28$
$4x = 196$
$x = 49$

8. $0.2 : 8 = 25 : x$
$0.2x = 200$
$x = 1,000$

9. $5 : 7 = x : 28$
$7x = 140$
$x = 20$

10. $\frac{1}{10} x : 2,000 = 1 : 100$
$10x = 2,000$
$x = 200$

Practice Exercise O

1. $0.225 = 22.5\%$

2. $3.45 = 345\%$

3. $0.7 = 70\%$

4. $0.14 = 14\%$

5. $4.5 = 450\%$

6.
$$\begin{array}{r} 72 \\ \times\ .24 \\ \hline 17.28 \end{array}$$

7.
$$\begin{array}{r} 12 \\ \times\ .05 \\ \hline .60 \end{array}$$

8. $\dfrac{225}{300} = \dfrac{3}{4} = 4\overline{)3.00} = 75\%$
$$\begin{array}{r} .75 \\ \underline{28} \\ 20 \\ \underline{20} \\ 0 \end{array}$$

9. $\dfrac{24}{60} = \dfrac{2}{5} = 5\overline{)2.0} = 40\%$
$$\begin{array}{r} .4 \\ \underline{20} \\ 0 \end{array}$$

10. $\dfrac{135}{45} = 3. = 300\%$

Practice Exercise P

1. The correct answer is VIII.

2. The correct answer is XV.

3. The correct answer is L.

4. The correct answer is IV.

5. The correct answer is XXIII.

6. The correct answer is XLIV.

7. The correct answer is XCIII.

8. The correct answer is XXXVI.

9. The correct answer is LVI.

10. The correct answer is XIX.

11. The correct answer is XXV.

12. The correct answer is C.

13. The correct answer is XXXVII.

14. The correct answer is VII.

15. The correct answer is XVIII.

16. The correct answer is DXXVI.

17. The correct answer is XCIV.

18. The correct answer is XXXIX.

19. The correct answer is LXII.

20. The correct answer is MCMLXXX.

Practice Exercise Q

1. The correct answer is 24.

2. The correct answer is 17.

3. The correct answer is 50.

4. The correct answer is 40.

5. The correct answer is 5.

6. The correct answer is 3.

7. The correct answer is 1,000.

8. The correct answer is 19.

9. The correct answer is 30.

10. The correct answer is 29.

11. The correct answer is 6.

12. The correct answer is 70.

13. The correct answer is 100.

14. The correct answer is 92.

15. The correct answer is 69.

16. The correct answer is 17.

17. The correct answer is 22.

18. The correct answer is 11.

19. The correct answer is 204.

20. The correct answer is 1,115.

ARITHMETIC AND MATHEMATICS ANSWER SHEETS

Arithmetic Test 1

Fill in your answers in the spaces provided on the test.

Arithmetic Test 2

1. Ⓐ Ⓑ Ⓒ Ⓓ   5. Ⓐ Ⓑ Ⓒ Ⓓ   9. Ⓐ Ⓑ Ⓒ Ⓓ   13. Ⓐ Ⓑ Ⓒ Ⓓ   17. Ⓐ Ⓑ Ⓒ Ⓓ

2. Ⓐ Ⓑ Ⓒ Ⓓ   6. Ⓐ Ⓑ Ⓒ Ⓓ   10. Ⓐ Ⓑ Ⓒ Ⓓ   14. Ⓐ Ⓑ Ⓒ Ⓓ   18. Ⓐ Ⓑ Ⓒ Ⓓ

3. Ⓐ Ⓑ Ⓒ Ⓓ   7. Ⓐ Ⓑ Ⓒ Ⓓ   11. Ⓐ Ⓑ Ⓒ Ⓓ   15. Ⓐ Ⓑ Ⓒ Ⓓ   19. Ⓐ Ⓑ Ⓒ Ⓓ

4. Ⓐ Ⓑ Ⓒ Ⓓ   8. Ⓐ Ⓑ Ⓒ Ⓓ   12. Ⓐ Ⓑ Ⓒ Ⓓ   16. Ⓐ Ⓑ Ⓒ Ⓓ   20. Ⓐ Ⓑ Ⓒ Ⓓ

answer sheet

ARITHMETIC TEST 1

30 Questions • 30 Minutes

Directions: Work out each problem and fill in your answer in the space provided.

Reduce to lowest terms:

1. $\dfrac{3}{6} =$ _____

2. $\dfrac{10}{12} =$ _____

3. $\dfrac{40}{1,000} =$ _____

4. $\dfrac{15}{50} =$ _____

5. $\dfrac{75}{90} =$ _____

Change to improper fractions:

6. $2\dfrac{3}{5} =$ _____

7. $10\dfrac{3}{5} =$ _____

8. $6\dfrac{5}{6} =$ _____

9. $17\dfrac{1}{2} =$ _____

10. $9\dfrac{1}{3} =$ _____

Add:

11. $\quad \dfrac{2}{3}$

$\quad\ \dfrac{1}{4}$

$+\ \dfrac{5}{6}$

_____

12. $\quad \dfrac{5}{9}$

$\quad\ \dfrac{3}{8}$

$+\ \dfrac{1}{4}$

_____

13. $\quad \dfrac{4}{5}$

$\quad\ \dfrac{3}{8}$

$+\ \dfrac{1}{20}$

14. $\quad 17\dfrac{2}{3}$

$\quad\ \dfrac{8}{9}$

$+\ 2\dfrac{1}{12}$

_____

15. $\quad 1\dfrac{9}{10}$

$\quad\ 8\dfrac{4}{5}$

$+\ 9\dfrac{2}{3}$

_____

Subtract

16. $\quad \dfrac{7}{8}$

$-\ \dfrac{1}{3}$

17.
$$\frac{11}{18}$$
$$-\ \frac{2}{9}$$

_____

18.
$$7\frac{1}{3}$$
$$-\ 2\frac{3}{4}$$

_____

19.
$$2\frac{5}{6}$$
$$-\ \frac{8}{9}$$

_____

20.
$$17\frac{1}{3}$$
$$-\ 8\frac{5}{15}$$

Multiply:

21. $\frac{1}{5} \times \frac{25}{50} =$ _____

22. $\frac{1}{3} \times \frac{3}{4} =$ _____

23. $\frac{7}{10} \times \frac{5}{6} =$ _____

24. $15 \times 2\frac{1}{3} =$ _____

25. $\frac{2}{3} \times \frac{9}{16} =$ _____

Divide:

26. $\frac{1}{2} \div \frac{1}{50} =$ _____

27. $\frac{1}{2} \div 6 =$ _____

28. $2\frac{1}{4} \div 3\frac{1}{2} =$ _____

29. $2\frac{4}{5} \div 7 =$ _____

30. $\frac{1}{2} \div \frac{3}{50} =$ _____

STOP

IF YOU FINISH BEFORE TIME IS CALLED, YOU MAY CHECK YOUR WORK ON THIS SECTION ONLY. DO NOT TURN TO ANY OTHER SECTION IN THE TEST.

ARITHMETIC TEST 2

20 Questions • 20 Minutes

Directions: Read each question carefully, then decide which choice is the best. Fill in the corresponding space on your answer sheet.

1. $23 + 4.67 + 19.2 + 0.365 =$
   - (A) 1047.0
   - (B) 47.235
   - (C) 1172.4
   - (D) 46.235

2. $2.37 \times 0.6 =$
   - (A) 14.22
   - (B) 1.282
   - (C) 1.422
   - (D) 12.82

3. The freshman nursing class consists of 40 students. $\frac{7}{8}$ of the class are women. How many women are in the class?
   - (A) 35
   - (B) 38
   - (C) 21
   - (D) 24

4. What percentage of 20 is 12?
   - (A) 12 percent
   - (B) 60 percent
   - (C) 14 percent
   - (D) 8 percent

5. What is the value of x in the proportion $1 : 5 = x : 1,500$?
   - (A) 5
   - (B) $\frac{1}{3}$
   - (C) 750,000
   - (D) 300

6. 3 percent of the 900 students in a school went on a trip. How many students remained in school?
   - (A) 27
   - (B) 30
   - (C) 873
   - (D) 773

7. What is the fraction $\frac{7}{16}$ expressed as a decimal?
   - (A) .1120
   - (B) .2286
   - (C) .4850
   - (D) .4375

8. If 30 is divided by .06, what is the result?
   - (A) 5
   - (B) 50
   - (C) 500
   - (D) 5,000

9. What is most nearly the sum of 637.894, 8352.16, 4.8673, and 301.5?
   - (A) 8,989.5
   - (B) 9,021.35
   - (C) 9,294.9
   - (D) 9,296.4

10. What is the sum of $82.79, $103.06, and $697.85?
    - (A) $883.70
    - (B) $1,628
    - (C) $791
    - (D) $873

11. What is 1 percent of $23,000?

(A) $23

(B) $2.30

(C) $230

(D) $2,300

12. If $1\frac{1}{2}$ pounds of candy are required to fill an Easter basket, how many baskets can be filled with $10\frac{1}{2}$ pounds of candy?

(A) 7.5

(B) 2.5

(C) $5\frac{1}{2}$

(D) 7

13. If 1 t-shirt costs $5.60, how many t-shirts can be bought for $61.60?

(A) $8\frac{1}{2}$

(B) 10

(C) 9

(D) 11

14. The decimal 410.07 less 38.49 equals what?

(A) 372.58

(B) 371.58

(C) 381.58

(D) 382.68

15. The fraction $\frac{3}{10}$ written as a decimal is what?

(A) 0.3

(B) 0.03

(C) 0.003

(D) 0.0003

16. The decimal 12.5 written as a fraction is what?

(A) $\frac{1}{25}$

(B) $12\frac{1}{2}$

(C) $1\frac{1}{2}$

(D) $\frac{125}{100}$

17. The product of 8.3×80 is what?

(A) 6.64

(B) 66.4

(C) 664

(D) 6,640

18. The fraction equal to 0.0625 is what?

(A) $\frac{1}{16}$

(B) $\frac{1}{15}$

(C) $\frac{1}{14}$

(D) $\frac{1}{13}$

19. The number 0.03125 equals what fraction?

(A) $\frac{3}{64}$

(B) $\frac{1}{16}$

(C) $\frac{1}{64}$

(D) $\frac{1}{32}$

20. The quantity 21.70 divided by 1.75 equals what?

(A) 124

(B) 12.4

(C) 1.24

(D) .124

STOP

IF YOU FINISH BEFORE TIME IS CALLED, YOU MAY CHECK YOUR WORK ON THIS SECTION ONLY. DO NOT TURN TO ANY OTHER SECTION IN THE TEST.

ANSWER KEY AND EXPLANATIONS

Arithmetic Test 1

1. $\frac{1}{2}$	7. $\frac{53}{5}$	13. $1\frac{9}{40}$	19. $1\frac{17}{18}$	25. $\frac{3}{8}$
2. $\frac{5}{6}$	8. $\frac{41}{6}$	14. $20\frac{23}{36}$	20. 9	26. 25
3. $\frac{1}{25}$	9. $\frac{35}{2}$	15. $20\frac{11}{30}$	21. $\frac{1}{10}$	27. $\frac{1}{12}$
4. $\frac{3}{10}$	10. $\frac{28}{3}$	16. $\frac{13}{24}$	22. $\frac{1}{4}$	28. $\frac{9}{14}$
5. $\frac{5}{6}$	11. $1\frac{3}{4}$	17. $\frac{7}{18}$	23. $\frac{7}{12}$	29. $\frac{2}{5}$
6. $\frac{13}{5}$	12. $1\frac{13}{72}$	18. $4\frac{7}{12}$	24. 35	30. $8\frac{1}{3}$

1. $\frac{3}{6} = \frac{1}{2}$

2. $\frac{10}{12} = \frac{5}{6}$

3. $\frac{40}{1,000} = \frac{1}{25}$

4. $\frac{15}{50} = \frac{3}{10}$

5. $\frac{75}{90} = \frac{5}{6}$

6. $2\frac{3}{5} = \frac{13}{5}$

7. $10\frac{3}{5} = \frac{53}{5}$

8. $6\frac{5}{6} = \frac{41}{6}$

9. $17\frac{1}{2} = \frac{35}{2}$

10. $9\frac{1}{3} = \frac{28}{3}$

11. $\frac{2}{3} = \frac{8}{12}$

$\frac{1}{4} = \frac{3}{12}$

$\frac{5}{6} = \frac{10}{12}$

$\overline{}$

$\frac{21}{12} = 1\frac{9}{12} = 1\frac{3}{4}$

12. $\frac{5}{9} = \frac{40}{72}$

$\frac{3}{8} = \frac{27}{72}$

$+\frac{1}{4} = \frac{18}{72}$

$\overline{}$

$\frac{85}{72} = 1\frac{13}{72}$

13. $\frac{4}{5} = \frac{32}{40}$

$\frac{3}{8} = \frac{15}{40}$

$\frac{1}{20} = \frac{2}{40}$

$\overline{}$

$\frac{49}{40} = 1\frac{9}{40}$

14. $17\frac{2}{3} = 17\frac{24}{36}$

$\frac{8}{9} = \frac{32}{36}$

$2\frac{1}{12} = 2\frac{3}{36}$

$\overline{}$

$19\frac{59}{36} = 20\frac{23}{36}$

15. $1\frac{9}{10} = 1\frac{27}{30}$

$8\frac{4}{5} = 8\frac{24}{30}$

$9\frac{2}{3} = 9\frac{20}{30}$

$\overline{}$

$18\frac{71}{30} = 20\frac{11}{30}$

16.
$$\frac{7}{8} = \frac{21}{24}$$
$$-\frac{1}{3} = \frac{8}{24}$$
$$\frac{13}{24}$$

17.
$$\frac{11}{18} = \frac{11}{18}$$
$$-\frac{2}{9} = \frac{4}{18}$$
$$\frac{7}{18}$$

18.
$$7\frac{1}{3} = 7\frac{4}{12} = 6\frac{16}{12}$$
$$2\frac{3}{4} = 2\frac{9}{12} = 2\frac{9}{12}$$
$$4\frac{7}{12}$$

19.
$$2\frac{5}{6} = 2\frac{15}{18} = 1\frac{33}{18}$$
$$\frac{8}{9} = \frac{16}{18} = \frac{16}{18}$$
$$1\frac{17}{18}$$

20.
$$17\frac{1}{3} = 17\frac{5}{15}$$
$$8\frac{5}{15} = 8\frac{5}{15}$$
$$9$$

21. $\frac{1}{5} \times \frac{\overset{1}{\cancel{25}}}{\underset{2}{\cancel{50}}} = \frac{1}{10}$

22. $\frac{1}{\underset{1}{\cancel{3}}} \times \frac{\overset{1}{\cancel{3}}}{4} = \frac{1}{4}$

23. $\frac{7}{\underset{2}{\cancel{10}}} \times \frac{\overset{1}{\cancel{5}}}{6} = \frac{7}{12}$

24. $15 \times 2\frac{1}{3} = \overset{5}{\cancel{15}} \times \frac{7}{\underset{1}{\cancel{3}}} = \frac{35}{1}$

25. $\frac{\overset{1}{\cancel{2}}}{\underset{1}{\cancel{3}}} \times \frac{\overset{3}{\cancel{9}}}{\underset{8}{\cancel{16}}} = \frac{3}{8}$

26. $\frac{1}{2} \div \frac{1}{50} = \frac{1}{\underset{1}{\cancel{2}}} \times \frac{\overset{25}{\cancel{50}}}{1} = \frac{25}{1} = 25$

27. $\frac{1}{2} \div 6 = \frac{1}{2} \times \frac{1}{6} = \frac{1}{12}$

28. $2\frac{1}{4} \div 3\frac{1}{2} = \frac{9}{4} \div \frac{7}{2} = \frac{9}{\underset{2}{\cancel{4}}} \times \frac{\overset{1}{\cancel{2}}}{7} = \frac{9}{14}$

29. $2\frac{4}{5} \div 7 = \frac{14}{5} \div \frac{7}{1} = \frac{\overset{2}{\cancel{14}}}{5} \times \frac{1}{\underset{1}{\cancel{7}}} = \frac{2}{5}$

30. $\frac{1}{2} \div \frac{3}{50} = \frac{1}{\underset{1}{\cancel{2}}} \times \frac{\overset{25}{\cancel{50}}}{3} = \frac{25}{3} = 8\frac{1}{3}$

Arithmetic Test 2

1. B	5. D	9. D	13. D	17. C
2. C	6. C	10. A	14. B	18. A
3. A	7. D	11. C	15. A	19. D
4. B	8. C	12. D	16. B	20. B

1. The correct answer is (B).

$$\begin{array}{r} 23.0 \\ 4.67 \\ 19.2 \\ + 0.365 \\ \hline 47.235 \end{array}$$

2. The correct answer is (C).

$$\begin{array}{r} 2.37 \\ \times 0.6 \\ \hline 1.422 \end{array}$$

3. The correct answer is (A).

$$\frac{7}{\cancel{8}_1} \times \frac{\cancel{40}^5}{1} = 35$$

4. The correct answer is (B).

$$\frac{12}{20} = \frac{3}{5} = .6 = 60\%$$
$$x = 60\%$$

5. The correct answer is (D).

$$1 : 5 = x : 1,500$$
$$5x = 1,500$$
$$x = 300$$

6. The correct answer is (C).

$$\begin{array}{cc} 900 & 900 \\ \times\ .03 & -\ 27 \\ \hline 27.00 & 873 \end{array}$$

7. The correct answer is (D).

$$\frac{7}{16} = 16\overline{)7.0000}^{\,.4375}$$
$$\begin{array}{r} \underline{64} \\ 60 \\ \underline{48} \\ 120 \\ \underline{112} \\ 80 \\ \underline{80} \end{array}$$

8. The correct answer is (C).

$$.06\overline{)30.00}^{\,500.}$$
$$\begin{array}{r} \underline{30} \\ 00 \end{array}$$

9. The correct answer is (D).

$$\begin{array}{r} 637.8940 \\ 8352.1600 \\ 4.8673 \\ + 301.5000 \\ \hline 9296.4213 \end{array}$$

10. The correct answer is (A).

$$\begin{array}{r} \$\ 82.79 \\ 103.06 \\ + 697.85 \\ \hline \$883.70 \end{array}$$

11. The correct answer is (C).

$$\begin{array}{r} \$\,230.000 \\ \underline{\times\ 0.01} \\ \$230.00 \end{array}$$

12. The correct answer is (D).

$$\frac{1.5}{1} = \frac{10.5}{x}$$
$$1.5x = 10.5$$
$$x = 7$$

13. The correct answer is (D).

$$\begin{array}{r} 11. \\ 5.60)\overline{61.60} \\ \underline{560} \\ 560 \end{array}$$

14. The correct answer is (B).

$$\begin{array}{r} 410.07 \\ \underline{-\ 38.49} \\ 371.58 \end{array}$$

15. The correct answer is (A).

$$\frac{3}{10} = 0.3$$

16. The correct answer is (B).

$$12.5 = 12\frac{5}{10} = 12\frac{1}{2}$$

17. The correct answer is (C).

$$\begin{array}{r} 8.3 \\ \underline{\times\ 80} \\ 00 \\ \underline{664} \\ 664.0 \end{array}$$

18. The correct answer is (A).

$$.0625 = \frac{625}{10,000} = \frac{1}{16}$$

19. The correct answer is (D).

$$0.03125 = \frac{3125}{100,000} = \frac{1}{32}$$

20. The correct answer is (B).

$$\begin{array}{r} 12.4 \\ 1.75)\overline{21.700} \\ \underline{17.5} \\ 4.20 \\ \underline{3.50} \\ 700 \\ \underline{700} \end{array}$$

ANSWER SHEET

Final Arithmetic and Mathematics Test

1. Ⓐ Ⓑ Ⓒ Ⓓ   5. Ⓐ Ⓑ Ⓒ Ⓓ   9. Ⓐ Ⓑ Ⓒ Ⓓ   13. Ⓐ Ⓑ Ⓒ Ⓓ   17. Ⓐ Ⓑ Ⓒ Ⓓ

2. Ⓐ Ⓑ Ⓒ Ⓓ   6. Ⓐ Ⓑ Ⓒ Ⓓ   10. Ⓐ Ⓑ Ⓒ Ⓓ   14. Ⓐ Ⓑ Ⓒ Ⓓ   18. Ⓐ Ⓑ Ⓒ Ⓓ

3. Ⓐ Ⓑ Ⓒ Ⓓ   7. Ⓐ Ⓑ Ⓒ Ⓓ   11. Ⓐ Ⓑ Ⓒ Ⓓ   15. Ⓐ Ⓑ Ⓒ Ⓓ   19. Ⓐ Ⓑ Ⓒ Ⓓ

4. Ⓐ Ⓑ Ⓒ Ⓓ   8. Ⓐ Ⓑ Ⓒ Ⓓ   12. Ⓐ Ⓑ Ⓒ Ⓓ   16. Ⓐ Ⓑ Ⓒ Ⓓ   20. Ⓐ Ⓑ Ⓒ Ⓓ

answer sheet

FINAL ARITHMETIC AND MATHEMATICS TEST

20 Questions • 30 Minutes

Directions: Work out each of the following problems. Fill in the corresponding space on your answer sheet.

1. Add $\frac{1}{4}$, $\frac{3}{8}$, and $\frac{7}{16}$.

   (A) $\frac{11}{16}$

   (B) $1\frac{1}{16}$

   (C) $\frac{11}{28}$

   (D) $\frac{18}{16}$

2. Multiply 25.5 by 0.326.
   (A) 83.13
   (B) 25.826
   (C) 0.2805
   (D) 8.313

3. Subtract 25.246 from 307.401.
   (A) 282.155
   (B) 54.941
   (C) 549.41
   (D) 28.2155

4. Add 14.75, 15.1256, and 0.07.
   (A) 299.46
   (B) 36.8756
   (C) 29.946
   (D) 268.756

5. Divide 36.36 by 0.0606.
   (A) .06
   (B) 0.6
   (C) 60
   (D) 600

6. Write the fraction $\frac{1}{8}$ as a ratio.

   (A) 8 : 1
   (B) 0.18
   (C) 1 : 8
   (D) 0.125

7. Solve for x in $2 : 8 = 11 : x$.
   (A) 44

   (B) $2\frac{3}{4}$

   (C) $\frac{11}{16}$

   (D) 4.4

8. Change 85 percent to a fraction and reduce to lowest terms.

   (A) $\frac{85}{100}$

   (B) $\frac{17}{20}$

   (C) $\frac{100}{85}$

   (D) $\frac{20}{17}$

9. Change 0.12 to a percent.
   (A) 0.12%
   (B) 0.0012%
   (C) .12%
   (D) 12%

10. Subtract $\frac{1}{8}$ from $\frac{1}{6}$.

    (A) $\frac{2}{8}$

    (B) $\frac{3}{24}$

    (C) $\frac{1}{24}$

    (D) $\frac{1}{12}$

11. How many grains of codeine are there in $1\frac{1}{2}$ tablets of $\frac{1}{8}$ grain each?

    (A) $\frac{2}{8}$

    (B) $\frac{3}{16}$

    (C) $\frac{3}{8}$

    (D) $\frac{5}{8}$

12. Mary drank 8 ounces of milk from a quart containing 32 ounces of milk. What part of the quart had she consumed?

    (A) $\frac{1}{4}$

    (B) $\frac{1}{8}$

    (C) $\frac{1}{3}$

    (D) $\frac{1}{2}$

13. There are 75 nursing students in the freshman class, and 15 are men. What is the ratio of women to men?

    (A) $\frac{1}{4}$

    (B) $\frac{1}{5}$

    (C) $\frac{4}{1}$

    (D) $\frac{5}{1}$

14. If a recipe calls for 5 ounces of sugar for every 15 ounces of flour, what part of the mixture will be sugar?

    (A) $\frac{1}{2}$

    (B) $\frac{1}{5}$

    (C) $\frac{1}{3}$

    (D) $\frac{1}{4}$

15. If a suit is on sale for $120, and the original cost was $150, what percentage would you save by buying it on sale?

    (A) 40%

    (B) 30%

    (C) 10%

    (D) 20%

16. A seamstress bought $2\frac{2}{3}$ yards of wool material and $1\frac{3}{4}$ yards of crepe material. How many yards of material did she buy?

    (A) $4\frac{5}{12}$

    (B) $4\frac{2}{3}$

    (C) $5\frac{1}{4}$

    (D) $4\frac{1}{3}$

17. A sack contained 10 pounds of potatoes. The chef used $1\frac{3}{4}$ pounds for French fries yesterday and $2\frac{1}{3}$ pounds for a casserole today. How many pounds of potatoes does she have left?

    (A) $5\frac{1}{2}$

    (B) $5\frac{11}{12}$

    (C) $6\frac{2}{3}$

    (D) $6\frac{11}{12}$

18. How many ounces is $\frac{3}{8}$ of a pound if a pound equals 16 ounces?

    (A) 6 ounces

    (B) 12 ounces

    (C) 8 ounces

    (D) 10 ounces

19. If John receives $\frac{2}{5}$ of $10, how much does he receive?

    (A) $2
    (B) $4
    (C) $5
    (D) $3

20. If there are 3,000 registered voters in Center City and $\frac{3}{5}$ of them are democrats, how many democrats are there in Center City?

    (A) 500
    (B) 600
    (C) 1,800
    (D) 1,500

STOP

IF YOU FINISH BEFORE TIME IS CALLED, YOU MAY CHECK YOUR WORK ON THIS SECTION ONLY, DO NOT TURN TO ANY OTHER SECTION IN THE TEST.

ANSWER KEY AND EXPLANATIONS

Final Arithmetic and Mathematics Test

1. B	5. D	9. D	13. C	17. B
2. D	6. C	10. C	14. D	18. A
3. A	7. A	11. B	15. D	19. B
4. C	8. B	12. A	16. A	20. C

1. The correct answer is (B).

$$\frac{1}{4} = \frac{4}{16}$$

$$\frac{3}{8} = \frac{6}{16}$$

$$\frac{7}{16} = \frac{7}{16}$$

$$\frac{17}{16} = 1\frac{1}{16}$$

2. The correct answer is (D).

$$\begin{array}{r} 25.5 \\ \times\ .326 \\ \hline 1530 \\ 510 \\ 765 \\ \hline 8.3130 \end{array}$$

3. The correct answer is (A).

$$\begin{array}{r} 307.401 \\ -\ 25.246 \\ \hline 282.155 \end{array}$$

4. The correct answer is (C).

$$\begin{array}{r} 14.75 \\ 15.1256 \\ +\ \ 0.07 \\ \hline 29.9456 = 29.946 \end{array}$$

5. The correct answer is (D).

$$\begin{array}{r} 600. \\ 0.0606\overline{)36.3600} \\ 36.36 \\ \hline 00 \end{array}$$

6. The correct answer is (C).

$$\frac{1}{8} = 1:8$$

7. The correct answer is (A).

$$2:8 = 11:x$$
$$2x = 88$$
$$x = 44$$

8. The correct answer is (B).

$$85\% = 0.08 = \frac{85}{100} = \frac{17}{20}$$

9. The correct answer is (D).

$$0.12 = 12\%$$

10. The correct answer is (C).

$$\frac{1}{6} = \frac{4}{24}$$

$$-\frac{1}{8} = \frac{3}{24}$$

$$\frac{1}{24}$$

11. The correct answer is (B).

$$1\frac{1}{2} \times \frac{1}{8} = \frac{3}{2} \times \frac{1}{8} = \frac{3}{16}$$

12. The correct answer is (A).

$$\frac{8}{32} = \frac{1}{4}$$

13. **The correct answer is (C).**

$$\frac{60 \text{ women}}{15 \text{ men}} = \frac{4}{1}$$

14. **The correct answer is (D).**

$$\frac{5 \text{ oz. sugar}}{20 \text{ oz. total mixture}} = \frac{1}{4}$$

15. **The correct answer is (D).**

$$\frac{30}{150} = 150\overline{)30.00} = 20\%$$
$$\underline{300}$$
$$00$$

16. **The correct answer is (A).**

$$2\frac{2}{3} = 2\frac{8}{12}$$
$$\underline{1\frac{3}{4} = 1\frac{9}{12}}$$
$$3\frac{17}{12} = 4\frac{5}{12}$$

17. **The correct answer is (B).**

$$1\frac{3}{4} = 1\frac{9}{12}$$
$$\underline{+2\frac{1}{3} = 2\frac{4}{12}}$$
$$3\frac{13}{12} = 4\frac{1}{12}$$

$$10 \text{ lbs}$$
$$\underline{-4\frac{1}{12} \text{ lbs}}$$
$$5\frac{11}{12} \text{ lbs}$$

18. **The correct answer is (A).**

$$\frac{3}{\cancel{8}_1} \times \frac{\cancel{16}^2}{1} = 6 \text{ ounces}$$

19. **The correct answer is (B).**

$$\frac{2}{\cancel{5}_1} \times \frac{\cancel{10}^2}{1} = \$4.00$$

20. **The correct answer is (C).**

$$\frac{3}{\cancel{5}_1} \times \frac{\cancel{3000}^{600}}{1} = 1,800 \text{ Democrats}$$

Health and Science

OVERVIEW

- **Understanding Body Structure and Function**
- **The Principles of Nutrition**
- **Factors Affecting Health**
- **Health Glossary**

The practical nurse needs comprehensive knowledge of basic concepts in order to understand body structure and functions and to recognize deviations from the norm. This unit provides facts and principles related to body structure, how the body functions, nutrition, and factors affecting health.

UNDERSTANDING BODY STRUCTURE AND FUNCTION

Understanding the concepts of anatomy and physiology is an important foundation for nursing. This section gives an overview of the structure and function of cells and each biological system in the human body. Cells, tissue, and organs make up the structure of multicellular organisms such as humans. Structure refers to the arrangement of parts of the organism and function refers to the activity of each part of the organism.

The Cell

Like all living organisms, humans are made up of cells. A cell is the smallest functional and structural unit of a living organism. Some organisms are made up of just one cell, but the human body is composed of trillions of cells. Although there are many types of cells in the human body and each has a specific function and structure, there are basic structures that are common to almost all of the cells in the body.

Cell Membrane

The cell membrane is a protective layer that covers the cell's outer surface. The membrane acts as a protective barrier between the inside of the cell and the cell's environment. There are small channels in the cell membrane that allow for substances such as water, oxygen, sodium, potassium, proteins, and other macromolecules to pass into and out of the cell.

Be sure you are familiar with the words in the Glossary.

The Cytoplasm

The region inside the cell membrane that includes the cellular fluids and all the organelles except the nucleus is called the cytoplasm. The cytoplasm is a watery substance that helps to maintain the shape of the cell and the concentration of various substances, such as sodium and potassium, in the cell.

The Nucleus

The nucleus is the control center of the cell. It is a membrane-bound organelle that contains the genetic information of the cell. Genetic information is packaged into molecules of DNA (deoxyribonucleic acid) that provide instruction for all the cell's processes. The DNA is responsible for the cell's ability to reproduce itself. Inside the nucleus is another structure called the nucleolus, and this is where RNA (ribonucleic acid) is made.

The Organelles

An organelle is a small structure in the cell's cytoplasm that performs a specific function for the cell. The following are typical organelles found in human cells.

- **Ribosomes:** Ribosomes are structures that are assembled in the nucleolus from proteins and RNA and are then transported to the cytoplasm. Ribosomes are the sites of protein synthesis.

- **Endoplasmic reticulum (ER):** The ER is the site of protein production and transportation. Some ER organelles are coated with ribosomes. These are called rough ER and are the structures in which proteins are made. Another type of ER has a smooth outer surface and is called smooth ER. It functions to break down toxic chemicals in the body and make lipids (fats), steroids, and hormones.

- **Golgi apparatus:** The Golgi apparatus, or Golgi body, plays a role in protein synthesis by making modifications to proteins, processing and sorting them, and then packaging the final protein product in a small sac called a vesicle. The vesicle leaves the Golgi body and transports the protein to the cell membrane where it can leave the cell to carry out its function in the body.

- **Mitochondria:** The mitochondria are known as the powerhouse of the cell. Their function is to convert energy from organic molecules into ATP (adenosine triphosphate), which is a form of energy that can be used by the cell.

- **Lysosomes:** Lysosomes are the "clean-up" crew of cells. They are tiny sacs that contain enzymes that can digest other molecules and substances. In the lysosome, old worn-out organelles, cell debris, and large molecules are broken down and digested.

- **Cytoskeleton:** The cytoskeleton helps to maintain the shape of the cell. It is made up of a network of fibers called microtubules and microfilaments.

- **Vacuoles:** Vacuoles are storage sacs filled with fluid. They store water, food, salts, waste, and pigments.

- **Centrioles:** Centrioles are the center of microtubule production in animal and human cells.

The Respiratory System

The respiratory system exchanges oxygen from the air with carbon dioxide in the body. The exchange of gases takes place in the lungs. When a person inhales air in through the mouth or nose, it is drawn into the lungs. In the lungs, the oxygen is transferred into the blood. The oxygen-rich blood in the lungs leaves through capillaries and enters cells in the body. The oxygen is used in each cell for cellular respiration. During cellular respiration, energy that is stored in food molecules is released to form ATP. ATP is the energy that all cells can use to maintain function and growth. Therefore, without oxygen, cells would not be able to produce energy to survive.

When a person exhales air out of the lungs, carbon dioxide is released from the body. Carbon dioxide is a waste product of the process of cellular respiration and the body needs to rid itself of it. Blood containing carbon dioxide moves from the cells in the body into capillaries that carry the blood back to the lungs. As the lung relaxes, the carbon dioxide is expelled from the lungs.

Air flows through the respiratory system in the following pathway:

1. Air enters the body through the nose and mouth.

2. Air then flows through the nose and mouth into the pharynx. The pharynx is also called the throat.

3. The pharynx branches into two tubes: one tube, the esophagus, leads to the stomach, and another tube called the larynx is the part of the throat through which air passes. The larynx also holds the vocal cords, and when air passes across the vocal cords, they vibrate, making vocal sounds.

4. From the larynx, air passes into a tube called the trachea, or windpipe. As the trachea approaches the lungs, it splits into two branches called bronchi. One bronchus connects to each lung (right and left).

5. Each bronchus branches into smaller tubes within the lungs called bronchioles. Air passes through the bronchi and into the bronchioles in the lungs. The bronchioles lead to tiny grape-like sacs called alveoli.

6. Alveoli are surrounded by blood vessels (capillaries), and oxygen moves across the thin walls of the alveoli into the blood vessels.

7. As you breathe, air is sucked in and out of the alveoli. The mechanical process of breathing is carried out by the diaphragm, a dome-shaped muscle below the lungs. As you inhale, the diaphragm contracts and moves down, so the lungs expand. As you exhale, the diaphragm relaxes and moves back up as the volume in the lungs decreases.

8. Blood that contains a lot of carbon dioxide is carried back to the lungs through blood vessels, and carbon dioxide travels back across the membrane of the capillaries and the alveoli where it can be expelled out through the respiratory structures (trachea, larynx, pharynx, mouth, or nose).

The Circulatory System

The circulatory system includes the cardiovascular system (heart and blood) and the lymphatic system (lymph nodes and lymphatic organs). Both systems work in connection with each other to

TIP

Draw a diagram to help you remember the pathway.

move fluids around the body and protect the body from disease. Both systems are made up of a network of vessels, and both systems are part of the body's defense against bacteria, viruses, and other pathogens.

The Cardiovascular System

The heart, blood, and blood vessels make up the cardiovascular system. The heart is a four-chambered organ that pumps blood by contracting and creating a pressure that moves the blood through vessels. The upper chambers of the heart are called the right and left atrium, and the lower chambers are called the right and left ventricles. Flap-like structures called valves are located between the atria and the ventricles. These valves ensure that blood flows only in one direction. The left atrium of the heart receives oxygen-rich blood from the lungs. The left ventricle of the heart pumps oxygen-rich blood through the body. The right atrium receives oxygen-poor blood from the body, and the right ventricle pumps oxygen-poor blood to the lungs.

Blood is pumped through the body by muscular contraction of the heart. Blood consists of four components: plasma, platelets, red blood cells, and white blood cells. Plasma is the fluid part of blood. Platelets are tiny pieces of larger cells that are found in the bone marrow. When the body is cut and blood flows out of the wound, platelets clump together to form a clot that stops the bleeding. Red blood cells are disk-shaped cells that carry oxygen to cells. The small disc shape of red blood cells helps them to squeeze through capillaries to deliver oxygen. White blood cells keep the body healthy by fighting infection from pathogens such as bacteria and viruses. Some white blood cells are able to destroy pathogens, and others form antibodies against the pathogens.

Even though all humans have these four components in their blood, blood can be further characterized by blood type. There are four blood groups found in humans: A, B, AB, and O. These are based on the type of antigen found in the red blood cells. Knowing a person's blood type is important for two reasons: if he or she needs to receive blood, or if the person wishes to donate blood.

TIP

Be sure you know the possible donors and recipients for different blood types.

- A person with type A blood will have the A antigen and will have white blood cells that produce antibodies against B antigen (anti-B). People with this blood type can donate blood to others with type A blood or to someone with type AB blood. They can receive blood from type A or type O individuals.

- Blood type B contains B antigens and anti-A antibodies. A person with blood type B can donate to type B or AB individuals and can receive blood from type B and O donors.

- Type AB blood contains A and B antigens and no antibodies. These individuals can only donate blood to AB individuals and can receive blood from all blood types.

- Type O blood contains no antigens and has both anti-A and anti-B antibodies. Type O blood can be donated to others of any blood type and is called the universal donor. Individuals with type O blood can only receive type O blood.

Blood acts as a transport system for supplies for cells, chemical messages, and waste. In this way, blood helps the body to remain in homeostasis. Blood carries gases such as oxygen and carbon dioxide, nutrients, and wastes through the body. The blood flowing through the body also helps keep the body at a constant temperature. The cardiovascular system forms a closed loop in the body.

Blood flows through this circuit from the heart, to the lungs, through the body, back to the lungs, and then back to the heart.

There are three types of blood vessels that carry blood through the body: arteries, capillaries, and veins. An artery is a blood vessel that has thick walls containing a layer of smooth muscle and carries blood away from the heart. Blood is pumped into the arteries at high pressure, when the heart contracts. This is known as blood pressure. The pressure pushes blood through the arteries. The walls of arteries are strong and able to stretch, so that they can withstand the pressure. A capillary is a tiny, thin-walled blood vessel that allows an exchange of gases between the blood and cells. Capillaries lead to veins. Veins are blood vessels that carry blood back to the heart. When the blood reaches the veins, it is not under the same high pressure as it was when it flowed from the heart into the arteries. Therefore, veins are thin-walled and do not have a lining of muscle. The contraction of skeletal muscles surrounding the veins helps blood to move through the veins and back to the heart. Valves in the veins keep the blood from flowing backwards.

The Lymphatic System

The lymphatic system is a group of tissue and organs that collect fluid that leaks from the blood and returns it back into the blood stream. The fluid that leaks out of the blood is called lymph. The lymphatic system—unlike the cardiovascular system—is an open circulatory system. As a result, lymph can move in and out of vessels. The lymphatic system together with the immune system helps the body to fight disease and pathogens. Other lymph vessels in the body are able to move fats from the intestine into the blood so they can be carried to cells.

Every time the heart pumps blood at high pressure, a small amount of fluid is forced out of the capillary walls. Most of this fluid is reabsorbed by the capillaries, and the remaining fluid is collected by lymph capillaries. Lymph capillaries absorb fluids, dead cell particles, pathogens, and toxic substances. Lymph capillaries carry this fluid called lymph to larger lymph vessels. The lymph vessels return the fluid to the cardiovascular system when the fluid drains into blood vessels at the base of the neck. White blood cells mature in the lymphatic system, and some can then attack pathogens picked up by the lymph.

There are also organs and tissue associated with the lymph system.

- **Lymph nodes:** Lymph nodes are small bean-shaped organs that remove pathogens and dead cell material from the lymph. Lymph nodes are concentrated in the neck, armpits, and groin areas of the body. Infection-fighting white blood cells called B-lymphocytes are found in lymph nodes. When bacteria or other pathogens cause an infection, the number of B-lymphocytes increases. As lymph nodes fill with B-lymphocytes, they may become swollen and tender to the touch. Thus, swollen lymph nodes are a good indicator of infection in the body.

- **Bones:** Bone, in particular bone marrow, is another important part of the lymphatic system. Bone marrow is the soft tissue in the center of a bone where blood cells are produced. Bone marrow produces the white blood cells of the lymphatic system.

- **Tonsils:** Tonsils are small lymphatic organs at the back of the throat that help to defend against infection. White blood cells in the tonsils help to trap pathogens from entering the body cavity. When tonsils take up pathogens, they become swollen and sore.

- **Thymus:** The thymus is an organ found in the chest region that is part of the lymphatic system. Some of the white blood cells that are produced in bone marrow are processed and developed in the thymus. White blood cells leave the thymus and travel through the lymphatic system to lymph nodes and other areas of the body. The thymus shrinks as a person ages.

- **Spleen:** The spleen is the largest lymphatic organ in the body. It stores white blood cells and allows them to mature. As blood flows through the spleen, white blood cells attack or mark any pathogens that might be in the blood. If pathogens cause an infection in another area of the body, the spleen can release white blood cells into the bloodstream as it passes through.

The Immune System

The immune system helps to keep the body healthy and free from disease. There are a series of processes that are carried out by the immune system to help prevent the spread of disease through the body. Several types of cells play roles in the immune system:

- **Phagocyte cells:** Phagocyte cells are activated and float around the body. This type of cell includes neutrophils, monocytes, and macrophages. They seek out and "eat," or engulf, foreign antigens from pathogens or diseased cells.

- **Basophils and eosinophils:** These types of cells release chemicals that respond to inflammation due to infection.

- **Natural killer cells (NKCs):** These cells are released to attack foreign antigens.

- **Cytokines and interferons:** These are chemicals in the immune system that are released to block viruses from replicating and activate surrounding cells that have antiviral functions.

- **B-cells:** B-cells or B-lymphocytes produce antibodies against disease-specific antigens. Some B-cells can become memory B-cells that produce plasma cells after an infection has been overcome by the immune system. These plasma cells produce antibodies that help with long-term immunity to a specific virus or bacteria.

- **T-cells:** When T-cells encounter infected cells, they are activated and multiply. Some T-cells become memory T-cells, and others become helper T-cells. Memory T-cells recognize a bacteria or virus that has previously infected the body. These cells help with long-term immunity. Helper T-cells activate B-lymphocytes and other T-cells. Other T-cells called cytotoxic T-cells recognize and kill infected cells.

Active immunity occurs when the immune system is exposed to an antigen of a particular virus or pathogen. Antibodies are created and stored permanently in the immune system to prevent a future infection by the same virus or pathogen. Artificial active immunity can be obtained through immunization. This type of immunization involves the injection of a specific antigen so that the immune system can build up antibodies against it. Immunization in which a body is injected with antibodies to fight against specific infections is called passive immunity. This type of immunity is immediate, but short-lived.

The Digestive System

The digestive system breaks down the food you eat into nutrients that the body can use for growth and energy. The digestive system interacts with other body systems to utilize the energy obtained from food consumed. Blood transports nutrients through the circulatory system once food has been digested. The respiratory system provides oxygen to cells so that they can produce energy from the nutrients that travel through the circulatory system to the cells. In addition, the nervous system controls and regulates the functioning of the digestive system.

The human digestive process occurs in five steps: ingestion, digestion, secretion, absorption, and defecation. The digestive system consists of the following:

- **Alimentary canal:** The alimentary canal is a long muscular tube that starts at the mouth and ends at the anus. Digestion begins in the mouth through the process of mechanical and chemical digestion. Teeth break down and crush the food ingested. Saliva is secreted from glands in the mouth. The saliva contains many substances, including many enzymes that begin the chemical digestion of food.

- **Esophagus:** As food is swallowed, it moves through the throat (pharynx) and into the esophagus. The esophagus is a long tube that moves the food through a wave of muscle contractions called peristalsis.

- **Stomach:** Both mechanical and chemical digestion also take place in the stomach. The stomach is a muscular bag that contracts to crush and mix up food with acids and enzymes. The acids and the enzymes form what is called gastric juice. Acids act to kill some bacteria that may be swallowed with food, and enzymes break down proteins. A thick layer of mucous protects the lining of the stomach from the acidic gastric juice.

- **Small intestine:** After digestion in the stomach, food is reduced to a soupy mixture called chyme. Chyme leaves the stomach and moves to the small intestine. The small intestine is a long, muscular tube of narrow diameter where most chemical digestion takes place, and most nutrients are absorbed. After nutrients are broken down, they are absorbed into the bloodstream.

- **Large intestine:** After food moves through the small intestine and some nutrients from the food are absorbed, food moves into the large intestine. In the large intestine, water and vitamins are absorbed. The solid material remaining in the large intestine is waste, which is compacted and stored in the rectum and eventually eliminated through the anus.

- **Accessory organs:** The digestion of nutrients in the small intestine takes place with the aid of three other organs: the pancreas, the liver, and the gall bladder. The pancreas produces fluids that break down proteins, carbohydrates, fats, and nucleic acids. The liver makes and releases a mixture called bile. Bile is stored in the gall bladder. The bile acts to break down fats into small droplets.

The Excretory System

As your cells perform the chemical activities to keep the body functioning, waste products such as carbon dioxide and ammonia are produced. These waste products are toxic to cells and must be removed in order to keep cells and the body healthy. The excretory system eliminates cellular wastes from the body through the lungs, skin, kidneys, and the digestive system.

Waste products are filtered through the blood by the kidneys and eliminated in urine. Urine is made by three processes: filtration, reabsorption, and secretion. Urine is made up of urea, uric acid, and creatinine. Urea is a waste product formed from the breakdown of amino acids (proteins). Uric acid is a waste product from the breakdown of nucleic acids (DNA, RNA), and creatinine is a waste product formed by muscle metabolism.

The excretory system that makes up the urinary system is composed of the following structures:

- **Kidneys:** The kidneys are a pair of organs that act to remove waste product from blood. Microscopic structures called nephrons fill the inside of the kidneys. Fluids and waste product are filtered through the blood into the nephron through a structure called the glomerulus. Filtered blood leaves the glomerulus and circulates around the nephrons. Valuable salts and ions are returned to the blood, and another tube in the kidneys called a final collecting duct collects the waste from the nephrons. Concentrated fluid (urine) in the collecting ducts then moves from the kidneys into the ureters.

- **Ureters:** Urine that leaves the kidneys flows into the ureters. These are the tubes that connect the kidneys to the bladder.

- **Bladder:** The bladder is a sac-like organ in the body that functions to store urine. As the bladder fills with urine, it is able to stretch. This stretching stimulates neurons in the bladder wall that send a message to the brain that gives an individual the urge to urinate, or void. Voluntary muscles in the bladder hold the urine inside until it is ready to be released. At that time, muscles contract and squeeze urine out of the bladder.

- **Urethra:** Urine exits the body by traveling through a narrow tube called the urethra.

Other waste products such as excess salts and water are released from the body through the pores in the skin. Carbon dioxide is a waste product of the respiratory system, and lungs release water and carbon dioxide during exhalation.

The Integumentary System

The intergumentary system is composed of skin, hair, nails, and sweat and sebaceous glands. It functions to protect the body from injury and dehydration, to maintain a constant temperature in the body, to produce vitamin D, to excrete waste materials and toxins, and to react to microorganisms and chemicals.

The skin and all of its associated structures, such as hair, nails, sweat and oil glands, and sensory receptors, make up the largest organ of the body. The skin is the body's first line of defense against infection or injury, heat and water loss, and UV radiation. It also assists with vitamin D production and sensory input.

The skin is composed of three layers of tissue:

1. **Epidermis:** The epidermis is a thin layer of cells on the body's outer surface. The epidermis has the fibrous protein keratin that helps keep water from entering or exiting the skin layers. Another layer of the epidermis is thin and clear and made up mostly of dead skin cells. It is found on the palms of hands and the soles of feet. Below this layer is the epidermis layer that will form scabs when the skin is wounded. This layer has special cells that contain granules in the cytoplasm. Below this layer is a layer of the epidermis that serves as a protective skin layer. The innermost layer of the epidermis is a single layer of melanocytes, or cells that contain melanin. Melanin protects the body from harmful UV rays and gives skin its pigment, or color.

This is the layer of the epidermis in which mitosis (cell division) takes place and epidermis cells are replaced.

2. **Dermis:** The dermis is a thick layer of dense connective tissue that lies beneath the epidermis layer. The connective tissue is made up of collagen fibers. This is the region of the skin where nerve endings are located. Therefore, this is the skin layer that is sensitive to touch, heat, and pain. The dermis layer also contains hair follicles, sweat glands, and blood vessels. The upper layer of the dermis is called the papillary layer. This is the layer of skin that is textured with fingerprint markings. Fibers from the dermis layer extend deep into skin tissue to help anchor the skin to the body.

3. **Hypodermis:** The hypodermis is a deep layer of fat that helps to protect and insulate the body.

The Musculoskeletal System

The muscular and skeletal systems are tightly linked together and function to supply structure and movement for the body. The skeletal system gives shape and support to the body and helps to prevent injury to internal organs. The rib cage protects the heart and lungs, the vertebrae protect the spinal cord, and the skull protects the brain. Bones also function to store important minerals such as calcium in their hard outer layer and produce red blood cells in their spongy center. Muscles contract to provide movement, and the bones act as levers for this movement. Muscle tissue is made of special proteins called microfilaments that shorten and lengthen to provide movement.

The Skeletal System

The skeletal system is composed of bones, cartilage, and ligaments. There are two parts to the skeletal system: the axial skeleton and the appendicular skeleton. The axial skeleton consists of the skull, the vertebrae, and the ribs. This system provides protection to organs and supports body weight. The appendicular skeletal system is composed of the arms, legs, shoulders, and pelvis. This system allows for movement of the body.

* **Bones:** Bones are hard organs made of minerals and connective tissue. Calcium is the most abundant mineral in bone tissue. The minerals in bones are deposited by bone cells called osteoblasts. Bone is deposited in proportion to the compressional load, or weight, that the bone must support. Bone tissue containing calcium and phosphorus is also continually absorbed by other cells called osteoclasts. Connective tissue in bone is made mostly of the fibrous protein collagen. Collagen allows bones to be flexible so that they don't break every time they are struck or bumped.

  Compact bone tissue is dense, is what makes bones hard and rigid, and is the outer layer of bones. Tiny channels in the compact bone contain blood capillaries. Spongy bone tissue has many open spaces, and it provides strength and support for the bone. In long bones, such as those in the arm or leg, an outer layer of compact bone surrounds a layer of spongy bone. Inside the spongy bone is the marrow. There are two types of bone marrow: red marrow and yellow marrow. Red marrow is the site of red and white blood cell production. Red marrow is found in the center of flat bones such as the ribs. Yellow marrow is found in the center of long bones, and it stores fat cells.

- **Ligaments:** Ligaments are tough, flexible strands of connective tissue that connect bones to one another. Ligaments hold together joints between bones. They allow for the movement and flexibility of the body. Some ligaments such as those along the vertebrae prevent too much movement of the bones.

  The places where bones connect are called joints. Joints can be fixed to restrict movement or movable to allow bones to move independently of each other. Some examples of movable joints are ball and socket joints, gliding joints, and hinge joints.

- **Cartilage:** Cartilage is a strong, flexible, smooth connective tissue that is found at the ends of bones. Cartilage allows for bones to move smoothly across each other. Cartilage like that found at the tip of the nose and the ears is soft and bendable. Cartilage does not contain any blood vessels. Growth plates are areas of cartilage at the ends of bones that continue to make new bone tissue as the body grows. Osteoclasts move into the cartilage and harden it, turning it into bone tissue. Most bones harden completely after they stop growing, but osteoclasts are still present to repair bone if it breaks.

The Muscular System

TIP

If you are not sure of an answer, your first idea is probably correct.

The muscular system is mostly composed of muscles that allow the body to move and function. Muscles pump blood through the body, cause the lungs to expand and relax, hold the body upright, and allow for mobility. Muscle tissue is made up of muscle cells, and there are the following three types of muscle tissue in the body:

1. **Skeletal muscle:** Skeletal muscles allow for voluntary movement of the body and are attached to bones by tendons. Skeletal muscle may be striated or striped. Both are composed of microfilaments called actin (thin filaments) and myosin (thick filaments), which slide past each other as muscles contract to provide movement. As a muscle contracts, or shortens, the attached bones are pulled closer to one another and this allows for movement. Most skeletal muscles work in pairs around a joint. One muscle in the pair is called the flexor, and it bends a joint. The other is the extensor, and it straightens the joint. When one muscle in the pair contracts, the other relaxes to allow movement.

2. **Cardiac muscle:** Cardiac muscle is the tissue that makes up the heart. The movement of cardiac muscle is involuntary, so that the heart contracts and relaxes without humans being conscious of it. Blood is continually pumped through the body, and in order to continually contract and relax the heart, muscle tissue requires a great amount of energy. In order to supply so much energy, cardiac muscle cells have a huge number of mitochondria. Mitochondria are the powerhouse of the cell and produce ATP.

3. **Smooth muscle:** Smooth muscle is found lining the walls of organs such as the stomach, the intestines, and the bladder. It is also found in the lining of blood vessels. Smooth muscle functions to help move materials such as blood and food through the body. Like cardiac muscle, it is involuntary.

Muscles contract when nerve impulses are sent to skeletal muscle tissue from the brain. This impulse causes the actin and myosin filaments to slide past each other, and the muscle shortens, or contracts. As the muscle relaxes, the filaments slide back to their original positions, and the muscle lengthens again.

The Nervous System

The nervous system is made of structures, cells, and organs that control the actions and reactions of the body in response to stimuli either from the environment or from inside the body. The nervous system is made up of two parts, that is, the central nervous system and the peripheral nervous system.

The Central Nervous System

The central nervous system (CNS) is composed of the brain and the spinal cord, along with the cranial nerves. The brain is the central command organ of the nervous system. It is made up of several parts: the cerebrum (cerebral cortex), cerebellum, midbrain, hypothalamus, and pons. The cerebrum is divided into right and left hemispheres and consists of grey matter and white matter. It is the area of the brain where sensory information is processed, and it controls voluntary movement. The cerebellum processes information that comes from inside the body. This allows the brain to keep track of body movements and position. The rest of the brain makes up what is called the brain stem. The brain stem connects the brain to the spinal cord. The medulla in the brain stem controls involuntary processes, such as blood pressure, body temperature, heart rate, and breathing. The spinal cord allows your brain to communicate with the rest of the body. The spinal cord is composed of a bundle of nerves and is surrounded by protective vertebrae. Sensory information travels to the spinal cord, and the spinal cord sends impulses to the brain.

The Peripheral Nervous System

The peripheral nervous system (PNS) connects the CNS to the rest of the body. The PNS has two main components, namely, sensory neurons and motor neurons. Neurons are the smallest functional units of the nervous system. They are excitable cells that conduct and transmit electrical signals that send sensory information to and from the brain. Neurons are composed of a cell body called a soma, dendrites that are like fingers projecting out of the cell body toward other neurons so that the neuron can receive signals from other cells, and a single long axon along which the electrical signal travels to other neurons. At the end of each axon is an axon terminal. At the axon terminal, the electrical signal is converted to a chemical signal. This chemical signal is called a neurotransmitter, and it is released into the gap between two neurons called a synaptic cleft. The neurotransmitter crosses the synaptic cleft to the dendrites of another neuron.

Neurons are classified into three categories:

1. **Sensory neurons:** Sensory, or afferent, neurons receive impulses from the environment or inside the body and send them to the CNS.

2. **Motor neurons:** Motor, or efferent, neurons transmit nerve signals from the CNS to muscles or glands to produce a response to the initial stimulus. This causes a contraction of muscles or a secretion of hormones.

3. **Interneurons:** Interneurons, or association neurons, are neurons that link sensory neurons to motor neurons. They are found in the brain and the spinal cord.

Signals move through the CNS and the PNS with the help of special cells called glial cells. Glial cells act to protect and support neurons.

Some actions of the nervous system are involuntary. This means that these actions occur without a conscious decision. There is no control over the body to perform these actions. Actions that can be consciously controlled by the brain are called voluntary actions.

The Endocrine System

The endocrine system controls body functions and helps to maintain homeostasis through the use of hormones. Hormones are chemical messengers that are made in a specific organ called an endocrine gland and can cause a change in another cell or tissue in a different part of the body. Signals sent by endocrine glands are indirect because they cycle through the whole body.

Hormones have multiple functions, including regulating growth, behavior, development, and reproduction. Hormones travel through the bloodstream and can only affect specific cells that have receptors for a given hormone. Cells that have receptors for a hormone are called target cells. The hormones bind to the receptors on the target cells and carry out their function.

The endocrine glands in the human body include:

- **Pituitary gland:** The pituitary gland secretes hormones that affect all other glands. Therefore, it is called the master gland. It also stimulates growth and sexual development.

- **Hypothalamus:** The hypothalamus gland is a gland in the brain stem that controls the release of hormones found in the pituitary gland.

- **Thyroid gland:** The thyroid gland is located in the neck. It secretes two hormones; one controls the metabolism in the body, and the other controls blood calcium levels by removing calcium from the bloodstream and depositing it back into bone tissue.

- **Parathyroid gland:** The parathyroid gland secretes a hormone that increases blood calcium levels. It works together with the thyroid to regulate blood calcium levels.

- **Pineal gland:** The pineal gland is in the brainstem and produces hormones that are essential for the control of sleep, aging, reproduction, and body temperature.

- **Adrenal glands:** The two adrenal glands sit atop the kidneys. Each adrenal gland has two parts. One part promotes the release of glucose from the liver, promotes water retention in the kidneys, and helps to regulate metabolism. The other part of the adrenal gland secretes hormones involved in the "fight-or-flight" mechanism of most animals.

- **Pancreas:** The pancreas helps to regulate blood sugar (glucose) levels in the body.

- **Gonads:** The gonads are endocrine glands that regulate the function of sex hormones and the process of reproduction.

The mechanism of hormone activity depends upon whether the hormone is a steroid hormone or a protein hormone. A steroid hormone can diffuse across the membrane of a target cell where it binds to a receptor protein in the cell nucleus. In the nucleus, the hormone will activate specific genes in the cell's DNA. If the hormone is a protein, it must bind to a receptor on the surface of the target cell. This triggers the production of a second messenger called cyclic AMP (cAMP). The cAMP activates enzymes in cells to initiate changes.

TIP

Use the process of elimination if you are not sure about an answer. Rule out answers you know are incorrect. If you can eliminate at least two answers, you have a fifty-fifty chance of being right.

The endocrine system helps to keep the body in homeostasis by increasing or decreasing the amount of hormones found in the bloodstream. This process is a feedback mechanism. Information from one action controls or affects another action or process.

The Reproductive System

Sexual reproduction in humans involves the creation of offspring by the fusion of a male and female sex cell, or gamete. The male gamete is the sperm, and the female gamete is the ovum (egg). Sex cells contain half the number of chromosomes (23) as other cells in the body, and when the sperm and ovum fuse during the process of fertilization, their chromosomes combine to form a fertilized egg (zygote) with the normal number of chromosomes (46). The male and female reproductive systems have distinctly different components.

The Male Reproductive System

The male reproductive system functions to produce sperm and deliver them to the female reproductive system. Sperm are male sex cells, or gametes, and each sperm contains 23 chromosomes, which is half the number of other types of cells in the body. The male reproductive system also produces hormones involved in growth and development of males and gamete production. Male hormones are continually secreted throughout the life of a male.

There are several organs and structures in the male reproductive system.

- **Testes:** Testes are the main organ of the male reproductive system. They produce testosterone, which is the male sex hormone. Testosterone is the hormone responsible for many male traits, including facial and body hair and a deep voice. These traits are known as secondary sex characteristics. The testes are also the site of sperm production. Immature sperm cells are called spermatids. Testes are located within the scrotum, which are sac-like structures that keep the testes outside the body so that they remain slightly cooler than body temperature.

- **Epididymis:** The epididymis is where sperm are stored after they have matured. The spermatids travel to the epididymis and mature into sperm cells.

- **Vas deferens:** When sperm leave the epididymis, they enter a tube called the vas deferens. In the vas deferens, sperm mix with fluid that comes from seminal vesicles and the prostate gland. The seminal vesicles provide sperm with fructose (sugar) and nutrients, and the prostate gland secretes a watery and alkaline fluid. The mixture of sperm and fluid is called semen. Semen acts to neutralize the acidic vaginal fluids during fertilization.

- **Urethra:** In leaving the body, sperm pass through a narrow tube called the urethra. Urine also passes through this tube.

- **Penis:** The penis is the organ that delivers semen into the female reproductive system.

The Female Reproductive System

The female reproductive system produces ova, or eggs, and hormones. It also provides a protective environment to nourish a developing fetus. The ovum, or egg, is the female gamete, and, therefore, like sperm, it only contains 23 chromosomes, or half the number of chromosomes of other cells in the body. The hormones secreted in the female reproductive system are estrogen and progesterone.

These hormones control the development of female sex characteristics such as breasts and wide hips. They are also responsible for the development and release of eggs in a regulated cycle called the menstrual cycle and the preparation of the reproductive system for pregnancy.

There are several organs and structures in the female reproductive system.

- **Ovaries:** The ovaries are the reproductive organs in which eggs are produced. At sexual maturity, females have hundreds and thousands of immature eggs (follicles) in the ovaries. During a lifetime, about 400 eggs will be released during the menstrual cycle of a female. The rest of the follicles will not leave the ovaries. Eggs are released about midway through the menstrual cycle, and a typical cycle lasts 28 days.

- **Fallopian tubes:** When eggs are released from the ovaries during a process called ovulation, they travel through the fallopian tubes. These are tubes that connect the ovaries to the uterus. Fertilization of an egg occurs in the upper third of the fallopian tube. During intercourse, a few hundred sperm travel up into the fallopian tubes. The sperm release an enzyme that helps to dissolve the outer covering of eggs. When one sperm enters the egg, the membrane is altered so that no other sperm can enter and the process of embryo formation begins. The egg and sperm combine to form one cell (now with 46 chromosomes), and this cell divides to form an embryo. The genetic material from the sperm and the egg combine, and a unique individual develops.

- **Uterus:** The egg travels through the fallopian tube and into the uterus. This process takes about five to six days. A fertilized egg will implant itself in the thickened lining of the uterus and develop into an embryo and then a fetus. A developing fetus will release a hormone called human chorionic gonadotropin (HCG) that helps to maintain the protective uterine lining throughout pregnancy. A fetus matures and develops for about 38 weeks in the uterus.

    An unfertilized ovum will not be implanted into the uterine lining and will be released from the uterus during a process of menstruation. During menstruation, the uterine lining is shed from the body. When menstruation ends, the lining of the uterus thickens, and the cycle begins again. Rising estrogen levels stimulate the development of a new lining in the uterus. Other hormones called follicle stimulating hormone (FSH) and luteinizing hormone (LH) also play a role in the menstrual cycle. FSH stimulates activity in the ovaries (and in the testes of males), and LH stimulates the release of an ovum (and the production of testosterone in males).

- **Vagina:** When a fetus is fully developed, it passes through the vagina during birth. The vagina is the canal between the uterus and outside the body. It is sometimes referred to as the birth canal.

The Stages of Fetal Development

A normal pregnancy spans about nine months. This time is measured from the date of the last start of menstruation to the birth of a fully developed baby. These nine months are broken down into three segments called trimesters. Each trimester spans a three-month period.

1. **First trimester:** The first trimester spans the first three months of development. The embryo implants in the first trimester. Soon after the first trimester begins, the placenta begins to grow. The placenta is a network of blood vessels that provides the embryo with oxygen and nutrients from the mother's blood. The placenta also carries waste away from the developing embryo. During the first trimester, the embryo becomes surrounded by amnion, a sac filled with fluid (amniotic fluid) that protects the embryo. The embryo is connected to the placenta through

the umbilical cord. After ten weeks of development, the embryo becomes a fetus. During the first trimester, many organs such as the heart, liver, and brain form. Arms, legs, fingers, and toes also begin to develop.

2. **Second trimester:** The second trimester spans months four through six of development. During the second trimester, bones and joints begin to form. Muscles develop and the fetus becomes stronger. It is during this trimester that fetal movement is detected. The fetus triples in size, and its brain rapidly develops and grows. Eventually, the fetus can make facial expressions. The fetus has the ability to hear, and it can make breathing movements and swallow. A protective coating called vernix forms on the skin.

3. **Third trimester:** The third trimester spans months seven through nine. During this trimester, the senses of sight, sound, taste, and touch are developed. The eyes can open and close, and the suck-swallow coordination is developed. The brain develops further and organs become fully functional. Bones grow and harden, and the lungs completely develop. The skin thickens with brown fat that provides nutrition and insulation, helping to regulate body temperature in newborns. Amniotic fluid is absorbed during the eighth month. Antibodies from the mother are transferred to the baby. Eventually, the fetus is fully developed and ready to be born.

THE PRINCIPLES OF NUTRITION

Humans and other animals have three basic nutritional needs.

1. Fuel is required for all body activities.

2. Organic molecules are required to build molecules that are essential for proper body functions.

3. All animals must obtain essential nutrients, or substances that are not produced in the body, from foods.

Digestion breaks down the larger molecules of food into essential molecules of proteins, carbohydrates, and lipids (fats). Cells can then oxidize these smaller molecules for energy or assemble the smaller molecules into other proteins, carbohydrates, lipids, or nucleic acids that are essential to maintain cell structure and function. Eating too much or too little food, or the wrong kinds of food, can endanger our health.

Chemical Energy

Chemical energy obtained from food is used to power the body. Every activity that the body performs requires fuel in the form of chemical energy. The process of cellular metabolism produces ATO, which is a usable form of energy for all of the body's cells. The process of cellular metabolism involves the breakdown, or oxidizing, of large molecules (macromolecules) found in food, such as carbohydrates, lipids, and proteins. Usually, cells rely on carbohydrates and fats (lipids) as a source of readily usable fuel. If these molecules are in short supply, then proteins can be used as an energy source. Fats are the macromolecules that are the most energy-rich. One gram of fat gives off twice as much energy when it is oxidized than one gram of carbohydrate or protein.

The energy content of food is given in units of kilocalories. One kilocalorie is equal to 1,000 calories. In fact, the amount of calories listed on food labels is actually kilocalories, but is written as Calories (with a capital C).

The rate of energy consumption by the body is called its metabolic rate. The metabolic rate is equal to the sum of all of the energy-requiring reactions over a given period of time. The process of cellular metabolism must constantly drive chemical reactions in the cell in order for an organism to stay alive and for all body systems to function properly. The number of kilocalories that a resting body requires to maintain these functions—such as cellular maintenance, breathing, heartbeat, and regulation of body temperature—is called the basal metabolic rate (BMR). The BMR for healthy adult females is about 1300 to 1500 kcal per day, and about 1600 to 1800 kcal per day for a healthy adult male. Any activity performed beyond those activities essential to sustain bodily functions consumes more kilocalories of energy. The more strenuous the activity, the greater the energy demand. For example, running uses up more energy than walking.

If more energy is taken in, in the form of food, than the body requires to maintain its activity level, the energy is stored in various forms. The liver and muscles store energy in the form of glycogen. Most healthy bodies have enough glycogen stored to perform a day's worth of basic activities. Cells store extra energy as fat. The liver can convert carbohydrates and proteins to fat for storage. Most healthy humans have enough fats stored to provide energy to the body for several weeks without food. Undernourishment is a condition that results in a diet that is too low in calories.

Essential Nutrients

In addition to providing fuel in the form of carbohydrates, fats, and proteins, food must also provide essential nutrients for the body. Animal cells cannot produce nutrients from raw material, so they must be ingested in their complete form. Malnourishment is the result of a long-term deficiency of essential nutrients in the diet. There are four types of essential nutrients.

1. **Essential fatty acids:** Essential fatty acids include omega-3 and omega-6 fatty acids as well as linoleic acid. Linoleic acid is important because it is needed by cells to make the phospholipids of the cell membrane. Most balanced diets provide a sufficient amount of essential fatty acids.

2. **Essential amino acids:** Twenty amino acids are required to make proteins, and there are eight amino acids that the human body cannot synthesize. These eight amino acids are known as essential amino acids and must be taken into the body through the foods we eat. The body cannot store excess amino acids, so a deficiency of a single amino acid limits the use of other amino acids, disrupts protein synthesis, and can lead to protein deficiency in the body. Protein deficiency is the most common form of malnutrition seen in humans. All essential amino acids can be provided by eating meat, eggs, milk, and cheese. Vegetarians and vegans must be especially careful to obtain all eight essential amino acids. The key is to eat a variety of plant foods that supply sufficient quantities of amino acids. A combination of beans and corn can provide all eight essential amino acids.

3. **Vitamins:** A vitamin is an essential nutrient that is required by the body in very small amounts. There are thirteen essential vitamins: vitamin B_1, vitamin B_2, niacin (B_3), pantothenic acid (B_5), vitamin B_6, folic acid (B_9), vitamin B_{12}, biotin, vitamin C, vitamin A, vitamin D, vitamin E (tocopherol), and vitamin K. These vitamins can be obtained from a variety of foods, and all

have essential functions in the body. For example, the B vitamins can function as coenzymes in the body during metabolic reactions, and vitamin C is required to produce connective tissue. Even though only a small amount is required, these vitamins are essential to good health. However, an excess of these vitamins can be harmful.

4. **Minerals:** Minerals are simple inorganic nutrients that are required by the body. Minerals like calcium and phosphorous are needed in relatively large amounts in order to construct and maintain healthy bone tissue. Calcium is also necessary for proper nerve and muscle function. Phosphorus is an essential component in ATP, DNA, and RNA. Iodine is required to make hormones produced in the thyroid that regulate the metabolic rate of the body. Sodium, potassium, and chloride are essential for nerve function and help to maintain the right amount of water in cells. Other essential minerals are magnesium, iron, fluorine, zinc, copper, manganese, cobalt, selenium, chromium, and molybdenum. Dietary source of minerals include dark green vegetables, legumes, proteins, and dairy products.

A normal and varied diet generally contains enough essential vitamins and minerals and is the best source of these nutrients. Certain people, however, can benefit from vitamin and mineral supplements. However, there is a concern that massive doses of certain vitamins can be harmful instead of beneficial and should therefore be avoided. An excess of fat-soluble vitamins (vitamins A, D, E, and K) can accumulate in the body to toxic levels, but an excess of water-soluble vitamins will be excreted in urine.

Food Labels

The Food and Drug Administration (FDA) requires that certain information be included on labels of packaged foods. Food labels include a list of ingredients listed in order from those used in the greatest amount to those used in the smallest amount.

Food labels also include nutrition facts. The serving size for the product is listed at the top of the label and is defined according to standards set by the FDA. The energy content of a single serving of the food product is listed in units of Calories (remember, this is actually in units of kilocalories).

Nutrients that are contained within one serving of the food product are listed as a percentage of the daily recommended amount based on a diet of 2,000 kcal per day. Emphasis is placed on informing consumers about nutrients that are linked to the risk of disease. These nutrients include fats (especially saturated and trans fats), cholesterol, and sodium. Other nutrients listed focus on those associated with a healthy diet, such as dietary fiber, protein, and certain vitamins and minerals (calcium, iron, vitamin A, B vitamins, and vitamin C).

Food labels allow consumers to compare nutrition facts of different brands and types of food choices. In this way, we can choose foods that will give us a balance of all the daily nutrition requirements. In a 2000-kcal/day diet, it is recommended that an adult consume less than 65 g of fat, less than 20 g of saturated fats, less than 300 mg cholesterol, less than 2400 mg sodium, 300 g of carbohydrates, and 25 g of dietary fiber.

Obesity and Weight Loss

Overnourishment, or consuming more food than is required to maintain all body functions and activities, leads to obesity. Obesity is the excessive accumulation of fat in cells, and it is now recognized by the World Health Organization (WHO) as a major global health problem.

Obesity can be brought on by a sedentary lifestyle, an increase in the availability of fattening foods, and oversized portions of certain foods. Over 30 percent of adults in the United States are considered obese, and another 35 percent are considered overweight. In addition, about 15 percent of all children and adolescents in the United States are overweight.

Obesity can contribute to many health problems, including diabetes, colon cancer, breast cancer, and cardiovascular disease. Some obese individuals may be predisposed to their overweight condition due to certain inherited factors. Scientists have isolated dozens of genes that are specific for weight-regulating hormones. For example, the hormone leptin is produced in adipose (fat) cells. As the amount of adipose tissue increases, leptin levels in the blood rise. This increase in leptin normally signals the brain to suppress appetite. Studies have shown that mice that inherit a defect in the gene for leptin become very obese because leptin does not accumulate in their bodies and signal the brain to stop eating.

Other research has been conducted to study the signaling pathways involved in regulating both long- and short-term appetite and the body's storage of fat. It is possible in the future that individuals with inheritable traits leading to obesity may be able to control the problem with effective and safe drugs.

Weight loss plans fall into several categories:

- **Low-carbohydrate diets:** Some low-carbohydrate diets promote eating high-protein, high-fat, and low carbohydrate food. Others encourage dieters to eat high-fiber fruits, vegetables, and beans and grains and to get about 40 percent of daily calories form carbohydrates. The danger in these diets is that too much fat is consumed, which can contribute to heart and kidney disease.

- **Low-fat diets:** Low-fat diets suggest taking in less than 10 percent of daily calories from fat. The focus is on an increase in vegetables, high-fiber fruits, and grains. These diets can lack sufficient amounts of fatty acids and protein that may make it difficult for the body to absorb fat-soluble vitamins.

- **Glycemic index diets:** These diets focus on eating carbohydrates with a low glycemic index in order to lower blood sugar levels.

- **Formula diets:** A formula diet is based on eating packaged products of a set number of calories, proteins, fats, and carbohydrates. These diets often involve consuming special nutritionally sound shakes or bars and can be expensive to follow.

- **Group-approach diets:** The group-approach diet involves group meetings, diet plans, exercise plans, and group support.

Scientific studies seem to indicate that an increase in exercise along with a restricted, but balanced diet that provides all essential nutrients and at least 1200-kcal per day is the healthiest way to approach weight loss. However, rather than on-again-off-again dieting, a change in eating habits and lifestyle to take weight off and keep it off is the better approach.

Diet and Disease Prevention

Diet, that is, what people eat, plays an important role in an individual's risk for developing certain diseases, including cardiovascular disease and cancer. Inheritable traits that predispose an individual to a certain disease are unavoidable, but diet is a controllable factor that can actually function to help prevent disease in some cases.

For example, high levels of low-density lipoproteins, or LDL cholesterol, generally correlate with blocked blood vessels (clogged arteries), high blood pressure, and subsequent heart attacks. In contrast, high-density lipoproteins (HDL cholesterol) may actually decrease the risk of blocked blood vessels because HDLs bring cholesterol to the liver, where it is broken down.

Diet seems to be linked to some forms of cancer. Some research suggests a link between diets high in carbohydrates and fats and an increase in the incidence of breast cancer. In addition, the incidence of colon and prostate cancer may be linked to diets rich in saturated fats or red meat. Some fruits and vegetable are rich in antioxidants that protect cells from damaging molecules called free radicals. Antioxidants may play a role in preventing cancer. As precautions to help lower the risk of cancer, the American Cancer Society recommends dietary guidelines that include eating five or more servings of fruits and vegetables a day, eating whole grains, limiting the consumption of red meats and alcoholic beverages, and increasing physical activity.

FACTORS AFFECTING HEALTH

Some aspects of health are uncontrollable. For example, age, gender, and genetic makeup are not something that an individual can change. Wellness, however, can be affected by several factors that are controllable such as diet, exercise, and personal relationships. Individuals can affect their own health by life-style choices that they make. Physical activity and a healthy, well-balanced diet can have a positive effect on health. Adequate sleep and preventative healthcare also have a positive effect on health. Other factors, such as obesity and alcohol and tobacco consumption, can have a negative effect on health. In fact, these three factors are some of the leading causes of death in the United States.

Wellness

A healthy lifestyle can be obtained by taking a holistic approach to health. A holistic approach includes understanding the importance of the following six dimensions of wellness: physical, emotional, spiritual, intellectual, interpersonal, and environmental.

1. **Physical wellness:** Physical wellness is determined by coordination, strength, and the command of the five senses (sight, hearing, taste, smell, and touch).

2. **Emotional wellness:** Emotional wellness reflects an individual's ability to understand and cope with various feelings and emotions in a healthy and positive way.

3. **Spiritual wellness:** Spiritual wellness involves developing a set of guided beliefs, principles, or values that give one's life meaning and purpose.

4. **Intellectual wellness:** Intellectual wellness involves engaging in pursuits that will continually challenge the mind and keep it active, including creative pursuits, problem solving, and processing information.

5. **Interpersonal wellness:** Interpersonal wellness involves the maintenance of healthy, supportive, and satisfying relationships with others.

6. **Environmental wellness:** Environmental wellness involves positive input from one's environment. A clean, safe environment contributes to wellness.

Stress

Another factor that can affect health is stress. Stress refers to both the stressor and the stress response. A stressor is the situation that triggers an emotional or physical reaction. The physical and emotional reactions that one exhibits are called the stress response. Stress responses are controlled by the nervous system and the endocrine system. The sympathetic division of the nervous system, which activates the "fight-or-flight" response, triggers signals that tell the body to stop storing energy and use it in response to a crisis. The nervous system triggers the endocrine system, which releases hormones and other chemical signals to the bloodstream. Some key hormones released in response to stress are cortisol and epinephrine. Stress can be managed by developing a healthy lifestyle, improving time management, learning to identify stressors, and changing unhealthy thought patterns. Relaxation is another method that is effective in dealing with stress.

Aging

In midlife, individuals may see a decline in health in terms of loss of bone mass, compression of vertebrae, loss of lean body mass, vision loss, hearing loss, fertility loss, and a loss of or decrease in sexual function. Women in particular experience loss of calcium in bones, a condition called osteoporosis, and a decline in their reproductive cycle (menopause). Both men and women can suffer from osteoarthritis due to the wearing down of joint tissue.

Through good health habits, it is possible to delay, lessen, prevent, and sometimes reverse changes in health associated with aging. Some of these habits include challenging the mind, developing a physical fitness regimen, establishing healthy eating habits, maintaining a healthy weight, controlling alcohol consumption and dependence on medication, refraining from smoking, and keeping up to date with preventative medical care. Physical examinations should include detection of treatable diseases or conditions.

Physical Fitness

The level of physical fitness practiced by an individual affects overall health. There are five basic components to physical fitness:

1. **Cardiorespiratory endurance:** Cardiorespiratory endurance is the ability to perform long, large-muscle, dynamic exercises at a moderate to high intensity level. This type of training increases the strength of the heart and affects positively other related body functions such as heart rate, blood pressure, metabolism, and certain chemical systems in the body.

2. **Muscular strength:** Strength training improves physical fitness and increases muscle mass. An increase in muscle mass means the body requires more energy to carry out life functions.

3. **Muscular endurance:** The development of muscular endurance involves developing the ability to contract a specific muscle group for a long period of time or to continually contract a muscle group for a long period of time.

4. **Flexibility:** Flexibility is the ability to move a joint through its full range of motion. Flexibility depends on the structure of a particular joint, the length and elasticity of the connective tissue, and the nervous system activity around the joint. Flexible and pain-free joints are an important part of maintaining good health. Stretching is a good way to improve and maintain flexibility.

5. **Body composition:** A healthy body composition includes a higher proportion of nonfat body mass than fat mass. This proportion varies by sex and age. Too high a concentration of body fat, especially in the abdominal region, can lead to issues such as high blood pressure, heart disease, stroke, joint problems, gall bladder disease, back pain, diabetes, and cancer.

For optimal fitness and health, twenty to sixty minutes of endurance exercise three to five times a week and strength training twice a week is recommended. Exercise lowers the risk of cardiovascular disease by lowering blood fat levels, reducing high blood pressure, and preventing the blocking of arteries. Exercise can also reduce the risk of some cancers, osteoporosis, and diabetes. Other benefits of exercise include an enhanced immune system, improved psychological health, and the prevention of injury and low back pain.

Nutrition

The body requires about forty-five essential nutrients to maintain a maximum level of health. Most foods provide one or more essential nutrients and act as fuel for the body.

In addition to essential nutrients, water is required for the body in order to digest and absorb food, transport substances to different regions of the body, and maintain cellular health and overall well-being.

Risk Factors, Disease, and Disease Prevention

A disease can be bacterial, viral, or fungal and can enter the body through the transfer of bodily fluids (saliva, semen, and blood), airborne droplets, or fecal materials. Other organisms such as mosquitoes or fleas can indirectly transfer disease from one host organism to another. A full-blown infection occurs when there is an environment in the body for the disease to "live" or reproduce. Infectious diseases also need an exit point in the body, so that they can leave and spread the infection to another host. Viral particles can leave the body through the nose via a sneeze or through the mouth via a cough and enter a second host. Some common infectious diseases include influenza, rhinitis (the common cold), pneumonia, tuberculosis, mononucleosis, Lyme disease, streptococcal infections, measles, mumps, rubella, pertussis, chicken pox, and herpes viruses.

Bacterial infections can be treated with oral antibiotics that act to kill the bacteria cells. The body can build up a defense against viral infections through the administration of vaccines. A vaccine will manipulate the immune system and cause the body to develop immunity to a specific viral disease agent. Vaccines protect against future infection from a specific virus, and they are administered through injection, oral medication, or a nasal spray.

Sexually Transmitted Diseases

There are seven sexually transmitted diseases (STDs) that can have a major affect on one's health. AIDS, or Acquired Immune Deficiency Syndrome, is the most serious and life-threatening sexually transmitted disease. It is caused by the HIV virus (Human Immunodeficiency Virus) and compromises the immune system of an infected individual. Chlamydia is an STD that causes painful urination. It can lead to another disorder called pelvic inflammatory disease if it is left untreated. This can lead to an increased risk of infertility in men and women, ectopic pregnancies in women, and inflammation of sperm-carrying ducts in men.

Gonorrhea causes urinary discomfort in men and a yellowish green discharge. Women infected with gonorrhea usually have no symptoms, but can experience painful urination, vaginal discharge, and severe cramps. Antibiotics are used to treat gonorrhea. Human papilloma virus, or HPV, causes genital warts, genital cancers, cervical cancer, penile cancer, and some forms of rectal cancers. A new vaccine has been developed to prevent the spread of HPV. Hepatitis B causes inflammation of the liver and can cause serious and permanent damage. There is a vaccine against this disease as well. Syphilis is caused by a bacterial infection and is treated with antibiotics. It causes ulcers, sore throat, and hair loss in its early stages; late stages of infection can cause permanent damage and death.

Cardiovascular Disease

There are six major preventable risk factors for cardiovascular disease (disease affecting the cardio-vascular system). These risk factors include smoking, high blood pressure, high LDL cholesterol levels, inactivity, overweight or obesity, and diabetes. Smoking lowers HDL levels, increases blood pressure and heart rate, and increases plaque formation and the chance of a blood clot. High blood pressure leads to hypertension, and high LDL levels contribute to clogged arteries. All of these risk factors can be reduced by good overall health and nutrition and exercise practices. Unavoidable risk factors are age, race, and family history.

Some common cardiovascular diseases include atherosclerosis (hardening of the arteries), heart attack, stroke, congestive heart failure, peripheral arterial disease (PAD), congenital heart disease, rheumatic heart disease, and heart valve malfunctions.

Cancer

Cancer can be found in all areas of the body, and treatment depends on the location of the tumor or tumors. The spreading of cancer cells from one area of the body to another is called metastasis. Cancer is caused by an uncontrolled growth of cells that cause an outgrowth, or tumor, of abnormal cell types. This uncontrolled growth can be due to genetics, exposure to agents that cause mutations in DNA (mutagens), viral infection, and chemical substances in food or the atmosphere. Cancer is categorized into five progressive stages (stage 0 to IV).

Some types of cancer are lung cancer, oral cancer, colon cancer, rectal cancer, skin cancer, prostate cancer, breast cancer, ovarian cancer, cervical cancer, uterine cancer, and testicular cancer. Tumors are classified according to the type of cells they have. Carcinomas form from epithelial cells, sarcomas are found in connective tissue, melanoma are found in skin cells, lymphomas are cancers of the lymph nodes, neuroblastomas occur in immature CNS cells, hepatomas are found in liver cells, and adenocarcinomas are found in endocrine glands.

Strategies for preventing cancer can include avoiding tobacco, eating a healthy and well-balanced diet, controlling weight, exercising, avoiding exposure to the sun, avoiding exposure to hazardous materials, and having routine cancer screening tests.

Immune Disorders

Immune disorders occur when the body comes under attack by its own cells. Often, the immune system can detect attacking cells such as cancer cells, and it is capable of destroying these harmful cells. If the immune system breaks down, due to infections such as HIV, age, chemotherapy, and other immune disorders, harmful cells can grow uncontrollably before the immune system is able to detect any danger.

In addition, some immune disorders cause the immune system to confuse its own cells with foreign organisms. Autoimmune diseases in which the immune system attacks the body's own cells include rheumatoid arthritis and lupus erythematosus.

Diabetes

Diabetes is a disease in which the pancreas does not produce insulin normally. There are three types of diabetes. Type I diabetes usually occurs in childhood and requires insulin injections to help the pancreas function. Type II diabetes can often be controlled by diet and exercise. Gestational diabetes is brought on during pregnancy and is a temporary condition that generally disappears at the end of pregnancy.

Other Factors Affecting Health

Asthma is caused by the inflammation of airways and a spasm of the muscles surrounding the airways. It can be linked to both biological and environmental factors. Asthma can be brought on by seasonal allergies, exercise, and occupational hazards. Anti-inflammatory drugs and muscle-relaxing medication can help relieve asthma symptoms.

Osteoarthritis is caused by the wear and tear of joints and is most common in older people. There is no cure for arthritis, but pain medication can help manage the symptoms.

Genetic disorders are inherited from biological parents. Parents pass one or two copies of a gene for an inheritable disease to an offspring. Some common inheritable, or genetic, diseases are hemophilia (blood disease), retinitis pitmentosa (eye disease), color blindness (eye disease), cystic fibrosis (lung disease), thalassemias (blood disorders), polydactyl (extra fingers or toes), achondroplasia (dwarfism), and polycystic kidney disease.

Some neurological disorders can also negatively affect health. Rett syndrome is a neurological disorder that affects brain development. It is similar to autism. Huntington's disease is characterized by the degeneration of brain cells in areas affecting intellect, emotional control, and muscle control.

Safety

Many injuries are caused by the interaction of humans with environmental factors or with other humans. Personal safety is necessary to protect oneself from harm or injury. It is necessary to be aware of one's surroundings and avoid atypical patterns in order to maintain safety. Residential safety, recreational safety, and motor vehicle safety are all ways to prevent injury.

Violence is defined as the intent to inflict harm on another person through physical force. Types of violence and intentional injury include assault, homicide, child abuse, sexual abuse, rape, gang-related violence, bullying, and terrorism. Alcohol and drug use often contribute to violence. Strategies for reducing violence include conflict resolution, developing social skills, and educational programs for victims and offenders.

Consumer awareness involves gathering information on health-related issues. As a nurse, you can provide materials for patient education, such as health reference publications and informational packets. In general, a patient should seek the help of a healthcare professional for symptoms that are severe, unusual, persistent, or recurrent.

Environmental health concerns include concern for air quality, global warming, various forms of pollution, and infectious diseases. Concern for water quality focuses on pathogenic organisms that can live in water, chemicals and hazardous waste that may contaminate a water supply, and water shortages (drought). Water can be polluted by animal waste, biological imbalance, pesticides, toxins, and other chemical waste that can cause mutations in DNA, cancer in certain cells, or birth defects in unborn offspring. Sewage and water treatment helps to prevent pathogens from polluting drinking water.

LAND POLLUTION IS CAUSED BY LANDFILLS THAT RELEASE CHEMICALS INTO THE GROUND, PESTICIDES, AUTOMOBILES, RADIATION, AND ACCIDENTAL CHEMICAL OR HAZARDOUS WASTE SPILLS. LAND POLLUTION CAN BE PREVENTED BY CONSERVATION EFFORTS IN AN EFFORT TO PREVENT CANCERS AND OTHER RELATED HEALTH PROBLEMS.

HEALTH GLOSSARY

TIP

This glossary is a helpful tool for those planning on taking the practical and vocational nursing school exam.

A

abductor A muscle that draws a part of the body away from the median line or normal position.

acetabulum The socket of the hip bone.

adductor A muscle that pulls a part of the body toward the median line.

adrenal glands The two small glands that are on the upper part of the kidneys.

adrenalin A hormone produced by the adrenal glands; a drug containing this hormone used to raise blood pressure.

alimentary canal The passageway in the body extending from the mouth to the anus.

alveolus An air cell of a lung; a tooth socket.

anatomy The science of the structure of plants and animals.

aorta The main artery of the body.

artery A blood vessel carrying blood away from the heart to all parts of the body.

atrium A chamber of the heart.

atrophy A wasting away or failure of an organ to grow.

auditory A term referring to the sense of hearing.

axilla The armpit.

B

backbone The column of bones (vertebrae) along the center of the back.

bile A substance produced by the liver and stored in the gallbladder.

brachial A term referring to the upper part of the forelimb of the vertebrae.

bronchus Either of the two main branches or tubes extending from the trachea (windpipe).

bursa A sac or cavity, especially between joints.

C

cardiac Of or near the heart.

caudal Near the tail.

cell The basic unit of protoplasm.

cephalic Of the head, skull, or cranium.

clavicle The collarbone.

clonus A series of muscle spasms.

colon The part of the large intestine extending from the cecum to the rectum.

conjunctiva The mucous membrane lining the inner surface of the eyelids and covering the front part of the eyeball.

cornea The transparent outer coating of the eyeball.

cranium The skull, especially that part containing the brain.

cutaneous Of or on the skin; affecting the skin.

D

dactyl A finger or toe.

dermis The layer of skin just below the epidermis.

digit A finger or toe.

duct A tube through which secretions or excretions pass through the body.

duodenum The first section of the small intestine below the stomach.

E

enamel The hard, white coating of the crowns of teeth.

endothelium A membrane that lines the heart, blood vessels, and lymphatic vessels.

epidermis The outermost layer of the skin.

esophagus The passage for food from the pharynx to the stomach; gullet.

eviscerate To remove the entrails from; disembowel.

extensor A muscle that straightens some part of the body.

F

fascia A thin layer of connective tissue.

femur The thighbone.

fibrin A protein formed in the clotting of blood.

flexor A muscle that bends a part of the body.

foramen A small opening.

G

ganglion A mass of nerve cells serving as a center from which nerve impulses are transmitted.

gastric In or near the stomach.

genitals The sexual organs.

glottis The opening between the vocal cords in the larynx.

gullet The esophagus.

H

hemoglobin The red coloring matter of the red blood cells.

humerus The bone of the upper arm or forelimb, extending from the shoulder to the elbow.

hyoid A U-shaped bone at the base of the tongue.

hypophysis The pituitary gland.

I

ileum The lowest part of the small intestine.

ilium The uppermost part of the three sections of the hipbone.

insulin A secretion of the pancreas that helps the body use sugar.

intestines The lower part of the alimentary canal, extending from the stomach to the anus.

J

jejunum The middle part of the small intestine.

jugular Two large veins in the neck carrying blood from the head to the heart.

K

kidney Either of a pair of organs that separate water and products from the blood and excrete them as urine through the bladder.

L

lacrimal Of, for, or producing tears.

larynx A structure serving as an organ of the voice.

ligament A band of tough tissue connecting bones or holding organs in place.

lumbar Pertaining to the small of the back.

lymph A clear, yellowish fluid found in the lymphatic system of the body.

lymphatic system A system of vessels and nodes that leads from the tissue spaces to large veins entering the heart.

M

mastication The act of chewing.

maxilla The upper jawbone.

membrane A thin, soft layer of tissue that covers or lines an organ or part.

meninges The three membranes that enclose the brain and spinal cord.

meningitis Inflammation of the meninges.

metacarpals The bones in the hand between the wrist and the fingers.

metatarsals The bones in the foot between the ankle and toes.

mucous A membrane lining cavities leading to the outside of the body, such as to the mouth, membrane anus, etc.

mucus The slimy secretion that moistens and protects the mucous membrane.

N

neural Pertaining to the nerves or the nervous system.

nutrition The series or processes by which an organism takes in and assimilates food for promoting growth and repairing tissues.

O

occiput The back of the skull or head.

ocular Pertaining to the eye.

olfactory A term referring to the sense of smell.

ophthalmic Of or connected with the eyes.

optic nerve The nerve running from the brain to the eye.

orbit The eye socket.

osteology The study of bones.

P

pancreas The gland that secretes insulin and other digestive juices.

parathyroid Four small glands embedded in the thyroid gland; their secretions increase the calcium content in the blood.

pathogenic Disease-producing.

pepsin An enzyme secreted in the stomach, aiding in the digestion of proteins.

pharynx The cavity extending from the mouth and nasal passages to the larynx and esophagus; throat.

placenta The structure through which the fetus is nourished.

protoplasm The essential living matter of animal and plant cells.

protozoa A one-celled microscopic animal.

pubis The bone that makes up the front part of the pelvis.

Q

quadrant A term referring to four or part of four.

quadruped A mammal or animal with four feet.

R

radius The bone of the forearm on the same side as the thumb.

rectum The lowest segment of the large intestine, ending at the anus.

retina The innermost coating of the back part of the eyeball.

riboflavin A factor of the vitamin B complex, found in milk, eggs, liver, fruits, leafy vegetables, etc.

S

scapula The shoulder blade.

semen The fluid secreted by the male reproductive organs containing sperm.

sphincter A round muscle that can open or close a natural opening in the body by expanding and contracting.

sternum The breastbone.

striated Streaked with fine lines.

T

tarsals The bones of the ankle.

tendons The connective tissue that joins muscles to bones.

thrombin A substance that aids in the clotting of blood.

thyroid gland A large ductless gland near the trachea that produces thyroxine, which regulates metabolism.

tibia The inner bone of the leg below the knee; shinbone.

trachea The windpipe; the tube that conveys air from the larynx to the bronchi.

U

ulna The bone of the forearm on the side opposite the thumb.

urea A soluble, crystalline solid, found in urine.

urine A yellowish fluid in mammals, containing urea and other waste products.

V

vagina In female mammals, the canal leading from the vulva to the uterus.

vermiform A small saclike appendage of the large intestine.

viscera The internal organs of the body, such as the heart, lungs, stomach, etc.

vomer A bone forming part of the nasal septum.

Z

zoology The branch of biology dealing with the classification of animals and the study of animal life.

ANSWER SHEET

Test 1

1. Ⓐ Ⓑ Ⓒ Ⓓ	9. Ⓐ Ⓑ Ⓒ Ⓓ	17. Ⓐ Ⓑ Ⓒ Ⓓ	25. Ⓐ Ⓑ Ⓒ Ⓓ	33. Ⓐ Ⓑ Ⓒ Ⓓ
2. Ⓐ Ⓑ Ⓒ Ⓓ	10. Ⓐ Ⓑ Ⓒ Ⓓ	18. Ⓐ Ⓑ Ⓒ Ⓓ	26. Ⓐ Ⓑ Ⓒ Ⓓ	34. Ⓐ Ⓑ Ⓒ Ⓓ
3. Ⓐ Ⓑ Ⓒ Ⓓ	11. Ⓐ Ⓑ Ⓒ Ⓓ	19. Ⓐ Ⓑ Ⓒ Ⓓ	27. Ⓐ Ⓑ Ⓒ Ⓓ	35. Ⓐ Ⓑ Ⓒ Ⓓ
4. Ⓐ Ⓑ Ⓒ Ⓓ	12. Ⓐ Ⓑ Ⓒ Ⓓ	20. Ⓐ Ⓑ Ⓒ Ⓓ	28. Ⓐ Ⓑ Ⓒ Ⓓ	36. Ⓐ Ⓑ Ⓒ Ⓓ
5. Ⓐ Ⓑ Ⓒ Ⓓ	13. Ⓐ Ⓑ Ⓒ Ⓓ	21. Ⓐ Ⓑ Ⓒ Ⓓ	29. Ⓐ Ⓑ Ⓒ Ⓓ	37. Ⓐ Ⓑ Ⓒ Ⓓ
6. Ⓐ Ⓑ Ⓒ Ⓓ	14. Ⓐ Ⓑ Ⓒ Ⓓ	22. Ⓐ Ⓑ Ⓒ Ⓓ	30. Ⓐ Ⓑ Ⓒ Ⓓ	38. Ⓐ Ⓑ Ⓒ Ⓓ
7. Ⓐ Ⓑ Ⓒ Ⓓ	15. Ⓐ Ⓑ Ⓒ Ⓓ	23. Ⓐ Ⓑ Ⓒ Ⓓ	31. Ⓐ Ⓑ Ⓒ Ⓓ	39. Ⓐ Ⓑ Ⓒ Ⓓ
8. Ⓐ Ⓑ Ⓒ Ⓓ	16. Ⓐ Ⓑ Ⓒ Ⓓ	24. Ⓐ Ⓑ Ⓒ Ⓓ	32. Ⓐ Ⓑ Ⓒ Ⓓ	40. Ⓐ Ⓑ Ⓒ Ⓓ

Test 2

1. Ⓐ Ⓑ Ⓒ Ⓓ	7. Ⓐ Ⓑ Ⓒ Ⓓ	13. Ⓐ Ⓑ Ⓒ Ⓓ	19. Ⓐ Ⓑ Ⓒ Ⓓ	25. Ⓐ Ⓑ Ⓒ Ⓓ
2. Ⓐ Ⓑ Ⓒ Ⓓ	8. Ⓐ Ⓑ Ⓒ Ⓓ	14. Ⓐ Ⓑ Ⓒ Ⓓ	20. Ⓐ Ⓑ Ⓒ Ⓓ	26. Ⓐ Ⓑ Ⓒ Ⓓ
3. Ⓐ Ⓑ Ⓒ Ⓓ	9. Ⓐ Ⓑ Ⓒ Ⓓ	15. Ⓐ Ⓑ Ⓒ Ⓓ	21. Ⓐ Ⓑ Ⓒ Ⓓ	27. Ⓐ Ⓑ Ⓒ Ⓓ
4. Ⓐ Ⓑ Ⓒ Ⓓ	10. Ⓐ Ⓑ Ⓒ Ⓓ	16. Ⓐ Ⓑ Ⓒ Ⓓ	22. Ⓐ Ⓑ Ⓒ Ⓓ	28. Ⓐ Ⓑ Ⓒ Ⓓ
5. Ⓐ Ⓑ Ⓒ Ⓓ	11. Ⓐ Ⓑ Ⓒ Ⓓ	17. Ⓐ Ⓑ Ⓒ Ⓓ	23. Ⓐ Ⓑ Ⓒ Ⓓ	29. Ⓐ Ⓑ Ⓒ Ⓓ
6. Ⓐ Ⓑ Ⓒ Ⓓ	12. Ⓐ Ⓑ Ⓒ Ⓓ	18. Ⓐ Ⓑ Ⓒ Ⓓ	24. Ⓐ Ⓑ Ⓒ Ⓓ	30. Ⓐ Ⓑ Ⓒ Ⓓ

Test 3

1. Ⓐ Ⓑ Ⓒ Ⓓ	7. Ⓐ Ⓑ Ⓒ Ⓓ	13. Ⓐ Ⓑ Ⓒ Ⓓ	19. Ⓐ Ⓑ Ⓒ Ⓓ	25. Ⓐ Ⓑ Ⓒ Ⓓ
2. Ⓐ Ⓑ Ⓒ Ⓓ	8. Ⓐ Ⓑ Ⓒ Ⓓ	14. Ⓐ Ⓑ Ⓒ Ⓓ	20. Ⓐ Ⓑ Ⓒ Ⓓ	26. Ⓐ Ⓑ Ⓒ Ⓓ
3. Ⓐ Ⓑ Ⓒ Ⓓ	9. Ⓐ Ⓑ Ⓒ Ⓓ	15. Ⓐ Ⓑ Ⓒ Ⓓ	21. Ⓐ Ⓑ Ⓒ Ⓓ	27. Ⓐ Ⓑ Ⓒ Ⓓ
4. Ⓐ Ⓑ Ⓒ Ⓓ	10. Ⓐ Ⓑ Ⓒ Ⓓ	16. Ⓐ Ⓑ Ⓒ Ⓓ	22. Ⓐ Ⓑ Ⓒ Ⓓ	28. Ⓐ Ⓑ Ⓒ Ⓓ
5. Ⓐ Ⓑ Ⓒ Ⓓ	11. Ⓐ Ⓑ Ⓒ Ⓓ	17. Ⓐ Ⓑ Ⓒ Ⓓ	23. Ⓐ Ⓑ Ⓒ Ⓓ	29. Ⓐ Ⓑ Ⓒ Ⓓ
6. Ⓐ Ⓑ Ⓒ Ⓓ	12. Ⓐ Ⓑ Ⓒ Ⓓ	18. Ⓐ Ⓑ Ⓒ Ⓓ	24. Ⓐ Ⓑ Ⓒ Ⓓ	30. Ⓐ Ⓑ Ⓒ Ⓓ

answer sheet

Test 4

1. Ⓐ Ⓑ Ⓒ Ⓓ	15. Ⓐ Ⓑ Ⓒ Ⓓ	29. Ⓐ Ⓑ Ⓒ Ⓓ	43. Ⓐ Ⓑ Ⓒ Ⓓ	57. Ⓐ Ⓑ Ⓒ Ⓓ
2. Ⓐ Ⓑ Ⓒ Ⓓ	16. Ⓐ Ⓑ Ⓒ Ⓓ	30. Ⓐ Ⓑ Ⓒ Ⓓ	44. Ⓐ Ⓑ Ⓒ Ⓓ	58. Ⓐ Ⓑ Ⓒ Ⓓ
3. Ⓐ Ⓑ Ⓒ Ⓓ	17. Ⓐ Ⓑ Ⓒ Ⓓ	31. Ⓐ Ⓑ Ⓒ Ⓓ	45. Ⓐ Ⓑ Ⓒ Ⓓ	59. Ⓐ Ⓑ Ⓒ Ⓓ
4. Ⓐ Ⓑ Ⓒ Ⓓ	18. Ⓐ Ⓑ Ⓒ Ⓓ	32. Ⓐ Ⓑ Ⓒ Ⓓ	46. Ⓐ Ⓑ Ⓒ Ⓓ	60. Ⓐ Ⓑ Ⓒ Ⓓ
5. Ⓐ Ⓑ Ⓒ Ⓓ	19. Ⓐ Ⓑ Ⓒ Ⓓ	33. Ⓐ Ⓑ Ⓒ Ⓓ	47. Ⓐ Ⓑ Ⓒ Ⓓ	61. Ⓐ Ⓑ Ⓒ Ⓓ
6. Ⓐ Ⓑ Ⓒ Ⓓ	20. Ⓐ Ⓑ Ⓒ Ⓓ	34. Ⓐ Ⓑ Ⓒ Ⓓ	48. Ⓐ Ⓑ Ⓒ Ⓓ	62. Ⓐ Ⓑ Ⓒ Ⓓ
7. Ⓐ Ⓑ Ⓒ Ⓓ	21. Ⓐ Ⓑ Ⓒ Ⓓ	35. Ⓐ Ⓑ Ⓒ Ⓓ	49. Ⓐ Ⓑ Ⓒ Ⓓ	63. Ⓐ Ⓑ Ⓒ Ⓓ
8. Ⓐ Ⓑ Ⓒ Ⓓ	22. Ⓐ Ⓑ Ⓒ Ⓓ	36. Ⓐ Ⓑ Ⓒ Ⓓ	50. Ⓐ Ⓑ Ⓒ Ⓓ	64. Ⓐ Ⓑ Ⓒ Ⓓ
9. Ⓐ Ⓑ Ⓒ Ⓓ	23. Ⓐ Ⓑ Ⓒ Ⓓ	37. Ⓐ Ⓑ Ⓒ Ⓓ	51. Ⓐ Ⓑ Ⓒ Ⓓ	65. Ⓐ Ⓑ Ⓒ Ⓓ
10. Ⓐ Ⓑ Ⓒ Ⓓ	24. Ⓐ Ⓑ Ⓒ Ⓓ	38. Ⓐ Ⓑ Ⓒ Ⓓ	52. Ⓐ Ⓑ Ⓒ Ⓓ	66. Ⓐ Ⓑ Ⓒ Ⓓ
11. Ⓐ Ⓑ Ⓒ Ⓓ	25. Ⓐ Ⓑ Ⓒ Ⓓ	39. Ⓐ Ⓑ Ⓒ Ⓓ	53. Ⓐ Ⓑ Ⓒ Ⓓ	67. Ⓐ Ⓑ Ⓒ Ⓓ
12. Ⓐ Ⓑ Ⓒ Ⓓ	26. Ⓐ Ⓑ Ⓒ Ⓓ	40. Ⓐ Ⓑ Ⓒ Ⓓ	54. Ⓐ Ⓑ Ⓒ Ⓓ	68. Ⓐ Ⓑ Ⓒ Ⓓ
13. Ⓐ Ⓑ Ⓒ Ⓓ	27. Ⓐ Ⓑ Ⓒ Ⓓ	41. Ⓐ Ⓑ Ⓒ Ⓓ	55. Ⓐ Ⓑ Ⓒ Ⓓ	69. Ⓐ Ⓑ Ⓒ Ⓓ
14. Ⓐ Ⓑ Ⓒ Ⓓ	28. Ⓐ Ⓑ Ⓒ Ⓓ	42. Ⓐ Ⓑ Ⓒ Ⓓ	56. Ⓐ Ⓑ Ⓒ Ⓓ	70. Ⓐ Ⓑ Ⓒ Ⓓ

TEST 1

40 Questions • 35 Minutes

Directions: Each question or incomplete statement below is followed by four suggested answers or completions. For each question, select the best choice and fill in the corresponding space on your answer sheet.

1. Muscles whose functions are to close off body openings are
   (A) flexors.
   (B) sphincters.
   (C) extensors.
   (D) adductors.

2. Bile aids in the digestion of
   (A) amino acids.
   (B) fats.
   (C) starches.
   (D) carbohydrates.

3. Urea is removed from the blood as it goes through the
   (A) bladder.
   (B) pancreas.
   (C) spleen.
   (D) kidney.

4. The blood group of a universal recipient is
   (A) AB
   (B) B
   (C) O
   (D) A

5. The stimulant in coffee is
   (A) tannic acid.
   (B) theobromine.
   (C) theophylline.
   (D) caffeine.

6. Which of the following foods is the most economical source of proteins?
   (A) Dried milk
   (B) Green leafy vegetables
   (C) Meats
   (D) Eggs

7. Connective tissue that attaches muscles to the bones is called
   (A) tendons.
   (B) ligaments.
   (C) cartilage.
   (D) osseous.

8. The hormone produced by the testes is
   (A) progesterone.
   (B) estrogen.
   (C) testosterone.
   (D) aldosterone.

9. The elbow joint is an example of
   (A) ball-and-socket joint.
   (B) hinge joint.
   (C) pivot joint.
   (D) saddle joint.

10. The movement that propels food down the digestive tract is called
    (A) pyloraspasm.
    (B) rugae.
    (C) mastication.
    (D) peristalsis.

11. In mumps, the gland affected is the
    (A) parathyroid.
    (B) pituitary.
    (C) parotid.
    (D) pineal.

12. The negative-charged particle found within the atom is the
    (A) proton.
    (B) electron.
    (C) nucleus.
    (D) neutron.

13. The exchange of nutrients and waste products occurs in the
    (A) venules.
    (B) capillaries.
    (C) arterioles.
    (D) arteries.

14. Hemoglobin is found in
    (A) basophils.
    (B) neutrophils.
    (C) monocytes.
    (D) erythrocytes.

15. Organic substances made up of several amino acids bound together are
    (A) carbohydrates.
    (B) fats.
    (C) proteins.
    (D) fatty acids.

16. The exchange of carbon dioxide and oxygen in the lungs occurs in the
    (A) venules.
    (B) alveoli.
    (C) bronchi.
    (D) bronchioles.

17. The pacemaker of the heart is the
    (A) Bundle of His.
    (B) AV node.
    (C) purkinje fibers.
    (D) SA node.

18. Mitral stenosis involves the
    (A) aortic valve.
    (B) pulmonary valve.
    (C) bicuspid valve.
    (D) tricuspid valve.

19. The smallest known microorganisms are
    (A) bacteria.
    (B) viruses.
    (C) fungi.
    (D) protozoa.

20. Which one of the following arteries carries deoxygenated blood?
    (A) Pulmonary
    (B) Coronary
    (C) Vena cava
    (D) Aorta

21. Electrolyte balance is maintained primarily by the action of the
    (A) testes.
    (B) kidney.
    (C) bladder.
    (D) liver.

22. The mineral that is necessary for the proper functioning of the thyroid gland is
    (A) sodium.
    (B) iodine.
    (C) calcium.
    (D) iron.

23. Vitamin C prevents
    (A) beriberi.
    (B) rickets.
    (C) pellagra.
    (D) scurvy.

24. The function of leukocytes is to
    (A) carry oxygen.
    (B) destroy bacteria.
    (C) carry food.
    (D) regulate metabolism.

25. Insulin is produced in the
    (A) pituitary gland.
    (B) thymus.
    (C) pancreas.
    (D) pineal gland.

26. The end product of protein metabolism is
    (A) amino acids.
    (B) glucose.
    (C) glycogen.
    (D) fatty acids.

27. Carbohydrates are absorbed into the blood as
    (A) glycogen.
    (B) amino acids.
    (C) glucose.
    (D) fatty acids.

28. When one muscle of a pair contracts, the opposing muscle must
    (A) also contract.
    (B) relax.
    (C) produce more energy.
    (D) remain in the same position.

29. The respiratory center is located in the part of the brain known as the
    (A) thalamus.
    (B) cerebrum.
    (C) pons.
    (D) medulla oblongata.

30. Rays pass through various parts of the eye in a process of bending called
    (A) refraction.
    (B) reflexion.
    (C) retraction.
    (D) retroversion.

31. The part of the eye commonly called the "window" is the
    (A) retina.
    (B) cornea.
    (C) lens.
    (D) pupil.

32. A calorie is a form of
    (A) light.
    (B) heat.
    (C) darkness.
    (D) sound.

33. The vitamin known as the "sunshine" vitamin is
    (A) vitamin E.
    (B) vitamin B.
    (C) vitamin K.
    (D) vitamin D.

34. The process by which the body changes food into substances that can be readily used by the body is
    (A) digestion.
    (B) deglutition.
    (C) micturition.
    (D) absorption.

35. The thyroid gland cannot function properly without
    (A) chloride.
    (B) iodine.
    (C) phosphorous.
    (D) iron.

36. The vitamin that is necessary for coagulation of the blood is
    (A) vitamin K.
    (B) vitamin C.
    (C) vitamin A.
    (D) vitamin E.

37. Another name for vitamin B_1 is
    (A) niacin.
    (B) thiamin.
    (C) riboflavin.
    (D) pyridoxine.

38. Food is moved through the alimentary canal by wave-like motions called
    (A) excretions.
    (B) mastication.
    (C) contractions.
    (D) peristalsis.

39. The femur is a bone located in the
(A) forearm.
(B) upper arm.
(C) thigh.
(D) lower leg.

40. The liquid portion of the blood is called
(A) serum.
(B) gamma globulin.
(C) plasma.
(D) lymph.

STOP

IF YOU FINISH BEFORE TIME IS CALLED, YOU MAY CHECK YOUR WORK ON THIS SECTION ONLY. DO NOT TURN TO ANY OTHER SECTION IN THE TEST.

TEST 2

30 Questions • 25 Minutes

Directions: For each question, choose the answer that you consider correct or most nearly correct. Fill in the corresponding space on your answer sheet.

1. The force of the blood exerted against the wall of the blood vessel is called
   (A) pulse deficit.
   (B) apical pulse.
   (C) blood pressure.
   (D) pulse pressure.

2. The relative amount of moisture in the air is the
   (A) evaporation factor.
   (B) temperature.
   (C) dew.
   (D) humidity.

3. A laboratory sample is called a(n)
   (A) collection.
   (B) agar.
   (C) specimen.
   (D) symptom.

4. Defecation means
   (A) swallowing.
   (B) eliminating solid waste.
   (C) irrigating the colon.
   (D) relieving flatus.

5. An object completely free of all microorganisms is
   (A) sterile.
   (B) clean.
   (C) septic.
   (D) contaminated.

6. Carbon dioxide is a
   (A) respiratory depressant.
   (B) circulatory stimulant.
   (C) respiratory stimulant.
   (D) circulatory depressant.

7. The presence of protein in the urine is called
   (A) polyuria.
   (B) anuria.
   (C) albuminuria.
   (D) hematuria.

8. The substance basic to life is
   (A) carbohydrates.
   (B) proteins.
   (C) starches.
   (D) fats.

9. In diseases of the gallbladder, which of the following nutrients is limited?
   (A) Starches
   (B) Proteins
   (C) Fats
   (D) Carbohydrates

10. Water-soluble vitamins include
    (A) vitamin A.
    (B) vitamin C.
    (C) vitamin D.
    (D) vitamin K.

11. Diets in the United States are most often deficient in
    (A) iron and calcium.
    (B) calcium and potassium.
    (C) iodine and sodium.
    (D) phosphorous and iron.

12. Tetany may be corrected by increasing the amount of
    (A) iron.
    (B) iodine.
    (C) calcium.
    (D) thiamine.

13. Which helps conserve body heat?

    (A) Increased sweat production

    (B) Increased respiratory activity

    (C) Dilation of the capillaries of the skin

    (D) Constriction of the capillaries of the skin

14. Milk is not a "perfect food" because it lacks

    (A) iron.

    (B) calcium.

    (C) phosphorous.

    (D) carbohydrates.

15. The body obtains most of its nitrogen from

    (A) carbohydrates.

    (B) proteins.

    (C) fats.

    (D) cellulose.

16. An ion is

    (A) one molecule of water.

    (B) one particle of hydrogen.

    (C) the same as a neutron.

    (D) an atom with an electric charge.

17. The basic unit of the living organism is

    (A) the brain.

    (B) the cell.

    (C) a tissue.

    (D) the nervous system.

18. The diffusion of water through a semipermeable membrane is known as

    (A) anabolism.

    (B) synthesis.

    (C) mitosis.

    (D) osmosis.

19. A physician who specializes in diseases of the heart is known as a

    (A) dermatologist.

    (B) cardiologist.

    (C) pediatrician.

    (D) neurologist.

20. A fracture that occurs without breaking through the skin is called

    (A) complex.

    (B) compound.

    (C) greenstick.

    (D) comminuted.

21. Smoking and pollution, which have a deadly effect upon the lungs and pulmonary function, are classified as

    (A) environmental factors.

    (B) biological factors.

    (C) sociological factors.

    (D) physiological factors.

22. In the digestive process, almost all of the water is reabsorbed by the

    (A) sigmoid.

    (B) cecum.

    (C) colon.

    (D) rectum.

23. In what structure does fertilization normally occur?

    (A) Vagina

    (B) Cervix

    (C) Ovary

    (D) Fallopian tube

24. The process in which carbon dioxide and water are combined under the influence of light in green plants is called

    (A) respiration.

    (B) fermentation.

    (C) assimilation.

    (D) photosynthesis.

25. The most abundant gas in the atmosphere is

    (A) oxygen.

    (B) nitrogen.

    (C) carbon dioxide.

    (D) chlorine.

26. A protein substance that initiates and accelerates a chemical reaction is called a(n)

    (A) gene.

    (B) enzyme.

    (C) hormone.

    (D) base.

27. Amino acids that cannot be manufactured by the body are called

    (A) essential amino acids.

    (B) synthetic amino acids.

    (C) basic amino acids.

    (D) dependent amino acids.

28. The instrument used to measure air pressure is called a

    (A) thermometer.

    (B) hydrometer.

    (C) barometer.

    (D) sphygmomanometer.

29. An elevation above normal body temperature is called

    (A) hypothermia.

    (B) pyrexia.

    (C) intermittent.

    (D) remittent.

30. The instrument used to examine the ears is called a(n)

    (A) ophthalmoscope.

    (B) stethoscope.

    (C) cystoscope.

    (D) otoscope.

STOP

IF YOU FINISH BEFORE TIME IS CALLED, YOU MAY CHECK YOUR WORK ON THIS SECTION ONLY. DO NOT TURN TO ANY OTHER SECTION IN THE TEST.

TEST 3

30 Questions • 25 Minutes

Directions: For each question, choose the answer that you consider correct. Fill in the corresponding space on your answer sheet.

1. The body's continuous response to changes in the external and internal environment is called
   (A) homeostasis.
   (B) diffusion.
   (C) osmosis.
   (D) filtration.

2. The ability of a cell to reproduce is called
   (A) osmosis.
   (B) crenation.
   (C) lysis.
   (D) mitosis.

3. The immunity that occurs when a person is given a substance containing antibodies or antitoxins is called
   (A) active.
   (B) autoimmune.
   (C) passive.
   (D) permanent.

4. The part of the cell necessary for reproduction is the
   (A) cytoplasm.
   (B) nucleus.
   (C) protoplasm.
   (D) cytoplasmic membrane.

5. The hormone that regulates the metabolic rate of the body cells is
   (A) oxytocin.
   (B) aldosterone.
   (C) thyroxin.
   (D) cortisone.

6. The sudoriferous glands secrete
   (A) sebum.
   (B) perspiration.
   (C) hormones.
   (D) synovial fluid.

7. Tanning of the skin is due to
   (A) keratin.
   (B) sebum.
   (C) sweat.
   (D) melanin.

8. The ovaries produce the hormones
   (A) estrogen and testosterone.
   (B) progesterone and testosterone.
   (C) estrogen and progesterone.
   (D) progesterone and prolactin.

9. The tissue that forms a protective covering for the body and lines the intestinal and respiratory tract is called the
   (A) periosteum.
   (B) pericardium.
   (C) epithelium.
   (D) connective tissue.

10. The hip joint is an example of a
    (A) ball and socket joint.
    (B) hinge joint.
    (C) pivot joint.
    (D) saddle joint.

11. The endocrine gland that prepares the body for the "fight or flight" response is the
    (A) adrenal cortex.
    (B) adrenal medulla.
    (C) pituitary.
    (D) thyroid.

12. Tears drain into the nose through the
    (A) ciliary body.
    (B) lacrimal gland.
    (C) eustachian tube.
    (D) nasolacrimal duct.

13. Respiration and heart rate are controlled
    by the
    (A) cerebellum.
    (B) cerebrum.
    (C) medulla oblongota.
    (D) pons.

14. The main function of the large intestine is
    to
    (A) absorb digested food.
    (B) absorb water from waste materials.
    (C) produce digestive enzymes.
    (D) secrete digestive enzymes.

15. The hormone produced by the adrenal
    glands is
    (A) progesterone.
    (B) estrogen.
    (C) testosterone.
    (D) aldosterone.

16. The sloughing off of the endometrium is
    called
    (A) menarche.
    (B) menopause.
    (C) menstruation.
    (D) myometritis.

17. The dorsal cavity has two subdivisions,
    namely
    (A) thoracic and abdominopelvic.
    (B) cranial and spinal.
    (C) thoracic and spinal.
    (D) medial and lateral.

18. The chamber of the heart that receives
    venous blood from body tissue is the
    (A) right atrium.
    (B) left atrium.
    (C) right ventricle.
    (D) left ventricle.

19. The major work of the heart is completed
    by the
    (A) right ventricle.
    (B) left ventricle.
    (C) right atrium.
    (D) left atrium.

20. The shape of the eyeball is maintained by
    the
    (A) aqueous humor.
    (B) vitreous humor.
    (C) eye muscles.
    (D) eyelid.

21. The inner lining of the heart is the
    (A) endocardium.
    (B) myocardium.
    (C) pericardium.
    (D) pleura.

22. The muscular structure that forms the floor
    of the pelvis is the
    (A) peritoneum.
    (B) perineum.
    (C) mons pubis.
    (D) rectus abdominis.

23. The large, round portion at the upper and
    lateral portion of the femur most often
    involved in hip fractures is the
    (A) acetabulum.
    (B) acromiom.
    (C) greater trochanter.
    (D) tricuspid valve.

24. One of the large muscles that is used in climbing stairs and that forms most of the buttocks is the
    (A) gluteus maximus.
    (B) gluteus medius.
    (C) vastus lateralis.
    (D) vastus medialis.

25. The basic unit of function of the kidney is the
    (A) medulla.
    (B) hilus.
    (C) nephron.
    (D) cortex.

26. Which of the following is abnormal for urine?
    (A) Clear, amber liquid
    (B) Nitrogenous waste products
    (C) Slightly aromatic
    (D) High specific gravity

27. The hormone that regulates blood composition and blood volume by acting on the kidney is
    (A) antidiuretic (ADH).
    (B) aldosterone.
    (C) parathormone.
    (D) oxytocin.

28. Composition of urine normally includes
    (A) creatinine, urea, and water.
    (B) creatinine, ammonia, and sugar.
    (C) nitrogen wastes, sugar, and hormones.
    (D) nitrogen wastes, water, and pus cells.

29. An injury to the left motor area of the cerebrum would cause paralysis of
    (A) the right side of the body.
    (B) the left side of the body.
    (C) both arms and legs.
    (D) both arms.

30. Electrolyte balance is maintained chiefly by the action of the
    (A) bladder.
    (B) kidney.
    (C) islets of Langerhans.
    (D) gonads.

STOP

IF YOU FINISH BEFORE TIME IS CALLED, YOU MAY CHECK YOUR WORK ON THIS SECTION ONLY. DO NOT TURN TO ANY OTHER SECTION IN THE TEST.

TEST 4

70 Questions • 70 Minutes

Directions: Read each question carefully and consider all possible answers. When you have decided which choice is best, fill in the corresponding space on your answer sheet. There is only one best answer for each question.

1. Diabetes mellitus initially results from
   (A) oversecretion of pancreatin.
   (B) undersecretion of insulin.
   (C) excessive intake of sugar.
   (D) inadequate intake of fats.

2. The so-called "bag of water," which breaks during labor in the pregnant female, is the
   (A) amniotic sac.
   (B) yolk sac.
   (C) placenta.
   (D) chorionic membrane.

3. Sebaceous glands are most numerous in areas where
   (A) there are small amounts of hair.
   (B) there are large amounts of hair.
   (C) the skin is thin.
   (D) sweat glands are located.

4. Hereditary determiners are found in
   (A) PKU.
   (B) RNA.
   (C) DNA.
   (D) SMA.

5. Skin color varies with the amount of
   (A) melanin.
   (B) matrix.
   (C) hair.
   (D) keratin.

6. The deciduous teeth contain no
   (A) cuspids.
   (B) bicuspids.
   (C) canines.
   (D) incisors.

7. The material covering the surface of the tooth below the gum line is
   (A) cementum.
   (B) dentine.
   (C) enamel.
   (D) pulp.

8. Hemoglobin is a molecule composed principally of
   (A) ferritin.
   (B) amino acids.
   (C) iron.
   (D) myosin.

9. The sex of a new individual is determined by
   (A) the female.
   (B) the male.
   (C) either the female or the male.
   (D) neither the female nor the male.

10. The umbilical cord is cut immediately after a baby is born because
    (A) of the need to stop circulation between the fetus and the placenta.
    (B) the mother's blood will contaminate the baby's blood.
    (C) the baby has less need for blood.
    (D) the mother will hemorrhage.

11. The major difference between plasma and blood is
    (A) cellular content.
    (B) acid-base balance.
    (C) anion-cation placement.
    (D) solute-solvent concentrations.

12. The blood cells that cause blood clotting are called
    (A) leucocytes.
    (B) erythrocytes.
    (C) thrombocytes.
    (D) lymphocytes.

13. The longest, strongest, and heaviest bone in the body is the
    (A) tibia.
    (B) spinal column.
    (C) femur.
    (D) radius.

14. Iron is needed for
    (A) development of nervous tissue.
    (B) formation of red blood cells.
    (C) growth of hair and nails.
    (D) utilization of vitamins.

15. Which of the following is necessary for digestion?
    (A) Transamination
    (B) Glucogenolysis
    (C) Krebs cycle
    (D) Peristalsis

16. Which of the following organs is vital to life?
    (A) Adrenal glands
    (B) Thymus
    (C) Liver
    (D) Spleen

17. Gram-negative bacterial pathogens are generally more difficult to treat clinically than grampositive due to differences in
    (A) cell wall compositions.
    (B) ribosomes.
    (C) nucleon regions.
    (D) mesosomes.

18. Three-dimensional vision is related to which of the following structures?
    (A) Iris
    (B) Pupil
    (C) Optic chiasma
    (D) Retina

19. Urea formation is the human body's method of eliminating excess
    (A) carbon.
    (B) hydrogen.
    (C) nitrogen.
    (D) phosphorus.

20. Which of the following hormones is predominant in females?
    (A) Androgen
    (B) Testosterone
    (C) Gonadotrophin
    (D) Estrogen

21. Proteins are polymers of
    (A) hydrocarbons.
    (B) amino acids.
    (C) heterocyclics.
    (D) alcohols.

22. Which one of the following statements is true?
    (A) Bone marrow produces red blood cells in the adult.
    (B) The spleen synthesizes vitamins in the child.
    (C) The liver manufactures glucose and stores bile.
    (D) The lymphatic system refines fats and stores water.

23. The most widely distributed of all tissues is
    (A) epithelial.
    (B) muscle.
    (C) connective.
    (D) nervous.

24. The chemical reaction that supplies immediate energy for muscular contractions can be summarized as

    (A) $ATP \rightarrow ADP + P$.
    (B) lactic acid $\rightarrow CO_2 + H_2O$.
    (C) lactic acid $\rightarrow$ glycogen.
    (D) glycogen $\rightarrow ATP$.

25. The body's reaction to stress includes which of the following mechanisms?

    (A) Conversion of carbohydrates into glycogen
    (B) Decreased pumping action of the heart
    (C) Secretion of adrenalin
    (D) Pooling of blood in the veins

26. After rigorous exercise, the body is depleted of

    (A) Na and H_2O.
    (B) glucose and H_2O.
    (C) H_2O and K.
    (D) H_2O and colloids.

27. Which of the following is related to the cause of heart disease?

    (A) Absence of serum transaminase
    (B) Accumulation of urea nitrogen
    (C) Decreased levels of bilirubin
    (D) Increased levels of blood cholesterol

28. The endocrine glands in the body have the function of

    (A) purifying the blood.
    (B) regulating bodily activities.
    (C) controlling the blood distribution.
    (D) preventing antigenic action.

29. Persons with overactive thyroids have which of the following changes in body functions?

    (A) Decrease in metabolic rate
    (B) Increase in metabolic rate
    (C) Loss of appetite
    (D) Gain in weight

30. The basic unit of the lung tissue is

    (A) lacuna.
    (B) nephron.
    (C) alveolus.
    (D) cyton.

31. Hemorrhoids, commonly called piles, affect which of the following structures?

    (A) Pyloric sphincter
    (B) Rectal sphincter
    (C) Urethral orifice
    (D) Mitral orifice

32. Before amino acids can be metabolized to release energy, which of the following must occur?

    (A) Fermentation
    (B) Hydrolysis
    (C) Deamination
    (D) Anabolism

33. A biochemical reaction, common to the digestion of carbohydrates, lipids, and proteins, is enzymatic

    (A) fermentation.
    (B) deamination.
    (C) glycogenolysis.
    (D) hydrolysis.

34. Fats yield more calories per gram and oxidize slower than carbohydrates, proteins, and nucleic acids due to excess atoms of

    (A) hydrogen.
    (B) oxygen.
    (C) nitrogen.
    (D) phosphorus.

35. In the circulatory system, oxygenated blood is pumped out of the heart from the

    (A) right ventricle.
    (B) left ventricle.
    (C) right atrium.
    (D) left atrium.

36. A person who escapes major infections and accidental death has an enhanced probability of living to age 100 if his or her apolipoprotein (E) allelic gene combination is
    (A) E-2/E-4
    (B) E-3/E-4
    (C) E-2/E-2
    (D) E-4/E-4

37. Smooth muscle tissue is found in the
    (A) heart.
    (B) kidneys.
    (C) intestines.
    (D) skeletal muscles.

38. The exchange of gases between the respiratory system and the circulatory system is by means of the pulmonary
    (A) arteries.
    (B) veins.
    (C) capillaries.
    (D) venules.

39. In the production of monoclonal antibodies, antigens and lymphocytes from an experimental animal are fused with myeloma tumor cells to form a cell-type known as which of the following?
    (A) Hydroma.
    (B) Polycloma.
    (C) Hybridoma.
    (D) None of the above

40. In systemic circulation, venous blood is different from arterial blood in that the
    (A) CO_2 concentration is lower than the O_2 concentration.
    (B) CO_2 concentration is higher than the O_2 concentration.
    (C) overall concentration is high and the rate of flow is low.
    (D) overall concentration is low and the rate of flow is high.

41. Sperm and egg cells have the haploid number of chromosomes as a result of
    (A) meiosis.
    (B) cleavage.
    (C) mitosis.
    (D) fertilization.

42. Fraternal twins develop from
    (A) one fertilized egg.
    (B) two fertilized eggs.
    (C) one egg fertilized by two sperms.
    (D) two eggs fertilized by the same sperm.

43. The term *restriction fragment length polymorphism (RFLP)* refers to differences in length between
    (A) chromosome fragments.
    (B) fragments of DNA.
    (C) ribosomal fragments.
    (D) fragments of protein molecules.

44. The "pacemaker" of the heart is located in the
    (A) left atrium.
    (B) left ventricle.
    (C) right atrium.
    (D) right ventricle.

45. Which generalization concerning sex determination is true?
    (A) The female determines the sex of the offspring.
    (B) The XY chromosomes are found in the male.
    (C) The sex of the offspring is first determined during maturation.
    (D) There is a greater chance of getting female offspring than male offspring.

46. A decrease in the number of red corpuscles would result in a corresponding decrease in the blood's ability to

(A) transport oxygen.

(B) destroy disease germs.

(C) form fibrinogen.

(D) absorb glucose.

47. Heat shock proteins (HSPs) may enable structural and functional proteins, under conditions of elevated temperatures, to

(A) expand their active sites.

(B) re-establish their molecular geometry.

(C) lower their optimal temperature.

(D) crystallize.

48. In the average person, the largest part of the central nervous system is the

(A) cerebrum.

(B) cerebellum.

(C) medulla.

(D) spinal cord.

49. Which one of the following terms is NOT directly associated with the same sense organ as the three others?

(A) Stapes

(B) Cochlea

(C) Tympanic membrane

(D) Cornea

50. Human activity on the earth's biodiversity has caused

(A) more species to occupy the total available space.

(B) a decrease in biodiversity.

(C) no change in overall space-species relationship.

(D) an increase in biodiversity.

51. If the order of strength of the following bases is: $HCO_3 > C_2H_3O_2 > HSO_4 > Cl$, the weakest acid is

(A) HC_1 $(H+ + C_1-)$.

(B) $HC_2H_3O_2$ $(H+ + C_2H_3O_2-)$.

(C) H_2SO_4 $(H+ + HSO_4)$.

(D) H_2CO_3 $(H+ + HCO_3-)$.

52. In a chemical reaction, [A] and [B] combine to form [C] and [D], as expressed by the reaction [A][B] = [C][D]. Select the statement that best describes the equilibrium condition.

(A) Reaction is shifted to the right.

(B) Concentrations of reactants and products are constant.

(C) Reaction is shifted to the left.

(D) Concentration of products is greater than the concentration reactants.

53. Down Syndrome is a genetic disorder caused by

(A) an extra copy of chromosome 21.

(B) a defective gene on chromosome 21.

(C) fragmentation of one copy of chromosome 23.

(D) a missing copy of chromosome 23.

54. In cellular metabolism, glycolysis

(A) requires O_2.

(B) does not require O_2.

(C) occurs only in animal cells.

(D) produces $CO_2 + H_2O$.

55. If 5×10^5 lbs. of NaCl were dumped into a 0.5-acre pond, what would happen to the water concentration inside a frog's body cells?

(A) It would not change.

(B) It would increase.

(C) It would decrease.

(D) It would approach boiling.

56. An astronaut, without a pressurized suit and with a blood pressure of 120/70, is accidentally sucked out of a spacecraft, halfway between the Earth and the moon. He or she would
    (A) experience a collapse of blood vessels.
    (B) rapidly develop cancer.
    (C) experience an expansion of blood vessels.
    (D) experience no adverse medical effect.

57. Which of the following viruses have been associated with cancer in animals?
    (A) Adenovirus
    (B) Retrovirus
    (C) Papovavirus
    (D) All of the above

58. The major contributions of whole wheat or enriched bread or cereal to the diet are
    (A) carbohydrate and vitamin B complex.
    (B) protein and iron.
    (C) calcium and riboflavin.
    (D) protein and vitamin B complex.

59. A good label for canned goods always includes
    (A) picture of product to give idea of color, size, and appearance.
    (B) net contents, number of portions, and quality of product.
    (C) brief but specific instructions or directions for use.
    (D) brand name.

60. Caloric needs are highest during
    (A) infancy.
    (B) childhood.
    (C) adulthood.
    (D) middle age.

61. Isolated genes shown to initiate malignancies are known as
    (A) carcinogens.
    (B) oncogenes.
    (C) prions.
    (D) None of the above

62. One of the most contentious current problems relative to science ethics involves
    (A) organ transplants.
    (B) blood transfusion.
    (C) human embryonic stem cell research.
    (D) hospitalization time.

63. In the life cycle of the AIDS-causing virus (HIV), the pathogens bind to lymphocyte membrane receptors by their surface
    (A) glycoproteins.
    (B) capsids.
    (C) reverse transcriptase molecules.
    (D) prions.

64. After an AIDS virus enters a lymphocyte, it synthesizes viral DNA from a template composed of
    (A) double-stranded DNA.
    (B) double-stranded RNA.
    (C) single-stranded DNA.
    (D) single-stranded RNA.

65. In patients with cystic fibrosis, the accumulation of mucus around the membranes of cells in the lungs, liver, and pancreas has been shown to be caused by the blockage of ionic channels for
    (A) CA^{++}
    (B) Cl^-
    (C) K^+
    (D) Na^+

66. Choose the correct statement, relative to the distribution of sodium (Na^+) and potassium (K^+), on opposites of cell membranes.

    (A) High Na+ outside

    (B) High K+ outside

    (C) Low Na+ outside

    (D) Low K+ inside

67. Which of the following are requirements for cloning a gene?

    (A) An enzyme to fragment DNA

    (B) A vector (a bacterial plasmid or a virus)

    (C) A host cell or organism

    (D) All of the above

68. Small circular self-duplicating DNA molecules found in bacterial cells are

    (A) microbodies.

    (B) oligaproteins.

    (C) plasmids.

    (D) None of the above

69. Enzymes necessary for fragmenting genes to be cloned are

    (A) restriction enzymes.

    (B) splicing enzymes.

    (C) recombinases.

    (D) polymerases.

70. In the formation of recombinant DNA, the DNA from two different sources is spliced by an enzyme

    (A) polymerase.

    (B) DNA ligase.

    (C) recombinant dehydrogenase.

    (D) None of the above

STOP

IF YOU FINISH BEFORE TIME IS CALLED, YOU MAY CHECK YOUR WORK ON THIS SECTION ONLY. DO NOT TURN TO ANY OTHER SECTION IN THE TEST.

ANSWER KEY AND EXPLANATIONS

Test 1

1. B	9. B	17. D	25. C	33. D
2. B	10. D	18. C	26. A	34. A
3. D	11. C	19. B	27. C	35. B
4. A	12. B	20. A	28. B	36. A
5. D	13. B	21. B	29. D	37. B
6. A	14. D	22. B	30. A	38. D
7. A	15. C	23. D	31. B	39. C
8. C	16. B	24. B	32. B	40. C

1. **The correct answer is (B).** Sphincters are circular muscles that contract when stimulated.

2. **The correct answer is (B).** Bile is released into the duodenum and breaks down the undigested fats into small droplets.

3. **The correct answer is (D).** Urea is filtered from the blood by the kidneys and excreted in urine.

4. **The correct answer is (A).** Group AB blood contains both group A and B antigens and neither A nor B antibodies; therefore, it cannot clump any donor red cells containing A and B antigens.

5. **The correct answer is (D).** Caffeine is a stimulant found in coffee.

6. **The correct answer is (A).** Dried milk is an inexpensive but valuable source of protein.

7. **The correct answer is (A).** Tendons, connective tissue made of dense fibers in the shape of a cord, have great strength.

8. **The correct answer is (C).** Testosterone is the hormone that regulates male sex characteristics.

9. **The correct answer is (B).** Hinge joints allow movement in only two directions.

10. **The correct answer is (D).** Peristalsis is the progressive, wavelike movement that occurs involuntarily to force food forward.

11. **The correct answer is (C).** The parotid gland is a large salivary gland that is affected by mumps.

12. **The correct answer is (B).** The electron is the unit of negative electricity.

13. **The correct answer is (B).** Capillaries connect arterioles with venules and function as exchange vessels.

14. **The correct answer is (D).** Erythrocytes (red blood cells) contain hemoglobin.

15. **The correct answer is (C).** Proteins are nutrients essential for growth and repair of tissue.

16. **The correct answer is (B).** The diffusion of gas occurs across the thin, squamous epithelium lining of the alveoli.

17. **The correct answer is (D).** The SA node, located in the right atrium, starts each heart beat.

18. **The correct answer is (C).** The mitral valve, located between the left atrium and left ventricle of the heart, is also called the bicuspid valve.

19. **The correct answer is (B).** Viruses are so small that they can be seen only through special electron microscopes.

20. **The correct answer is (A).** The pulmonary artery carries deoxygenated blood from the heart.

21. **The correct answer is (B).** When water intake is excessive, the kidneys excrete generous amounts of urine; if water intake is lost, they produce less urine. The process is regulated by hormones.

22. **The correct answer is (B).** Iodine makes up about 65 percent of thyroxine, a hormone secreted by the thyroid gland.

23. **The correct answer is (D).** Scurvy is a disease caused by a deficiency of vitamin C.

24. **The correct answer is (B).** Leukocytes (white blood cells) destroy bacteria when there is an infection in the body.

25. **The correct answer is (C).** The islets of Langerhans are located in the pancreas and produce insulin.

26. **The correct answer is (A).** Gastric and intestinal enzymes gradually break down the protein molecule into its separate amino acids.

27. **The correct answer is (C).** Glucose is the end product of carbohydrate digestion.

28. **The correct answer is (B).** When one muscle contracts, the opposing muscle must relax; in this way, movements are coordinated and normal functions are carried out.

29. **The correct answer is (D).** The medulla oblongata is located between the pons and the spinal cord, and the vital centers are located in it.

30. **The correct answer is (A).** Rays pass through a series of transparent, colorless eye parts. On the way, they undergo a process of bending called refraction, which makes it possible for light from a large area to focus on the retina.

31. **The correct answer is (B).** The cornea is referred to frequently as the "window" of the eye.

32. **The correct answer is (B).** A calorie is the unit of measure of heat—the amount of heat required to raise the temperature of 1 kilogram of water by 1°C.

33. **The correct answer is (D).** Vitamin D is referred to as the "sunshine" vitamin because it is formed in the body by the action of the sunshine on the cholesterol products in the skin.

34. **The correct answer is (A).** Digestion is the process whereby the enzymes in the body change food into simple substances that can be readily used by the body.

35. **The correct answer is (B).** The thyroid gland needs iodine for the formation of thyroxine.

36. **The correct answer is (A).** Vitamin K helps the liver to produce substances necessary for the clotting of blood.

37. **The correct answer is (B).** Thiamine is another name for vitamin B1.

38. **The correct answer is (D).** Peristalsis is a wave-like progression of muscular contractions that moves food through the alimentary canal.

39. **The correct answer is (C).** The thigh bone is the femur. It is the longest and strongest bone in the body.

40. **The correct answer is (C).** Plasma is the liquid portion of the blood in which corpuscles are suspended.

Test 2

1. C	7. C	13. D	19. B	25. B
2. D	8. B	14. A	20. C	26. B
3. C	9. C	15. B	21. A	27. A
4. B	10. B	16. D	22. C	28. C
5. A	11. A	17. B	23. D	29. B
6. C	12. C	18. D	24. D	30. D

1. **The correct answer is (C).** Blood pressure is the force of the blood exerted against the wall of the blood vessel.

2. **The correct answer is (D).** Relative humidity refers to the amount of moisture in the air in relation to the temperature.

3. **The correct answer is (C).** A specimen is a laboratory sample used to help the physician make a diagnosis.

4. **The correct answer is (B).** Defecation means the act of having a bowel movement or removing solid waste materials from the body.

5. **The correct answer is (A).** Sterile means that an object is completely free of all microorganisms. Steam under pressure (autoclave) will give complete sterilization.

6. **The correct answer is (C).** Carbon dioxide stimulates the respiratory center in the brain (medulla oblongata).

7. **The correct answer is (C).** Protein substance in the urine is called albuminuria. It results from the failure of the kidneys to filter.

8. **The correct answer is (B).** Protein, the body's vital building material, makes up the basic structure of all cells.

9. **The correct answer is (C).** The gallbladder stores and concentrates bile, which is used to break down fats into droplets and aids in the absorption of fatty acids and glyceral.

Therefore, fats are restricted when there are diseases of the gallbladder.

10. **The correct answer is (B).** Water-soluble vitamins include vitamin C and vitamin B complex.

11. **The correct answer is (A).** Iron and calcium are the minerals most often deficient in the American diet.

12. **The correct answer is (C).** Tetany, which is due to lack of calcium, may be corrected by increasing the consumption of milk or milk products, which are rich in calcium salts. Drugs containing high amounts of calcium may be given intravenously in emergencies.

13. **The correct answer is (D).** Constriction of the blood vessels prevents loss of heat from the blood through the skin.

14. **The correct answer is (A).** Milk contains only about 0.1 milligram of iron per cup. The recommended daily amount is 15–18 milligrams.

15. **The correct answer is (B).** Food proteins supply our bodies with nitrogen to replace that lost in urine, feces, and perspiration.

16. **The correct answer is (D).** The electrical charge results when a neutral atom or group of atoms loses or gains one or more electrons during chemical reactions.

17. **The correct answer is (B).** The cell is the unit of structure and function of all living

things. The simplest organisms consist of only one cell.

18. **The correct answer is (D).** Osmosis is the diffusion of water through a semi-permeable membrane from a region of greater concentration to a region of lesser concentration.

19. **The correct answer is (B).** Cardiologist comes from the word cardiology, meaning the study of the heart's physiology and pathology.

20. **The correct answer is (C).** Greenstick fractures are incomplete fractures with a longitudinal split of the shaft. They usually occur in long bones of children.

21. **The correct answer is (A).** Environmental factors are the relationships of living things to their surroundings.

22. **The correct answer is (C).** The fluid-like residue of digestion found in the colon contains valuable water, which is absorbed into the bloodstream.

23. **The correct answer is (D).** After ovulation, the egg travels into the fallopian tube. If sperms are present, the union of the sperm and the egg (fertilization) takes place in the fallopian tube.

24. **The correct answer is (D).** Photosynthesis is the process by which certain living plant cells combine carbon dioxide and water, in the presence of chlorophyll and light energy, to form carbohydrates and release oxygen as a waste product.

25. **The correct answer is (B).** The atmosphere is composed of about 78 percent nitrogen.

26. **The correct answer is (B).** Enzymes are protein substances that act as biochemical catalysts. They affect the rate at which a specific reaction occurs.

27. **The correct answer is (A).** Essential amino acids are those that cannot be manufactured by the body and, therefore, must be included in the daily diet.

28. **The correct answer is (C).** The barometer is an instrument used to measure air pressure and forecast weather.

29. **The correct answer is (B).** An elevation of body temperature above normal is referred to as fever or pyrexia.

30. **The correct answer is (D).** The otoscope is a lighted instrument used to examine the ear canal, eustachian tube, eardrum, and the middle ear.

Test 3

1. A	7. D	13. C	19. B	25. C
2. D	8. C	14. B	20. B	26. D
3. C	9. C	15. D	21. A	27. B
4. B	10. A	16. C	22. B	28. A
5. C	11. B	17. B	23. C	29. A
6. B	12. D	18. A	24. A	30. B

1. **The correct answer is (A).** The body is constantly stabilizing and equalizing its environment to prevent any sudden or severe changes.

2. **The correct answer is (D).** The DNA molecules in the nucleus of a cell duplicate themselves and the cell divides, forming two cells.

3. **The correct answer is (C).** In acquiring passive immunity, the body of the recipient plays an active part in response to an antigen.

4. **The correct answer is (B).** The functional unit is suspended near the center of the cell and has the property of division.

5. **The correct answer is (C).** Produced by the thyroid gland, thyroxin controls the rate at which glucose is burned and converts it to heat and energy.

6. **The correct answer is (B).** Sweat glands are distributed in the skin and produce perspiration, primarily water.

7. **The correct answer is (D).** Melanin, a brown pigment, increases when exposed to sun.

8. **The correct answer is (C).** Estrogen and progesterone promote development of female sex characteristics and regulate menstruation.

9. **The correct answer is (C).** Epithelial tissue has many forms—flat and irregular, square, long and narrow—that are arranged in single or multiple layers to form a protective covering and lining.

10. **The correct answer is (A).** The ball-shaped head of the femur fits into the concave socket of the hipbone and allows for a wide range of motion.

11. **The correct answer is (B).** Adrenaline is released from the adrenal medulla to prepare the body for emergency situations.

12. **The correct answer is (D).** A small opening into the nose at the inner corner of the eye allows the fluid to drain through.

13. **The correct answer is (C).** Many gray-matter areas that form the cranial nerves are located in the medulla oblongota and are involved in the control of vital activities.

14. **The correct answer is (B).** As peristalsis moves content along, water is absorbed through the walls into the circulation, and the remaining cellulose passes on to the rectum.

15. **The correct answer is (D).** Aldosterone is the hormone released from the adrenal cortex that helps regulate sodium and potassium balance.

16. **The correct answer is (C).** The shedding of the lining of the uterus occurs if the egg has not been fertilized by the sperm.

17. **The correct answer is (B).** Dorsal pertains to the back; the cranial and spinal cavities contain the brain and the spinal cord.

18. **The correct answer is (A).** Deoxygenated blood returns from the body tissues via the superior and inferior vena cava into the right atrium.

19. **The correct answer is (B).** The left ventricle has the major responsibility for pumping blood into the aorta to be dispersed throughout the body.

20. **The correct answer is (B).** The jelly-like substance prevents the eyeball from collapsing inward.

21. **The correct answer is (A).** The endocardium is a smooth lining, which helps blood flow smoothly through the heart.

22. **The correct answer is (B).** The perineum, which forms the pelvic floor, is the external region between the vulva and anus in the female or between the scrotum and anus in the male.

23. **The correct answer is (C).** The greater trochanter is the ball-like head that articulates with the hipbone.

24. **The correct answer is (A).** The gluteus maximus is part of the hips and buttocks.

25. **The correct answer is (C).** Nephrons are responsible for the processes of filtration, absorption, and secretion.

26. **The correct answer is (D).** Normal urine has a low specific gravity.

27. **The correct answer is (B).** Aldosterone is released by the adrenal cortex in response to decreased blood volume, decreased blood sodium ions, or increased potassium ions.

28. **The correct answer is (A).** Water plus creatinine and urea, which are nitrogenous wastes, are normal substances in urine.

29. **The correct answer is (A).** The left motor control center in the brain controls the right side of the body because of the crossing of the nerve tracts within the brain.

30. **The correct answer is (B).** When the water intake is excessive, the kidneys excrete generous amounts of urine; if the water intake is lost, they produce less urine. The process is regulated by hormones.

Test 4

1. B	15. D	29. B	43. B	57. D
2. A	16. C	30. C	44. C	58. A
3. B	17. A	31. B	45. B	59. B
4. C	18. C	32. C	46. A	60. A
5. A	19. C	33. D	47. B	61. B
6. B	20. D	34. A	48. A	62. C
7. A	21. B	35. B	49. D	63. A
8. B	22. A	36. C	50. B	64. D
9. B	23. C	37. C	51. D	65. B
10. A	24. A	38. C	52. B	66. A
11. A	25. C	39. C	53. A	67. D
12. C	26. A	40. B	54. B	68. C
13. C	27. D	41. A	55. C	69. A
14. B	28. B	42. B	56. C	70. B

1. **The correct answer is (B).** Insulin increases the permeability of the cell membrane to glucose, thus enhancing the uptake of glucose from the blood by the cells. If insulin is deficient, glucose is not removed from the blood and utilized by the cells, resulting in an excess of glucose in the blood and leading to other symptoms of diabetes.

2. **The correct answer is (A).** The amnion is one of the extraembryonic structures formed during embryonic development. It surrounds the embryo and becomes filled with fluid in which the embryo floats. The amniotic fluid probably provides protection from mechanical shock for the embryo.

3. **The correct answer is (B).** Sebaceous glands are associated with hair follicles: the cells lining the glands form the secretion, and the entire cellular lining, plus the fatty secretion, form sebum, which is expelled into the hair follicle. Sebum serves to keep the hair and skin pliable.

4. **The correct answer is (C).** DNA (deoxyribonucleic acid) is found in the nucleus of each cell and "stores" genetic information, or the genetic code. DNA replicates itself before mitosis or meiosis begins, and genetic information is distributed equally to the daughter nuclei. RNA (ribonucleic acid), transcribed on DNA, translates the genetic or hereditary information.

5. **The correct answer is (A).** Melanin is a dark pigment found in the cells of the basal layers of the skin. Skin color varies with the size and density of the melanin particles: the more melanin present, the darker the skin.

6. **The correct answer is (B).** Each person has a set of 20 deciduous teeth, as contrasted to 32 permanent or nondeciduous teeth. The set of deciduous teeth contains no bicuspids, and only two molars per quad-

rant rather than three. A set per quadrant of deciduous teeth includes two incisors, one canine, and two molars; a set per quadrant of nondeciduous teeth includes two incisors, one canine, two premolars (bicuspids), and three molars.

7. **The correct answer is (A).** Cementum covers the surface of roots of teeth; enamel covers the surface of the crowns of teeth.

8. **The correct answer is (B).** The bulk of a hemoglobin molecule consists of 4 subunits, each one of which is a chain of amino acids. Iron is also present in hemoglobin but does not comprise as large a part of the entire molecule as the 4 chains of amino acids. Ferritin is an iron-containing molecule stored in the liver. Myosin is a major component of muscle cells.

9. **The correct answer is (B).** The XY chromosomes are found in the male, while the female carries XX. As a result of meiosis, a sperm will carry either an X or Y chromosome; all eggs will carry one X. Fertilization of an X-bearing egg by a Y-bearing sperm produces an XY zygote, which develops into a male. Fertilization of an X-bearing egg by an X-bearing sperm produces an XX zygote, which develops into a female.

10. **The correct answer is (A).** The fetus and the mother have independent circulatory systems. Fetal blood passing to and from the placenta by way of the umbilical blood vessels is separated from the mother's blood in the placenta by thin tissues; food, gases, and metabolic wastes can diffuse through these tissues between the two bloodstreams. After birth, the placenta's function has ended, and as the baby's systems become "active," there is no longer an exchange of materials between the two bloodstreams.

11. **The correct answer is (A).** Plasma is the liquid portion of the blood. Whole blood consists of plasma with its dissolved materials and the blood cells.

12. **The correct answer is (C).** Thrombocytes disintegrate when blood flows from a blood vessel, releasing a phospholipid, thrombokinase, that acts to convert prothrombin in the plasma to thrombin. Thrombin acts enzymatically on fibrinogen in the plasma, converting it to fibrin, which is insoluble and forms a mesh, trapping blood cells. This mesh is the blood clot.

13. **The correct answer is (C).** The femur is the thigh bone of the leg. It is the longest, strongest, and heaviest bone of the body.

14. **The correct answer is (B).** Iron is a part of the hemoglobin molecule, the red, oxygen-carrying pigment of red blood cells. If iron is deficient, hemoglobin cannot be produced, and the formation of red blood cells is inhibited.

15. **The correct answer is (D).** Peristalsis is the wave of muscular contractions that pushes food through the esophagus into the stomach and through the intestine. Food must reach the digestive sites, the stomach and small intestine, for digestion to occur. The other possible answer choices are involved in metabolic processes, not in digestion.

16. **The correct answer is (C).** The liver is the largest glandular organ of vertebrates and has the important function of regulating organic materials such as wastes, glucose, and proteins in the blood. It can also perform other essential functions, such as fat digestion and storage functions, immune responses, protein metabolism, and detoxifying blood by converting toxic substances into harmless wastes. It is essential for life.

17. **The correct answer is (A).** The cell walls of gram-negative bacteria are more complex than gram-positives—with less peptidoglycan and more lipopolysaccharides—which renders them more difficult for drugs to cross.

18. **The correct answer is (C).** Nerve fibers from the retina of the eye form the optic nerve of the eye; at the crossover point

(optic chiasma), fibers from the nasal halves (inner halves) of each retina cross to the opposite side of the brain, while fibers of the temporal halves (outer halves) of each retina remain uncrossed. Thus, each optic nerve, after the chiasma, contains fibers from both retinas. This means that objects in one field of vision (either left or right) produce effects in two eyes that are transmitted to one side of the brain. In other words, the two halves of the retina of each eye are represented on opposite sides of the brain, producing a stereoscopic effect and permitting perception of depth.

19. **The correct answer is (C).** Many aquatic animals excrete ammonia as their nitrogenous waste, egg-laying animals excrete uric acid, and intra-uterine animals excrete urea.

20. **The correct answer is (D).** Estrogen is a complex of female sex hormones responsible for the appearance of secondary sex characteristics, such as widening of the pelvis, breasts, etc. Estrogen also functions in the menstrual cycle, preparing the uterus for implantation of the embryo.

21. **The correct answer is (B).** A polymer is a large, chain-like organic molecule formed by bonding together many smaller organic molecules of the same kind. A protein is a chain of many amino acid molecules joined to one another by peptide bonds. The amino acid molecules present, and the sequence in which they are joined, are considered the primary structure of the protein and determine its physical or chemical properties.

22. **The correct answer is (A).** Red blood cells are produced in the bone marrow in the adult. The other statements are incorrect as follows: vitamins typically are consumed with food (two possible exceptions); glucose is a product of digestion, and bile is stored in the gallbladder; water is a part of almost all tissues; and fats are refined by the bile from the liver.

23. **The correct answer is (C).** Connective tissues are those whose cells are not contigu-

ous but scattered throughout a noncellular matrix. Connective tissues can bind and support other tissues; therefore, they are widely distributed. Some examples of connective tissues are blood, bone, cartilage, adipose, and tissues composing tendons or ligaments.

24. **The correct answer is (A).** The limited amount of ATP stored in muscle tissue supplies immediate energy for contraction when the ATP is converted to ADP. When the ATP is used up, it is recreated by energy from a reserve, creatine phosphate. When the creatine phosphate is consumed, oxidation of glucose to CO2 and water provides energy for muscle contraction and for the resynthesis of creatine phosphate. Lactic acid can form anaerobically during severe muscle exertion, and its accumulation is partly responsible for the feeling of fatigue. Lactic acid diffuses out of the muscle tissue into the bloodstream and thus to the liver, where some of it is oxidized to produce further energy, and some can be converted to glycogen for carbohydrate storage.

25. **The correct answer is (C).** Adrenalin, or epinephrine, secreted by the adrenal medulla, is normally released in small quantities and helps to regulate blood circulation and carbohydrate metabolism. Under stressful conditions, the adrenal medulla is stimulated to release larger amounts of adrenalin, which increases blood pressure, heart rate, carbohydrate metabolism, and conversion of glycogen to sugar, thus raising the blood sugar level, etc. This prepares the body to cope with the stressful situation—hence, the "flight or fight" response.

26. **The correct answer is (A).** Exercise will cause perspiration, which evaporates from the skin. Perspiration is a liquid composed of water, salt, and a small amount of urea and is drawn from the bloodstream (from capillaries in the sweat glands) and released to the body surface through pores. Thus, rigorous exercise will cause the body to lose sodium (salt) and water.

27. **The correct answer is (D).** Cholesterol is a lipid that is insoluble in fluids such as blood; therefore, it is bound to protein-aceous carriers for transport. Evidence indicates that cholesterol is involved in the fatty deposits in arteries, even infiltrating cells and the intercellular spaces of arterial walls, if carried by certain carriers. This can lead to plaque and clot formation, blocking off the arteries and interfering with blood circulation. This same plaque and clot formation can occur in the coronary artery supplying heart muscle, causing a heart attack.

28. **The correct answer is (B).** The endocrine glands secrete hormones directly into the bloodstream. The hormones are transported throughout the body, but only specific "target" cells or tissues can pick up a specific hormone. Thus, the hormone may regulate cellular activities in tissues some distance from the cells that secreted it. By regulating cellular activities of tissues, hormones regulate bodily activities.

29. **The correct answer is (B).** The thyroid hormone controls the rate of cellular metabolism for the release of energy. An overactive gland secretes an excess of hormone, which will increase the metabolic rate. A deficiency of thyroid hormone causes the rate of metabolism to be lowered.

30. **The correct answer is (C).** The alveolus is a small, thin-walled sac of the lung; it is the blind end of the smallest bronchioles. Each alveolus (approximately 300 million are present in human lungs) is surrounded by, or adjacent to, small capillaries. It is here that gaseous exchange between the blood and lungs occur. Carbon dioxide passes into the alveolus from the blood, and oxygen passes from the alveolus into the bloodstream through the capillary walls.

31. **The correct answer is (B).** A hemorrhoid is a dilation of veins in the anal region. This can lead to an enlargement of tissue, especially the rectal sphincter, which is a ring-shaped muscle controlling the anal opening.

32. **The correct answer is (C).** The amino nitrogen must be removed from amino acids in order to give them the basic hydrocarbon skeleton similar to carbohydrates. After the amino group is removed, the resulting compounds may enter the same metabolic pathways used by carbohydrates.

33. **The correct answer is (D).** The chemistry of life is closely dependent upon the chemistry of water. Water, in the presence of the proper enzymes, must be added to the bonds that bind monosaccharides in carbohydrates, amino acids in proteins, and fatty acids and glycerol in fats to degrade these polymers to their subunits.

34. **The correct answer is (A).** Energy production, in the degradation of foods, is associated with the release of hydrogen (oxidation). The ratio of hydrogen to oxygen is significantly greater in fats than in carbohydrates and proteins.

35. **The correct answer is (B).** Oxygenated blood passes from the lungs to the left atrium of the heart by way of the pulmonary veins. From the left atrium, blood moves to the left ventricle, from which it is pumped through the aorta to the arterial system of the body, and thus throughout the body, where oxygen is diffused into the cells and carbon dioxide is picked up by the blood. The carbon-dioxide-laden blood is returned to the heart, entering the right atrium, and passing to the right ventricle. From the right ventricle, it is pumped to the lungs through the pulmonary arteries, where it becomes oxygenated again.

36. **The correct answer is (C).** Studies conducted by Dr. Allan Roses and D. Warren Stuttmatter at the Duke University Medical Center and reported in the Wall Street Journal (October 19, 1995) indicated that the apoliprotein (**E**) gene occurs as E-2, E-3, and E-4 subtypes. The potential of gene E for promoting cell maintenance and protection against Alzheimer's, heart disease, and diabetes is in order of potency of E-2 > E-3 > E-4. Therefore, E-2 is the good gene and E-4 is the bad form.

37. **The correct answer is (C).** The three basic kinds of muscle tissue are smooth, skeletal, and cardiac. Smooth muscle is characteristic of the digestive tract and arteries, organs not under voluntary control. Cardiac muscle is found in the heart. Skeletal muscle (striated) makes up the muscles associated with voluntary movement. The kidney is nonmuscular.

38. **The correct answer is (C).** Gaseous exchange between the respiratory system and the circulatory system occurs by means of the capillaries present in the lungs surrounding alveoli. These are referred to as the pulmonary capillaries.

39. **The correct answer is (C).** The hybridoma, formed by fusing lymphocytes with cancer cells, produces a single type of antibody. The hybridoma can be injected into a mouse or cultured, in vitro, to increase production of the single antibody type.

40. **The correct answer is (B).** Blood in systemic veins is returning to the right atrium of the heart from the cells of the body. Therefore, it is high in concentrations of carbon dioxide and metabolic wastes that were received from the cells as a result of cellular metabolism. Venous blood of the pulmonary system is returning to the left atrium of the heart from the lungs, where it gave up carbon dioxide to be expelled from the body and acquired oxygen. Therefore, it has a higher concentration of oxygen.

41. **The correct answer is (A).** The first division of meiosis results in a reduction of the number of chromosomes, because the members of each pair of chromosomes are separated from one another. Each daughter nucleus resulting from meiosis receives only one chromosome of each pair present in the parent nucleus, or one half the number of chromosomes of the parent nucleus. Nuclei resulting from meiosis are haploid, as contrasted to the diploid condition of the parent nucleus.

42. **The correct answer is (B).** Fraternal, or nonidentical, twins result from two fertilized eggs, or zygotes. If two eggs are released during ovulation and both are fertilized (one sperm per egg), fraternal twins result. These twins are like ordinary siblings, whereas identical twins resulting from a single zygote are genetically identical.

43. **The correct answer is (B).** Restriction fragment length polymorphisms are differences in the lengths of fragments of DNA produced by exposing DNA from genetically different individuals to a bacterial restriction enzyme that cuts DNA at specific points.

44. **The correct answer is (C).** Specialized muscle cells, known as the "pacemaker" of the heart, make up a region of the right atrium. When these cells are excited, the atria are stimulated to contract, emptying the blood into the ventricles. Certain muscle fibers then carry the excitation stimulus, by way of the atrio-ventricular node, to muscles of the ventricles, stimulating them to contract and force blood from the heart.

45. **The correct answer is (B).** The XY chromosomes are found in the male, while the female carries XX. As a result of meiosis, a sperm will carry either an X or a Y chromosome; all eggs will carry an X. Fertilization of an X-bearing egg by a Y-bearing sperm produces an XY zygote, which develops into a male. Fertilization of an X-bearing egg by an X-bearing sperm produces an XX zygote, which develops into a female.

46. **The correct answer is (A).** Red blood cells contain the pigment hemoglobin, which has as its function the transport of oxygen. If the number of red blood cells is decreased, the ability of the blood to transport oxygen is decreased.

47. **The correct answer is (B).** Temperatures greater than 40°C will denature (destroy) the molecular geometry of most proteins. In many plant and animal cells, special proteins (heat shock proteins) are synthesized to prevent denaturation at these temperatures.

48. The correct answer is (A). The cerebrum is the largest division of the central nervous system of humans. It originates thinking and controls learning, memory, thought, some voluntary movements, and the senses. In the animal kingdom, observations indicate that intelligence increases with cerebrum size. Humans have the largest cerebrum, in proportion to body size, in the animal kingdom.

49. The correct answer is (D). The stapes, cochlea, and tympanic membrane are all parts of the ear. The stapes is one of the vibrating bones of the middle ear, the cochlea is the receptor portion of the inner ear from which electrical impulses ("messages") are transmitted to the brain through the auditory nerve, and the tympanic membrane is the eardrum. The cornea, on the other hand, is the transparent covering over the front of the lens of the eye.

50. The correct answer is (B). Human activities (e.g., agricultural and industrial) generally destroy food and alter physical conditions required to complete the life cycle in some species. The overall effect is a reduction in the total number of species that occupy a habitat.

51. The correct answer is (D). Acidity is determined by the concentration of hydrogen ion H+s per unit of volume. Strong bases allow fewer H+s to escape in aqueous solution than weak bases, producing weaker acids (e.g., Cl– is a weak base, making HCl a strong acid, whereas HCO3 is a strong base, making H2CO3 a weak acid).

52. The correct answer is (B). The arrows directed to the right in chemical equations represent products generated from the forward reaction, and those directed to the left represent reactants produced by the reverse reaction. The arrow length symbolizes the concentration of the substances on both sides of the equation.

53. The correct answer is (A). In humans and other animals, it is normal for an individual to have two copies of each type of chromosome in the nucleus of any body cell, except an egg or a sperm. There are 23 different types of chromosomes in humans; therefore, the normal complement of chromosomes in human cells is 46. Individuals with Down Syndrome receive an extra copy of chromosome 21 from one of their parents. They have three copies of chromosome 21 and a total of 47 chromosomes in the nuclei of their cells.

54. The correct answer is (B). In cellular metabolism, glycolysis is an anaerobic process (requires no O2), produces reduced nicotinamide adeninedinucleotide (NADH2) and small amounts of ATP, and occurs in all types of cells.

55. The correct answer is (C). Osmosis is the movement of water across cell membranes from solutions of low solute concentration to solutions with higher concentrations of solute. The salt gives the water a higher solute concentration than the frog's intracellular fluids. Therefore, the water concentration inside the cells would decrease as water flowed to the outside.

56. The correct answer is (C). The air (atmosphere) around the earth exerts a normal pressure of 760 mmHg (1.0 atmosphere). The pressure in interplanetary space is zero (a vacuum). Since the pressure inside the astronaut's blood vessels is greater than zero, the vessels would push outward.

57. The correct answer is (D). All of these viruses have been associated with cancer: adenoviruses (respiratory tract tumors), retroviruses (leukemia and AIDS), and papovaviruses (cervical cancer).

58. The correct answer is (A). Cereals (grains) are rich in certain members of the vitamin B complex; because of the starchy endosperm in seeds, cereals also are high in carbohydrates.

59. The correct answer is (B). Labels on canned goods may include a variety of information about the product, but the net contents by weight or volume and the quality should always be included. The number of portions may vary per net contents, according to the nature of the product, so knowledge of the number of servings is useful information. Other information may also be included on the label.

60. **The correct answer is (A).** Caloric needs vary with age as well as with physiological state, activity, and the size of the individual. Both physical and mental growth and development are more rapid during infancy and early childhood than at any other time in one's life. Therefore, more food is needed in proportion to size to provide the needed calories of energy and to provide the materials for growth. A proper diet is essential for normal development.

61. **The correct answer is (B).** Genes shown to cause cancerous growths are called oncogenes.

62. **The correct answer is (C).** Many individuals believe that the use of tissues from aborted fetuses is ethically unacceptable.

63. **The correct answer is (A).** The AIDS virus uses its surface glycoproteins to bind to membrane receptors of host cells, initiating the infection by infusing viral RNA into the host cell.

64. **The correct answer is (D).** The AIDS virus uses an enzyme—reverse transcriptase—as the normal pattern of synthesis (using DNA as a template to produce RNA) to a reverse method (using RNA as a template to form DNA).

65. **The correct answer is (B).** The inability to pass Cl– to the outside of cells in cystic fibrosis patients causes water to enter the cells by osmosis, making the intercellular mucus thicker than normal.

66. **The correct answer is (A).** Cell membranes maintain their high external Na+ and high internal K+ concentrations by using ATP to energize membrane carrier proteins that form the sodium-potassium pump. This is an active transport mechanism, which moves both ions against concentration gradients.

67. **The correct answer is (D).** The general procedure for cloning includes: isolating DNA plasmid from a bacterium, isolating the DNA comprising the gene of interest from a different cell type, mixing the gene of interest with the plasmid to form a hybrid type of DNA called recombinant DNA, infecting a vector (bacteria or virus) with the recombinant DNA, and culturing the vector (containing the recombinant DNA) to produce many identical copies of itself (clones).

68. **The correct answer is (C).** Plasmids—small, circular self-duplicating DNA molecules isolated from bacteria—are major requirements for recombinant DNA technology.

69. **The correct answer is (A).** The restriction enzymes recognize and fragment the DNA (at the proper location) of the genes to be cloned.

70. **The correct answer is (B).** The splicing of DNA from two different sources is accomplished by the enzyme, DNA ligase, which catalyzes bonding by the complementarity of base pairing.

READING COMPREHENSION ANSWER SHEETS

Test 1

1. Ⓐ Ⓑ Ⓒ Ⓓ   2. Ⓐ Ⓑ Ⓒ Ⓓ   3. Ⓐ Ⓑ Ⓒ Ⓓ   4. Ⓐ Ⓑ Ⓒ Ⓓ   5. Ⓐ Ⓑ Ⓒ Ⓓ

Test 2

1. Ⓐ Ⓑ Ⓒ Ⓓ   3. Ⓐ Ⓑ Ⓒ Ⓓ   4. Ⓐ Ⓑ Ⓒ Ⓓ   5. Ⓐ Ⓑ Ⓒ Ⓓ   6. Ⓐ Ⓑ Ⓒ Ⓓ

2. Ⓐ Ⓑ Ⓒ Ⓓ

Test 3

1. Ⓐ Ⓑ Ⓒ Ⓓ   3. Ⓐ Ⓑ Ⓒ Ⓓ   4. Ⓐ Ⓑ Ⓒ Ⓓ   5. Ⓐ Ⓑ Ⓒ Ⓓ   6. Ⓐ Ⓑ Ⓒ Ⓓ

2. Ⓐ Ⓑ Ⓒ Ⓓ

Test 4

1. Ⓐ Ⓑ Ⓒ Ⓓ   2. Ⓐ Ⓑ Ⓒ Ⓓ   3. Ⓐ Ⓑ Ⓒ Ⓓ   4. Ⓐ Ⓑ Ⓒ Ⓓ   5. Ⓐ Ⓑ Ⓒ Ⓓ

Test 5

1. Ⓐ Ⓑ Ⓒ Ⓓ   2. Ⓐ Ⓑ Ⓒ Ⓓ   3. Ⓐ Ⓑ Ⓒ Ⓓ   4. Ⓐ Ⓑ Ⓒ Ⓓ   5. Ⓐ Ⓑ Ⓒ Ⓓ

answer sheet

Reading
Comprehension

OVERVIEW

- Reading comprehension test 1
- Reading comprehension test 2
- Reading comprehension test 3
- Reading comprehension test 4
- Reading comprehension test 5
- Answer key and explanations

READING COMPREHENSION TEST 1

5 Questions • 8 Minutes

Review Unit 4, Reading Comprehension, before attempting this test.

Directions: Following the passage below, you will find a number of incomplete statements about the passage. Select the word or expression that most satisfactorily completes each statement. Fill in the corresponding space on your answer sheet.

How can we know that the birds we see in the South in the winter are the same ones that come north in the spring? John J. Audubon, a bird lover, wondered about this. Every year, he watched a pair of little phoebes nesting in the same place. He wondered if they were the same birds and so decided to put tiny silver bands on their legs. The next spring, back came the birds with the bands to build their nests on the walls of farm buildings in the neighborhood. The phoebe, it was learned, wintered wherever it was warm enough to find flies. In summer, phoebes could be seen from Georgia to Canada; in winter, anywhere from Georgia to Florida and Mexico. The phoebe was the first kind of bird to be banded, and Mr. Audubon was the first birdbander. Today there are thousands of birdbanders all over America, people who band all kinds of birds.

The government of the United States has a special birdbanding department that makes all the birdbands. The bands do not hurt the birds because they are made of aluminum and are very light. They come in different sizes for different-sized birds. Each band has a special number and the words, "Notify Fish and Wildlife Service, Washington, DC." Anyone who finds a dead bird with a band on one of its legs is asked to send the band to Washington with a note telling where and when the bird was found. In this way naturalists add to their knowledge of the habits and needs of birds.

1. The title below that best expresses the main theme or subject of this selection is
   (A) "The Migration of Birds."
   (B) "The Work of John Audubon."
   (C) "The Habits and Needs of Birds."
   (D) "Studying Bird Life Through Birdbanding."

2. According to the selection, Audubon proved his theory that
   (A) birds prefer a diet of flies.
   (B) birds return to the same nesting place each spring.
   (C) silver is the best material for birdbands.
   (D) phoebes are the most interesting birds to study.

3. Audubon's purpose in banding the phoebes was to
   (A) satisfy his curiosity.
   (B) notify the government.
   (C) start a birdbanding department.
   (D) gain fame as the first birdbander.

4. The migration habits of phoebes depend upon
   (A) nesting places.
   (B) the help of bird lovers.
   (C) the available food supply.
   (D) the number of young birds.

5. Which statement is true according to the selection?
   (A) Residents of Georgia may expect to see phoebes all year long.
   (B) The weight of a band causes a bird considerable discomfort.
   C) The government offers a reward for information about dead birds.
   (D) Phoebes are more plentiful in the East than any other kind of bird.

STOP

IF YOU FINISH BEFORE TIME IS CALLED, YOU MAY CHECK YOUR WORK ON THIS SECTION ONLY. DO NOT TURN TO ANY OTHER SECTION IN THE TEST.

READING COMPREHENSION TEST 2

6 Questions • 10 Minutes

Review Unit 4, Reading Comprehension, before attempting this test.

Directions: Following the passage below, you will find a number of incomplete statements about the passage. Select the word or expression that most satisfactorily completes each statement. Fill in the corresponding space on your answer sheet.

It is important to understand just what we mean when we talk about stress, and theoretical definitions of stress abound. Probably the best definition was offered by the renowned stress researcher Hans Selye, who summarized stress as ". . . any bodily change produced as a response to a perceived demand being placed upon the individual." This definition highlights the notion that there are two important facets to stress: the psychological (or menial) and the physiological (or physical).

Stress can be typically negative events, called "distress," as well as the more positive happenings in life that nonetheless demand change and adjustment. After a demand is perceived, bodily or physical changes occur as a reaction. These biological responses typically include increased heart rate, respiration rate, rising blood pressure, and muscular tension, shallow (rather than deep) breathing, and the increased release of certain so-called stress hormones such as adrenaline and cortisol.

Such bodily changes occur for what is commonly known as the "fight-or-flight" response. The fight-or-flight response served a purpose ages ago, when acute, sudden stressors such as animal predators immediately threatened a person's existence. Successfully fighting off or fleeing from the threat greatly increased one's chance of survival. And, as with other creatures, our fight-or-flight stress reaction became "wired in" as a protective mechanism.

Stress continues to serve us today, as mild to moderate levels of stress can sharpen our alertness and motivate positive growth, spur the need to accept challenges, and promote change in our lives. Stress becomes a problem only when you consider the nature of some of our stressors. Unlike the saber-tooth tigers of long age, today's stressors tend to be more chronic in nature. Most people struggle with the demands of health problems, interpersonal difficulties, financial worries, and negative or critical self-imaging, to name just a few. These concerns have a propensity to stick around. When you begin to experience any one of them, your body reacts with predictable changes. However, because these stressors usually stay around and dominate parts of our existence for long stretches of time, the bodily changes that get "turned on," stay "turned on," which can cause or influence numerous undesirable consequences.

Chronic stress can contribute to such physical problems as migraine headaches, lower back pain, ulcers, digestive disorders, TMJ (temporomandibular joint) syndrome, suppressed immunity, and, of particular concern to people with diabetes, difficulty controlling rising blood sugar. There is even some evidence that cardiovascular disease, high blood pressure, and certain types of cancer can be adversely affected by stress. Chronic stress also appears to contribute to many psychological and behavioral disorders such as depression, anxiety disorders, and low self-esteem.

Everyone attempts to cope with the stress in his or her life, whether doing so consciously and deliberately or not. Unfortunately, many of the strategies people use to deal with stress actually produce additional sources of stress. Overeating, excessive alcohol consumption, cigarette smoking, and drug use are examples of stress management attempts gone awry.

Any effective strategy of stress management needs to do more than just distract you from that which is causing the stress. It needs to address both the physical and the psychological aspects of stress. Everyone attempts to cope with the stress in his or her life, whether doing so consciously and deliberately or not..

—"Women and Diabetes: Strategies for Handling Stress"
Reprinted with permission from Diabetes Self-Management.
Copyright © 1997 R.A. Rapaport Publishing, Inc.

1. According to Hans Selye, stress is stimulated by a(n)

   (A) environmental change.
   (B) bodily change.
   (C) perceived demand.
   (D) physiological and psychological conflict.

2. The physiological symptoms of stress are a result of

   (A) secretion of adrenalin and cortisol.
   (B) suppression of adrenaline.
   (C) accumulation of cortisol.
   (D) absence of adrenaline and cortisol.

3. The main problem presented by stress in diabetics is that the

   (A) blood sugar rises.
   (B) blood pressure drops.
   (C) immune system is suppressed.
   (D) stomach develops ulcers.

4. The theoretical basis for the effects of stress is based on the

   (A) interaction of the physiological and psychological self.
   (B) interaction of the self with the environment.
   (C) relationship between change and coping.
   (D) relationship between change and growth.

5. An effective method of coping with stress would be

   (A) focusing on the pleasure of eating.
   (B) inducing relaxation by drinking alcoholic beverages.
   (C) delaying stopping smoking.
   (D) adapting to change.

6. According to this passage,

   (A) stress causes cancer.
   (B) stress can be controlled.
   (C) all stress is harmful.
   (D) all stress is continuous.

STOP

IF YOU FINISH BEFORE TIME IS CALLED, YOU MAY CHECK YOUR WORK ON THIS SECTION ONLY. DO NOT TURN TO ANY OTHER SECTION IN THE TEST.

READING COMPREHENSION TEST 3

6 Questions • 10 Minutes

Review Unit 4, Reading Comprehension, before attempting this test.

Directions: Following the passage below, you will find a number of incomplete statements about the passage. Select the word or expression that most satisfactorily completes each statement. Fill in the corresponding space on your answer sheet.

Since 1910, more American women have died of heart disease than of any other cause. But for most of this century, physicians and researchers treated heart disease almost exclusively as a man's problem. When the American Heart Association held its first public conference for women in 1964, it focused on how women could help protect their husbands' hearts.

How could doctors and scientists overlook such a clear threat to women's health for so long?

For many years, heart-disease researchers concerned themselves primarily with premature heart attacks—heart attacks that strike down the young or middle-aged rather than the elderly. When women get heart disease, however, they tend to develop it 10 to 15 years later than men; thus, they are more likely to have heart attacks when they are past middle age.

For much of their lives, the sex hormone estrogen offers women substantial protection from heart disease. Only around age 55 does the rate of heart disease in women start to climb, both because estrogen levels drop after menopause and because other risk factors for heart disease become more common at the same age.

The age difference makes heart disease appear a more dramatic problem in men than in women; it's somehow more shocking when a heart attack hits a 50-year-old than when a 65-year-old is the victim. Indeed, the fact that men develop heart disease earlier than women means the disease may have a greater impact on their lives, and offers some justification for putting a greater emphasis on studying heart disease in men than in women. But until recently, researchers have done much more than that: They have systematically and almost completely excluded women from studies of all aspects of coronary heart disease. One major heart-disease study did include women in virtually equal numbers with men, but the data were misinterpreted in a way that actually added to the confusion over women's risks. The Framingham Heart Study has been following more than 5,000 men and women since 1948 to chart the causes and course of heart disease. Among other factors, the researchers identified people with chest pain, and assumed that they were suffering from angina, a symptom indicating that narrowed coronary arteries are supplying inadequate amounts of oxygen to the heart muscle.

Angina often precedes a heart attack. But in the mid-1950s, the Framingham researchers found that men with chest pain were much more likely than women with chest pain to have a heart attack within five years. They concluded that heart disease was simply not much of a threat to women.

There are two problems with that conclusion. First, many women with chest pain turn out not to have angina at all. A major study published in 1982 revealed that fully half of all women with chest pain who underwent coronary angiography—an X-ray procedure for visualizing the arteries of the heart—did not have blockages. (The same was true of only 17 percent of the men.) And second, in the 1950s most of Framingham's women were still too young to be at high risk for heart attack. A later analysis of the Framingham data showed that heart disease in women develops more gradually than in men. Women are more likely to experience angina for an extended period of time before suffering a heart attack.

Clinical trials—studies that test the effects of different treatments on a disease, rather than simply trying to understand the factors that lead to illness—have also tended to exclude women. Investigators have traditionally steered clear of testing any new treatments on women of childbearing age to avoid the confounding effects their hormonal cycles might have on test results, and to avoid unwittingly exposing a fetus by giving a drug to a woman who doesn't yet know she is pregnant. Many researchers have also excluded people over age 65, the age when women have the greatest heart-disease risk, out of concern that other illnesses in these older people would muddy the data. In clinical trials conducted over the past 30 years to evaluate treatments for heart attack, fewer than 20 percent of the total 151,000 subjects were women, according to a recent analysis in the Journal of the American Medical Association.

As a result, physicians have proceeded on the assumption that a treatment tested in men will work about equally well in women. Not necessarily. It is now clear, for instance, that the drug propranolol (Inderal), a beta-blocker commonly prescribed for high blood pressure and angina, is broken down far more slowly in women's bodies—an important consideration for dosage. Moreover, the potential of estrogen treatment to prevent heart disease in postmenopausal women is only now being tested in large clinical trials.

In 1985, the U.S. Public Health Service Task Force on Women's Health Issues ordered the National Institutes of Health to include more women in research, particularly research on heart disease. After several years of foot-dragging, the NIH established an office to ensure that women are appropriately represented in NIH-funded studies. Several large-scale clinical trials including women are now in the planning stage or underway. The clinical trial portion of the Women's Health Initiative—a $600 million, 14-year effort—will study the effects of a low-fat diet and hormonal therapy in preventing cardiovascular disease (as well as cancer and osteoporosis). It may be many years, however, before the decades of neglect are overcome.

—"Heart Disease: Women at Risk"
Reprinted by permission from Consumer Reports, May 1993.
Copyright © 1993 by Consumers Union of U.S., Inc., Yonkers, NY 10703-1057

1. The theory that estrogen protects women from heart disease is supported by the fact that

   (A) the rate of heart disease in women drops after age 55.

   (B) the rate of heart disease in women increases after age 55.

   (C) the incidence of heart disease in women is far less than in men.

   (D) only post-menopausal women have heart disease.

2. Physicians and researchers have placed emphasis on heart disease in men more than in women because

   (A) men develop heart disease earlier than women.

   (B) more men die from heart disease than women.

   (C) men are more prone to heart disease than women.

   (D) men respond to treatment more readily than women.

3. When comparing the occurrence of angina in men and women,

   (A) women rather than men have angina for a longer period of time before a heart attack.

   (B) angina usually proceeds a heart attack in both men and women.

   (C) the occurrence is more frequent in females.

   (D) the occurrence is less frequent in males.

4. The age when women are at greatest risk for heart disease is

(A) 45-49.

(B) 50-59.

(C) 60-65.

(D) over 65.

5. It is important to conduct clinical research on both men and women because

(A) preventive techniques are the same for both men and women.

(B) age differences in occurrence of heart disease indicate differences in causes.

(C) physiological differences lead to differences in responses to treatment.

(D) the impact of heart disease on an individual's life is the same for men and women.

6. The focus of the NIH clinical trials for Women's Health Initiative is to study the

(A) relationship between the aging process and the occurrence of heart disease.

(B) factors that lead to high risk for heart disease.

(C) female responses to drugs used to treat heart disease.

(D) effects of diet and hormonal therapy on prevention of heart disease.

STOP

IF YOU FINISH BEFORE TIME IS CALLED, YOU MAY CHECK YOUR WORK ON THIS SECTION ONLY. DO NOT TURN TO ANY OTHER SECTION IN THE TEST.

READING COMPREHENSION TEST 4

5 Questions • 8 Minutes

Review Unit 4, Reading Comprehension, before attempting this test.

Directions: Following the passage below, you will find a number of incomplete statements about the passage. Select the word or expression that most satisfactorily completes each statement. Fill in the corresponding space on your answer sheet.

Can creativity evolve with aging—maybe even flower with aging? If you belong to the "can't teach an old dog new tricks" school of thought, you may think that unless you have been an artist or writer or musician your whole life you are unlikely to be one in midlife—that increased creativity isn't compatible with growing old.

But research into fields as varied as neurology, behavioral science and art history says otherwise. So do the thousands of people who are finding that different types of creativity can accompany aging.

There is the artistic creativity of people like Bill Traylor, a folk art painter who did not pick up a paintbrush until he was 85 years old.

There is the exhilaration of the 81-year-old whose late-life burst of creativity led to her discovery of literature, a discovery she felt changed her life.

Then there is social creativity, a deftness with interpersonal relationships, that older people, the keepers of the culture, have traditionally offered.

The point is not that every older person can or should be a Picasso, but that aging precludes neither productivity nor creative energy. Moreover, creative capacity after age 65 is considerably more common than most people realize.

Creativity at older ages is not just a matter of anecdote; science has shown that the potential for intellectual growth with aging has biological underpinnings. Studies of the brain show that, in response to a more stimulating or challenging environment, brain cells sprout new extensions, improving their communication with other brain cells.

The same studies, along with behavioral research, indicate that brain cells respond to mental exercise just as muscle cells respond to physical exercise. Science, in short, supports the maxim "use it or lose it" when it comes to the aging brain.

There are several ways of categorizing the creative impulses of older persons:

- creativity that continues with aging;
- creativity that commences with aging;
- creativity that changes with aging;
- creativity in response to late-life loss.

There are famous examples of older people exuding creativity throughout their lives—Picasso experimenting with new styles of painting in his 90s, Verdi composing new operas in his 80s, George Bernard Shaw writing new plays in his 90s.

—"Contemplating Creativity"
by Dr. Gene Cohen Reprinted with permission from
AARP Bulletin, April 1997 Copyright © 1997 by AARP

1. According to this passage, the relationship between aging and creativity can be

   (A) direct.

   (B) indirect.

   (C) mutually exclusive.

   (D) unpredictable.

2. Bill Traylor is an example of which one of the following types of creativity?

   (A) Composing music

   (B) Social creativity

   (C) Literature discovery

   (D) Folk art painting

3. A theoretical basis for creativity at older ages is that

   (A) intercommunication among brain cells expands in response to physical exercise.

   (B) intercommunication among brain cells expands in response to stimulating environments.

   (C) intellectual growth increases in the aging brain.

   (D) intellectual growth decreases in the aging brain.

4. The point of this article is to explain

   (A) different types of creativity.

   (B) the scientific and behavioral research studies about creativity and aging.

   (C) that aging and creativity are compatible.

   (D) the different stages related to creativity and aging.

5. Which one of the following statements is true?

   (A) All aged people are creative.

   (B) Only people who have been creative in younger life can be creative in older life.

   (C) The first sign of creativity may occur in older life.

   (D) Only one type of creativity is seen in aged people.

STOP

IF YOU FINISH BEFORE TIME IS CALLED, YOU MAY CHECK YOUR WORK ON THIS SECTION ONLY. DO NOT TURN TO ANY OTHER SECTION IN THE TEST.

READING COMPREHENSION TEST 5

5 Questions • 9 Minutes

Review Unit 4, Reading Comprehension, before attempting this test.

Directions: Following the passage below, you will find a number of incomplete statements about the passage. Select the word or expression that most satisfactorily completes each statement. Fill in the corresponding space on your answer sheet.

A nearby flow of water is a very convenient place to dispose of waste materials, and people have been doing this for many years. If the right chemicals are dumped into the water, it can be beneficial. Lakes tend to follow a course from being deep, clear, nutrient-poor lakes to becoming shallow and more productive nutrient-rich lakes. This is the natural course of most lakes, and the addition of chemicals such as phosphates and nitrates can actually accelerate this process. To a certain extent, this is beneficial, and it has been done intentionally in some cases: but when carried to extremes, it can lead to a human-caused natural disaster. The water produces so much algae that most other forms of life cannot exist, and the lake chokes to death. In most cases, factories and sewage drains have carried this addition of chemicals too far.

Another consequence of dumping waste material into waterways, especially lakes, occurs when the waste contains metals, such as copper. Some metals literally cover the lake bottom and kill off all the bottom-dwelling organisms. Since many of these organisms are responsible for the decomposition of organic material on the bottom, the removal of these animals results in a great deal of the organic material remaining undecomposed, decreasing the nutrient content of the environment.

The dumping of waste materials from combustion into the air is quite obvious every time you look at the skyline of any major industrial area. Dumping poisonous materials into the environment has resulted in the destruction of many of our oxygen-producing plants and has driven many animals from our immediate environment. Another result that strikes perhaps closer to home is the increase in lung disease attributed to air pollution. Moreover, the propellants from aerosol cans cause problems by deteriorating the ozone layer of the atmosphere. This depletion allows greater amounts of ultraviolet radiation to reach the surface of the Earth. This higher level of radiation reputedly causes an increase in skin cancer.

Both air and water pollution are a retaliation by nature to human abuse. We assume that the dumping of wastes into the environment is a one-way process, and we do not count on any repercussions. But the cost of dumping garbage into the environment is slowly coming back to haunt us. Whether it be by the return of mercury and DDT to us in our food, or the destruction of shields in the atmosphere that protect us from being burned by the sun's radiation, we will pay for our assaults on the environment.

1. The title that best expresses the main idea of this section is
   (A) "Save Our Lakes."
   (B) "Humans' Responsibility Toward Nature"
   (C) "Air Pollution."
   (D) "How Pollution Causes Cancer."

2. According to this passage, one of the negative results of dumping waste chemicals into lakes is the
   (A) increased growth of algae, which kills other organisms.
   (B) discoloration of water.
   (C) limitation of recreational activities.
   (D) increased temperature in the water.

3. Two causes of air pollution are
   (A) smoke and copper.
   (B) aerosol cans and recycling of waste materials.
   (C) decomposition of organisms and deoxygenation of plants.
   (D) dumping of waste materials and use of aerosol cans.

4. The author's attitude toward environmental protection is
   (A) complacency.
   (B) pro-conservation.
   (C) indifference.
   (D) apathy

5. The author's reference to the driving of animals from our immediate environment implies
   (A) migration.
   (B) extinction.
   (C) destruction.
   (D) poaching.

STOP

IF YOU FINISH BEFORE TIME IS CALLED, YOU MAY CHECK YOUR WORK ON THIS SECTION ONLY. DO NOT TURN TO ANY OTHER SECTION IN THE TEST.

ANSWER KEY AND EXPLANATIONS

Test 1

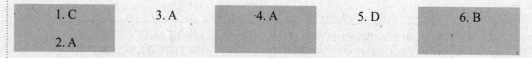

| 1. D | 2. B | 3. A | 4. C | 5. A |

1. **The correct answer is (D).** The title of a piece typically reflects the main idea of that piece. Only choice (D) is broad enough to cover the range of information in the passage. Choices (A), (B), and (C) focus on just one detail in the passage.

2. **The correct answer is (B).** The answer is found in sentence 5 of paragraph 1.

3. **The correct answer is (A).** The answer is found in sentence 4 of paragraph 1.

4. **The correct answer is (C).** The answer is found in sentence 6 of paragraph 1.

5. **The correct answer is (A).** The answer can be inferred by putting together the information in the two clauses in sentence 7 of paragraph 1.

Test 2

| 1. C | 3. A | 4. A | 5. D | 6. B |
| 2. A | | | | |

1. **The correct answer is (C).** The answer is stated in sentence 2 of paragraph 1.

2. **The correct answer is (A).** The answer is stated in the last sentence in paragraph 2.

3. **The correct answer is (A).** The answer is stated in sentence 1 in paragraph 5.

4. **The correct answer is (A).** The answer can be found by integrating information in sentence 1 and sentence 3 in paragraph 1.

5. **The correct answer is (D).** The answer can be inferred from information in paragraphs 6 and 7.

6. **The correct answer is (B).** The answer can be inferred from information in paragraphs 6 and 7.

Test 3

| 1. B | 3. A | 4. D | 5. C | 6. D |
| 2. A | | | | |

1. **The correct answer is (B).** The answer is stated in sentence 2 of paragraph 4.

2. **The correct answer is (A).** The answer is stated in sentence 1 of paragraph 3.

3. **The correct answer is (A).** The answer is stated in the last sentence in paragraph 8.

4. **The correct answer is (D).** The answer is stated in sentence 3 in paragraph 9.

5. **The correct answer is (C).** The answer can be inferred from information in paragraph 10.

6. **The correct answer is (D).** The answer is stated in sentence 4 in the last paragraph.

Test 4

| 1. A | 2. D | 3. B | 4. C | 5. C |

1. **The correct answer is (A).** That there is a direct relationship between aging and creativity is the main idea of the entire passage.

2. **The correct answer is (D).** The answer is stated in paragraph 2.

3. **The correct answer is (B).** The answer is stated in sentence 2 in paragraph 7.

4. **The correct answer is (C).** When a question asks about the point of a passage, it's asking for the main idea of the passage. Look for the broadest, that is, the most general answer. In this case, it's choice (C). The other answer choices give just one detail of the passage, not the general idea of what the passage is about.

5. **The correct answer is (C).** The answer is found in the second bullet point in paragraph 9.

Test 5

1. B	2. A	3. D	4. B	5. A

1. **The correct answer is (B).** Any question that asks you to choose the best title for a passage is really asking you to identify the main idea of the piece. Look for the title that is the broadest, the most general. In this set of answers, it's choice (B). The other choices focus on just one detail in the passage.

2. **The correct answer is (A).** The answer is stated in sentence 6 in paragraph 1.

3. **The correct answer is (D).** The answer is stated in sentences 1 and 4 in paragraph 3.

4. **The correct answer is (B).** All the information in the passage suggests that the author supports conservation, so his or her attitude, or tone, is pro-conservation. Choice (A) is incorrect because *complacency* means "a feeling of self-satisfaction," which doesn't fit the information chosen by the author to include in the passage. Choice (C), *indifference*, is also incorrect because the word means "lacking concern or care for something." Choice (D) is incorrect because *apathy* means "a lack of interest, being indifferent."

5. **The correct answer is (A).** The answer can be inferred from sentence 2 in paragraph 3. If the sentence didn't have the phrase "our immediate environment," then either choice (B) or choice (C) could be correct. Choice (D) is incorrect because there is no indication that illegal shooting of animals is involved.

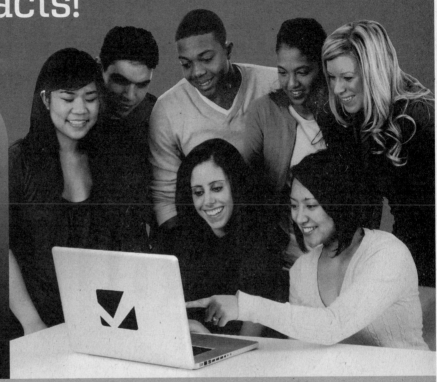

College Portraits
No rankings, no spin... just the facts!

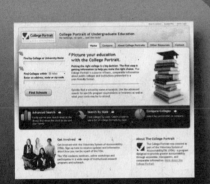

Free access and use—no fees, no log in required!

Visit a website with reliable and user-friendly information on more than 300 public colleges and universities:

>> Learn about the student experience on campus

>> Compare admissions, majors, campus life, class size, and more

>> Calculate your cost to attend a participating university

>> Search by state, distance from home, size, and more

>> Find links and contact information for each campus

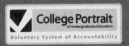

Sponsored by the Association of Public and Land-grant Universities and the American Association of State Colleges and Universities

www.collegeportraits.org

Save 10% on the cost of college

Visit
simpletuition.com/smarterstudent
to find out how!

simpletuition
plan · pay less · pay back

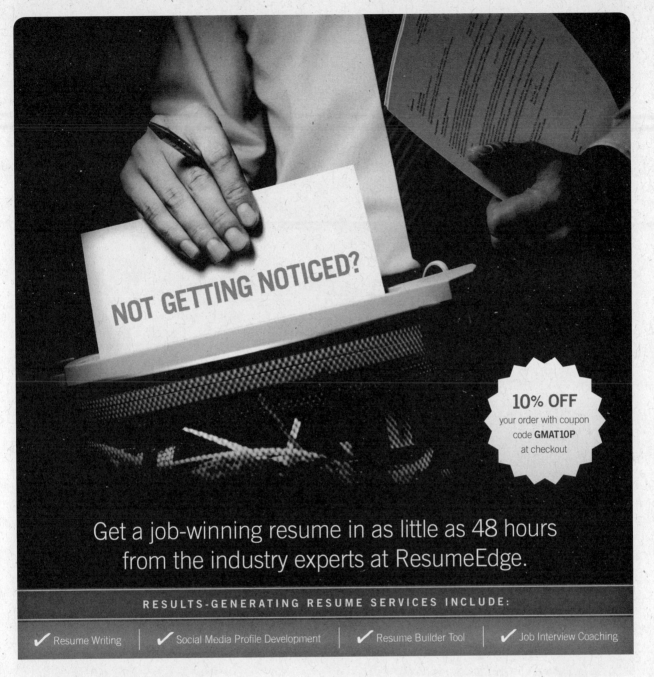

NOT GETTING NOTICED?

10% OFF
your order with coupon
code **GMAT10P**
at checkout

Get a job-winning resume in as little as 48 hours
from the industry experts at ResumeEdge.

RESULTS-GENERATING RESUME SERVICES INCLUDE:

✓ Resume Writing | ✓ Social Media Profile Development | ✓ Resume Builder Tool | ✓ Job Interview Coaching

The ResumeEdge Difference

- Certified Professional Resume Writers
- One-on-one contact with your writer
- 98% customer satisfaction rating
- Experts in more than 40 industries
- As little as 48-hour turnaround for most orders
- An established business since 2001
- Resume writing partner to leading sites such
  as **Dice.com**

*"I received calls from every potential
employer that I sent my resume to.
I was offered a fantastic position and
feel that it was due, in no small part,
to the great resume that [my editor]
put together for me!"* —N.G.

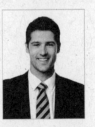

LEARN MORE—visit ResumeEdge.com or call 888.438.2633

ResumeEdge
A **nelnet** SERVICE

NOTES

NOTES

NOTES

NOTES

NOTES

NOTES

NOTES

NOTES

NOTES

NOTES

NOTES

NOTES

NOTES

NOTES